Pharmacology in Rehabilitation

Third Edition

Contemporary Perspectives in Rehabilitation

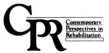

Steven L. Wolf, PhD, FAPTA, Editor-in-Chief

The Biomechanics of the Foot and Ankle, 2nd Edition
Robert Donatelli, MA, PT, OCS

Wound Healing: Alternatives in Management, 3rd Edition
Luther C. Kloth, MS, PT, CWS, FAPTA, and Joseph M. McCulloch, PhD, PT, CWS

Thermal Agents in Rehabilitation, 3rd Edition
Susan L. Michlovitz, MS, PT, CHT

Electrotherapy in Rehabilitation
Meryl Roth Gersh, MMSc, PT

Dynamics of Human Biologic Tissues
Dean P. Currier, PhD, PT, and Roger M. Nelson, PhD, PT

Concepts in Hand Rehabilitation
Barbara G. Stanley, PT, CHT, and Susan M. Tribuzi, OTR, CHT

Cardiopulmonary Rehabilitation: Basic Theory and Application, 3rd Edition
Frances J. Brannon, PhD, Margaret W. Foley, RN, MN, Julie Ann Starr, MS, PT, CCS, and Lauren M. Saul, MSN, CCRN

Vestibular Rehabilitation, 2nd Edition
Susan J. Herdman, PhD, PT

Fundamentals of Orthopedic Radiology
Lynn McKinnis, PT, OCS

Evaluation and Treatment of the Shoulder: An Integration of the *Guide to Physical Therapist Practice*
Brian J. Tovin, MMSc, PT, SCS, ATC, and Bruce H. Greenfield, MMSc, PT, OCS

Pharmacology in Rehabilitation

Third Edition

Charles D. Ciccone, PhD, PT
Professor
Department of Physical Therapy
School of Health Sciences and Human Performance
Ithaca College
Ithaca, New York

F. A. DAVIS COMPANY • **Philadelphia**

F. A. Davis Company
1915 Arch Street
Philadelphia, PA 19103
www.fadavis.com

Copyright © 2002 by F. A. Davis Company

Printed in the United States of America

Last digit indicates print number: 10 9 8 7 6 5 4 3 2 1

Acquisitions Editor: Margaret M. Biblis
Developmental Editor: Maryann Foley
Production Editor: Jack C. Brandt
Cover Designer: Louis J. Forgione

As new scientific information becomes available through basic and clinical research, recommended treatments and drug therapies undergo changes. The author and publisher have done everything possible to make this book accurate, up to date, and in accord with accepted standards at the time of publication. The author, editors, and publisher are not responsible for errors or omissions or for consequences from application of the book, and make no warranty, expressed or implied, in regard to the contents of the book. Any practice described in this book should be applied by the reader in accordance with professional standards of care used in regard to the unique circumstances that may apply in each situation. The reader is advised always to check product information (package inserts) for changes and new information regarding dose and contraindications before administering any drug. Caution is especially urged when using new or infrequently ordered drugs.

Library of Congress Cataloging-in-Publication Data

Ciccone, Charles D., 1953–
  Pharmacology in rehabilitation / Charles D. Ciccone.— Ed. 3
    p. cm.—(Contemporary perspectives in rehabilitation)
  Includes bibliographical references and index.
  ISBN 0-8036-0779-2 (alk. paper)
  1. Pharmacology.   2. Medical rehabilitation.   I. Series.
RM301 .C515 2002
615.5'8—dc21
                            2001047232

Dedicated to Penny, Kate, and Alex for providing constant faith, support, and inspiration.

Foreword

When one reflects upon the growth of this text over its first two editions and its continued popularity, a fundamental question arises, "Why has Dr. Ciccone's book become a gold standard for students learning about rehabilitation and clinicians engaged in the provision of excellent care to patients with such diverse diagnoses that impact one or several physiologic systems?" Perhaps the answer lies in part in Chuck's attention to detail and obsession with providing the most current information available with the dynamic transformations that characterize pharmacology. The task is far more daunting than simply keeping up with the *PDR* (*Physicians' Desk Reference*).

The most unique attribute of Dr. Ciccone's effort is his ability to make complex information easy to comprehend and relevant to the needs of all rehabilitation students and clinicians. This challenge becomes far more profound when one considers the increasing number of specialty areas in which health care professionals take interest. Certainly, physical therapists who have interests in the management of patients with female health issues or in the use of aquatic therapies, for example, have as much need to understand the interactions of medications with physical interventions as does the clinician specializing in the care of patients with cardiopulmonary problems. This diversity demands attention to recognizing the treatment areas subsumed within each specialty area, the medications that patients with unique systemic problems might be taking, the interactions of these drugs, and the implications that such intake might have on the treatments we provide.

So, against this background, one might ask why we even consider another edition. The answer is relatively simple. Dr. Ciccone delivers the most recent information about new medications in a comprehensible manner, and this information influences our decisions in delivering treatment plans and assists us in channeling our efforts in a defensible and logical manner. If the fundamental basis for justification of service resides in the emergent properties of *evidence*, then any factor influencing that evidence must be considered. In this vein, can there be a more relevant variable to impact evidence and justification for provision of treatment than the interaction between the approach we defend and the pharmacokinetics that might influence that approach? The merit in this question takes the third edition of *Pharmacology in Rehabilitation* to a new dimension, one that transcends simply knowing about drugs to reevaluating the evidence for successful treatment against the impact that these medications might have on successful outcomes.

Consequently, students and clinicians are urged to explore this edition in a contemporary light—one that demands we view pharmacologic interactions with treatment, not just as a checklist, but also as an exercise to help us justify our treatments or explain why our services might not be as effective as we wish. In either event, the thought processes are totally compatible with the acquisition and analyses of evidence to support treatment efficacy or effectiveness. If the reader maintains this perspective, then the recognition of Chuck Ciccone's contribution to clinical practice becomes all the more obvious.

Steven L. Wolf, PhD, PT, FAPTA
Series Editor

Preface

Pharmacology continues to be an exciting and dynamic aspect of health care. It seems that important and innovative breakthroughs in drug therapy are being made almost daily. Drug therapy is likewise an important intervention for almost all patients receiving physical therapy and occupational therapy. Therefore, as therapists, we must have some understanding of how medications affect our patients. The third edition of this text follows the principles established in previous editions: to provide a comprehensive, relevant, and up-to-date compendium of how pharmacology interacts with physical rehabilitation.

While writing this edition, I was again amazed by how quickly pharmacology has changed in only a few short years. New drugs appear on the market on a regular basis, and we are constantly refining the way that we use existing drugs. It was a somewhat daunting task to consider all the basic and clinical aspects of pharmacotherapeutics and also consider all the changes and innovations that occurred over the last 5 or 6 years. As with previous editions, this edition focuses primarily on the major drug groups and how these groups are used therapeutically. Each chapter, however, has been updated and revised extensively to give readers the most current information about the indications, effects, and potential problems associated with each drug group. Special emphasis has been placed on the major pharmacologic issues pertaining to physical therapists and occupational therapists. This edition also draws heavily on current literature to provide an overview of recent advances in various aspects of pharmacology.

The first section of this book (Chapters 1 through 4) addresses some general pharmacologic concepts, including basic issues concerning drug approval and safety and those related to drug pharmacokinetics and drug-receptor interactions. The remainder of the book focuses on specific drug applications, with drugs organized according to their effect on specific physiologic systems and pathologic conditions. Chapters are designed to provide background information on each system or disorder, followed by detailed descriptions of how these drugs work, how they exert beneficial and adverse effects, and how drug therapy can impact physical therapy and occupational therapy.

It is my fervent hope that this edition serves as a useful resource for students and clinicians. Pharmacology is a complex but important topic, and therapists must realize that drug therapy will influence the responses we see in our patients. This book is designed to give therapists insight into how pharmacology interacts with physical rehabilitation so that we can ultimately provide the best care for our patients.

Charles D. Ciccone

Acknowledgments

I would like to thank everyone who provided insight and guidance to the third edition of this text. In particular, Peter Panus was especially helpful in making suggestions about revising this edition, and many substantive changes in this text were based on Dr. Panus's ideas. Additionally, this edition is the culmination of all of the input from reviewers of past editions: Barbara MacDermott Costa, Linda D. Crane, John F. Decker, Mark Greve, Sandra B. Levine, Donald L. Merrill, Grace Minerbo, and Jeffrey Rothman.

I would also like to thank Bonnie DeSombre, Fred Estabrook, and Cheryl Tarbell for their help in preparing various tables and figures appearing in this text.

Finally, my thanks go to Steve Wolf, editor of the CPR series, for his continued encouragement and support and to the staff of F. A. Davis Company for their help and expertise in developing this text. In particular, I want to thank Jean-François Vilain for his patience, guidance, and tireless efforts in bringing this book to publication and making this resource available to students and clinicians.

Contents

Chapter 35.   Treatment of Infections III: Antifungal and Antiparasitic Drugs

General Principles of Pharmacology

CHAPTER **1**

Basic Principles of Pharmacology

Pharmacology is the study of drugs. In its broadest definition, a drug can be described as "any chemical agent that affects processes of living."[2] In this sense, a drug includes any substance that alters physiologic function in the organism, regardless of whether the effect is beneficial or harmful. In terms of clinical pharmacology, it has traditionally been the beneficial or therapeutic effects that have been of special interest. Throughout history, certain naturally occurring chemicals have been used to relieve pain or treat disease in humans. Within the past century, the use of natural, semisynthetic, and synthetic chemical agents has expanded to the point where many diseases can be prevented or cured, and the general health and well-being of many individuals have improved dramatically through the use of therapeutic drugs.

Because of the extensive clinical use of therapeutic medications, members of the medical community must have some knowledge of the basic types of drugs and the mechanisms of their actions. Although this has always been true for individuals who prescribe and administer drugs (i.e., physicians and nurses), it is now recognized that members of other health-related professions must also have a fundamental knowledge of pharmacology.

An understanding of basic drug mechanisms can help practitioners such as physical therapists, occupational therapists, and other rehabilitation specialists better understand the patient's response to the drug. In addition, the knowledge of how certain rehabilitative procedures may interact with the medication will be helpful in getting the optimal response from the patient to both the drug and the therapy treatment. For instance, scheduling the patient for therapy when certain drugs reach their peak effect may improve the therapy session dramatically. This may be true for drugs that decrease pain (analgesics) or improve the patient's motor skills (antiparkinsonian drugs). Conversely, some therapy sessions that require the patient's active participation may be rendered useless if scheduled when medications such as sedatives reach their peak effect. Also, any adverse responses that may occur because of a direct interaction between the therapy treatment and certain medications may be avoided or controlled by understanding the pharmacologic aspects of specific drugs. For example, the patient taking a peripheral vasodilator may experience a profound decrease in blood pressure when he or she

3

is placed in a hot whirlpool. By understanding the implications of such an interaction, the therapist can be especially alert for any detrimental effects on the patient, or a different therapy treatment may be instituted in some patients.

In order to help the reader have a more focused approach to the study of drugs, pharmacology is often divided into several areas of concern (Fig. 1–1). **Pharmacotherapeutics** is the area of pharmacology that refers to the use of specific drugs to prevent, treat, or diagnose disease. For the purposes of this text, the effects of drugs on humans will be of primary concern, with animal pharmacology mentioned only in reference to drug testing and research in animals.

When drugs are used therapeutically in humans, the way that the body interacts with the drug and what specific effect the drug has on the individual must be known. Consequently, pharmacotherapeutics is divided into two functional areas: pharmacokinetics and pharmacodynamics (see Fig. 1–1). **Pharmacokinetics** is the study of how the body deals with the drug in terms of the way the drug is absorbed, distributed, and eliminated. **Pharmacodynamics** is the analysis of what the drug does to the body, including the mechanism by which the drug exerts its effect. In this text, the basic principles of pharmacokinetics will be outlined in Chapters 2 and 3, and the pharmacodynamics and pharmacokinetics of specific drugs will be discussed in their respective chapters.

Toxicology is the study of the harmful effects of chemicals. Although it can be viewed as a subdivision of pharmacology, toxicology has evolved into a separate area of study because of the scope of all the adverse effects of therapeutic agents, as well as environmental toxins and poisons. However, because virtually every medication can produce some adverse effects, a discussion of toxicology must be included in pharmacotherapeutics. For the purposes of this text, discussions of drug toxicity are limited to the unwanted effects that occur when therapeutic drugs reach excessively high (toxic) levels. The toxic side effects of individual drugs are covered in the chapter describing the therapeutic effects of that drug.

Pharmacy deals with the preparation and dispensing of medications. Although pharmacy is also frequently considered a subdivision of pharmacology, this area has evolved

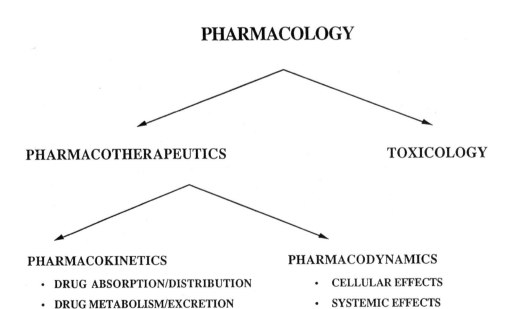

FIGURE 1–1. Areas of study within pharmacology.

into a distinct professional discipline. Care must be taken not to use the terms "pharmacy" and "pharmacology" interchangeably, because these are quite different areas of study.

DRUG NOMENCLATURE

One of the most potentially confusing aspects of pharmacology is the variety of names given to different drugs or even to the same compound. Students of pharmacology as well as clinicians are often faced with myriad terms that represent the same drug.[10,14] Most of the problems in drug terminology arise from the fact that each drug can be identified according to its *chemical, generic,* or *trade* name[1] (Table 1–1). **Chemical names** refer to the specific structure of the compound and are usually fairly long and cumbersome. The **generic name** (also known as the "official" or "nonproprietary" name) tends to be somewhat shorter and is often derived from the chemical name. A **trade name** (also known as the "brand" name) is assigned to the compound by the pharmaceutical company and may or may not bear any reference at all to the chemical and generic terminology. An additional problem with trade names is that several manufacturers may be marketing the same compound under different names, thus adding to the confusion. If there is no existing patent for that compound or if the patent has expired, the same drug may be marketed by separate drug companies.[6] For practical purposes, the generic name is often the easiest and most effective way to refer to a drug, and this terminology will be used most frequently in this text.

Drug nomenclature also influences the prescribing of many medications. Generic forms are typically less expensive than their brand-name counterparts, and substitution of a generic drug can help reduce health-care costs.[14] The generic equivalent should produce the same effects as the brand-name drug if the generic form has been tested and found to have the same pharmacokinetic profile as the brand-name drug; that is, the generic form has been shown to have the same variables for absorption, distribution, metabolism, and so forth.[6,14] There are, however, other safety and ethical issues that should be considered before a generic drug is substituted, and practitioners may want to prescribe a specific brand-name drug based on the pharmacologic profile of that drug and the specific way that the drug may affect a given patient.

WHAT CONSTITUTES A DRUG: DEVELOPMENT AND APPROVAL OF THERAPEUTIC AGENTS

In the United States, the **Food and Drug Administration (FDA)** is responsible for monitoring the use of existing drugs as well as the development and approval of new drugs.[3,30] The analogous body in Canada is the Drugs Directorate of Health Protection

TABLE 1–1 Examples of Drug Nomenclature

Chemical	Generic (Nonproprietary)	Trade (Proprietary)
N-Acetyl-p-aminophenol	Acetaminophen	Tylenol, Panadol, many others
3,4-Dihydroxyphenyl-l-alanine	Levodopa	Larodopa
5,5-Phenylethylbarbituric acid	Phenobarbital	Luminal, Solfoton
7-Chloro-1,3-dihydro-1-methyl-5-phenyl-2H-1,4-benzodiazepin-2-one	Diazepam	Valium

Branch, Department of Health and Welfare. The two primary concerns of these agencies are (1) whether the drug is effective in treating a certain condition and (2) whether the drug is reasonably safe for human use.

Drug Approval Process

The development of a new drug involves extensive preclinical (animal) and clinical (human) studies.[3,30] The basic procedure for testing a new drug is outlined here and is summarized in Table 1–2.

PRECLINICAL STUDIES

Drugs are tested initially in animals, often several different species. Initial information on the basic pharmacokinetic and pharmacodynamic properties of the compound is obtained. Information on dosage and toxicity is also obtained from these animal trials.

HUMAN (CLINICAL) STUDIES

If the results from animal trials are favorable, the drug sponsor files an investigational new drug (IND) application with the FDA. If the drug is approved as an IND, the sponsor may begin testing the drug in humans. Human or "clinical" testing is divided into three primary phases.

Phase I: The drug is tested in a relatively small number of healthy volunteers. Initial information about the possible toxic effects of the drug on humans is determined.

TABLE 1–2 Drug Development and Approval

Testing Phase	Purpose	Subjects	Usual Time Period
Preclinical testing	Initial laboratory tests to determine drug effects and safety	Laboratory animals	1–2 yr
Investigational New Drug (IND) Application			
Human (clinical) testing:			
Phase I	Determine effects, safe dosage, pharmacokinetics	Small number of healthy volunteers	<1 yr
Phase II	Assess drug's effectiveness in treating a specific disease/disorder	Limited number (10–150) of patients with target disorder	2 yr
Phase III	Assess safety and effectiveness in a larger patient population	Large number (1000–3000) of targeted patients	3 yr
New Drug Application (NDA) Approval			
Phase IV (postmarketing surveillance)	Monitor any problems that occur after NDA approval	General patient population	Indefinite

Phase II: The drug is tested in a small, select patient population (10 to 150 subjects) to evaluate the effect of the drug and the appropriate dosage range needed to treat a specific disease or pathologic condition.

Phase III: Clinical evaluation is expanded to include more patients (several hundred to several thousand) as well as more evaluators. Additional information is obtained regarding the drug's safety and effectiveness in a large patient population.

At the end of phase III, the drug sponsor applies for a new drug application (NDA). Results from clinical testing are reviewed extensively by the FDA, and if found favorable, the NDA is approved. At this point, the drug can be marketed and prescribed for use in the general population.

A fourth phase known as "postmarketing surveillance" should be instituted after the NDA is approved. Postmarketing surveillance refers to all the methods used to continue to monitor drug safety and effectiveness after the drug is approved for public use.[11] These methods often consist of reports from health-care providers that describe specific rare adverse effects that were not discovered during clinical testing.[23] A certain drug, for example, could cause a specific adverse effect in only 1 in 10,000 patients taking the drug.[3] It is very likely that such an adverse effect could be missed during phase I through phase III of the clinical trials because the drug is typically tested in only a few thousand subjects (e.g., 1000 to 3000 people). In addition to monitoring adverse effects, postmarketing surveillance can use more formal research methods to obtain information about how a specific drug is used in clinical practice and how that drug compares with similar drugs on the market.[11] Hence, postmarketing surveillance has been advocated as critical in ensuring that the safety and efficacy of the drug continue to be monitored when the drug is actually being used by the general patient population.[11,20,23,27]

The development of a new drug in the United States is an extremely expensive and time-consuming process. The time course for the entire testing process from the beginning of animal trials to the end of phase III human testing may be as long as 7 to 9 years. The FDA has made provisions, however, to shorten the review process if the drug shows exceptional promise or there is a critical need for the immediate clinical use of the drug.[13,17] For example, certain drugs that have shown promise in treating conditions such as cancer or acquired immunodeficiency syndrome (AIDS) may be made available for patient use even before clinical testing is completed.[3,31] Likewise, the approval process can be expedited if a drug has already received approval for treating one condition, but the drug is now being considered for use in other "supplemental" conditions.[7,29]

The process of drug testing and approval does seem to be fairly rigorous in its ability to screen out ineffective or potentially harmful drugs. Of every 10,000 compounds, it is estimated that only 10 make it to the stage of human clinical trials. Of the 10 tested clinically, only 1 will ever be released as a prescription drug.[9]

Prescription versus Over-the-Counter Medications

In the United States, pharmacotherapeutic agents are divided into those requiring a prescription for use and those available as nonprescription, **over-the-counter (OTC) drugs.**[15] Nonprescription drugs can be purchased directly by the consumer, whereas prescription medications may be ordered or dispensed only by an authorized practitioner (i.e., physician, dentist, or other appropriate health-care provider). The classification as a prescription or a nonprescription drug falls under the jurisdiction of the FDA.[15,16] In general, OTC medications are used to treat relatively minor problems and to make the consumer more comfortable until the condition is resolved. These medications have been judged to be safe for use by the consumer without direct medical supervision, and the chances of toxic effects are usually small when the medications are taken in the recommended amounts.[15] Of course, the patient may ingest more than the recommended amount, and in the case of an overdose, the danger always exists for potentially harmful effects, even if the drug is nonprescription in nature.[22,26]

The role of OTC products in the health-care market has expanded dramatically in recent years.[21,24] Many drugs that were formerly available only by prescription are now available in a nonprescription form. Transition of a prescription drug to an OTC product usually occurs when the marketing company applies to the FDA and receives approval to develop and market the drug in a nonprescription form. FDA approval is based on the drug's having an adequate safety profile, and the FDA may require other stipulations, such as lowering the drug dosage in the OTC product.

The fact that more and more prescription drugs are now available in a nonprescription form offers some obvious benefits. Increased availability of OTC products can make it easier for consumers to obtain important medications and decrease the costs associated with obtaining prescription drugs.[21,24,28] There are, however, some obvious concerns about increased OTC drug use. Consumers must realize that these products are important therapeutic medications, and they must use these products appropriately.[25,26] There is also the chance that indiscriminate use of OTC products can cause serious interactions with the patient's prescription medications.[5,12,18] The impact of such OTC compounds is discussed in this text in the appropriate chapters.

There has therefore been considerable debate about the recent increase in the use of OTC products and the increased emphasis on self-care that permeates today's health-care market. It is clear that consumers need to be educated about the use of such medications and reminded that OTC products can produce substantial benefits and adverse effects. All health-care providers, including physical therapists and occupational therapists, need to be in a position to help educate and counsel their patients about the benefits and drawbacks of such medications. Although therapists should not directly prescribe or administer OTC products, therapists can provide information about the proper use and potential benefits of these medications.

Controlled Substances

In 1970, federal legislation was enacted to help control the abuse of legal and illegal drugs. The Comprehensive Drug Abuse Prevention and Control Act (or Controlled Substances Act, as it is also known) placed drugs into specific categories, or "schedules," according to their potential for abuse.[1,16] Descriptions of these schedules for controlled drugs follow.

Schedule I: These drugs are regarded as having the highest potential for abuse, and the legal use of agents in this category is restricted to approved research studies or therapeutic use in a very limited number of patients (e.g., use of marijuana as an antiemetic). Examples of schedule I drugs include heroin, lysergic acid diethylamide (LSD), psilocybin, mescaline, peyote, marijuana, tetrahydrocannabinols, and several other hallucinogens.

Schedule II: Drugs in this category are approved for specific therapeutic purposes but still have a high potential for abuse and possible addiction. Examples include opioids such as morphine and meperidine, barbiturates such as pentobarbital and secobarbital, and drugs containing amphetamines.

Schedule III: Although these drugs have a lower abuse potential than those in schedules I and II, there is still the possibility of developing mild to moderate physical dependence or strong psychologic dependence, or both. Drugs in schedule III include opioids (e.g., codeine, hydrocodone) that are combined in a limited dosage with nonopioid drugs. Other drugs in this category are certain barbiturates and amphetamines that are not included in schedule II.

Schedule IV: These drugs supposedly have a lower potential for abuse than schedule III drugs, with only a limited possibility of physical dependence or psychologic dependence, or both. Examples include the benzodiazepines (diazepam, chlordiazepoxide), certain opioids (pentazocine, propoxyphene), barbiturates not included in other schedules, and a variety of other depressants and stimulants.

Schedule V: These drugs have the lowest relative abuse potential. Drugs in this category consist primarily of low doses of opioids that are used in cough medications and antidiarrheal preparations.

Several other criteria relate to the different controlled substance schedules, such as restrictions on prescription renewal and penalties for illegal possession of drugs in different schedules. For further discussion of controlled substances, the reader is referred to another source.[1]

BASIC CONCEPTS IN DRUG THERAPY

All drugs exert their beneficial effects by reaching some specific target cell or tissue. On the cellular level, the drug in some way changes the function of the cell either to help restore normal physiologic function or to prevent a disease process from occurring. In general, the **dose** of the drug must be large enough to allow an adequate concentration to reach the target site, thus producing a beneficial response. However, the administered **dosage** must not be so excessive that toxicologic effects are produced. Some aspects of the relationship between dosage and response are discussed here.

Dose-Response Curves and Maximal Efficacy

The relationship between the dosage of a drug and a specific response to the drug is illustrated in Figure 1–2. Typically, very low doses do not produce any observable effect. At some threshold dose, the response begins to occur and continues to increase in magnitude before reaching a plateau. The plateau in the response indicates that there will be no further increment in the response even if the dosage continues to be increased. The point at which there is no further increase in the response is known as **ceiling effect,** or **maximal efficacy,** of the drug.[4]

Dose-response curves are used to provide information about the dosage range over which the drug is effective, as well as the peak response that can be expected from the drug. In addition, the characteristic shape of the dose-response curve and the presence of the plateau associated with maximal efficacy can be used to indicate specific information about the binding of the drug to cellular receptors. The relevance of dose-response curves to drug-receptor interactions is discussed further in Chapter 4.

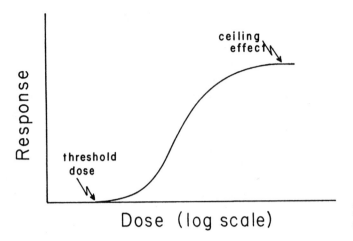

FIGURE 1–2. Dose-response curve.

Potency

One criterion used frequently to compare drugs is the concept of **potency.** Potency is related to the dosage that produces a given response in a specific amplitude.[4,8] When two drugs are compared, the more potent drug requires a lower dosage to produce the same effect as a higher dose of the second drug. For instance, in Figure 1–3, a dosage of 10 mg of drug A would lower blood pressure by 25 percent, whereas 80 mg of drug B would be required to produce the same response. Consequently, drug A would be de-

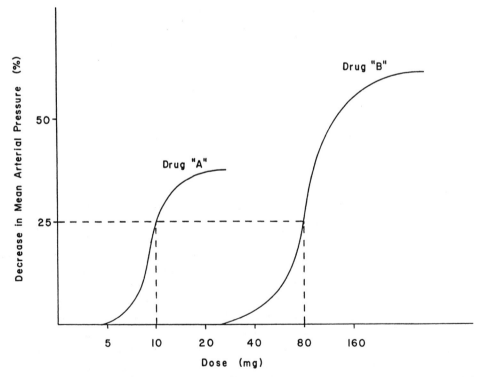

FIGURE 1–3. Relative potency and maximal efficacy of two drugs. Drug A is more potent, and drug B has a greater maximal efficacy.

scribed as the more potent drug. It should be noted that potency is not synonymous with maximal efficacy. Drug B is clearly able to exert a greater maximal effect than drug A. Consequently, the term "potency" is often taken to be much more significant than it really is. The potency of a drug is often misinterpreted by the layperson as an indication of the drug's overall therapeutic benefits, whereas potency really just refers to the fact that less of the compound is required to produce a given response. In fact, neither potency nor maximal efficacy fully indicates a drug's therapeutic potential. Other factors such as the therapeutic index (discussed later) and drug selectivity (see Chap. 4) are also important in comparing and ultimately choosing the best medication for a given problem.

ELEMENTS OF DRUG SAFETY

Quantal Dose-Response Curves and the Median Effective Dose

The dose-response curves shown in Figures 1–2 and 1–3 represent the graded response to a drug as it would occur in a single individual or in a homogeneous population. In reality, variations in the response to a drug that are caused by individual differences in the clinical population need to be considered in trying to assess whether a drug is safe as well as effective. Consequently, the relationship between the dose of the drug and the occurrence of a certain response is measured in a large group of people (or animals if the drug is being tested preclinically). When plotted, this relationship yields a cumulative, or *quantal*, dose-response curve (Fig. 1–4).[4,8] This curve differs from the dose-

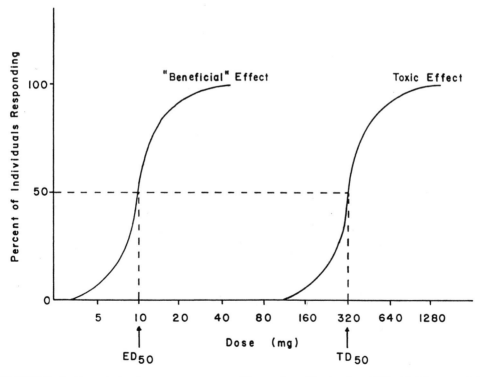

FIGURE 1–4. Cumulative dose-response curve. The median effective dose (ED_{50}) is 10 mg, and the median toxic dose (TD_{50}) is 320 mg. The therapeutic index (TI) for this drug is 32.

response curve discussed previously in that it is not the magnitude of the response that increases with increasing dosage, but the percentage of the population that exhibits a specific response as the dose is increased. The response is not graded; it is either present or absent in each member of the population. For example, a headache medication is administered in an increasing dosage to 1000 people. At some dose, some of the individuals will begin to respond to the drug by reporting the absence of their headaches. As the dosage is increased, more and more individuals will experience pain relief because of the medication, until finally 100 percent of the population reports pain relief. Again, it is the percentage of the population that responds in a specific way (e.g., reporting loss of their headaches) that is measured relative to the dose of the drug. An important reference point in this type of cumulative dose-response curve is the **median effective dose (ED$_{50}$).** This is the dose at which 50 percent of the population responds to the drug in a specified manner.

Median Toxic Dose

In the aforementioned example, relief from pain was the desired response, which is often termed the "beneficial" effect. As doses of the drug continue to be increased, however, adverse or toxic effects may become apparent. To continue the earlier example, higher doses of the same medication may be associated with the appearance of a specific toxic effect, such as acute gastric hemorrhage. As the dosage is increased, more and more individuals will then begin to exhibit that particular adverse effect. The dosage at which 50 percent of the group exhibits the adverse effect is termed the **median toxic dose (TD$_{50}$).** In animal studies, the toxic effect studied is often the death of the animal. In these cases, high doses of the drug are used to determine the **median lethal dose (LD$_{50}$),** the dose that causes death in 50 percent of the animals studied. Of course, the LD$_{50}$ is not a relevant term in clinical use of the drug in humans, but it does serve to provide some indication of the drug's safety in preclinical animal trials.

Therapeutic Index

The median effective and toxic doses are used to determine the **therapeutic index (TI).**[8] The TI is calculated as the ratio of the TD$_{50}$ to the ED$_{50}$:

$$TI = \frac{TD_{50}}{ED_{50}}$$

In animal studies in which the median lethal dose is known, the TI is often calculated by using the LD$_{50}$ in place of the TD$_{50}$. In either human or animal studies, the TI is used as an indicator of the drug's safety.[4,8] The greater the value of the TI, the safer the drug is considered to be. In essence, a large TI indicates that it takes a much larger dose to evoke a toxic response than it does to cause a beneficial effect.

It should be noted, however, that the TI is a relative term. Acetaminophen, a nonprescription analgesic, has a TI of approximately 27 (i.e., the ratio of the median toxic dose to the median effective dose equals 27). Prescription agents tend to have lower TIs. For instance, the narcotic analgesic meperidine (Demerol) has a TI of 8, and the sedative-hypnotic diazepam (Valium) has a TI equal to 3. Other prescription agents such as the cancer chemotherapeutic agents (methotrexate, vincristine, and so on) may have a very low TI, some being close to 1. However, a low TI is often acceptable in these agents, considering the critical nature of cancer and similar serious conditions. The consequences of not using the drug outweigh the risks of some of the toxic effects.

To help keep the risk of toxicity to a minimum with low-TI drugs, it is generally advisable to periodically monitor blood levels of the drug. This helps prevent concentrations from quickly reaching toxic levels. This precaution is usually not necessary with high-TI drugs, because there is a greater margin of error (i.e., blood levels can rise quite a lot above the therapeutic concentration before becoming dangerous).

SUMMARY

In its broadest sense, pharmacology is the study of the effects of chemicals on living organisms. Most discussions of clinical pharmacology deal primarily with the beneficial effects of specific drugs on humans and the manner in which these drugs exert their therapeutic effects. Because all drugs have the potential to produce unwanted or toxic responses, some discussion of the adverse effects of drugs is also essential in pharmacology. Drugs used therapeutically are subjected to extensive testing prior to approval for use in humans and are classified as either prescription or over-the-counter, depending on their dosage, effectiveness, and safety profile. Finally, certain characteristic relationships exist between the dosage of a drug and the response or effect it produces. Such relationships can provide useful information about drug efficacy and potency and about the relative safety of different compounds.

REFERENCES

 1. Benet, LZ: Appendix I. Principles of prescription order writing and patient compliance instructions. In Hardman, JG, et al (eds): The Pharmacological Basis of Therapeutics, ed 9. McGraw Hill, New York, 1996.
 2. Benet, LZ: Introduction. In Hardman, JG, et al (eds): The Pharmacological Basis of Therapeutics, ed 9. McGraw Hill, New York, 1996.
 3. Berkowitz, BA and Katzung, BG: Basic and clinical evaluation of new drugs. In Katzung, BG (ed): Basic and Clinical Pharmacology, ed 7. Appleton & Lange, Stamford, CT, 1998.
 4. Bourne, HR: Drug receptors and pharmacodynamics. In Katzung, BG (ed): Basic and Clinical Pharmacology, ed 7. Appleton & Lange, Stamford, CT, 1998.
 5. Bradley, JG: Nonprescription drugs and hypertension. Which ones affect blood pressure? Postgrad Med 89:195, 1991.
 6. Chow, SC and Liu, J: Meta-analysis for bioequivalence review. J Biopharm Stat 7:97, 1997.
 7. DiMasi, JA, et al: New indications for already approved drugs: An analysis of regulatory review times. J Clin Pharmacol 31:205, 1991.
 8. Fleming, WW: Mechanisms of drug action. In Craig, CR and Stitzel, RE (eds): Modern Pharmacology with Clinical Applications, ed 5. Little Brown, Boston, 1997.
 9. Grabowski, HG and Vernon, JM: The regulation of pharmaceuticals: Balancing the benefits and risks. American Enterprise Institute for Public Policy Research, Washington, DC, 1983.
10. Hemminki, E, et al: Trade names and generic names: Problems for prescribing physicians. Scand J Prim Health Care 2:84, 1984.
11. Hennessy, S: Postmarketing drug surveillance: An epidemiologic approach. Clin Ther 20(Suppl C):C32, 1998.
12. Honig, PK and Gillespie, BK: Drug interactions between prescribed and over-the-counter medication. Drug Saf 13:296, 1995.
13. Kaitlin, KI, et al: Therapeutic ratings and end-of-phase II conferences: Initiatives to accelerate the availability of important new drugs. J Clin Pharmacol 31:17, 1991.
14. Keith, LG, et al: Generics: What's in a name? Int J Fertil Womens Med 43:139, 1998.
15. Koda-Kimble, MA: Therapeutic and toxic potential of over-the-counter agents. In Katzung, BG (ed): Basic and Clinical Pharmacology, ed 7. Appleton & Lange, Stamford, CT, 1998.
16. Kuhn, MA and Moraca-Sawicki, AM: Pharmacology and the nurse's role. In Kuhn, MA (ed): Pharmacotherapeutics: A Nursing Process Approach, ed 4. FA Davis, Philadelphia, 1997.
17. Kupecz, D: Keeping up with current drug approvals. Nurse Pract 24:44, 1999.
18. Lake, KD, et al: Over-the-counter medications in cardiac transplant recipients: Guidelines for use. Ann Pharmacother 26:1566, 1992.

19. Leach, EE: Nurses' guide to the drug development process and the current regulatory environment. Dermatol Nurs 5:351, 1993.
20. Mellinger, GD, et al: Survey method for post-marketing drug surveillance: A demonstration. J Clin Psychopharmacol 8:168, 1988.
21. Morgan, PP and Cohen, L: Off the prescription pad and over the counter: The trend toward drug deregulation grows. CMAJ 152:387, 1995.
22. Murray, S and Brewerton, T: Abuse of over-the-counter dextromethorphan by teenagers. South Med J 86:1151, 1993.
23. Schafer, H: Post-approval drug research: Objectives and methods. Pharmacopsychiatry 30(Suppl):4, 1997.
24. Schmid, B: The safety assessment of over-the-counter (OTC) products. Arch Toxicol Suppl 17:305, 1995.
25. Schulke, DG: American Pharmaceutical Association review of literature on prescription to over-the-counter drug switches. Clin Ther 20(Suppl C):C124, 1998.
26. Sheftell, FD: Role and impact of over-the-counter medications in the management of headache. Neurol Clin 15:187, 1997.
27. Smart, AJ and Walters, L: The importance of postmarketing drug surveillance. S Afr Med J 82:383, 1992.
28. Soller, RW: Evolution of self-care with over-the-counter medications. Clin Ther 20(Suppl C):C134, 1998.
29. Spivey, RN, Lasagna, L, and Trimble, AG: New applications for already approved drugs: Time trends for the new drug application review phase. Clin Pharmacol Ther 41:368, 1987.
30. Stitzel, RE and McPhillips, JJ: Transitions and progress in therapeutics. In Craig, CR and Stitzel, RE (eds): Modern Pharmacology with Clinical Applications, ed 5. Little Brown, Boston, 1997.
31. Vanchieri, C: Speedier drug approval modeled after FDA's cancer drug review system. J Natl Cancer Inst 84:666, 1992.

CHAPTER 2

Pharmacokinetics I: Drug Administration, Absorption, and Distribution

Pharmacokinetics is the study of the way that the body deals with pharmacologic compounds. In other words, what does the body do to the drug? It includes the manner in which the drug is administered, absorbed, distributed, and eventually eliminated from the body. These topics are discussed in this chapter and the next.

ROUTES OF ADMINISTRATION

In general, drugs can be administered via two primary routes: through the alimentary canal (**enteral administration**) or through nonalimentary routes (**parenteral administration**). Each major route has several variations, and each offers distinct advantages and disadvantages (Table 2–1). The primary features of some of the major routes are discussed here. For a more detailed description of the specific methodology involved in drug administration, the reader is referred to several excellent discussions of this topic.[7,8,10,46]

Enteral

ORAL

The primary way drugs are given enterally is through the oral route. This is the most common method of administering most medications and offers several distinct advantages. Oral administration is the easiest method of taking medications, especially when self-administration is necessary or desired. The oral route is also relatively safe because drugs enter the system in a fairly controlled manner. This avoids the large, sudden increase in plasma drug levels that can occur when the drug is administered by other methods, such as intravenous injection. Most medications administered orally are ab-

TABLE 2–1 Routes of Drug Administration

Route	Advantages	Disadvantages	Examples
		Enteral	
Oral	Easy, safe, convenient	Limited or erratic absorption of some drugs; chance of first-pass inactivation in liver	Analgesics, sedative-hypnotics, many others
Sublingual	Rapid onset; not subject to first-pass inactivation	Drug must be easily absorbed from oral mucosa	Nitroglycerin
Rectal	Alternative to oral route; local effect on rectal tissues	Poor or incomplete absorption; chance of rectal irritation	Laxatives, suppository forms of other drugs
		Parenteral	
Inhalation	Rapid onset; direct application for respiratory disorders; large surface area for systemic absorption	Chance of tissue irritation; patient compliance sometimes a problem	General anesthetics; antiasthmatic agents
Injection	Provides more direct administration to target tissues; rapid onset	Chance of infection if sterility is not maintained	Insulin, antibiotics, anticancer drugs, narcotic analgesics
Topical	Local effects on surface of skin	Only effective in treating outer layers of skin	Antibiotic ointments, creams used to treat minor skin irritation and injury
Transdermal	Introduces drug into body without breaking the skin	Drug must be able to pass through dermal layers intact	Nitroglycerin, motion sickness medications, drugs used with phonophoresis and iontophoresis

sorbed from the small intestine, thus utilizing the large surface area of the intestinal microvilli to enhance entry into the body.

Several disadvantages may preclude drugs from being given orally. Drugs that are administered by mouth must have a relatively high degree of lipid solubility to pass through the gastrointestinal mucosa into the bloodstream. Large, non–lipid-soluble compounds are absorbed very poorly from the alimentary canal and will eventually be lost from the body in the feces. Absorption of some non–lipid-soluble substances (peptides, small proteins) can be enhanced to some extent by encapsulating these agents in lipid vesicles (liposomes), and this technique has been developed recently to enable oral administration of drugs that were formerly administered only by injection or some other parenteral route.[28] Other drawbacks to the oral route include the fact that certain medications may irritate the stomach and cause discomfort, vomiting, or even damage to the gastric mucosa. The acidic environment and presence of digestive proteases in the stomach may also cause various compounds to be degraded and destroyed prior to absorption from the gastrointestinal tract.

Drugs that are given orally are subject to a phenomenon known as the **first-pass effect**.[8,42] After absorption from the alimentary canal, the drug is transported directly to the liver via the portal vein, where a significant amount of the drug may be metabolized and destroyed prior to reaching its site of action. The dosage of the orally administered drug must be sufficient to allow an adequate amount of the compound to survive hepatic degradation and eventually reach the target tissue.[12] Some drugs such as nitroglycerin undergo such extensive inactivation from the first-pass effect that it is usually preferable to administer them by nonoral routes.

A final limitation of the oral route is that the amount and rate at which the drug eventually reaches the bloodstream tend to be somewhat less predictable with oral administration than with more direct routes such as injection. Factors that affect intestinal absorption (intestinal infection, presence of food, rate of gastric emptying, amount of visceral blood flow, and so on) can alter the usual manner in which a drug is absorbed into the body from the gastrointestinal tract.[4,8,30,40,58]

SUBLINGUAL AND BUCCAL

Drugs are administered sublingually by placing the drug under the tongue. Buccal administration occurs when the drug is placed between the cheek and gums. A drug that is administered sublingually or buccally is then absorbed through the oral mucosa into the venous system draining the mouth region. These veins eventually carry blood to the superior vena cava, which in turn carries blood to the heart. Consequently, a drug administered sublingually or buccally can reach the systemic circulation without being subjected to first-pass inactivation in the liver. This provides an obvious advantage for drugs such as nitroglycerin that would be destroyed in the liver when absorbed from the stomach or intestines. These routes also offer a means of enteral administration to people who have difficulty swallowing or to patients who cannot be given drugs rectally.[33,53] The restrictions of the sublingual and buccal routes are that the amount of drug that can be administered is somewhat limited and that the drug must be able to pass easily through the oral mucosa in order to reach the venous drainage of the mouth.

RECTAL

A final method of enteral administration is via the rectum. Many drugs are available as rectal suppositories to allow administration through this route. This method is less favorable because many drugs are absorbed poorly or incompletely, and irritation of the rectal mucosa may occur.[8] Rectal administration does offer the advantage of allowing drugs to be given to a patient who is unconscious, or when vomiting prevents drugs from being taken orally. However, the rectal route is used most often for treating local conditions such as hemorrhoids.

Parenteral

All methods of drug administration that do not use the gastrointestinal tract are termed *parenteral*. Parenteral administration generally allows the drug to be delivered to the target site more directly, and the quantity of the drug that actually reaches the target site is often more predictable.[8,71] Also, drugs given parenterally are not usually subject to first-pass inactivation in the liver. Other advantages and disadvantages of various parenteral routes are discussed further on.

INHALATION

Drugs that exist in a gaseous or volatile state or that can be suspended as tiny droplets in an aerosol form may be given via inhalation. Pulmonary administration offers the advantage of a large (alveolar) surface area for diffusion of the drug into the pulmonary circulation and is generally associated with rapid entry of the drug into the bloodstream.[32,73] This method is used extensively in administering the volatile general anesthetics (e.g., halothane) and is also advantageous for applying medications directly to the bronchial and alveolar tissues for the treatment of specific pulmonary pathologies. The pulmonary route may also be a potential way to administer larger non-lipid-soluble agents such as peptides, small proteins, and DNA.[56,73]

One limitation of the inhalation route is that the drug must not irritate the alveoli or other areas of the respiratory tract. Also, some patients have trouble administering drugs by this route, and drug particles tend to be trapped by cilia and mucus in the respiratory tract. Both of these factors tend to limit the ability to predict exactly how much drug eventually reaches the lungs.

INJECTION

Various types of injection can be used to introduce the drug either systemically or locally. If sterility is not maintained, all types of injection have the disadvantage of possible infection, and certain types of injection are more difficult, if not impossible, for the patient to self-administer. Specific types of injection include the following routes.

Intravenous. The bolus injection of a medication into a peripheral vein allows an accurate, known quantity of the drug to be introduced into the bloodstream over a short period of time, frequently resulting in peak levels of the drug appearing almost instantaneously in the peripheral circulation and thus reaching the target site rapidly. This is advantageous in emergency situations when it is necessary for the medication to exert an immediate effect. Of course, adverse reactions may also occur because of the sudden appearance of large titers of the drug in the plasma. Any unexpected side effect or miscalculation in the amount of the administered drug is often difficult to deal with after the full dosage has been injected. In certain situations, an indwelling intravenous cannula (IV "line") can be used to allow the prolonged, steady infusion of a drug into the venous system. This method prevents large fluctuations in the plasma concentration of the drug and allows the dose of the drug to be maintained at a specific level for as long as desired.

Intra-arterial. The injection of a drug directly into an artery is understandably a difficult and dangerous procedure. This method permits a large dose of the medication to reach a given site, such as a specific organ, and may be used to focus the administration of drugs into certain tissues. Intra-arterial injections are used occasionally in cancer chemotherapy to administer the anticancer drug directly to the tumor site with minimal exposure of the drug to healthy tissues. This route may also be used to focus the administration of other substances such as radiopaque dyes for various diagnostic procedures.

Subcutaneous. Medications are injected directly beneath the skin when a local response is desired, such as in certain situations requiring local anesthesia. Also, a slower, more prolonged release of the medication into the systemic circulation can be achieved in situations where this is the desired effect. A primary example is insulin injection in the patient with diabetes mellitus. Subcutaneous administration provides a relatively easy route of parenteral injection that can be performed by patients themselves, provided they are properly trained. Some limitations are that the amount of drug that can be injected in this fashion is fairly small and that the injected drug must not irritate or inflame the subcutaneous tissues. The subcutaneous route can also be used when certain types of drug preparations are implanted surgically beneath the skin so that the drug is slowly dispersed from the implanted preparation and absorbed into the bloodstream for prolonged periods.[22] An example of this form of subcutaneous administration is the use of implanted hormonal contraceptive products (Norplant). The use of this drug is discussed in more detail in Chapter 30.

Intramuscular. The large quantity of skeletal muscle in the body makes this route an easily accessible site for parenteral administration. Intramuscular injections can be used to treat a problem located directly in the injected muscle or as a method for a relatively steady, prolonged release of the drug into the systemic circulation.

Intramuscular injection offers the advantage of providing a relatively rapid effect (i.e., within a few minutes), while avoiding the sudden, large increase in plasma levels seen with intravenous injection. The major problem with intramuscular administration is that many drugs injected directly into a muscle cause a significant amount of local pain and prolonged soreness, tending to limit the use of this route for repeated injections.

Intrathecal. Intrathecal injections are given by injecting the medication within a sheath. The term frequently refers to injections within the spinal subarachnoid space. This particular type of intrathecal route allows drugs such as narcotic analgesics, local anesthetics, and antispasticity drugs to be applied directly to the spinal cord. Also, intrathecal injections allow certain drugs such as antibiotics and anticancer drugs to bypass the blood-brain barrier and reach the central nervous system (see Chap. 5). Other intrathecal injections include administration of the drug within a tendon sheath or bursa, which may be used to treat a local condition such as an inflammation within those structures.[60]

TOPICAL

Drugs given topically are applied to the surface of the skin or mucous membranes. Most medications applied directly to the skin are absorbed fairly poorly through the epidermis and into the systemic circulation and are used primarily to treat problems that exist on the skin itself. Topical application to mucous membranes is also used frequently to treat problems on the membrane itself. Significant amounts of the drug, however, can be readily absorbed through the mucous membrane and into the bloodstream. Topical application of drugs to mucous membranes can therefore provide a fairly easy and convenient way to administer drugs systemically. Certain medications, for example, can be administered to the nasal mucosa (via nasal spray), to the ocular membranes (via eye drops), or to other mucous membranes to facilitate systemic absorption and treat disorders throughout the body. Nonetheless, the potential for adverse systemic effects must also be considered if large amounts of topically administered drugs are inadvertently absorbed into the body.[64,70]

TRANSDERMAL

Unlike topical administration, transdermal administration consists of applying drugs directly to the surface of the skin with the intent that they *will* be absorbed through the dermal layers and into either the subcutaneous tissues or the peripheral circulation. A transdermally administered drug must possess two basic properties: (1) it must be able to penetrate the skin, and (2) it must not be degraded to any major extent by drug-metabolizing enzymes located in the dermis.[29,44] Absorption may be enhanced by mixing the drug in an oily base, thus increasing solubility and permeability through the dermis.

Transdermal administration provides a slow, controlled release of the drug into the body that is effective in maintaining plasma levels of the drug at a relatively constant level for prolonged periods of time.[13,35] Drugs that can be administered transdermally are often delivered through medicated "patches" that adhere to the skin much like a small adhesive bandage. This method has been used for some time to allow the prolonged administration of drugs such as nitroglycerin and some anti–motion sickness medications, including scopolamine. The use of transdermal patches has been expanded recently to include other medications such as hormonal agents (estrogen)[5,19,39] and opioid analgesics (fentanyl).[3,17,72] Likewise, transdermal nicotine patches have received a great deal of attention for their use in helping people quit smoking cigarettes.[23,34,35] Researchers continue to explore the use of the transdermal route, and transdermal patches continue to gain acceptance as a safe and effective method of administering many medications.

The transdermal route also includes the use of iontophoresis and phonophoresis to administer the drug. In iontophoresis, electric current is used to "drive" the ionized form of the medication through the skin.[6,16,20] Phonophoresis uses ultrasound waves to enhance transmission of the medication through the dermis.[14] Both phonophoresis and iontophoresis are often used to treat pain and inflammation by transmitting specific medications to a subcutaneous tissue such as a muscle, tendon, or bursa. These forms of transdermal administration are important in a rehabilitation setting because they are often administered by a physical therapist following prescription by a physician. Specific medications that can be administered via iontophoresis or phonophoresis are listed in Appendix A. For a more detailed description of how these transdermal routes are employed, the reader is referred to several additional sources.[14,16,20,41,52]

DRUG ABSORPTION AND DISTRIBUTION: BIOAVAILABILITY

Although several routes exist for the administration of drugs, merely introducing the drug into the body does not ensure that the compound will reach all tissues uniformly or even that the drug will reach the appropriate target site. For instance, oral administration of a drug that affects the myocardium will not have any pharmacologic effect unless the drug is absorbed from the gastrointestinal tract into the bloodstream. The extent to which the drug reaches the systemic circulation is referred to as **bioavailability,** which is a parameter that is expressed as the percentage of the drug administered that reaches the bloodstream.[8,15] For instance, if 100 g of a drug is given orally, and 50 g eventually makes it to the systemic circulation, the drug is said to be 50 percent bioavailable. If 100 g of the same compound were injected intravenously, the drug would be 100 percent bioavailable by that route.

Consequently, bioavailability depends on the route of administration as well as the drug's ability to cross membrane barriers. Once in the systemic circulation, further distribution into peripheral tissues may also be important in allowing the drug to reach the target site. Many drugs must eventually leave the systemic capillaries and enter other cells. Thus, drugs have to move across cell membranes and tissue barriers to get into the body and be distributed within the body. In this section, the ability of these membranes to affect the absorption and distribution of drugs is discussed.

Membrane Structure and Function

Throughout the body, biologic membranes act as barriers that permit some substances to pass freely, whereas others pass through with difficulty or not at all. This differential separation serves an obvious protective effect by not allowing certain substances to enter the body or by limiting the distribution of the substance within the body. In effect, the body is separated into various "compartments" by these membranes. In the case of pharmacotherapeutics, there is often the need for the drug to cross one or more of these membrane barriers to reach the target site.

The ability of the membrane to act as a selective barrier is related to the membrane's normal structure and physiologic function. The cell membrane is composed primarily of lipids and proteins. Membrane lipids are actually *phospholipids,* which are composed of a polar, hydrophilic "head" (which contains a phosphate group) and a lipid, hydrophobic "tail" (Fig. 2–1). The phospholipids appear to be arranged in a bilayer, with the hydrophobic tails of the molecule oriented toward the membrane's center, and the hydrophilic heads facing away from the center of the membrane.[65] Interspersed throughout the lipid bilayer are membrane proteins, which can exist primarily in the outer or inner portion of the membrane or can span the entire width of the cell membrane (see Fig. 2–1).

The lipid bilayer that composes the basic structure of the cell membrane acts as a water barrier. The lipid portion of the membrane is essentially impermeable to water and other non–lipid-soluble substances (electrolytes, glucose). Lipid-soluble compounds (including most drugs) are able to pass directly through the membrane by becoming dissolved in the lipid bilayer. Non–lipid-soluble substances, including water, may be able to pass through the membrane because of the presence of membrane pores. Small holes or channels appear to exist in the membrane, thereby allowing certain substances to pass from one side of the membrane to the other. These channels are thought to be formed by some of the membrane proteins that span the width of the membrane.[47,55] The ability of a substance to pass through a specific pore depends primarily on the size, shape, and electrical charge of the molecule. Also, in excitable membranes (nerve, muscle) some of these pores are dynamic in nature and appear to have the ability to "open" and "close," thus regulating the flow of certain ions in and out of the cell.[1,47,49,61,67]

Movement across Membrane Barriers

Drugs and other substances that pass through biologic membranes usually do so via passive diffusion, active transport, facilitated diffusion, or some "special" process such as endocytosis (Fig. 2–2). Each of these mechanisms is discussed here.

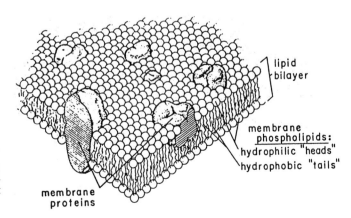

FIGURE 2–1. Schematic diagram of the cell membrane. (Adapted from Singer and Nicolson,[65] p 723. Copyright 1972 by the AAAS.)

lipid bilayer

membrane phospholipids: hydrophilic "heads" hydrophobic "tails"

membrane proteins

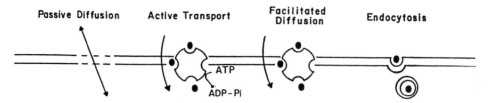

FIGURE 2–2. Schematic diagram summarizing the ways in which substances may cross the cell membrane. Energy is expended during active transport by hydrolyzing adenosine triphosphate (ATP) into adenosine diphosphate (ADP) and inorganic phosphate (Pi). The three other mechanisms do not require any net energy expenditure. See text for further discussion of how and when each mechanism is utilized.

PASSIVE DIFFUSION

Drugs and other substances will pass through a membrane by way of diffusion, providing two essential criteria are met. First, there must be some type of difference or "gradient" on one side of the membrane compared with the other. A concentration gradient, for example, occurs when the concentration of substance differs on one side of the membrane compared with that on the other side. When this gradient occurs, the diffusing substance can move "downhill" from the area of high concentration to that of low concentration. In addition to a concentration difference, diffusion can also occur because of the presence of a pressure gradient or, in the case of charged particles, an electrical potential gradient. The rate of the diffusion is dependent on several factors, including the magnitude of the gradient, the size of the diffusing substance, the distance over which diffusion occurs, and the temperature at which diffusion occurs.[47] The term "passive diffusion" is often used to emphasize the fact that this movement occurs without any energy being expended. The driving force in passive diffusion is the electrical, chemical, and pressure difference on the two sides of the membrane.

For passive diffusion through a membrane to occur, the second essential factor is that the membrane must be permeable to the diffusing substance. As mentioned earlier, non–lipid-soluble compounds can diffuse through the membrane via specific pores. Some non–lipid-soluble drugs such as lithium are small enough to diffuse through these pores. Many drugs, however, are able to diffuse directly through the lipid bilayer; hence, they must be fairly lipid soluble. Passive lipid diffusion is nonselective, and a drug with a high degree of lipid solubility can gain access to many tissues because of its ability to pass directly through the lipid portion of the cell membrane.

Effect of Ionization on Lipid Diffusion. Passive lipid diffusion of certain drugs is also dependent on whether the drug is ionized. Drugs will diffuse more readily through the lipid layer if they are in their neutral, nonionized form. Most drugs are weak acids or weak bases,[37,45] meaning that they have the potential to become positively charged or negatively charged, depending on the pH of certain body fluids. In the plasma and in most other fluids, most drugs remain in their neutral, nonionized form because of the relatively neutral pH of these fluids. In specific fluids, however, a drug may exist in an ionized state, and the absorption of the drug will be affected because of the decreased lipid solubility associated with ionization. For instance, when a weak acid is in an acidic environment (e.g., gastric secretions of the stomach), it tends to be in its neutral, nonionized form. The same drug will become positively charged if the pH of the solution increases and becomes more basic (e.g., the digestive fluids in the duodenum). A weak acid such as aspirin, for example, will be nonionized and therefore absorbed fairly easily from the stomach because of its lipid solubility (Fig. 2–3). This same drug will be poorly absorbed

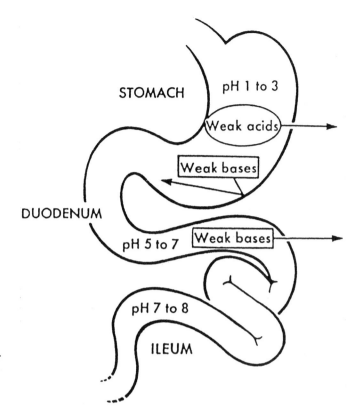

FIGURE 2–3. Effect of pH and ionization on absorption of drugs from the gastrointestinal tract. Weak acids and bases are absorbed from the stomach and duodenum, respectively, when they are in their neutral, nonionized form. (From Clark, JB, Queener, SF, and Karb, VB: Pharmacological Basis of Nursing Practice, ed 4. CV Mosby, St. Louis, 1993, p 8, with permission.)

if it reaches the basic pH of the duodenum and becomes ionized. Conversely, a drug that is a weak base will be ionized and poorly absorbed from the acidic environment of the stomach. The same drug will be nonionized and therefore lipid soluble when it reaches the duodenum, allowing it to be absorbed from the proximal small intestine.

Diffusion Trapping. Changes in lipid solubility caused by ionization can also be important when the body attempts to excrete a drug in the urine. Here the situation becomes slightly more complex because the urine can sometimes be acidic and other times basic in nature. In either situation, it is often desirable for the drug to remain ionized while in the urine so that the drug will be excreted from the body. If the drug becomes nonionized while in the nephron, it may be reabsorbed back into the body because of its increased lipid solubility. An ionized form of the drug will remain "trapped" in the nephron and will eventually be excreted in the urine.[45] Thus, if the urine is basic, weak acids will become trapped in the nephron and will be excreted more readily. Weak bases will be excreted better if the urine is acidic. The importance of the kidneys in excreting drugs from the body is discussed further in Chapter 3.

Diffusion between Cell Junctions. So far, the diffusion of drugs and other substances through individual cell membranes has been discussed. Often groups of cells join together to form a barrier that separates one body compartment from another. In some locations, cells form "tight junctions" with each other and do not allow any appreciable space to exist between adjacent cells. In these cases, the primary way a drug may diffuse across the barrier is by diffusing first into and then out of the other side of the cells comprising the barrier. Such locations include the epithelial lining of the gastrointestinal tract and the capillary endothelium of the brain (one of the reasons for the **blood-brain barrier**). In other tissues, such as peripheral capillaries, there may be relatively large gaps between adjacent cells. Here, relatively large substances with molecular weights as high as 30,000 may be able to diffuse across the barrier by diffusing between adjacent cells.

Osmosis. Osmosis refers to the special case of diffusion in which the diffusing substance is water. In this situation, water moves from an area where it is highly concentrated to an area of low concentration. Of course, permeability is still a factor when osmosis occurs across a membrane or tissue barrier. During osmosis, certain drugs may simply travel with the diffusing water, thus crossing the membrane by the process of "bulk flow." This is usually limited to osmosis through the gaps between adjacent cells because membrane pores are often too small to allow the passage of the drug molecule along with the diffusing water.

ACTIVE TRANSPORT

Active or carrier-mediated transport involves using membrane proteins to transport substances across the cell membrane (see Fig. 2–2). Membrane proteins that span the entire membrane may serve as some sort of carrier that shuttles substances from one side of the membrane to the other.[37,47] Characteristics of active transport include the following:

Carrier specificity: The protein carrier exhibits some degree of specificity for certain substances, usually discriminating among different compounds according to their shape and electrical charge. This specificity is not absolute, and some compounds that resemble one another will be transported by the same group of carriers.

Expenditure of energy: The term "active transport" implies that some energy must be used to fuel the carrier system. This energy is usually in the form of adenosine triphosphate (ATP) hydrolysis.

Ability to transport substances against a concentration gradient: Carrier-mediated active transport may be able to carry substances "uphill," that is, from areas of low concentration to areas of high concentration.

The role of active transport in moving drugs across cell membranes is somewhat limited. Essentially, the drug has to bear a good deal of resemblance to the endogenous substance that the transport system routinely carries. However, some drugs, such as theophylline, are apparently absorbed from the intestine via active transport,[43] and active transport systems in the kidney may be important in the excretion of certain drugs into the urine.[9] Also, some drugs may exert their effect by either facilitating or inhibiting endogenous transport systems that affect cellular homeostasis.

FACILITATED DIFFUSION

Facilitated diffusion, as the name implies, bears some features of both active transport and passive diffusion. A protein carrier is present in facilitated diffusion, but no net energy is expended in transporting the substance across the cell membrane.[47] As a result, in most cases of facilitated diffusion there is an inability to transport substances "uphill" against a concentration gradient. The entry of glucose into skeletal muscle cells via facilitated diffusion is probably the best example of this type of transport in the body. As in active transport, the movement of drugs across membranes through facilitated diffusion is fairly infrequent, but certain medications may affect the rate at which endogenous facilitated diffusion occurs.

SPECIAL PROCESSES

Certain cells have the ability to transport substances across their membranes through processes such as endocytosis. Here the drug is engulfed by the cell via an invagination of the cell membrane. Although limited in scope, this method does allow certain large non–lipid-soluble drugs to enter the cell.

DISTRIBUTION OF DRUGS WITHIN THE BODY

Factors Affecting Distribution

Following administration, the extent to which a drug is uniformly distributed throughout the body or sequestered in a specific body compartment depends on several factors:

1. *Tissue permeability:*   As discussed earlier, the ability to pass through membranes radically affects the extent to which a drug moves around within the body. A highly lipid-soluble drug can potentially reach all the different body compartments and enter virtually every cell it reaches.[57,68] A large non–lipid-soluble compound will remain primarily in the compartment or tissue to which it is administered. Also, certain tissues such as the brain capillary endothelium have special characteristics that limit the passage of drugs. This so-called blood-brain barrier limits the movement of drugs out of the bloodstream and into the central nervous system tissue.
2. *Blood flow:*   If a drug is circulating in the bloodstream, it will gain greater access to tissues that are highly perfused. More of the drug will reach organs that receive a great deal of blood flow, such as the brain, kidneys, and exercising skeletal muscle, than less active tissues such as adipose stores.[37]
3. *Binding to plasma proteins:*   Certain drugs will form reversible bonds to circulating proteins in the bloodstream such as albumin.[8,37] This fact is significant because only the unbound or "free" drug is able to reach the target tissue and exert a pharmacologic effect. Basically, the fraction of the drug that remains bound to the circulating proteins is sequestered within the vascular system and not available for therapeutic purposes in other tissues and organs.
4. *Binding to subcellular components:*   In a situation similar to plasma protein binding, drugs that are bound within specific cells are unable to leave the cell and be distributed throughout other fluid compartments. An example of this is the antimalarial drug quinacrine, which binds to nucleoproteins located within liver and muscle cells.[8]

Volume of Distribution

The distribution of a given drug within the body is often described by calculating the **volume of distribution (V_d)** for that drug.[8,15,37] V_d is the ratio of the amount of drug administered to the concentration of drug in the plasma:

$$V_d = \text{amount of drug administered} \div \text{concentration of drug in plasma}$$

V_d is used to estimate a drug's distribution by comparing the calculated V_d with the total amount of body water in a normal person. A normal 70-kg man has a total body fluid content of approximately 42 L (5.5 L blood, 12.0 L extracellular fluid, 24.5 L intracellular fluid). If the calculated V_d of a drug is approximately equal to the total amount of body water, then the drug is distributed uniformly throughout all of the body fluids. If the V_d of the drug is far less than 42 L, then the drug is being retained in the bloodstream because of factors such as plasma protein binding. A V_d much greater than 42 L indicates that the drug is being concentrated in the tissues. It should be noted that V_d is not a "real" value; that is, it does not indicate the actual amount of fluid in the body but is merely an arbitrary figure that reflects the apparent distribution of a drug by using total body water as a reference point. Table 2–2 gives some examples of the calculation of the V_d for three different types of drugs.

DRUG STORAGE

Storage Sites

Following administration and absorption, many drugs are "stored" to some extent at certain locations in the body[8]; that is, prior to drug elimination, the drug may be sequestered in its active form in a relatively inert tissue that may be different from the target site of the drug. Some storage sites include the following:

1. *Adipose:* The primary site for drug storage in the body is adipose tissue. Because many drugs are lipid soluble, fat deposits throughout the body can serve as a considerable reservoir for these compounds. In some individuals, the amount of fat in the body can reach as high as 50 percent of body weight, thus creating an extensive storage compartment. Once drugs have been stored in adipose tissue, they tend to remain there for long periods because of the low metabolic rate and poor blood perfusion of these tissues. Examples of drugs that tend to be stored in fat include the highly lipid-soluble anesthetics such as the barbiturates (thiopental) and inhalation anesthetics (halothane).
2. *Bone:* Bone acts as a storage site for several toxic agents, especially the heavy metals like lead. Also, drugs such as the tetracyclines, which bind to and form molecular complexes with the crystal components within the skeletal matrix, are stored within bone.
3. *Muscle:* Binding of drugs to components within the muscle may create the long-term storage of these compounds. Various agents may be actively transported into the muscle cell and may form reversible bonds to intracellular structures such as proteins, nucleoproteins, or phospholipids. An example is the antimalarial drug quinacrine.
4. *Organs:* Drugs are often stored within certain organs such as the liver and kidneys. As in muscle cells, the drug may enter the cell passively or by active transport and then form bonds to subcellular components. Examples include the antimicrobial aminoglycoside agents (such as gentamicin and streptomycin), which accumulate in renal proximal tubular cells.

Adverse Consequences of Drug Storage

High concentrations of drugs, drug metabolites, and toxic compounds within tissues can cause local damage to the tissues in which they are stored. This event is particularly true for toxic compounds that are incorporated and stored in the matrix of bone

TABLE 2-2 Examples of Volume of Distribution

Drug	Amount Administered	Plasma Concentration	Volume of Distribution	Indication	Examples
A	420 mg	0.01 mg/mL	$\dfrac{420\ mg}{0.01\ mg/mL} = 42{,}000\ mL = 42\ L$	Uniform distribution	Erythromycin, lithium
B	420 mg	0.05 mg/mL	$\dfrac{420\ mg}{0.05\ mg/mL} = 8{,}400\ mL = 8.4\ L$	Retained in plasma	Aspirin, valproic acid
C	420 mg	0.001 mg/mL	$\dfrac{420\ mg}{0.001\ mg/mL} = 420{,}000\ mL = 420\ L$	Sequestered in tissues	Morphine, quinidine

or that are highly concentrated within specific organs. Lead poisoning, for example, causes several well-known and potentially devastating effects when this metal accumulates in the central nervous system (CNS), bone, gastrointestinal tract, and several other tissues. Exposing various organs to high concentrations of therapeutic drugs can also result in myriad problems. Acetaminophen, for example, is normally metabolized in the liver to form several highly reactive by-products or metabolites (see Chap. 15). When normal doses of acetaminophen are metabolized in a reasonably healthy liver, these metabolites are rapidly inactivated in the liver and subsequently excreted by the kidneys. Very high doses of acetaminophen, however, result in the formation of excessive amounts of a toxic metabolite that can react with hepatic proteins and cause severe liver damage.[69] Hence, organs such as the liver and kidneys are often subjected to local damage when these organs must deal with high concentrations of therapeutic and toxic agents.

Another problem of drug storage occurs when the storage site acts as a reservoir that "soaks up" the drug and prevents it from reaching the target site. For instance, a highly lipid-soluble drug such as a general anesthetic must be administered in a sufficient dose to ensure that there will be enough drug available to reach the CNS, despite the tendency for much of the drug to be sequestered in the body's fat stores. Storage sites may also be responsible for the redistribution of drugs. This is seen when the drug begins to leak out of the storage reservoir after plasma levels of the drug have begun to diminish. In this way, the drug may be reintroduced to the target site long after the original dose should have been eliminated. This redistribution may explain why certain individuals experience prolonged effects of the drug or extended adverse side effects.

NEWER TECHNIQUES FOR DRUG DELIVERY

Controlled-Release Preparations

Controlled-release preparations, also known as *timed-release* or *extended-release preparations*, are generally designed to permit a slower and more prolonged absorption of the drug from the gastrointestinal tract and other routes of administration.[18] This technique may offer several advantages, such as decreasing the number of doses needed each day, preventing large fluctuations in the amount of drug appearing in the plasma, and sustaining plasma levels throughout the night.[8] This type of preparation has been used successfully with several types of drugs, including cardiovascular medications (beta blockers, calcium channel blockers),[28,31] narcotic analgesics such as morphine,[25,36] and antiparkinsonian medications that contain L-dopa.[50,62] Controlled-release preparations will probably continue to gain popularity as a means for administering these and other medications in the future.[18]

Implanted Drug Delivery Systems

Several techniques have been developed whereby some type of drug "reservoir" is implanted surgically within the body and the drug is then released in a controlled fashion from the implanted reservoir.[22,54,59,63] These drug reservoirs typically consist of a small container placed under the skin in the abdomen. These containers are often programmed to allow a small, measured dose of the drug to be released periodically from the reservoir. Alternatively, the reservoir can be controlled electronically from outside the body through the use of small remote-control devices, thus allowing the patient to regulate release of the drug as needed. In some cases, the drug reservoir may be connected by a small cannula to a specific body compartment, such as the subarachnoid space or epidural space, and the drug can be delivered directly into that space. This type of system appears to be very helpful in applying certain drugs such as analgesics, anesthetics, and muscle relaxants to the spinal cord.[54,59,63]

Another type of implantable system has been developed recently that incorporates the drug into some type of biodegradable or nonbiodegradable substance such as a polymer matrix or gel.[2,48,51,66] The drug-polymer complex is then implanted in the body, and the drug is slowly released into the surrounding tissues (nonbiodegradable), or the drug is released as the matrix gradually dissolves (biodegradable). This type of system is probably best known for administering contraceptive hormones such as progesterone (Norplant, see Chap. 30), and these implants have also shown promise in being able to deliver other medications such as local anesthetics, insulin, and vaccines.[38,48,51]

Hence, implantable drug delivery systems are being considered as a potential means of administering several drugs, including analgesics, muscle relaxants, and hormones. Improvements in the technology of this type of drug delivery will hopefully permit increased clinical applications of these systems in the near future. The use of implantable drug delivery systems with specific types of medications will be discussed in more detail when these medications are addressed in subsequent chapters in this book.

Targeting Drug Delivery to Specific Cells and Tissues

Some very innovative approaches have been attempted on a molecular level to try to target the drug specifically to the cells that require treatment. For instance, specific types of antibodies (monoclonal antibodies) can be synthesized and attached to drugs such as the cytotoxic agents often used in cancer chemotherapy.[11,24] The antibodies are then attracted to antigens located on the surface of the tumor cells. This offers the distinct advantage of focusing the drug more directly on the cancerous cells rather than on healthy human tissues. Other cellular techniques have been investigated that could also help direct the drug to the affected tissues. It may be possible, for example, to link a drug to a modified virus so that the virus transports and helps insert the drug directly into specific tissues[21]; the virus, of course, must be modified so that it will not cause viral infection. Other nonviral techniques include encapsulating the drug in a certain type of fat particle (liposome) or attaching the drug to certain proteins that will be attracted to the surface receptors of specific cells.[21,26] These viral and nonviral techniques have been particularly important in helping to deliver DNA to specific cells in order to modify the genetic regulation of those cells (gene-based therapy).[21,26]

The idea of targeting drugs to specific tissues through various cellular and molecular mechanisms is still fairly experimental at this time. These techniques have shown considerable promise, however, and may ultimately be extremely useful in increasing the effectiveness of certain drugs while decreasing their side effects.

SUMMARY

For any drug to be effective, it must be able to reach specific target tissues. The goal of drug administration is to deliver the drug in the least complicated manner that will still allow sufficient concentrations of the active form of the drug to arrive at the desired site. Each route of administration has certain advantages and disadvantages that will determine how much and how fast the drug is delivered to specific tissues. In addition to the route of administration, the distribution of the drug within the body must be taken into account. Simply introducing the drug into certain body fluids such as the bloodstream does not ensure its entry into the desired tissues. Factors such as tissue permeability and protein binding may influence how the drug is dispersed within the various fluid compartments within the body. Finally, some drugs have a tendency to be stored in certain tissues for prolonged periods of time. This storage may produce serious toxic effects if high concentrations of the compound damage the cells in which it is stored.

REFERENCES

1. Agnew, WS: Voltage-regulated sodium channel molecules. Annu Rev Physiol 46:517, 1984.
2. Anderson, JM and Langone, JJ: Issues and perspectives on the biocompatibility and immunotoxicity evaluation of implanted controlled release systems. J Controlled Release 57:107, 1999.
3. Ashburn, MA and Stanley, TH: Non-invasive drug delivery systems for the management of postoperative pain. Prog Anesth 5:146, 1991.
4. Bailey, DG, et al: Interaction of citrus juices with felodipine and nifedipine. Lancet 337:268, 1991.
5. Balfour, JA and McTavish, D: Transdermal estradiol: A review of its pharmacological profile, and therapeutic potential in the prevention of postmenopausal osteoporosis. Drugs Aging 2:487, 1992.
6. Banga, AK, Bose, S, and Ghosh, TK: Iontophoresis and electroportion: Comparisons and contrasts. Int J Pharm 179:1, 1999.
7. Bauer, LA: Clinical pharmacokinetics and pharmacodynamics. In DiPiro, JT, et al (eds): Pharmacotherapy: A Pathophysiologic Approach, ed 4. Appleton & Lange, Stamford, CT, 1999.
8. Benet, LZ, Kroetz, DL, and Sheiner, LB: Pharmacokinetics: The dynamics of drug absorption, distribution and elimination. In Hardman, JG, et al (eds): The Pharmacological Basis of Therapeutics, ed 9. McGraw Hill, New York, 1996.
9. Berndt, WO and Stitzel, RE: Excretion of drugs. In Craig, CR and Stitzel, RE (eds): Modern Pharmacology with Clinical Applications, ed 5. Little Brown, Boston, 1997.
10. Beyssac, E: The unusual routes of administration. Eur J Drug Metab Pharmacokinet 21:181, 1996.
11. Blakely, DC: Drug targeting with monoclonal antibodies: A review. Acta Oncol 31:91, 1992.
12. Brockmeier, D and Ostrowski, J: Mean time and first pass metabolism. Eur J Clin Pharmacol 29:45, 1985.
13. Brown, L and Langer, R: Transdermal delivery of drugs. Annu Rev Med 39:221, 1988.
14. Byl, NN: The use of ultrasound as an enhancer for transcutaneous drug delivery: Phonophoresis. Phys Ther 75:539, 1995.
15. Ciccone, CD: Basic pharmacokinetics and the potential effect of physical therapy interventions on pharmacokinetic variables. Phys Ther 75:343, 1995.
16. Ciccone, CD: Iontophoresis. In Robinson, AJ and Snyder-Mackler, L (eds): Clinical Electrophysiology, ed 2. Williams & Wilkins, Baltimore, 1994.
17. Collins, JJ, et al: Transdermal fentanyl in children with cancer pain: Feasibility, tolerability, and pharmacokinetic correlates. J Pediatr 134:319, 1999.
18. Colombo, P, et al: Controlled release dosage forms: From ground to space. Eur J Drug Metab Pharmacokinet 21:87, 1996.
19. Corson, SL: A decade of experience with transdermal estrogen replacement therapy: Overview of key pharmacologic and clinical findings. Int J Fertil 38:79, 1993.
20. Costello, CT and Jeske, AH: Iontophoresis: Applications in transdermal medication delivery. Phys Ther 75:554, 1995.
21. Dachs, GU, et al: Targeting gene therapy to cancer: A review. Oncol Res 9:313, 1997.
22. Dash, AK and Cudworth, GC: Therapeutic applications of implantable drug delivery systems. J Pharmacol Toxicol Methods 40:1, 1998.
23. Davidson, M, et al: Efficacy and safety of an over-the-counter transdermal nicotine patch as an aid for smoking cessation. Arch Fam Med 7:569, 1998.
24. Denny, WA and Wilson, WR: The design of selectively-activated anti-cancer prodrugs for use in antibody-directed and gene-directed enzyme-prodrug therapies. J Pharm Pharmacol 50:387, 1998.
25. Deschamps, M, et al: The evaluation of analgesic effects in cancer patients as exemplified by a double-blind, cross-over study of immediate-release versus controlled-release morphine. J Pain Symptom Manage 7:384, 1992.
26. Eck, SL and Wilson, JM: Gene-based therapy. In Hardman, JG, et al (eds): The Pharmacological Basis of Therapeutics, ed 9. McGraw Hill, New York, 1996.
27. Fasano, A: Innovative strategies for the oral delivery of drugs and peptides. Trends Biotechnol 16:152, 1998.

28. Feliciano, NR, et al: Pharmacokinetic and pharmacodynamic comparison of an osmotic release oral metoprolol tablet and the metoprolol conventional tablet. Am Heart J 120(2, suppl):483, 1990.
29. Finnen, MJ, Herdman, ML, and Shuster, S: Distribution and subcellular localization of drug metabolizing enzymes in the skin. Br J Dermatol 113:713, 1985.
30. Fleisher, D, et al: Drug, meal and formulation interactions influencing drug absorption after oral administration. Clinical implications. Clin Pharmacokinet 36:233, 1999.
31. Frishman, WH: A new extended-release formulation of diltiazem HCl for the treatment of mild-to-moderate hypertension. J Clin Pharmacol 33:612, 1993.
32. Gillis, CN: Pharmacologic aspects of metabolic processes in the pulmonary microcirculation. Ann Rev Toxicol 26:183, 1986.
33. Gong, L and Middleton, RK: Sublingual administration of opioids. Ann Pharmacother 26:1525, 1992.
34. Gora, ML: Nicotine transdermal systems. Ann Pharmacother 27:742, 1993.
35. Gorsline, J, et al: Steady-state pharmacokinetics and dose relationship of nicotine delivered from Nicoderm. J Clin Pharmacol 33:161, 1993.
36. Gourlay, GK: Sustained relief of chronic pain. Pharmacokinetics of sustained release morphine. Clin Pharmacokinet 35:173, 1998.
37. Gram, TE: Drug absorption and distribution. In Craig, CR and Stitzel, RE (eds): Modern Pharmacology with Clinical Applications, ed 5. Little Brown, Boston, 1997.
38. Gupta, RK, Chang, AC, and Siber, GR: Biodegradable polymer microspheres as vaccine adjuvants and delivery systems. Dev Biol Stand 92:63, 1998.
39. Harrison, LI, et al: Comparative serum estradiol profiles from a new once-a-week transdermal estradiol patch and a twice-a-week transdermal estradiol patch. Ther Drug Monit 19:37, 1997.
40. Hebbard, GS, et al: Pharmacokinetic considerations in gastrointestinal motor disorders. Clin Pharmacokinet 28:41, 1995.
41. Henley, EJ: Transcutaneous drug delivery: Iontophoresis, phonophoresis. CRC Crit Rev Phys Rehabil Med 2:139, 1991.
42. Holford, NHG and Benet, LZ: Pharmacokinetics and pharmacodynamics: Dose selection and the time course of drug action. In Katzung, BG (ed): Basic and Clinical Pharmacology, ed 7. Appleton & Lange, Stamford, CT, 1998.
43. Johansson, O, Lindberg, T, and Melander, A: In-vivo absorption of theophylline and salicylic acid from rat small intestine. Acta Pharmacol Toxicol 55:335, 1984.
44. Kao, J, Patterson, FK, and Hall, J: Skin penetration and metabolism of topically applied chemicals in six mammalian species, including man: An in-vitro study with benzo(a)pyrene and testosterone. Toxicol Appl Pharmacol 81:502, 1985.
45. Katzung, BG: Introduction. In Katzung, BG (ed): Basic and Clinical Pharmacology, ed 7. Appleton & Lange, Stamford, CT, 1998.
46. Kuhn, MA (ed): Pharmacotherapeutics: A Nursing Process Approach, ed 4. FA Davis, Philadelphia, 1997.
47. Kutchai, HC: Cellular membranes and transmembrane transport of solutes and water. In Berne, RM and Levy, MN (eds): Principles of Physiology, ed 3. Mosby, St Louis, 2000.
48. Kwon, IC, Bae, YH, and Kim, SW: Electrically erodible polymer gel for controlled release of drugs. Nature 354:291, 1992.
49. Latore, R and Alvarez, O: Voltage-dependent channels in lipid bilayer membranes. Physiol Rev 61:77, 1981.
50. Manyam, BV, et al: Evaluation of equivalent efficacy of Sinemet and Sinemet CR in patients with Parkinson's disease applying levodopa dosage conversion formula. Clin Neuropharmacol 22:33, 1999.
51. Masters, DB, et al: Prolonged regional nerve blockade by controlled release of local anesthetic from a biodegradable polymer matrix. Anesthesiology 79:340, 1993.
52. McDiarmid, T, Ziskin, MC, and Michlovitz, SL: Therapeutic ultrasound. In Michlovitz, SL (ed): Thermal Agents in Rehabilitation, ed 3. FA Davis, Philadelphia, 1996.
53. Mercadante, S and Fulfaro, F: Alternatives to oral opioids for cancer pain. Oncology 13:215, 1999.
54. Meythaler, JM, et al: Continuous intrathecal baclofen in spinal cord spasticity: A prospective study. Am J Phys Med Rehabil 71:321, 1992.
55. Miller, C: Integral membrane channels: Studies in model membranes. Physiol Rev 63:1209, 1983.
56. Niven, RW: Delivery of biotherapeutics by inhalation aerosol. Crit Rev Ther Drug Carrier Syst 12:151, 1995.
57. Ochs, HR, et al: Cerebrospinal fluid uptake and peripheral distribution of centrally acting drugs: Relation to lipid solubility. J Pharm Pharmacol 37:428, 1985.
58. Oguey, D, et al: Effect of food on the bioavailability of low-dose methotrexate in patients with rheumatoid arthritis. Arthritis Rheum 35:611, 1992.
59. Penn, SD, et al: Intrathecal baclofen for severe spinal spasticity. N Engl J Med 320:1517, 1989.
60. Rizk, TE, Pinals, RS, and Talaiver, AS: Corticosteroid injections in adhesive capsulitis: Investigation of their value and site. Arch Phys Med Rehabil 72:20, 1991.
61. Rogart, R: Sodium channels in nerve and muscle membranes. Annu Rev Physiol 43:711, 1981.
62. Sage, JI and Mark, MH: Pharmacokinetics of continuous-release carbidopa/levodopa. Clin Neuropharmacol 17(Suppl 2):S1, 1994.
63. Shaw, HL: Treatment of the patient with cancer using parenteral electrical drug administration. Cancer 70(4, suppl):993, 1992.

64. Shohat, M, et al: Adrenocortical suppression by topical application of glucocorticoids in infants with seborrheic dermatitis. Clin Pediatr (Phila) 25:209, 1986.
65. Singer, SJ and Nicolson, GL: The fluid-mosaic model of the structure of membranes. Science 175:720, 1972.
66. Sinha, VR and Khosla, L: Bioabsorbable polymers for implantable therapeutic systems. Drug Dev Ind Pharm 24:1129, 1998.
67. Standen, NB and Quayle, JM: K$^+$ channel modulation in arterial smooth muscle. Acta Physiol Scand 164:549, 1998.
68. Theodorsen, L and Brors, O: The importance of lipid solubility and receptor selectivity of beta-adrenoceptor blocking drugs for the occurrence of symptoms and side effects in out-patients. J Intern Med 226:17, 1989.
69. Thomas, SH: Paracetamol (acetaminophen) poisoning. Pharmacol Ther 60:91, 1993.
70. Urtti, A and Salminen, L: Minimizing systemic absorption of topically administered ophthalmic drugs. Surv Ophthalmol 37:435, 1993.
71. Weiss, M: On pharmacokinetics in target tissues. Biopharm Drug Dispos 6:57, 1985.
72. Yee, LY and Lopez, JR: Transdermal fentanyl. Ann Pharmacother 26:1393, 1992.
73. Yu, J and Chien, YW: Pulmonary drug delivery: Physiologic and mechanistic aspects. Crit Rev Ther Drug Carrier Syst 14:395, 1997.

CHAPTER **3**

Pharmacokinetics II: Drug Elimination

All drugs must eventually be eliminated from the body to terminate their effect and to prevent excessive accumulation of the drug. Drugs are usually eliminated by chemically altering the original compound while it is still in the body so that it is no longer active (*biotransformation*), by excreting the active form of the drug from the body (*excretion*), or by a combination of biotransformation and excretion. These methods of drug elimination will be discussed here.

BIOTRANSFORMATION

Drug metabolism, or **biotransformation,** refers to chemical changes that take place in the drug following administration. Enzymes located within specific tissues are responsible for catalyzing changes in the drug's structure and subsequently altering the pharmacologic properties of the drug. The location of these enzymes and the reactions involved in biotransformation are discussed later in this chapter.

Biotransformation usually results in an altered version of the original compound known as a **metabolite,** which is usually inactive or has a greatly reduced level of pharmacologic activity. Occasionally, the metabolite has a higher level of activity than the original compound. If the metabolite has a higher level of activity, the drug may be given in an inactive, or "prodrug," form that will be activated via biotransformation following administration. However, termination of the drug after it has exerted its pharmacologic effect is the primary function of drug biotransformation.[48]

Inactivation of a drug and termination of its effect once the drug is no longer needed are often essential. For instance, the effects of general and local anesthetics must eventually wear off and allow the patient to resume normal function. Although termination of drug activity can occur when the active form of the drug is excreted from the body via organs such as the kidneys, excretory mechanisms are often too slow to effectively terminate the activity of most drugs within a reasonable time period. If excretion was the only way to terminate drug activity, some compounds would continue to exert their effects for several days or even weeks. Biotransformation of the drug into an inactive form usually occurs within a matter of minutes or hours, thus reducing the chance for toxic effects caused by drug accumulation or prolonged drug activity.

Cellular Mechanisms of Drug Biotransformation

The chemical changes that occur during drug metabolism are usually caused by oxidation, reduction, hydrolysis, or conjugation of the original compound.[6,27] Examples of each type of reaction are listed in Table 3–1. Each type of reaction and the location of the enzymes catalyzing the reaction are also discussed here.

1. *Oxidation:* Oxidation occurs because of the addition of oxygen or the removal of hydrogen from the original compound. Oxidation reactions are the predominant

TABLE 3–1 Examples of Drug Biotransformation Reactions

	Examples
I. Oxidation	
A. Side chain (aliphatic) hydroxylation	
$\overset{\displaystyle [O]}{RCH_2CH_3 \rightarrow} \overset{\displaystyle OH}{\underset{\displaystyle \vert}{R}CHCH_3}$	Ibuprofen
B. N-oxidation	
$(R)_2NH \overset{[O]}{\rightarrow} (R)_2NOH$	Acetaminophen
C. Deamination	
$RCH_2NH_2 \overset{[O]}{\rightarrow} RCHO + NH_3$	Diazepam
II. Reduction	
A. Nitro reductions	
$RNO_2 \rightarrow RNH_2$	Dantrolene
B. Carbonyl reduction	
$\overset{O}{\underset{\Vert}{R}}CR' \rightarrow \overset{OH}{\underset{\vert}{R}}CHR'$	Methadone
III. Hydrolysis	
A. Esters	
$\overset{O}{\underset{\Vert}{R}}COR' \rightarrow RCOOH + R'OH$	Aspirin
B. Amides	
$\overset{O}{\underset{\Vert}{R}}CNR' \rightarrow RCOOH + R'NH_2$	Lidocaine
IV. Conjugation	
A. Acetylation	
$RNH_2 + AcetylCoA \rightarrow RNH\overset{O}{\underset{\Vert}{C}}CH_3 + CoA\text{-}SH$	Clonazepam
B. Glycine conjugation	
$RCOOH \rightarrow R\overset{O}{\underset{\Vert}{C}}SCoA + NH_2CH_2COOH \rightarrow$	
$R\overset{O}{\underset{\Vert}{C}}NHCH_2COOH + CoA\text{-}SH$	Benzoic acid

Parent drug compounds are represented by the letter "R." Examples are types of drugs that undergo biotransformation via the respective type of chemical reaction.

method of drug biotransformation in the body, and the primary enzymes that catalyze these reactions are known collectively as the cytochrome P450 mono-oxygenases.[27,48] These enzymes are located primarily on the smooth endoplasmic reticulum of specific cells and are sometimes referred to as the **drug microsomal metabolizing system (DMMS).** The general scheme of drug oxidation as catalyzed by the DMMS is shown in Figure 3–1.

2. *Reduction:* Reduction reactions remove oxygen or add hydrogen to the original compound. Enzymes that are located in the cell cytoplasm are usually responsible for reducing the drug.

3. *Hydrolysis:* The original compound is broken into separate parts. The enzymes responsible for hydrolysis of the drug are located at several sites within the cell (i.e., the endoplasmic reticulum and cytoplasm) as well as extracellularly (e.g., circulating in the plasma).

4. *Conjugation:* In conjugation reactions, the intact drug, or the metabolite of one of the reactions described earlier, is coupled to an endogenous substance such as acetyl coenzyme A (acetyl CoA), glucuronic acid, or an amino acid. Enzymes that catalyze drug conjugations are found in the cytoplasm and on the endoplasmic reticulum.

The chemical reactions involved in drug biotransformation are also classified as either phase I or phase II reactions.[6,16] Phase I reactions use oxidation, reduction, or hydrolysis. Phase II reactions involve conjugation of the parent drug or the metabolite of a drug that was already metabolized using a phase I reaction.

Regardless of the type of chemical reaction used, biotransformation also helps in the excretion of the metabolite from the body by creating a more polar compound.[48] After one or more of the reactions just described, the remaining drug metabolite usually has a greater tendency to be ionized in the body fluids. The ionized metabolite is more water soluble and thus more easily transported in the bloodstream to the kidneys. Upon reaching the kidneys, the polar metabolite can be excreted from the body in the urine. The contribution of biotransformation toward renal excretion is discussed in a later section.

Organs Responsible for Drug Biotransformation

The primary location for drug metabolism is the liver.[6,48,50] Enzymes responsible for drug metabolism such as the cytochrome P450 enzymes are abundant on hepatic smooth endoplasmic reticulum, and liver cells also contain other cytoplasmic enzymes responsible for drug reduction and hydrolysis. Other organs that contain metabolizing enzymes and exhibit considerable drug transformation ability include the lungs, kidneys, gastrointestinal epithelium, and skin. Drug metabolism can be radically altered if these tissues are damaged. For instance, inactivation of certain drugs may be significantly de-

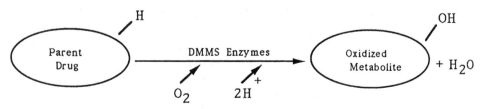

FIGURE 3–1. Drug oxidation catalyzed by drug microsomal metabolizing system (DMMS) enzymes.

layed in the patient with hepatitis or cirrhosis of the liver.[23,61,66] As would be expected, dosages in these patients must be adjusted accordingly to prevent drug accumulation and toxicity.

Enzyme Induction

A frequent problem in drug metabolism is the phenomenon of **enzyme induction**.[16,27,51] Prolonged use of certain drugs "induces" the body to be able to enzymatically destroy the drug more rapidly, usually because either more of the metabolizing enzymes are being manufactured or less are being degraded. Enzyme induction may cause drugs to be metabolized more rapidly than expected, thus decreasing their therapeutic effect. This may be one reason that **tolerance** to some drugs occurs when the drug is used for extended periods (tolerance is the need for increased dosages of the drug to produce the same effect). Long-term ingestion or inhalation of other exogenous compounds such as alcohol, cigarette smoke, or environmental toxins may also cause enzyme induction.[19,21,51,58] When this occurs, medicinal drugs may be more rapidly metabolized even when they are first administered because of the pre-existing enzyme induction.

DRUG EXCRETION

The kidneys are the primary site for drug excretion.[6,10] The functional unit of the kidney is the nephron (Fig. 3–2), and each kidney is composed of approximately 1 million nephrons. Usually the metabolized or conjugated version of the original drug reaches the nephron and is then filtered at the glomerulus. Following filtration at the glomerulus, the compound traverses the proximal convoluted tubule, loop of Henle, and distal convoluted tubule before reaching the collecting ducts. If a compound is not reabsorbed while moving through the nephron, it will ultimately leave the body in the urine. As discussed earlier, biotransformation plays a significant role in creating a polar, water-soluble metabolite that is able to reach the kidneys through the bloodstream. Only drugs or their metabolites that are relatively polar will be excreted in significant amounts by the kidney because the ionized metabolite has a greater tendency to remain in the nephron and not be reabsorbed into the body.[6,48] Nonpolar compounds that are filtered by the kidneys are relatively lipophilic and can easily be passively reabsorbed back into the body by diffusing through the wall of the nephron. However, the polar metabolite is relatively impermeable to the epithelium lining the nephron and tends to remain "trapped" in the nephron following filtration; it will eventually be excreted in the urine (see Fig. 3–2).

In addition to filtration, some drugs may be secreted into the nephron by active transport mechanisms located in the proximal convoluted tubule. Two basic transport systems exist, one for the secretion of organic acids (e.g., uric acid) and one for the secretion of organic bases (e.g., choline, histamine).[6,9] A third transport system that actively secretes the chelating agent EDTA (ethylenediaminetetra-acetic acid, an agent that binds to heavy metals and is sometimes used to treat lead poisoning) has also been identified, but its significance is unclear. Certain drugs may be transported by one of these carrier systems so that they are actively secreted into the nephron. For example, penicillin G is actively secreted via the transport system for organic acids, and morphine is secreted by the organic base transport system. In these specific cases, elimination of the drug is enhanced by the combined effects of tubular secretion and filtration in delivering the drug to the urine.

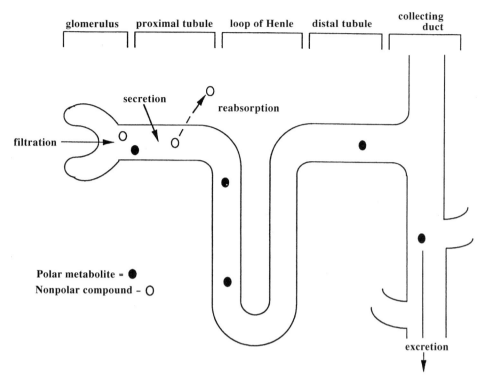

FIGURE 3-2. Drug excretion at the nephron. Compounds reach the nephron by filtration and/or secretion. Polar metabolites remain trapped in the nephron and are eventually excreted. Nonpolar compounds are able to diffuse back into the body (reabsorption).

Other routes for drug excretion include the lungs and gastrointestinal tract. The lungs play a significant role in excreting volatile drugs, that is, drugs that are usually administered by inhalation. Consequently, the lungs serve as the route of both administration and excretion for drugs such as the gaseous anesthetics. The gastrointestinal tract usually plays only a minor role in drug excretion. Certain drugs can be excreted by the liver into the bile and subsequently reach the duodenum via the bile duct. If the drug remains in the gastrointestinal tract, it will eventually be excreted in the feces. However, most of the secreted bile is reabsorbed, and drugs contained in the bile are often reabsorbed simultaneously. Other minor routes for drug excretion include the sweat, saliva, and breast milk of lactating mothers. Although drugs excreted via lactation are considered a relatively minor route with regard to loss from the mother, the possibility exists that the infant may imbibe substantial concentrations of the drug. Careful consideration for the welfare of the nursing infant must always be a factor in administering medications to the lactating mother.[44,45,53]

DRUG ELIMINATION RATES

The rate at which a drug is eliminated is significant in determining the amount and frequency of the dosage of the drug. If a drug is administered much faster than it is eliminated, the drug will accumulate excessively in the body and reach toxic levels. Conversely, if elimination greatly exceeds the rate of delivery, the concentration in the body may never reach therapeutic levels. Several parameters are used to indicate the rate at which a drug is usually eliminated so that dosages may be adjusted accordingly. Two of the primary measurements are *clearance* and *half-life*.[7]

Clearance

Clearance of a drug (CL) can be described in terms of the ability of all organs and tissues to eliminate the drug (systemic clearance) or in terms of the ability of a single organ or tissue to eliminate the drug.[6,14] To calculate clearance from a specific organ, two primary factors must be considered. First, the blood flow to the organ (Q) determines how much drug will be delivered to the organ for elimination. Second, the fraction of drug removed from the plasma as it passes through the organ must be known. This fraction, termed the *extraction ratio*, is equal to the difference in the concentration of drug entering (Ci) and exiting (Co) the organ, divided by the entering concentration (Ci). Clearance by an individual organ is summarized by the following equation:

$$CL = Q \times \frac{Ci - Co}{Ci}$$

The calculation of clearance using this equation is illustrated by the following example. Aspirin is metabolized primarily in the liver. Normal hepatic blood flow (Q) equals 1500 mL/min. If the blood entering the liver contains 200 μg/mL of aspirin (Ci) and the blood leaving the liver contains 134 μg/mL (Co), hepatic clearance of aspirin is calculated as follows:

$$CL_{hepatic} = Q \times \frac{Ci - Co}{Ci}$$

$$= 1500 \text{ mL/min} \times \frac{200 \text{ μg/mL} - 134 \text{ μg/mL}}{200 \text{ μg/mL}}$$

$$= 495 \text{ mL/min}$$

This example illustrates that clearance is actually the amount of plasma from which the drug can be totally removed per unit of time. As calculated here, the liver would be able to completely remove aspirin from 495 mL of blood each minute. Tetracycline, a common antibacterial drug, has a clearance equal to 130 mL/min, indicating that this drug would be completely removed from approximately 130 mL of plasma each minute.

Clearance is dependent on the ability of the organ or tissue to extract the drug from the plasma as well as on the perfusion of the organ. Some tissues may have an excellent ability to remove the drug from the bloodstream, but clearance is limited because only a small amount of blood reaches the organ. Conversely, highly perfused organs may be ineffective in removing the drug, thus prolonging its activity.

In terms of the elimination of the drug from the entire body, systemic clearance is calculated as the sum of all the individual clearances from all organs and tissues (i.e., systemic CL = hepatic CL + renal CL + lung CL, and so on). Note that the elimination of the drug includes the combined processes of loss of the drug from the body (excretion) as well as inactivation of the drug through biotransformation.[14]

Half-Life

In addition to clearance, the **half-life** of the drug is important in describing the length of activity of the compound. Half-life is defined as the amount of time required for 50 percent of the drug remaining in the body to be eliminated.[6] Most drugs are eliminated in a manner such that a fixed portion of the drug is eliminated in a given time period. For example, acetaminophen's half-life of 2 hours indicates that in each 2-hour period, 50 percent of the acetaminophen still in the body will be eliminated (Fig. 3–3).

Half-life is a function of both clearance and volume of distribution (V_d)[6]; that is, the time it takes to eliminate 50 percent of the drug depends not only on the ability of the organ(s) to remove the drug from the plasma but also on the distribution or presence of the drug in the plasma. A drug that undergoes extensive inactivation in the liver may have a long half-life if it is sequestered intracellularly in skeletal muscle. Also, disease states that affect either clearance or V_d will affect the half-life of the drug, so dosages must be altered accordingly.

DOSING SCHEDULES AND PLASMA CONCENTRATION

With most medications, it is desirable to bring plasma concentrations of the drug up to a certain level and maintain them at that level. If the drug is given by continuous intravenous administration, this can be done fairly easily by matching the rate of administration with the rate of drug elimination (clearance), once the desired plasma concentration is achieved (Fig. 3–4). If the drug is given at specific intervals, the dosage must be adjusted to provide an average plasma concentration over the dosing period. Figure

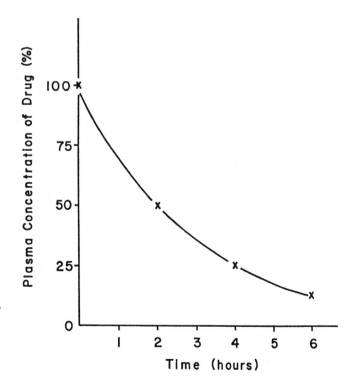

FIGURE 3–3. Elimination of a drug with a half-life of 2 hours. Fifty percent of the drug remaining in the bloodstream is eliminated in each 2-hour period.

3–4 illustrates that if the dosing interval is relatively long (e.g., 12 hours), the dose must be considerably larger to provide the same relative plasma concentration that would exist in a shorter dosing interval (e.g., 8 hours). Note also that larger doses given further apart result in greater plasma fluctuations, that is, greater maximum and minimum plasma levels over the dosing period. Giving smaller doses more frequently provides an equivalent average concentration without the extreme peaks and valleys associated with longer intervals (see Fig. 3–4).

VARIATIONS IN DRUG RESPONSE AND METABOLISM

The fact that different people may react differently to the same relative dosage of a drug is an important and often critical aspect of pharmacology.[50] Two individuals who are given the same drug may exhibit different magnitudes of a beneficial response as well as different adverse effects. Several of the primary factors responsible for variations in the response to drugs are discussed here.

1. *Genetic factors:* Genetic differences are often a major factor in the way in which individuals metabolize specific compounds.[35,57,64,68] Genetic variations may result in

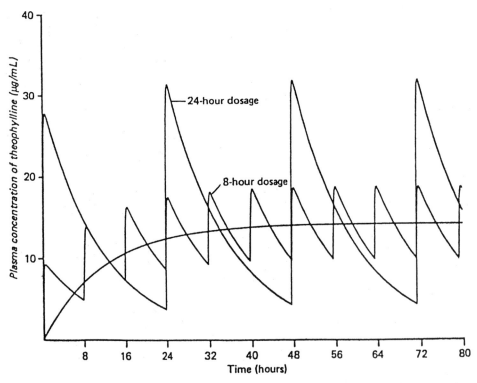

FIGURE 3–4. Relationship between dosing interval and plasma concentrations of the antiasthmatic drug theophylline. A constant intravenous infusion (shown by the smoothly rising line) yields a desired plasma level of 15 µg/ml. The same *average* plasma concentration is achieved when a dose of 340 mg is taken every 8 hours, or a dose of 1020 mg every 24 hours. Note, however, the fluctuations in plasma concentration seen when doses are taken at specific hourly intervals. (From Katzung, BG: Basic and Clinical Pharmacology, ed 4. Appleton & Lange, East Norwalk, CT, 1989, with permission.)

abnormal or absent drug-metabolizing enzymes.[15,43,47,48] This can be harmful or even fatal if the drug is not metabolized and begins to exert toxic effects because of accumulation or prolonged pharmacologic activity. For example, some individuals lack the appropriate plasma cholinesterase that breaks down circulating acetylcholine and acetylcholine-like compounds. Succinylcholine is a neuromuscular blocking agent that is usually administered during general anesthesia to ensure muscular relaxation during surgery. Normally, the succinylcholine is quickly degraded by plasma cholinesterase. However, individuals lacking the appropriate form of the cholinesterase may suffer respiratory paralysis because the succinylcholine exerts its effect much longer than expected.

2. *Disease:* Structural or functional damage to an organ or tissue responsible for drug metabolism or excretion presents an obvious problem in pharmacology. Diseases that initiate changes in tissue function or blood flow to specific organs such as the liver and kidneys can dramatically affect the elimination of various drugs.[6,22,39,42,52,63] Certain diseases may also impair the absorption and distribution of the drug, further complicating the problem of individualized response.[6,33,39,42,63] The significance of disease in affecting the patient's response is crucial because the response to the medication may be affected by the very same pathology that the drug is being used to treat. For instance, renal excretion of antibiotics such as the aminoglycosides is altered radically in many types of bacterial infection, but these drugs are typically administered to treat the same infections that alter their own excretion.[2] Consequently, great care must be taken to adjust the dosage accordingly if drug elimination may be altered.[33,42,52,63]

3. *Drug interactions:* When two or more drugs are present in the body at the same time, the chance exists that they may interact and alter each other's effects and metabolism.[10,17,30,34] Two similar compounds may act synergistically to produce a cumulative effect that is greater than each drug would produce alone. In some situations, this cumulative effect may be desirable if the augmented response is anticipated and well controlled.[11,60] However, two or more drugs with similar actions may lead to an adverse response even if each individual drug is given in a nontoxic dose. For instance, taking two central nervous system (CNS) depressants simultaneously (e.g., barbiturates and alcohol) may cause such severe CNS inhibition that the additive effects are lethal. In contrast to an additive effect, drugs with opposite actions may essentially cancel each other out, thus negating or reducing the beneficial effects of one or both medications. A drug that causes bronchodilation (i.e., for the treatment of asthma) will be negated by an agent that constricts the bronchioles.

Some of the most serious problems occurring in drug interactions have to do with one drug delaying the biotransformation of the other. If the enzymes that normally metabolize a drug are inhibited by a second compound, the original drug will exert its effect for prolonged periods, possibly leading to toxic effects.[8,32] For instance, the antiulcer drug cimetidine (Tagamet) inhibits the hepatic metabolism of oral anticoagulants such as warfarin (Coumadin). Taking these two drugs together tends to cause elevated plasma levels of the anticoagulant, which may lead to prolonged blood clotting and possible hemorrhage. Another type of interaction occurs when two or more drugs alter each other's absorption and distribution, such as when they compete for the same active transport carrier or bind to the same plasma proteins. An example is the interaction between aspirin and methotrexate, a drug used to treat cancer and rheumatoid arthritis. Aspirin can displace methotrexate from its binding site on plasma proteins, thus allowing relatively higher amounts of unbound or "free" methotrexate to exist in the bloodstream. The increased levels of "free" methotrexate may lead to toxic effects.

Considering the large number of drugs on the market, it is well beyond the scope of this text to discuss all of the clinically relevant drug interactions. The potential for drug interactions, however, must be carefully evaluated by the prescribing physician and pharmacist. Likewise, physical therapists, occupational therapists, and other individuals dealing with the patient must be alert for any abnormal symptoms or untoward effects because these effects may indicate a possible drug interaction.

4. *Age:* In general, older patients are more sensitive to most drugs.[13] Many drugs are not metabolized as quickly in the elderly, resulting in higher plasma levels than those that would occur in younger adults given equivalent doses.[4,12,28,40] The cause may simply be that changes in organ structure and function are part of the aging process. Children are also subject to problems and variability in drug metabolism.[49,54,56] Adjusting the dosage appropriately for the smaller body mass of a child is often difficult. Newborns may totally lack specific drug-metabolizing enzymes, thus prolonging the effects of certain drugs in the very young patient.[46,49] In the elderly and the young person, the combined effects of age *and* disease dramatically increase the complexity of pharmacokinetic variability, so special care must be taken in prescribing appropriate dosages in these situations.

5. *Diet:* Diet has been shown to affect the absorption, metabolism, and response to many drugs.[26,67] Animal and human studies have indicated that total caloric input as well as the percentage of calories obtained from different sources (carbohydrates, proteins, and fats) will influence drug pharmacokinetics.[18,31,37,62,65] Specific dietary constituents such as cruciferous vegetables and charcoal-broiled beef can also alter drug metabolism.[1]

Fortunately, most food-drug interactions are not serious and will not alter the clinical effects of the drug. There are, however, a few well-known food-drug combinations that should be avoided because of their potentially serious interaction. For instance, certain foods such as fermented cheese and wine should not be ingested with drugs that inhibit the monoamine oxidase enzyme (MAO inhibitors). These foods contain high amounts of tyramine, which stimulates the release of catecholamines (norepinephrine, epinephrine) within the body. MAO-inhibiting drugs work by suppressing the destruction of catecholamines, thus allowing higher levels of norepinephrine and epinephrine to occur. (MAO inhibitors are frequently used in the treatment of depression; see Chapter 7.) Consequently, when MAO inhibitors are taken with tyramine-containing foods, excessive levels of catecholamines may develop, leading to a dangerous increase in blood pressure (hypertensive crisis). Another food-drug interaction involving grapefruit juice was discovered recently.[3,25] Grapefruit juice inhibits drug-metabolizing enzymes in the gastrointestinal mucosa, thus allowing more of the active form of certain drugs to be absorbed into the bloodstream. Combining these drugs with grapefruit juice should be avoided because plasma levels (bioavailability) of the drug will be much higher than expected and this increased bioavailability will increase the risk of side effects and adverse reactions. Clinicians should therefore be aware of these well-known interactions and be on the alert for other such interactions as new drugs arrive on the market.

6. *Gender:* Men and women may have distinct differences in the way that certain drugs are absorbed, distributed, and metabolized.[24] This idea makes sense when one considers that gender-related differences in body composition, gastrointestinal function, enzyme activity, and various other systems can potentially affect pharmacokinetic variables.[24] Drug disposition may also be influenced in women by the cyclic hormonal variations that occur during the menstrual cycle, whereas men do not typically undergo such routine hormonal fluctuations.[38] Pharmacokinetics can clearly differ

between men and women, and future research is needed to determine how gender-related differences affect the therapeutic outcomes of specific drugs.[24]

7. *Other factors:*   A number of additional factors may alter the predicted response of the patient to a drug. As discussed earlier, environmental and occupational hazards may produce certain toxins that alter drug absorption and metabolism.[21,48] Factors such as cigarette smoking and alcohol consumption have been shown to influence the metabolism of specific compounds.[19,51,58] Drug distribution and metabolism may be altered in the obese patient[5,41,55] or in response to chronic and acute exercise.[14,20] Individuals with spinal cord injuries have a decreased ability to absorb certain drugs from their gastrointestinal tract, presumably because of a general decrease in gastrointestinal motility in these people.[29,59] Conversely, patients with extensive burn injuries may have increased gastrointestinal absorption and therefore increased bioavailability to certain drugs, although the reason for this effect is not clear.[36] Clearly, the way each individual responds to a medication is affected by any number of factors, and these must be taken into account whenever possible.

SUMMARY

Drug elimination occurs because of the combined effects of drug metabolism and excretion. Elimination is essential in terminating drug activity within a reasonable and predictable time frame. Various tissues and organs (especially the liver and kidneys) are involved in drug elimination, and injury to or disease of these tissues can markedly alter the response to certain drugs. In cases of disease or injury, dosages must frequently be adjusted to prevent adverse side effects due to altered elimination rates. Many other environmental, behavioral, and genetic factors may also alter drug metabolism and disposition, and possible variability in the patient's response should always be a matter of concern when the type and amount of the drug are selected.

REFERENCES

1. Anderson, KE, et al: Nutrient regulation of chemical metabolism in humans. Fed Proc 44:130, 1985.
2. Aronson, JK and Reynolds, DJM: ABC of monitoring drug therapy: Aminoglycoside antibiotics. BMJ 305:1421, 1992.
3. Bailey, DG, et al: Grapefruit juice–drug interactions. Br J Clin Pharmacol 46:101, 1998.
4. Baillie, SP, et al: Age and the pharmacokinetics of morphine. Age Ageing 18:258, 1989.
5. Benedek, IH, Blouin, RA, and McNamara, PJ: Serum protein binding and the role of increased alpha-acid glycoprotein in moderately obese male subjects. Br J Clin Pharmacol 18:941, 1984.
6. Benet, LZ, Kroetz, DL, and Sheiner, LB: Pharmacokinetics: The dynamics of drug absorption, distribution, and elimination. In Hardman, JG, et al (eds): The Pharmacological Basis of Therapeutics, ed 9. McGraw-Hill, New York, 1996.
7. Benet, LZ and Zia-Amirhosseini, P: Basic principles of pharmacokinetics. Toxicol Pathol 23:115, 1995.
8. Bergstrom, RF, Peyton, AL, and Lemberger, L: Quantification and mechanism of the fluoxetine and tricyclic antidepressant interaction. Clin Pharmacol Ther 51:239, 1992.
9. Berndt, WO and Stitzel, RE: Excretion of drugs. In Craig, CR and Stitzel, RE (eds): Modern Pharmacology with Clinical Applications, ed 5. Little Brown, Boston, 1997.
10. Bonate, PL, Reith, K, and Weir, S: Drug interactions at the renal level. Implications for drug development. Clin Pharmacokinet 34:375, 1998.
11. Caranasos, GJ, Stewart, RB, and Cluff, LE: Clinically desirable drug interactions. Annu Rev Pharmacol Toxicol 25:67, 1985.
12. Chutka, DS, et al: Symposium on geriatrics—Part I: Drug prescribing for elderly patients. Mayo Clin Proc 70:685, 1995.
13. Ciccone, CD: Geriatric pharmacology. In Guccione, AA (ed): Geriatric Physical Therapy, ed 2. CV Mosby, St. Louis, 2000.

14. Ciccone, CD: Basic pharmacokinetics and the potential effect of physical therapy interventions on pharmacokinetic variables. Phys Ther 75:343, 1995.
15. Cohen, LJ and De Vane, CL: Clinical implications of antidepressant pharmacokinetics and pharmacogenetics. Ann Pharmacother 30:1471, 1996.
16. Correia, MA: Drug biotransformation. In Katzung, BG (ed): Basic and Clinical Pharmacology, ed 7. Appleton & Lange, Stamford, CT, 1998.
17. Crowther, NR, et al: Drug interactions among commonly used medications. Chart simplifies data from critical literature review. Can Fam Physician 43:1972, 1997.
18. Cuddy, PG, et al: Theophylline disposition following parenteral feeding of malnourished patients. Ann Pharmacother 27:846, 1993.
19. Djordjevic, D, Nikolic, J, and Stefanovic, V: Ethanol interactions with other cytochrome P450 substrates including drugs, xenobiotics, and carcinogens. Pathol Biol (Paris) 46:760, 1998.
20. Dossing, M: Effect of acute and chronic exercise on hepatic drug metabolism. Clin Pharmacokinet 10:426, 1985.
21. Dossing, M: Changes in hepatic microsomal function in workers exposed to mixtures of chemicals. Clin Pharmacol Ther 32:340, 1982.
22. Elston, AC, Bayliss, MK, and Park, GR: Effect of renal failure on drug metabolism by the liver. Br J Anaesth 71:282, 1993.
23. Fenyves, D, Gariepy, L, and Villeneuve, JP: Clearance by the liver in cirrhosis. Relationship between propranolol metabolism in vitro and its extraction by the perfused liver in the rat. Hepatology 17:301, 1993.
24. Fletcher, CV, Acosta, EP, and Strykowski, JM: Gender differences in human pharmacokinetics and pharmacodynamics. J Adolesc Health 15:619, 1994.
25. Fuhr, U: Drug interactions with grapefruit juice. Extent, probable mechanism and clinical relevance. Drug Saf 18:251, 1998.
26. Gauthier, I and Malone, M: Drug-food interactions in hospitalized patients. Methods of prevention. Drug Saf 18:383, 1998.
27. Gram, TE: Metabolism of drugs. In Craig, CR and Stitzel, RE (eds): Modern Pharmacology with Clinical Applications, ed 5. Little Brown, Boston, 1997.
28. Groen, K, et al: The relationship between phenazone (antipyrine) metabolite formation and theophylline metabolism in healthy and frail elderly women. Clin Pharmacokinet 25:136, 1993.
29. Halstead, LS, et al: Drug absorption in spinal cord injuries. Arch Phys Med Rehabil 66:298, 1985.
30. Hansten, PD: Appendix I. Important drug interactions. In Katzung, BG (ed): Basic and Clinical Pharmacology, ed 7. Appleton & Lange, Norwalk, CT, 1998.
31. Hathcock, JN: Metabolic mechanisms of drug-nutrient interactions. Fed Proc 44:124, 1985.
32. Honig, PK, et al: Terfenadine-ketoconazole interaction: Pharmacokinetic and electrocardiographic consequences. JAMA 269:1513, 1993.
33. Hoyer, J, Schulte, KL, and Lenz, T: Clinical pharmacokinetics of angiotensin converting enzyme (ACE) inhibitors in renal failure. Clin Pharmacokinet 24:230, 1993.
34. Ito, K, et al: Prediction of pharmacokinetic alterations caused by drug-drug interactions: Metabolic interaction in the liver. Pharmacol Rev 50:387, 1998.
35. Iyer, L and Ratain, MJ: Pharmacogenetics and cancer chemotherapy. Eur J Cancer 34:1493, 1998.
36. Jaehde, U and Sorgel, F: Clinical pharmacokinetics in patients with burns. Clin Pharmacokinet 29:15, 1995.
37. Jung, D: Pharmacokinetics of theophylline in protein-calorie malnutrition. Biopharm Drug Dispos 6:291, 1985.
38. Kashuba, AD and Nafziger, AN: Physiological changes during the menstrual cycle and their effects on the pharmacokinetics and pharmacodynamics of drugs. Clin Pharmacokinet 34:203, 1998.
39. Keller, F and Czock, D: Pharmacokinetic studies in volunteers with renal impairment. Int J Clin Pharmacol Ther 36:594, 1998.
40. Kinirons, MT and Crome, P: Clinical pharmacokinetic considerations in the elderly. An update. Clin Pharmacokinet 33:302, 1997.
41. Kotlyar, M and Carson, SW: Effects of obesity on the cytochrome P450 enzyme system. Int J Clin Pharmacol Ther 37:8, 1999.
42. Lam, YW, et al: Principles of drug administration in renal insufficiency. Clin Pharmacokinet 32:30, 1997.
43. Lennard, MS: Oxidative phenotype and the metabolism and action of beta-blockers. Klin Wochenschr 63:285, 1985.
44. Llewellyn, A and Stowe, ZN: Psychotropic medications in lactation. J Clin Psychiatry 59(Suppl 2):41, 1998.
45. Lobstein, R, Lalkin, A, and Koren, G: Pharmacokinetic changes during pregnancy and their clinical relevance. Clin Pharmacokinet 33:328, 1997.
46. Mannering, GJ: Drug metabolism in the newborn. Fed Proc 44:2302, 1985.
47. Meier, UT, et al.: Mephenytoin hydroxylation polymorphism: Characterization of the enzymatic deficiency in liver microsomes of poor metabolizers phenotyped in-vivo. Clin Pharmacol Ther 38:488, 1985.
48. Meyer, UA: Overview of enzymes of drug metabolism. J Pharmacokinet Biopharm 24:449, 1996.
49. Milsap, RL and Jusko, WJ: Pharmacokinetics in the infant. Environ Health Perspect 102(Suppl 11):107, 1994.
50. Pang, KS, Xu, X, and St. Pierre, MV: Determinants of metabolite disposition. Annu Rev Pharmacol Toxicol 32:623, 1992.

51. Park, BK, et al: Relevance of induction of human drug-metabolizing enzymes: Pharmacological and toxicological implications. Br J Clin Pharmacol 41:477, 1996.
52. Perucca, E, Grimaldi, R, and Crema, A: Interpretation of drug levels in acute and chronic disease states. Clin Pharmacokinet 10:498, 1985.
53. Pons, G, Rey, E, and Matheson, I: Excretion of psychoactive drugs into breast milk. Pharmacokinetic principles and recommendations. Clin Pharmacokinet 27:270, 1994.
54. Prandota, J-J: Clinical pharmacokinetics of changes in drug elimination in children. Dev Pharmacol Ther 8:311, 1985.
55. Prather, RD, et al: Nicotine pharmacokinetics of Nicoderm (nicotine transdermal system) in women and obese men compared with normal-sized men. J Clin Pharmacol 33:644, 1993.
56. Routledge, PA: Pharmacokinetics in children. J Antimicrob Chemother 34(Suppl A):19, 1994.
57. Salva Lacombe, P, et al: Causes and problems of nonresponse or poor response to drugs. Drugs 51:552, 1996.
58. Schein, JR: Cigarette smoking and clinically significant drug interactions. Ann Pharmacother 29:1139, 1995.
59. Segal, JL and Brunnemann, SR: Clinical pharmacokinetics in patients with spinal cord injuries. Clin Pharmacokinet 17:109, 1989.
60. Tallarida, RJ: Statistical analysis of drug combinations for synergism: A review. Pain 49:93, 1992.
61. Teunissen, MWE, et al: Antipyrine clearance and metabolite formation in patients with alcohol cirrhosis. Br J Clin Pharmacol 18:707, 1984.
62. Thomas, JA and Burns, RA: Important drug-nutrient interactions in the elderly. Drugs Aging 13:199, 1998.
63. Verbeeck, RK and Horsmans, Y: Effect of hepatic insufficiency on pharmacokinetics and drug dosing. Pharm World Sci 20:183, 1998.
64. Vesell, ES: Pharmacogenetic perspectives: Genes, drugs and disease. Hepatology 4:959, 1984.
65. Walter-Sack, I and Klotz, U: Influence of diet and nutritional status on drug metabolism. Clin Pharmacokinet 31:47, 1996.
66. Williams, RL: Drug administration in hepatic disease. N Engl J Med 309:1616, 1983.
67. Yamreudeewong, W, et al: Drug-food interactions in clinical practice. J Fam Pract 40:376, 1995.
68. Zhou, H-H, et al: Racial differences in drug response: Altered sensitivity to and clearance of propranolol in men of Chinese descent as compared with American whites. N Engl J Med 320:565, 1989.

CHAPTER 4

Drug Receptors

A **receptor** is the component of the cell to which the drug binds and through which a chain of biochemical events is initiated.[3] Most drugs exert their effect by binding to and activating such a receptor, which subsequently brings about some change in the physiologic function of the cell. These receptors can be any cellular macromolecule, but many receptors have been identified as proteins that are located on or within the cell.[3,20,33] The general mechanisms of receptor function in conjunction with their cellular location are discussed here.

RECEPTORS LOCATED ON THE CELL'S SURFACE

Proteins that are located on the outer surface of the cell may act as receptors for endogenous and exogenous compounds.[35] These receptors are responsive primarily to specific amino acid, peptide, or amine compounds. Surface receptors can affect cell function (1) by acting as an ion channel and directly altering membrane permeability, (2) by acting enzymatically to directly influence function within the cell, or (3) by being linked to regulatory proteins that control other chemical and enzymatic processes within the cell. Each of the three basic ways that surface receptors can affect cell function is addressed here.

Surface Receptors Linked Directly to Ion Channels

Membrane receptors may be directly involved in the cellular response to the drug by acting as an ion pore and thus changing the membrane permeability.[31,40] An example is the acetylcholine receptor located on the postsynaptic membrane of the neuromuscular junction (Fig. 4–1). When bound by acetylcholine molecules, the receptor increases the permeability of the muscle cell to sodium, which results in depolarization of the cell because of sodium influx. Another important example of a receptor–ion channel system is the **gamma-aminobutyric acid (GABA)**–benzodiazepine–chloride ion channel complex found on neuronal membranes in the central nervous system.[7,45] In this situation, the membrane's permeability to chloride is increased by the binding of both the neurotransmitter GABA and the benzodiazepine drugs such as diazepam (Valium) and

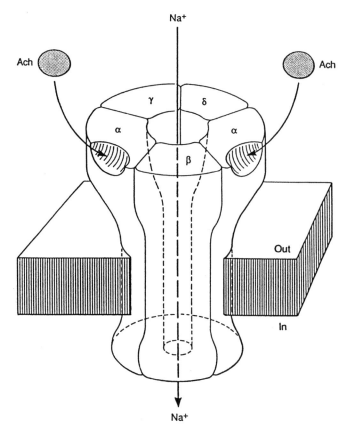

FIGURE 4–1. Schematic model of the acetylcholine receptor, an example of a surface receptor that is linked directly to an ion channel. Binding of two acetylcholine (ACh) molecules to the outer surface of the receptor protein induces opening of a central ion channel, thus allowing sodium (Na^+) to enter the cell. (From Bourne, HR and Roberts, JM: Drug receptors and pharmacodynamics. In Katzung, BG (ed): Basic and Clinical Pharmacology, ed 5. Appleton & Lange, Norwalk, CT, 1992, p 21, with permission.)

chlordiazepoxide (Librium). The function of this chloride ion channel complex is discussed in more detail in Chapter 6.

Surface Receptors Linked Directly to Enzymes

Some proteins that span the entire width of the cell membrane may have an extracellular receptor site (binding domain) as well as an intracellular enzymatic component (catalytic domain) (Fig. 4–2). Drugs and endogenous chemicals that bind to the receptor site can change the enzyme activity of the intracellular catalytic component, thus altering the biochemical function within the cell.[39] Receptor-enzyme systems in this category are often referred to as *protein tyrosine kinases* because binding of an appropriate substance to the outer (receptor) component initiates the phosphorylation of certain tyrosine amino acids on the inner (catalytic) component of the protein, which in turn increases the enzyme activity of the intracellular component (see Fig. 4–2). The activated enzymatic component of the receptor then catalyzes the activation of other substrates within the cell.

It appears that insulin and certain growth factors may exert their effects by acting through this type of tyrosine kinase receptor-enzyme system.[3,10] Insulin, for example, binds to the extracellular component of a protein located on skeletal muscle cells, thereby initiating activation of this protein's enzymatic activity on the inner surface of the cell membrane. This change in enzyme function causes further changes in cell activ-

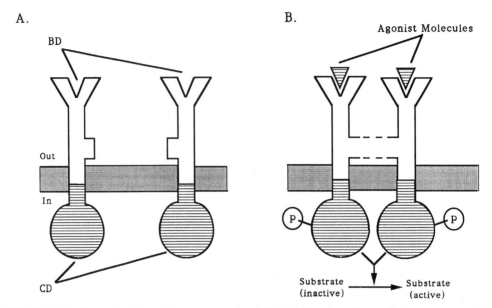

FIGURE 4–2. Example of a surface receptor that is linked directly to intracellular enzyme activity. (*A*) The receptor exists in an inactive state as two subunits: Each subunit has a binding domain (BD) on the outer surface and a catalytic domain (CD) on the inner surface. (*B*) Binding of agonist molecules to the BDs causes the subunits to join together and induces phosphorylation (P) of tyrosine receptors on the CD. Tyrosine phosphorylation initiates enzymatic activity of the catalytic units, which then causes substrate activation within the cell.

ity, which ultimately result in increased glucose uptake in the muscle cell. The function of insulin receptors and their role in the cause and treatment of diabetes mellitus are discussed in more detail in Chapter 32.

Surface Receptors Linked to Regulatory (G) Proteins: Role of the Second Messenger

Rather than directly affecting membrane permeability or directly influencing enzyme activity, other membrane receptors affect cell function by being linked to an intermediate regulatory protein that is located on the inner surface of the cell's membrane.[14,43] Because these regulatory proteins are activated by binding guanine nucleotides, they are often termed **G proteins.**[2,23] When an appropriate substance binds to the surface receptor, the receptor in turn activates the regulatory G protein. The activated G protein then alters the activity of some type of intracellular effector (such as an enzyme or ion channel), which then leads to a change in cell function.[21,43]

Receptors that are linked to G proteins (also called "G protein–coupled receptors") represent the primary way that signals from the surface receptor are transduced into the appropriate response within the cell.[14,17] There appear to be two types of regulatory G proteins: a stimulatory protein (G_s), which increases the cellular response, and an inhibitory protein (G_i), which decreases that response (Fig. 4–3). The two types of G proteins (stimulatory and inhibitory) are linked to different receptors, and the two receptors are responsive to different drugs. Certain drugs affect the cell by binding to a receptor that is linked to a G_s protein. The activated receptor activates the G_s protein,

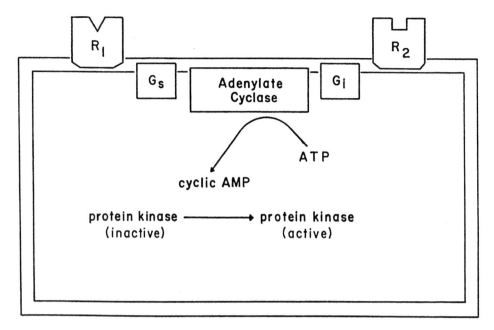

FIGURE 4–3. Schematic diagram of a surface receptor–second messenger system. In this example, the second messenger is cyclic adenosine monophosphate (cAMP), which is synthesized from adenosine triphosphate (ATP) by the adenylate cyclase enzyme. The enzyme is linked to surface receptors (R_1 and R_2) by regulatory G proteins. G_S stimulates the enzyme and G_i inhibits enzyme activity. Thus, a drug binding to R_1 will increase production of cAMP, and a different drug binding to R_2 will inhibit cAMP production.

which in turn activates the effector system, which consists of opening an ion channel or activating a specific enzyme. Conversely, a drug that binds to a receptor that is linked to a G_i protein inhibits channel opening or intracellular enzyme activity.

Hence, these regulatory G proteins help account for how drugs can bind to one type of receptor and stimulate cell function, whereas drugs that bind to a different receptor on the same cell can inhibit cell activity. G proteins also seem to be important in mediating other responses of the cell to stimulation or inhibition. For instance, cell function may continue to be affected through the action of G proteins even after the drug has left the binding site on the cell's surface[3]; that is, the drug may bind to the cell for only a short period of time, but this binding is sufficient to initiate the interaction of the G protein with the intracellular effector system. The sustained influence of the G protein on the effector system can help explain why the cell may continue to exhibit a response even after the drug has dissociated from the cell or even after the drug has been eliminated from the body.

As indicated earlier, many G protein–coupled receptors are linked directly to an intracellular enzyme. Drugs and other substances that exert their effects through this type of receptor–G protein–enzyme system often lead to the formation (or inhibition of the formation) of an intracellular compound known as a **second messenger**. In effect, the drug acts as the first messenger, which triggers a biochemical change in the cell, but the drug itself does not enter the cell. The second messenger, which is the substance produced inside the cell, actually mediates the change in function.

The primary example of this type of second messenger strategy is the **adenylate cyclase–cyclic adenosine monophosphate (cAMP)** system present in many cells[6,21,27] (see

Fig. 4–3). Adenylate cyclase, which is an enzyme that is located on the inner surface of the cell membrane, is responsible for hydrolyzing adenosine triphosphate (ATP) into cAMP. Cyclic AMP acts as the second messenger in this system by activating other enzymes (i.e., protein kinases) throughout the cell. Thus, drugs that bind to a surface receptor that is linked to a G_s protein will increase adenylate cyclase activity, resulting in increased production of cAMP within the cell. Other drugs that bind to a different receptor that is linked to a G_i protein will inhibit adenylate cyclase activity, resulting in decreased production of cAMP.

The adenylate cyclase–cAMP system is associated with specific membrane receptors such as the beta-adrenergic receptors.[5,6,16,27] Other surface receptors may also be linked to this particular effector–second messenger system, or they may be linked to other intracellular processes that use different second messengers. Additional second messengers that have been identified in various cells include cyclic guanosine monophosphate (cGMP), diacylglycerol, phosphoinositides, calcium ions, and intracellular peptides.[1,3,4,17,30]

Finally, alterations in the synthesis and function of G proteins have been identified in certain pathologic conditions, including alcoholism, diabetes mellitus, heart failure, and certain tumors.[13,19] This illustrates the fact that G proteins seem to play an integral role in mediating the cell's response to various substances in both normal and disease states. The importance of these regulatory proteins will almost certainly continue to emerge as additional information about their structure and function becomes available.

INTRACELLULAR RECEPTORS

Receptors have been identified at intracellular locations such as the cytoplasm and the nucleus.[29] Certain drugs exert their effect by entering the cell directly and then binding with one of these receptors. For instance, steroid and steroidlike compounds usually interact with a receptor that is located in the cytoplasm.[9] Certain hormones such as thyroxine appear to act by binding primarily with a receptor that is located on the chromatin in the cell's nucleus.[29] In either case, cell function is altered because the drug-receptor complex binds directly to specific genes in the DNA and causes changes in gene expression and messenger RNA transcription. Altered transcription of specific genes results in altered cellular protein synthesis that ultimately results in altered cell function.[25,29] The role of intracellular receptors is discussed further in this text in the chapters that deal with specific drugs that bind to these intracellular components.

DRUG-RECEPTOR INTERACTIONS

The ability of a drug to bind to any receptor is dictated by factors such as the size and shape of the drug relative to the configuration of the binding site on the receptor. The electrostatic attraction between the drug and the receptor may also be important in determining the extent to which the drug binds to the receptor. This drug-receptor interaction is somewhat analogous to a key fitting into a lock. The drug acts as a "key" that will fit into only certain receptors. Once inserted into a suitable receptor, the drug activates the receptor much as a key would be able to turn and "activate" the appropriate lock. To carry this analogy one step further, unlocking a door to a room would increase the "permeability" of the room in a manner similar to the direct effect of certain activated membrane receptors (e.g., the acetylcholine receptor on the neuromuscular junction).

Other types of key-lock interactions would be "linked" to some other event, such as using a key to start an automobile engine. This situation is analogous to linking a surface receptor to some intracellular enzymatic process that would affect the internal "machinery" of the cell.

Although the key-lock analogy serves as a crude example of drug-receptor interactions, the attraction between a drug and any receptor is much more complex. Binding a drug to a receptor is not an all-or-none phenomenon but is graded depending on the drug in question. Some drugs will bind readily to the receptor, some moderately, and others very little or not at all. The term **affinity** is used to describe the amount of attraction between a drug and a receptor.[37] Affinity is actually related to the amount of drug that is required to bind to the unoccupied receptors.[24] A drug with high affinity binds readily to the open receptors, even if the concentration of drug is relatively low. Drugs with moderate or low affinity require a higher concentration in the body before the receptors become occupied.

In addition to the relative degree of affinity of different drugs for a receptor, apparently the status of the receptor may also vary under specific conditions. Receptors may exist in variable affinity states (super-high, high, low), depending on the influence of local regulators such as guanine nucleotides, ammonium ions, and divalent cations.[8,36,42] Membrane receptors may also be influenced by the local environment of the lipid bilayer. The amount of flexibility or "fluidity" of the cell membrane is recognized as critical in providing a suitable environment in which membrane constituents such as receptors can optimally function. Physical and chemical factors (including other drugs) may change the fluidity and organization of the membrane, thereby disrupting the normal orientation of the receptor and subsequently altering its affinity state and ability to interact with a drug.[12,32]

The exact way in which a drug activates a receptor has been the subject of considerable debate. Binding of a drug to the receptor is hypothesized to cause the receptor to undergo some sort of temporary change in its shape or conformation. The change in structure of the activated receptor then mediates a change in cell function, either directly or by being linked to some effector system. Some studies have suggested that certain receptor proteins do undergo a change in structure after binding with specific chemicals.[5] This event certainly seems plausible because most receptors have been identified as protein molecules, and proteins are known to be able to reversibly change their shape and conformation as part of normal physiologic function.[22,33] This fact should not, however, rule out other possible ways in which an activated receptor may mediate changes in cell function. Future research will continue to clarify the role of conformational changes as well as other possible mechanisms of receptor activation.

FUNCTIONAL ASPECTS OF DRUG-RECEPTOR INTERACTIONS

The interaction between the drug and the receptor dictates several important aspects of pharmacology, including those discussed here.

Drug Selectivity

A drug is said to be *selective* if it affects only one type of cell or tissue and produces a specific physiologic response. For instance, a drug that is cardioselective affects heart function without affecting other tissues such as the gastrointestinal tract or respiratory system. The selectivity of a particular drug is a function of the ability of that drug to interact with specific receptors on the target tissue, and not with other receptors on the target tissue or receptors on other tissues (Fig. 4–4). In reality, drug selectivity is a relative term because no drug produces only one effect. Drugs can be compared, however, with the more selective drug being able to affect one type of tissue or organ with only a minimum of other responses.

Dose-Response

The shape of the typical dose-response curve discussed in Chapter 1 is related to the number of receptors that are bound by the drug (see Fig. 1–2), because within certain limits of the drug concentration, the response is proportional to the number of receptors occupied by the drug.[41] At low dosages, for example, only a few receptors are bound by the drug; hence, the effect is relatively small. As dosage (and drug concentration) increases, more receptors become occupied, and the response increases. Finally, at some dosage, all available receptors are occupied, and the response is maximal. Increasing the dosage beyond the point at which the maximal effect is reached will not produce any further increase in response because all the receptors are bound by the drug. It should be noted, however, that the relationship between drug receptors and drug response is not a simple linear relationship for many drugs. A drug that occupies half the available

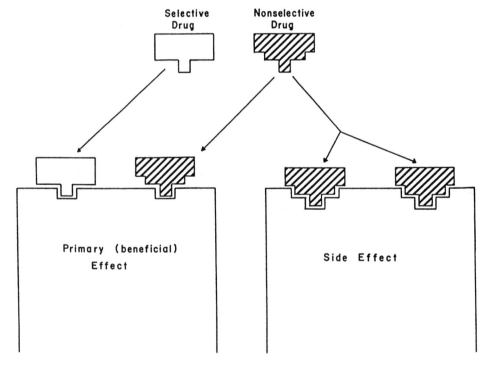

FIGURE 4–4. Drug selectivity. The diagram represents an ideal situation in which the selective drug produces only beneficial effects and the nonselective drug exerts both beneficial and side effects. Drug selectivity is actually a relative term, because all drugs produce some side effects; however, a selective drug produces fewer side effects than a nonselective agent.

receptors, for example, may produce a response that is greater than 50 percent of the maximal response.[37,46] Clearly, other factors influence the absolute magnitude of the response, including how well the occupied receptor can transmit the signal to the cell's effector mechanisms. It is, nonetheless, essentially true that increasing or decreasing the amount of drug available to the appropriate receptors will bring about a concomitant increase or decrease in the response to that drug.[41]

Classification of Drugs: Agonist versus Antagonist

So far, drug-receptor interactions have been used to describe the process by which a drug occupies a receptor and in some way activates the receptor. The activated receptor then brings about a change in cell function. Such a drug that binds to a receptor and initiates a change in the function of the cell is referred to as an **agonist.** An agonist is identified as having affinity and efficacy.[3] As discussed earlier, *affinity* refers to the fact that there is an attraction, or desire, for the drug to bind to a given receptor. The second characteristic, *efficacy*, indicates that the drug will activate the receptor and subsequently lead to a change in the function of the cell. Whereas an agonist has both affinity and efficacy, an **antagonist** has only affinity. This means that the drug will bind to the receptor, but it will not cause any change in the function of the receptor or cell (Fig. 4–5). Antagonists are significant because, by occupying the receptor, they prevent the agonistic compound from having any effect on the cell. Antagonists are often referred to as *blockers* because of this ability to block the effect of another chemical. The primary pharmacologic significance of these antagonists has been their use in blocking the effects of certain endogenous compounds. A classic example of this is the use of the so-called beta blockers, which occupy specific receptors on the myocardium, thus preventing circulat-

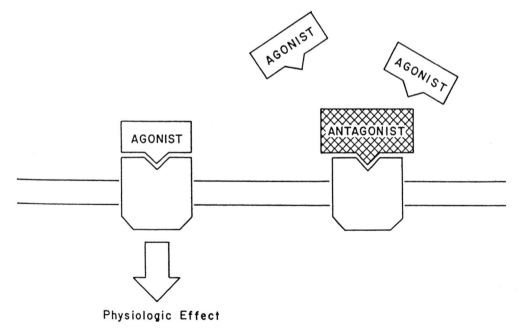

FIGURE 4–5. Drug classification: agonist versus antagonist. The antagonist (blocker) prevents the agonist from binding to the receptor and exerting a physiologic effect.

ing catecholamines from increasing heart rate and contractility. Other examples of antagonistic drugs are discussed in their appropriate chapters.

Competitive versus Noncompetitive Antagonists

Pharmacologic antagonists are generally divided into two categories, depending on whether they are competing with the agonist for the receptor.[3,37] *Competitive antagonists* are so classified because they seem to be vying for the same receptor as the agonist. In other words, both the agonist and antagonist have a more or less equal opportunity to occupy the receptor. For practical purposes, whichever drug is present in the greater concentration tends to have the predominant effect. If the number of competitive antagonist molecules far exceeds the number of agonist molecules, the antagonists will occupy most of the receptors and the overall effect will be inhibition of the particular response. Conversely, a high concentration of agonist relative to antagonist will produce a pharmacologic effect, because the agonist will occupy most of the receptors. In fact, raising the concentration of agonist in the presence of a competitive antagonist can actually overcome the inhibition that was originally present, because the competitive antagonists form rather weak bonds with the receptor and can be displaced from the receptor by a sufficient concentration of agonist molecules.[3,37] This is an important advantage of competitive antagonists because, if necessary, the inhibition caused by the antagonist can be overcome simply by administering high concentrations of the agonist.

In contrast to competitive antagonists, *noncompetitive antagonists* form strong, essentially permanent, bonds to the receptor. Noncompetitive antagonists have either an extremely high affinity for the receptor or actually form irreversible covalent bonds to the receptor.[3,37] Once bound to the receptor, the noncompetitive antagonist cannot be displaced by the agonist, regardless of how much agonist is present. Thus the term *noncompetitive* refers to the inability of the agonist to compete with the antagonist for the receptor site. The obvious disadvantage to this type of receptor blocker is that the inhibition cannot be overcome in cases of an overdose of the antagonist. Also, noncompetitive antagonists often remain bound for the life of the receptor, and their effect is terminated only after the receptor has been replaced as part of the normal protein turnover within the cell. Consequently, the inhibition produced by a noncompetitive blocker tends to remain in effect for long periods (i.e., several days).

Partial Agonists

Drugs are classified as *partial agonists* when they do not evoke a maximal response as compared with a strong agonist. This classification is used even though the partial agonist occupies all available receptors.[3] In fact, partial agonists can be thought of as having an efficacy that lies somewhere between that of a full agonist and a full noncompetitive antagonist. The lack of a maximal response is not caused by decreased drug-receptor affinity. On the contrary, partial agonists often have a high affinity for the receptor. The decreased efficacy may be caused by the fact that the partial agonist does not completely activate the receptor after it binds, and that binding results in a lower level of any postreceptor events (e.g., less activation of G proteins, smaller changes in enzyme function).

The realization that certain drugs act as partial agonists has led to the idea that a range of efficacy can exist, depending on how specific drugs interact with their respective receptors.[37] At one end of this range are drugs that bind strongly and produce a high degree of efficacy (strong agonists), and the other end of the spectrum contains drugs that bind strongly and produce no effect (strong antagonists). Agents that fall between these two extremes (partial agonists) can have varying degrees of agonistic activity. These partial agonists can also have certain clinical advantages. For instance, certain antianxiety drugs that function as partial agonists may provide adequate anxiolytic effects without excessive side effects.[15] Other examples of how partial agonists can be used clinically are discussed elsewhere in this text.

RECEPTOR REGULATION

Receptor responses are not static but are regulated by endogenous and exogenous factors. In general, a prolonged increase in the stimulation of various receptors will lead to a *decrease* in receptor function, and decreased stimulation will lead to an *increase* in receptor numbers or sensitivity (Fig. 4–6). The mechanisms and significance of these receptor changes are described here.

Receptor Desensitization and Down-Regulation

As presented in Figure 4–6, overstimulation of postsynaptic receptors by endogenous substances (neurotransmitters, hormones) or by exogenous agonists (drugs) may lead to a functional decrease in the appropriate receptor population.[11,16,27] In effect, the cell becomes less responsive to the prolonged stimulation by decreasing the number of active receptors. The term **desensitization** is used to describe a fairly brief and transient

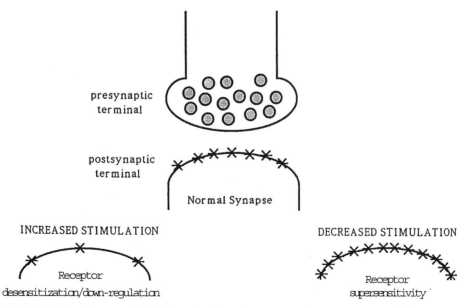

FIGURE 4–6. Receptor regulation. Functionally active receptor sites are represented by an "X." Increased stimulation results in a decrease in receptor sensitivity and numbers (desensitization and down-regulation), and decreased stimulation causes increased receptor sensitivity and numbers (supersensitivity and up-regulation).

decrease in responsiveness.[11,16,18,38] Desensitization is believed to occur because of the addition of phosphate residues (phosphorylation) or some other chemical modification to the receptor protein.[11,16,26] Adding a phosphate molecule seems to cause some membrane receptors to uncouple from their intermediate regulatory proteins and consequently from the rest of the cell's biochemical machinery.[16,18,28] Receptor desensitization helps account for the decrease in response that may be seen even though the agonist remains present in high concentration in the body. The decrease in responsiveness caused by desensitization is fairly brief, however, and a return to normal response may occur within a few minutes after the agonist is removed.

Receptor **down-regulation** describes a slower, more prolonged process in which the actual number of available receptors is diminished.[18,26,34,38] Although the exact mechanisms responsible for down-regulation are not fully understood, it appears that prolonged exposure of the agonist causes increased receptor removal, decreased receptor synthesis, or a combination of increased removal and decreased synthesis.[18] In any event, the cell undergoes a decrease in responsiveness that remains in effect long after the agonist is removed (i.e., several days). Normal sensitivity to the agonist will be reestablished only when the cell has the chance to replace and restore the receptors that were eliminated during down-regulation.

Receptor desensitization and down-regulation appear to be examples of a negative feedback system used by the cell to prevent overstimulation by an agonist. The cell appears to selectively decrease its responsiveness to a particular stimulus in order to protect itself from excessive perturbation. Receptor down-regulation is important pharmacologically because it may be one of the primary reasons that a decrease in drug responsiveness occurs when certain drugs are used for prolonged periods.[3] Conversely, some drugs, such as the antidepressants, may exert their beneficial effects by intentionally causing receptor down-regulation and desensitization in certain neural pathways that cause clinical depression. These drugs are discussed in detail in Chapter 7.

Receptor Supersensitivity and Up-Regulation

A prolonged decrease in the stimulation of the postsynaptic receptors can result in a functional increase in the number and sensitivity of these receptors. An increase in sensitivity of existing receptors is typically referred to as receptor **supersensitivity**, and an increase in receptor numbers is known as receptor up-regulation. These changes are the opposite of desensitization and down-regulation as described earlier; that is, supersensitivity is a fairly rapid and transient increase in receptor sensitivity, and receptor up-regulation represents a slower but longer-term increase in the number of functioning receptors. The best example of this phenomenon is the denervation supersensitivity and up-regulation seen when a peripheral nerve is severed.[44] In this situation, the lack of presynaptic neurotransmitter release results in a compensatory increase in the sensitivity and ultimately the number of postsynaptic receptors. A somewhat different type of denervation supersensitivity and up-regulation may occur when receptor antagonist drugs are used for prolonged periods. Here the postsynaptic receptors are blocked by the antagonistic drug, and they are unavailable for stimulation by the appropriate agonist. The postsynaptic neuron interprets this as if the synapse was denervated and responds by increasing the sensitivity of existing receptors and by eventually manufacturing more receptors, resulting in a compensatory increase in function at the synapse that was supposed to be blocked by the antagonist. Several problems may result from this pharmacologically induced supersensitivity and receptor up-regulation.

NONRECEPTOR DRUG MECHANISMS

Certain drugs do not appear to exert their effects by binding to a specific cellular component.[37] Certain cancer chemotherapeutic agents, for example, act as "antimetabolites" by becoming incorporated into the manufacture of specific cellular components. The drug acts as an improper ingredient in the biosynthesis of the component, so that the cell does not manufacture certain harmful or unwanted materials. In addition, many common antacids work by directly neutralizing stomach acid; that is, these drugs act via a chemical reaction rather than through a specific receptor molecule. Other drugs may affect cell function without first binding to a receptor by directly altering enzyme function or by acting as "chelating agents," which bind to harmful compounds such as the heavy metals and prevent them from exerting toxic effects. Additional nonreceptor-mediated mechanisms of specific compounds are discussed when those drugs are examined in their respective chapters.

SUMMARY

Many drugs and endogenous chemicals have been shown to exert their effects by first binding to and activating a cellular receptor. Cellular receptors seem to be proteins located on the cell surface or at specific locations within the cell. The primary role of the receptor is to recognize specific chemicals from the vast number of compounds that are introduced to the cell and to initiate a change in cell function by interacting with a specific agent. Activated receptors mediate a change in function by altering cell permeability or modifying the biochemical function within the cell, or both. The exact mechanism by which a receptor affects cell function depends on the type and location of the receptor.

Drug-receptor interactions are significant pharmacologically because they account for some of the basic pharmacodynamic principles such as drug selectivity and the relationship between drug dose and response. Also, the development of chemical agents that block specific receptors (antagonists) has been useful in moderating the effects of endogenous compounds on specific physiologic processes. Finally, changes in receptor number and sensitivity have been implicated as important in the altered response seen in certain drugs with prolonged use. Information about the relationship between drugs and cellular receptors has been, and will continue to be, critical to our understanding of how drugs work, as well as to helping researchers develop new compounds.

REFERENCES

1. Berridge, MJ: Inositol triphosphate and diacylglycerol as second messengers. Biochem J 220:345, 1984.
2. Birnbaumer, L: G proteins in signal transduction. Annu Rev Pharmacol Toxicol 30:675, 1990.
3. Bourne, HR and Roberts, JM: Drug receptors and pharmacodynamics. In Katzung, BG (ed): Basic and Clinical Pharmacology, ed 7. Appleton & Lange, Norwalk, CT, 1998.
4. Cheng, K and Larner, J: Intracellular mediators of insulin action. Annu Rev Physiol 47:405, 1985.
5. Contreras, ML, Wolfe, BB, and Molinoff, PB: Thermodynamic properties of agonist interactions with the beta adrenergic receptor-coupled adenylate cyclase system: II. Agonist binding to soluble beta adrenergic receptors. J Pharmacol Exp Ther 237:165, 1986.
6. Cooper, DMF: Receptor-mediated stimulation and inhibition of adenylate cyclase. In Kleinzeller, A (ed): Current Topics in Membranes and Transport, Vol 18: Membrane Receptors. Academic Press, New York, 1983.
7. Davies, M, Bateson, AN, and Dunn, SMJ: Molecular biology of the GABA-A receptor: Domains implicated by mutational analysis. Front Biosci 1:d214, 1996.
8. Eterovic, VA, et al: Positive modulators of muscle acetylcholine receptor. J Receptor Res 9:107, 1989.
9. Evans, RM: The steroid and thyroid hormone receptor superfamily. Science 240:889, 1988.

10. Fantl, WJ, Johnson, DE, and Williams, LT: Signalling by receptor tyrosine kinases. Annu Rev Biochem 62:453, 1993.
11. Freedman, NJ and Lefkowitz, RJ: Desensitization of G protein–coupled receptors. Recent Prog Horm Res 51:319, 1996.
12. Goldstein, DB: The effects of drugs on membrane fluidity. Annu Rev Pharmacol Toxicol 24:43, 1984.
13. Gordeladze, JO, et al: G-proteins: Implications for pathophysiology and disease. Eur J Endocrinol 131:557, 1994.
14. Gudermann, T, Schoneberg, T, and Schultz, G: Functional and structural complexity of signal transduction via G-protein-coupled receptors. Annu Rev Neurosci 20:399, 1997.
15. Haefely, W, Martin, JR, and Schoch, P: Novel anxiolytics that act as partial agonists at benzodiazepine receptors. Trends Pharmacol Sci 11:452, 1990.
16. Hausdorff, WP, Caron, MG, and Lefkowitz, RJ: Turning off the signal: desensitization of beta-adrenergic receptor function. FASEB J 4:2881, 1990.
17. Hebert, TE and Bouvier, M: Structural and functional aspects of G protein–coupled receptor oligomerization. Biochem Cell Biol 76:1, 1998.
18. Heck, DA and Byland, DB: Differential down-regulation of alpha-2 adrenergic receptor subtypes. Life Sci 62:1467, 1998.
19. Houslay, MD: Review: G-protein linked receptors—a family probed by molecular cloning and mutagenesis. Clin Endocrinol (Oxf) 36:525, 1992.
20. Jaffe, RC: Thyroid receptor hormones. In Conn, PM (ed): The Receptors, Vol 1. Academic Press, New York, 1984.
21. Karoor, V, et al: Regulating expression and function of G-protein-linked receptors. Prog Neurobiol 48:555, 1996.
22. Karplus, M and McGammon, JA: Dynamics of proteins: Elements of function. Annu Rev Biochem 52:263, 1983.
23. Kaziro, Y, et al: Structure and function of signal-transducing GTP-binding proteins. Annu Rev Biochem 60:349, 1991.
24. Kenakin, TP: The classification of drugs and drug receptors in isolated tissues. Pharmacol Rev 36:165, 1984.
25. Lamb, P and Rosen, J: Drug discovery using receptors that modulate gene expression. J Recept Signal Transduct Res 17:531, 1997.
26. Lefkowitz, RJ, Hausdorff, WP, and Caron, MG: Role of phosphorylation in desensitization of the beta-adrenoceptor. Trends Pharmacol Sci 11:190, 1990.
27. Lefkowitz, RJ, Stadel, JM, and Caron, MG: Adenylate cyclase-coupled beta-adrenergic receptors: Structure and mechanisms of activation and desensitization. Annu Rev Biochem 52:159, 1983.
28. Lohse, MJ, et al: G-protein-coupled receptor kinases. Kidney Int 49:1047, 1996.
29. McDonnell, DP, et al: The mechanism of action of steroid hormones: A new twist to an old tale. J Clin Pharmacol 33:1165, 1993.
30. McKinney, M and Richelson, E: The coupling of the neuronal muscarinic receptor to responses. Annu Rev Pharmacol Toxicol 24:121, 1984.
31. Montal, M: Molecular anatomy and molecular design of channel proteins. FASEB J 4:2623, 1990.
32. Muccioli, G, Ghe, D, and DiCarlo, R: Drug-induced membrane modifications differentially affect prolactin and insulin binding in the mouse liver. Pharmacol Res Commun 17:883, 1985.
33. Neubig, RR and Thomsen, WJ: How does a key fit a flexible lock? Structure and dynamics of receptor function. Bioessays 11:136, 1989.
34. Oakley, RH and Cidlowski, JA: Homologous down regulation of the glucocorticoid receptor: The molecular machinery. Crit Rev Eukaryot Gene Expr 3:63, 1993.
35. Raffa, RB and Tallarida, RJ: The concept of a changing receptor concentration: Implications for the theory of drug action. J Theor Biol 115:625, 1985.
36. Ransnas, L, Hjalmarson, A, and Jacobsson, B: Adenylate cyclase modulation by ammonium ion: GTP-like effect on muscarinic and alpha 2-adrenergic receptors. Acta Pharmacol Toxicol 56:382, 1985.
37. Ross, EM: Pharmacodynamics: Mechanisms of drug action and the relationship between drug concentration and effect. In Hardman, JG, et al (eds): The Pharmacological Basis of Therapeutics, ed 9. McGraw-Hill, New York, 1996.
38. Roth, BL, et al: 5-hydroxytryptamine2A receptor desensitization can occur without down-regulation. J Pharmacol Exp Ther 275:1638, 1995.
39. Schenk, PW and Snaar-Jagalska, BE: Signal perception and transduction: The role of protein kinases. Biochim Biophys Acta 1449:1, 1999.
40. Swope, SL, et al: Regulation of ligand-gated ion channels by protein phosphorylation. Adv Second Messenger Phosphoprotein Res 33:49, 1999.
41. Tallarida, RJ: Receptor discrimination and control of agonist-antagonist binding. Am J Physiol 269:E379, 1995.
42. Ukena, D, Poeschla, E, and Schwabe, U: Guanine nucleotide and cation regulation of radioligand binding to R(i) adenosine receptors of rat fat cells. Naunyn-Schmiedebergs Arch Pharmacol 326:241, 1984.
43. Wess, J: G-protein-coupled receptors: Molecular mechanisms involved in receptor activation and selectivity of G-protein recognition. FASEB J 11:346, 1997.
44. Woodcock, EA, et al: Specific increase in renal alpha 1-adrenergic receptors following unilateral renal denervation. J Recept Res 5:133, 1985.
45. Xue, H, et al: Fragment of GABA(A) receptor containing key ligand-binding residues overexpressed in *Escherichia coli*. Protein Sci 7:216, 1998.
46. Zhu, BT: The competitive and noncompetitive antagonism of receptor-mediated drug actions in the presence of spare receptors. J Pharmacol Toxicol Methods 29:85, 1993.

Pharmacology of the Central Nervous System

CHAPTER **5**

Central Nervous System Pharmacology: General Principles

The central nervous system (CNS) is responsible for controlling bodily functions as well as being the center for behavioral and intellectual abilities. Neurons within the CNS are organized into highly complex patterns that mediate information through synaptic interactions. CNS drugs often attempt to modify the activity of these neurons in order to treat specific disorders or to alter the general level of arousal of the CNS. This chapter presents a simplified introduction to the organization of the CNS and the general strategies that can be used with drugs to alter activity within the brain and spinal cord.

CNS ORGANIZATION

The CNS can be grossly divided into the brain and the spinal cord (Fig. 5–1). The brain is subdivided according to anatomic or functional criteria. The following is a brief overview of the general organization of the brain and spinal cord, with some indication of where particular CNS drugs tend to exert their effects, and is by no means intended to be an extensive review of neuroanatomy. A more elaborate discussion of CNS structure and function can be found in several excellent sources.[9,13,23]

Cerebrum

The largest and most rostral aspect of the brain is the *cerebrum* (see Fig. 5–1). The cerebrum consists of bilateral hemispheres, with each hemisphere anatomically divided into several lobes (frontal, temporal, parietal, and occipital). The outer cerebrum, or cerebral cortex, is associated with the highest order of conscious function and integration in the CNS. Specific cortical areas are responsible for sensory and motor functions, as well as intellectual and cognitive abilities. Other cortical areas are involved in short-

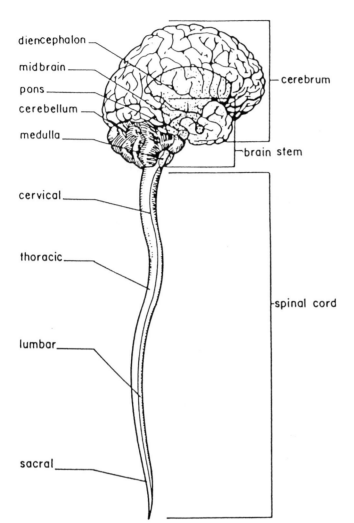

diencephalon

midbrain

pons

cerebellum

medulla

cervical

thoracic

lumbar

sacral

cerebrum

brain stem

spinal cord

FIGURE 5–1. General organization of the CNS. (From Crouch, JE: Essential Human Anatomy. Lea & Febiger, Philadelphia, 1982, with permission.)

term memory and speech. The cortex also seems to function in somewhat of a supervisory capacity regarding lower brain function and may influence the control of other activities such as the autonomic nervous system. With regard to CNS drugs, most therapeutic medications tend to affect cortical function indirectly by first altering the function of lower brain and spinal cord structures. An exception is the group of drugs used to treat epilepsy; these drugs are often targeted directly for hyperexcitable neurons in the cerebral cortex.

Basal Ganglia

A group of specific areas located deep within the cerebral hemispheres is collectively termed the *basal ganglia*. Components of the basal ganglia include the caudate nucleus, putamen, globus pallidus, lentiform nucleus, and substantia nigra. The basal ganglia are involved primarily in the control of motor activity, and deficits in this area are significant in movement disorders such as *Parkinson* disease and *Huntington* chorea. Certain medications used to treat these movement disorders exert their effects by interacting with basal ganglia structures.

Diencephalon

The area of brain enclosing the third ventricle is the *diencephalon.* This area consists of several important structures, including the thalamus and hypothalamus. The thalamus contains distinct nuclei that are crucial in the integration of certain types of sensation and the relay of these sensations to other areas of the brain, such as the somatosensory cortex. The hypothalamus is involved in the control of diverse body functions, including temperature control, appetite, water balance, and certain emotional reactions. The hypothalamus is also significant in its control over the function of hormonal release from the pituitary gland. Several CNS drugs affecting sensation and control of the body functions listed here manifest their effects by interacting with the thalamus and hypothalamus.

Mesencephalon and Brainstem

The *mesencephalon,* or *midbrain,* serves as a bridge between the higher areas (cerebrum and diencephalon) and the *brainstem.* The brainstem consists of the pons and the medulla oblongata. In addition to serving as a pathway between the higher brain and the spinal cord, the midbrain and brainstem are the location of centers responsible for controlling respiration and cardiovascular function (vasomotor center). The reticular formation is also located in the midbrain and brainstem. The reticular formation is a collection of neurons that extend from the reticular substance of the upper spinal cord through the midbrain and the thalamus. The reticular formation monitors and controls consciousness and is important in regulating the amount of arousal or alertness of the cerebral cortex. Consequently, CNS drugs that affect the state of arousal of the individual tend to exert their effects on the reticular formation. Sedative-hypnotics and general anesthetics tend to decrease activity in the reticular formation, whereas certain CNS stimulants (caffeine, amphetamines) may increase arousal through a stimulatory effect on reticular formation neurons.

Cerebellum

The *cerebellum* lies posterior to the brainstem and is separated from the brainstem by the fourth ventricle. Anatomically, it is divided into two hemispheres, with each hemisphere consisting of three lobes (anterior, posterior, and flocculonodular). The function of the cerebellum is to help plan and coordinate motor activity and assume responsibility for comparing the actual movement with the intended motor pattern. The cerebellum interprets various sensory input and helps modulate motor output so that the actual movement closely resembles the intended motor program. The cerebellum is also concerned with the vestibular mechanisms responsible for maintaining balance and posture. Therapeutic medications are not usually targeted directly for the cerebellum, but incoordination and other movement disorders may result if a drug exerts a toxic side effect on the cerebellum.

Limbic System

So far, all of the structures described have been grouped primarily by anatomic relationships with the brain. The *limbic system* is comprised of several structures that are dispersed throughout the brain but are often considered as a functional unit or system within the CNS. Major components of the limbic system include cortical structures (such as the amygdala, hippocampus, and cingulate gyrus), the hypothalamus, certain thalamic nuclei, mamillary bodies, septum pellucidum, and several other structures and tracts. These structures share the common function of being involved in the control of emotional and behavioral activity. Certain aspects of motivation, aggression, sexual activity, and instinctive responses may be influenced by activity within the limbic system. CNS drugs affecting these aspects of behavior, including some antianxiety and antipsychotic medications, are believed to exert their beneficial effects primarily by altering activity in the limbic structures.

Spinal Cord

At the caudal end of the brainstem, the CNS continues distally as the *spinal cord*. The spinal cord is cylindrically shaped and consists of centrally located gray matter that is surrounded by white matter. The gray matter serves as an area for synaptic connections between various neurons. The white matter consists of the myelinated axons of neurons, which are grouped into tracts that ascend or descend between the brain and specific levels of the cord. Certain CNS drugs exert some or all of their effects by modifying synaptic transmission in specific areas of the gray matter; other CNS drugs, such as the narcotic analgesics, may exert an effect on synaptic transmission in the gray matter of the cord as well as on synapses in other areas of the brain. Some drugs may be specifically directed toward the white matter of the cord. Drugs such as the local anesthetics can be used to block action potential propagation in the white matter so that ascending or descending information is interrupted (i.e., a spinal block).

THE BLOOD-BRAIN BARRIER

The *blood-brain barrier* refers to the unique structure and function of CNS capillaries.[8,11,15,16] Certain substances are not able to pass from the bloodstream into the CNS, despite the fact that these same substances are able to pass from the systemic circulation into other peripheral tissues. This fact suggests the existence of some sort of unique structure and function of the CNS capillaries that prevents many substances from entering the brain and spinal cord—hence the term **blood-brain barrier.** This barrier effect is caused primarily by the tight junctions between capillary endothelial cells; in fact, CNS capillaries lack the gaps and fenestrations that are seen in peripheral capillaries. Also, nonneuronal cells in the CNS (e.g., astrocytes) and the capillary basement membrane seem to contribute to the relative impermeability of this barrier. Functionally, the blood-brain barrier acts as a selective filter and seems to protect the CNS by limiting the entry of harmful substances into the brain and spinal cord.

The blood-brain barrier obviously plays an important role in clinical pharmacotherapeutics. To exert their effects, drugs that are targeted for the CNS must be able to pass from the bloodstream into the brain and spinal cord. In general, nonpolar, lipid-soluble drugs are able to cross the blood-brain barrier by passive diffusion.[8] Polar and lipophobic compounds are usually unable to enter the brain. Some exceptions occur because of the presence of carrier-mediated transport systems in the blood-brain barrier.[8,16] Some substances such as glucose are transported via facilitated diffusion; other compounds, including some drugs, may be able to enter the brain by active transport. However, these transport processes are limited to certain specific compounds, and the typical manner by which most drugs enter the brain is by passive lipid diffusion.[8]

CNS NEUROTRANSMITTERS

The majority of neural connections in the human brain and spinal cord are characterized as chemical synapses. The term *chemical synapse* indicates that some chemical neurotransmitter is used to propagate the nervous impulse across the gap that exists between two neurons. Several distinct chemicals have been identified as neurotransmitters within the brain and spinal cord (Table 5–1). Groups of neurons within the CNS tend to use one of these neurotransmitters to produce either excitation or inhibition of other neurons. Although each neurotransmitter can be generally described as either excitatory or inhibitory within the CNS, some transmitters may have different effects, depending on the nature of the postsynaptic receptor involved. As discussed in Chapter 4, the interaction of the transmitter and the receptor dictates the effect on the postsynaptic neuron.

The facts that several distinct neurotransmitters exist and that neurons using specific transmitters are organized functionally within the CNS have important pharmacologic implications. Certain drugs may alter the transmission in pathways using a specific neurotransmitter, while having little or no effect on other transmitter pathways. This allows the drug to exert a rather specific effect on the CNS, so many disorders may be rectified without radically altering other CNS functions. Other drugs may have a much more general effect and alter transmission in many CNS regions. To provide an indication of neurotransmitter function, the major categories of CNS neurotransmitters and their general locations and effects are discussed subsequently.

Acetylcholine

Acetylcholine is the neurotransmitter found in many areas of the brain as well as in the periphery (skeletal neuromuscular junction, some autonomic synapses). In the

TABLE 5–1 Central Neurotransmitters

Transmitter	Primary CNS Locations	General Effect
Acetylcholine	Cerebral cortex (many areas), basal ganglia, limbic and thalamic regions, spinal interneurons	Excitation
Norepinephrine	Neurons originating in brainstem and hypothalamus that project throughout other areas of brain	Inhibition
Dopamine	Basal ganglia, limbic system	Inhibition
Serotonin	Neurons originating in brainstem that project upward (to hypothalamus) and downward (to spinal cord)	Inhibition
GABA (gamma-aminobutyric acid)	Interneurons throughout spinal cord, cerebellum, basal ganglia, cerebral cortex	Inhibition
Glycine	Interneurons in spinal cord and brainstem	Inhibition
Glutamate, aspartate	Interneurons throughout brain and spinal cord	Excitation
Substance P	Pathways in spinal cord and brain that mediate painful stimuli	Excitation
Enkephalins	Pain suppression pathways in spinal cord and brain	Excitation

brain, neurons originating in the large pyramidal cells of the motor cortex and many neurons originating in the basal ganglia secrete acetylcholine from their terminal axons. In general, acetylcholine synapses in the CNS are excitatory in nature.

Monoamines

Monoamines such as the **catecholamines** (dopamine, norepinephrine) and 5-hydroxytryptamine (serotonin) have been recognized as transmitters in several brain locations.[3] Within the basal ganglia, **dopamine** is the transmitter secreted by neurons that originate in the substantia nigra and project to the corpus striatum. Dopamine may also be an important transmitter in areas within the limbic system such as the hypothalamus. In general, dopamine inhibits neurons onto which it is released.

Norepinephrine is secreted by neurons that originate in the locus caeruleus of the pons and project throughout the reticular formation. Norepinephrine is generally regarded as an inhibitory transmitter within the CNS, but the overall effect following activity of norepinephrine synapses is often general excitation of the brain, probably because norepinephrine directly inhibits other neurons that produce inhibition. This phenomenon of *disinhibition* causes excitation by removing the influence of inhibitory neurons.

Serotonin (also known as 5-hydroxytryptamine) is released by cells originating in the midline of the pons and brainstem and is projected to many different areas, including the dorsal horns of the spinal cord and the hypothalamus. Serotonin is considered a strong inhibitor in most areas of the CNS and is thought to be important in mediating the inhibition of painful stimuli. Serotonin is also involved in controlling many aspects of mood and behavior, and problems with serotonergic activity have been implicated in several psychiatric disorders, including depression and anxiety.[5] The roles of serotonin and the other monoamines in psychiatric disorders are discussed in Chapters 6 through 8.

Amino Acids

Several amino acids such as glycine and gamma-aminobutyric acid (GABA) are important inhibitory transmitters in the brain and spinal cord. Glycine seems to be the inhibitory transmitter used by certain interneurons located throughout the spinal cord.[1] Likewise, GABA is released by spinal cord inhibitory interneurons and seems to be the predominant transmitter used to mediate presynaptic inhibition in the cord.[6] GABA also has been identified as an inhibitory transmitter in areas of the brain such as the cortex and basal ganglia.[10] Other amino acids such as aspartate and glutamate have been found in high concentrations throughout the brain and spinal cord; these substances cause excitation of CNS neurons.[4,21] These excitatory amino acids have received a great deal of attention lately because they may also produce neurotoxic effects when released in large amounts during CNS injury and certain neurologic disorders (epilepsy, amyotrophic lateral sclerosis, and so forth).[19,22]

Peptides

Many peptides have already been established as CNS neurotransmitters.[18] One peptide that is important from a pharmacologic standpoint is substance P, which is an excitatory transmitter that is involved in spinal cord pathways that transmit pain impulses. Increased activity at substance P synapses in the cord serves to mediate the transmission of painful sensations, and certain drugs such as the opioid analgesics may decrease activity at these synapses. Other peptides that have important pharmacologic implications include three families of compounds, the endorphins, enkephalins, and dynorphins.[14] These peptides, also known as the endogenous opioids, are excitatory transmitters in certain brain synapses that inhibit painful sensations. Hence, endogenous opioids in the brain are able to decrease the central perception of pain. The interaction of these compounds with exogenous opioid drugs is discussed in Chapter 14. Finally, peptides such as galanin, neuropeptide Y, and vasoactive intestinal polypeptide (VIP) have been identified recently in various areas of the CNS. These peptides may affect various CNS functions, either by acting directly as neurotransmitters or by acting as co-transmitters that moderate the effects of other neurotransmitters.[7,18]

Other Transmitters

In addition to the well-known substances, other chemicals are continually being identified as potential CNS neurotransmitters. Recent evidence has implicated substances such as adenosine and ATP as transmitters or modulators of neural transmission in specific areas of the brain and in the autonomic nervous system.[2,20] Many other chemicals that are traditionally associated with functions outside the CNS are now being identified as possible CNS transmitters. Such chemicals include histamine, nitric oxide, and certain hormones (vasopressin, oxytocin). As the function of these chemicals and other new transmitters becomes clearer, the pharmacologic significance of drugs that affect these synapses will undoubtedly be considered.

CNS DRUGS: GENERAL MECHANISMS

The majority of CNS drugs work by modifying synaptic transmission in some way. Figure 5–2 shows a typical chemical synapse that would be found in the CNS. Most drugs that attempt to rectify CNS-related disorders do so by either increasing or decreasing transmission at specific synapses. For instance, psychotic behavior has been associated with overactivity in central synapses that use dopamine as a neurotransmitter (see Chap. 8). Drug therapy in this situation consists of agents that decrease activity at central dopamine synapses. Conversely, Parkinson disease results from a decrease in activity at specific dopamine synapses (see Chap. 10). Antiparkinsonian drugs attempt to increase dopaminergic transmission at these synapses and to bring synaptic activity back to normal levels.

A drug that modifies synaptic transmission must somehow alter the quantity of the neurotransmitter released from the presynaptic terminal or affect the stimulation of postsynaptic receptors, or both. In considering a typical synapse, such as the one shown in Figure 5–2, there are several distinct sites at which a drug may alter activity in the synapse. Specific ways in which a drug may modify synaptic transmission are presented here.

1. *Presynaptic action potential:* The arrival of an action potential at the presynaptic terminal initiates neurotransmitter release. Certain drugs such as the local anesthetics block propagation along neural axons so that the action potential fails to reach the

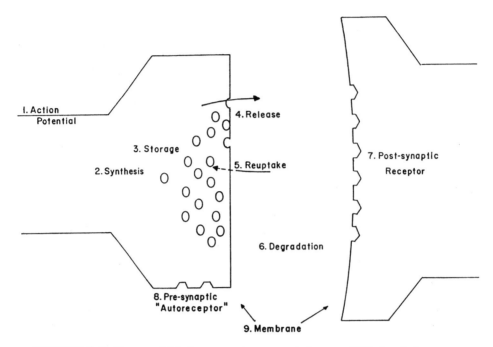

FIGURE 5–2. Sites at which drugs can alter transmission at a CNS chemical synapse.

presynaptic terminal, which effectively eliminates activity at that particular synapse. Also, the amount of depolarization or height of the action potential arriving at the presynaptic terminal is directly related to the amount of transmitter released. Any drug or endogenous chemical that limits the amount of depolarization occurring in the presynaptic terminal will inhibit the synapse because less neurotransmitter is released. In certain situations, this is referred to as presynaptic inhibition, because the site of this effect is at the presynaptic terminal. The endogenous neurotransmitter GABA is believed to exert some of its inhibitory effects via this mechanism.

2. *Synthesis of neurotransmitter:* Drugs that block the synthesis of neurotransmitter will eventually deplete the presynaptic terminal and impair transmission. For example, metyrosine inhibits an enzyme essential for catecholamine biosynthesis in the presynaptic terminal. Treatment with metyrosine results in decreased synthesis of transmitters such as dopamine and norepinephrine.

3. *Storage of neurotransmitter:* A certain amount of chemical transmitter is stored in presynaptic vesicles. Drugs that impair this storage will decrease the ability of the synapse to continue to transmit information for extended periods. An example of this is the antihypertensive drug reserpine, which impairs the ability of adrenergic terminals to sequester and store norepinephrine in presynaptic vesicles.

4. *Release:* Certain drugs will increase synaptic activity by directly increasing the release of neurotransmitter from the presynaptic terminal. Amphetamines appear to exert their effects on the CNS primarily by increasing the presynaptic release of catecholamine neurotransmitters (e.g., norepinephrine). Conversely, other compounds may inhibit the synapse by directly decreasing the amount of transmitter released during each action potential. An example is botulinum toxin, which can be used as a skeletal muscle relaxant because of its ability to impair the release of acetylcholine from the skeletal neuromuscular junction (see Chap. 13).

5. *Reuptake:*   After the neurotransmitter is released, some chemical synapses terminate activity primarily by transmitter reuptake. Reuptake involves movement of the transmitter molecule back into the presynaptic terminal. A drug that impairs the reuptake of transmitter allows more of the transmitter to remain in the synaptic cleft and continue to exert an effect. Consequently, blocking reuptake actually increases activity at the synapse. For instance, the tricyclic antidepressants (see Chap. 7) impair the reuptake mechanism that pumps amine neurotransmitters back into the presynaptic terminal, which allows the transmitter to continue to exert its effect, thus prolonging activity at the synapse.

6. *Degradation:*   Some synapses rely primarily on enzymatic breakdown of the released transmitter to terminate synaptic activity. Inhibition of the enzyme responsible for terminating the transmitter allows more of the active transmitter to remain in the synaptic cleft, thereby increasing activity at the synapse. An example is the use of a drug that inhibits the **cholinesterase** enzyme as a method of treating myasthenia gravis. In myasthenia gravis, there is a functional decrease in activity at the skeletal neuromuscular junction. Anticholinesterase drugs such as neostigmine and pyridostigmine inhibit acetylcholine breakdown, allowing more of the released neurotransmitter to continue to exert an effect at the neuromuscular synapse.

7. *Postsynaptic receptor:*   As discussed in Chapter 4, chemical antagonists can be used to block the postsynaptic receptor, thus decreasing synaptic transmission. The best-known example of this is the use of the so-called beta blockers. These agents are antagonists that are specific for the beta-adrenergic receptors on the myocardium, and they are used frequently to treat hypertension, cardiac arrhythmias, and angina pectoris. Other drugs may improve synaptic transmission by directly affecting the receptor so that there is a tendency for increased neurotransmitter binding or improved receptor-effector coupling, or both. For instance, the benzodiazepines (e.g., diazepam, chlordiazepoxide) appear to enhance the postsynaptic effects of the inhibitory neurotransmitter GABA.

8. *Presynaptic autoreceptors:*   In addition to postsynaptic receptors, there are also receptors on the presynaptic terminal of some types of chemical synapses. These presynaptic receptors seem to serve as a method of negative feedback in controlling neurotransmitter release.[12,17] During high levels of synaptic activity, the accumulation of neurotransmitter in the synaptic cleft may allow binding to these presynaptic receptors and limit further release of chemical transmitter. Certain drugs may also be able to attenuate synaptic activity through these presynaptic autoreceptors. Clonidine, for instance, may exert some of its antihypertensive effects by binding to presynaptic receptors on sympathetic postganglionic neurons and impairing the release of norepinephrine onto the peripheral vasculature. The use of drugs that alter synaptic activity by binding to these autoreceptors is still somewhat new, however, and the full potential for this area of pharmacology remains to be determined.

9. *Membrane effects:*   Drugs may alter synaptic transmission by affecting membrane organization and fluidity. Membrane fluidity is basically the amount of flexibility or mobility of the lipid bilayer. Drugs that alter the fluidity of the presynaptic membrane could affect the way that presynaptic vesicles fuse with and release their neurotransmitter. Drug-induced changes in the postsynaptic membrane would affect the receptor environment and thereby alter receptor function. Membrane modification will result in either increased or decreased synaptic transmission, depending on the drug in question and the type and magnitude of membrane change. For example, alcohol (ethanol) and general anesthetics may exert some of their effects by causing reversible changes in the fluidity and organization of the cell membranes of central neurons.

A CNS drug does not have to adhere specifically to only one of these methods of synaptic modification. Some drugs may affect the synapse in two or more ways. For example, the antihypertensive agent guanethidine impairs both the presynaptic storage and the release of norepinephrine. Other drugs such as the barbiturates may affect both the presynaptic terminal and the postsynaptic receptor in CNS synapses.

SUMMARY

Drugs affecting the brain and spinal cord usually exert their effects by somehow modifying synaptic transmission. In some instances, drugs may be targeted for specific synapses in an attempt to rectify some problem with transmission at that particular synapse. Other drugs may increase or decrease the excitability of CNS neurons in an attempt to have a more general effect on the overall level of consciousness of the individual. Specific categories of CNS drugs and their pharmacodynamic mechanisms are discussed in succeeding chapters.

REFERENCES

1. Breitinger, HG and Becker, CM: The inhibitory glycine receptor: Prospects for a therapeutic orphan? Curr Pharm Des 4:315, 1998.
2. Burnstock, G: Purinergic mechanisms broaden their sphere of influence. Trends Neurosci 8:5, 1985.
3. Carlsson, A: Perspectives on the discovery of central monoaminergic transmission. Annu Rev Neurosci 10:19, 1987.
4. Cunningham, MD, Ferkany, JW, and Enna, SJ: Excitatory amino acid receptors: A gallery of new targets for pharmacological intervention. Life Sci 54:135, 1994.
5. Graeff, FG: Serotonergic systems. Psychiatr Clin North Am 20:723, 1997.
6. Hevers, W and Luddens, H: The diversity of GABAA receptors. Pharmacological and electrophysiological properties of GABAA channel subtypes. Mol Neurobiol 18:35, 1998.
7. Hokfelt, T, et al: Galanin in ascending systems. Focus on coexistence with 5-hydroxytryptamine and noradrenaline. Ann N Y Acad Sci 863:252, 1998.
8. Jolliet-Riant, P and Tillement, JP: Drug transfer across the blood-brain barrier and improvement of brain delivery. Fundam Clin Pharmacol 13:16, 1999.
9. Kandel, ER, Schwartz, JH, and Jessell, TM (eds): Principles of Neural Science, ed 4. McGraw-Hill, New York, 2000.
10. Korpi, ER, et al: GABA(A)-receptor subtypes: Clinical efficacy and selectivity of benzodiazepine site ligands. Ann Med 29:275, 1997.
11. Laterra, J and Goldstein, GW: Appendix B: Ventricular organization of cerebrospinal fluid: Blood-brain barrier, brain edema, and hydrocephalus. In Kandel, ER, Schwartz, JH, and Jessell, TM (eds): Principles of Neural Science, ed 4. McGraw-Hill, New York, 2000.
12. Mercuri, NB, Bonci, A, and Bernardi, G: Electrophysiological pharmacology of the autoreceptor-mediated responses of dopaminergic cells to antiparkinson drugs. Trends Pharmacol Sci 18:232, 1997.
13. Nolte, J: The Human Brain, ed 4. CV Mosby, St Louis, 1999.
14. Reisine, T and Pasternak, G: Opioid analgesics and antagonists. In Hardman, JG, et al (eds): The Pharmacological Basis of Therapeutics, ed 9. McGraw-Hill, New York, 1996.
15. Rubin, LL and Staddon, JM: The cell biology of the blood-brain barrier. Annu Rev Neurosci 22:11, 1999.
16. Saunders, NR, Habgood, MD, and Dziegielewska, KM: Barrier mechanisms in the brain, I. Adult brain. Clin Exp Pharmacol Physiol 26:11, 1999.
17. Schlicker, E and Gothert, M: Interactions between the presynaptic alpha2-autoreceptor and presynaptic inhibitory heteroreceptors on noradrenergic neurones. Brain Res Bull 47:129, 1998.
18. Schwartz, JH: Neurotransmitters. In Kandel, ER, Schwartz, JH, and Jessell, TM (eds): Principles of Neural Science, ed 4. McGraw-Hill, New York, 2000.
19. Seal, RP and Amara, SG: Excitatory amino acid transporters: A family in flux. Annu Rev Pharmacol Toxicol 39:431, 1999.
20. Stiles, GL and Olah, ME: Adenosine receptors: Annu Rev Physiol 54:211, 1992.
21. Thomas, RJ: Excitatory amino acids in health and disease. J Am Geriatr Soc 43:1279, 1995.
22. Vandenberg, RJ: Molecular pharmacology and physiology of glutamate transporters in the central nervous system. Clin Exp Pharmacol Physiol 25:393, 1998.
23. Waxman, SG: Correlative Neuroanatomy, ed 24. McGraw-Hill, New York, 2000.

CHAPTER **6**

Sedative-Hypnotic and Antianxiety Agents

Drugs that are classified as sedative-hypnotics are used to relax the patient and promote sleep.[47] As the name implies, **sedative** drugs exert a calming effect and serve to pacify the patient. At a higher dose, the same drug tends to produce drowsiness and to initiate a relatively normal state of sleep (hypnosis). At still higher doses, some sedative-hypnotics (especially the barbiturates) will eventually bring on a state of general anesthesia. Because of their general central nervous system (CNS)–depressant effects, some sedative-hypnotic drugs are also used for other functions, such as treating epilepsy or producing muscle relaxation. However, the sleep-enhancing effects are of concern in this chapter.

By producing sedation, many drugs will also decrease the level of anxiety in the patient. Of course, these anxiolytic properties often occur at the expense of a decrease in the level of alertness in the individual. However, certain agents are available that can reduce anxiety without an overt sedative effect. Those medications that selectively produce antianxiety effects are discussed later in this chapter.

Even though sedative-hypnotic and antianxiety drugs are not used to directly treat any somatic disorders, many patients receiving physical therapy and occupational therapy take these agents to help decrease anxiety and enhance relaxation. A person who becomes ill or sustains an injury requiring rehabilitation certainly has some apprehension concerning his or her welfare. If necessary, this apprehension can be controlled to some extent by using sedative-hypnotic and antianxiety drugs during the course of rehabilitation. Consequently, an understanding of the basic pharmacology of these agents will be helpful to rehabilitation specialists such as the physical therapist and occupational therapist.

SEDATIVE-HYPNOTIC AGENTS

Sedative-hypnotics fall into two general categories: barbiturates and benzodiazepines (Table 6–1). Several other nonbarbiturate, nonbenzodiazepine drugs are available (see Table 6–1), but they are typically used on only a limited basis in selected patients.

71

TABLE 6–1 Common Sedative-Hypnotic Drugs

Generic Name	Trade Name	Oral Adult Dose (mg)	
		Sedative	Hypnotic*
Barbiturates			
Amobarbital	Amytal	25–150 BID	65–200
Aprobarbital	Alurate	40 TID	40–160
Butabarbital	Butalan, Butisol, others	15–30 TID or QID	50–100
Pentobarbital	Nembutal	20 TID or QID	100
Phenobarbital	Solfoton	15–40 BID or TID	100–320
Secobarbital	Seconal	30–50 TID or QID	100
Benzodiazepines†			
Estazolam	ProSom	———	1–2
Flurazepam	Dalmane	———	15–30
Quazepam	Doral	———	7.5–15
Temazepam	Restoril	———	7.5–30
Triazolam	Halcion	———	0.125–0.25
Others			
Chloral hydrate	(generic)	250 TID	500–1000
Ethchlorvynol	Placidyl	———	500–1000
Glutethimide	(generic)	———	250–500
Promethazine	Phenergan, Promacot, others	———	25–50

*Use of hypnotic agents typically involves a single dose administered at bedtime.

†Benzodiazepines listed here are indicated specifically as hypnotic agents and are not approved for other uses (antianxiety, anticonvulsant, and so forth). Virtually all benzodiazepines have sedative-hypnotic effects, and other benzodiazepines may be administered to produce sedation or sleep, depending on the patient.

The barbiturates are a group of CNS depressants that share a common chemical origin from barbituric acid. The potent sedative-hypnotic properties of these drugs have been recognized for some time, and their status as the premier medication used to promote sleep was unchallenged for many years. However, barbiturates are associated with a relatively small therapeutic index, with approximately 10 times the therapeutic dose often being fatal. These drugs are also addictive, and their prolonged use is often a problem in terms of drug abuse. Consequently, the lack of safety of the barbiturates and their strong potential for addiction and abuse necessitated the development of alternative nonbarbiturate drugs such as the benzodiazepines. Still, some barbiturates are occasionally used for their **hypnotic** properties; these drugs are listed in Table 6–1.

At present, the use of barbiturates as hypnotics has essentially been replaced by other drugs, with the benzodiazepines the current drugs of choice.[5] Several benzodiazepines are currently approved for use as hypnotics (Table 6–2). These agents exert hypnotic effects similar to those of the barbiturates, but they are generally regarded as safer because there is less chance of a lethal overdose.[5] However, benzodiazepines are not without their drawbacks, in that tolerance and physical dependence can also occur with their prolonged use (see "Benzodiazepines").[38,39]

Several other nonbarbiturate compounds may also be prescribed for their sedative-hypnotic properties (see Table 6–1). These compounds are chemically dissimilar but share the common ability to promote relaxation and sleep via their general ability to depress the CNS. Cyclic ethers and alcohols (including ethanol) can be included in this cat-

TABLE 6–2 Pharmacokinetic Properties of Benzodiazepine Sedative-Hypnotic Drugs

Generic Name (Trade Name)	Time to Peak Plasma Concentration (hr)*	Relative Half-Life	Comments
Estazolam (ProSom)	0.5–1.6	Intermediate	Rapid oral absorption
Flurazepam (Dalmane)	0.5–1.0	Long	Long elimination half-life because of active metabolites
Quazepam (Doral)	2.0	Long	Daytime drowsiness more likely than with other benzodiazepines
Temazepam (Restoril)	2–3	Short–intermediate	Slow oral absorption
Triazolam (Halcion)	Within 2	Short	Rapid oral absorption

*Adult oral hypnotic dose.

egory, but their use specifically as sedative-hypnotics is fairly limited at present. The recreational use of ethanol in alcoholic beverages is an important topic in terms of abuse and long-term effects. However, this area is much too extensive to be addressed here, so this presentation will focus on the clinical use of sedative-hypnotics.

PHARMACOKINETICS

Sedative-hypnotics are usually highly lipid soluble. They are typically administered orally and are absorbed easily and completely from the gastrointestinal tract. Distribution is fairly uniform throughout the body, and these drugs reach the CNS readily because of their high degree of lipid solubility. Sedative-hypnotics are metabolized primarily by the oxidative enzymes of the drug-metabolizing system in liver cells. Termination of their activity is accomplished either by hepatic enzymes or by storage of these drugs in non-CNS tissues; that is, by sequestering these drugs in adipose and other peripheral tissues, their CNS-depressant effects are not exhibited. However, when these drugs slowly leak out of their peripheral storage sites, they can be redistributed to the brain and can cause low levels of sedation. This occurrence may help explain the hangover-like feelings that are frequently reported the day after taking sedative-hypnotic drugs. Finally, excretion of these drugs takes place through the kidney after their metabolism in the liver. As with most types of drug biotransformation, metabolism of sedative-hypnotics is essential in creating a polar metabolite that is readily excreted by the kidney.

MECHANISM OF ACTION

Benzodiazepines

The benzodiazepines exert their effects by increasing the inhibitory effects at CNS synapses that use the neurotransmitter gamma-aminobutyric acid (GABA).[12,36,45] These inhibitory synapses are associated with a membrane protein complex containing three primary components: (1) a binding site for GABA, (2) a binding site for benzodiazepines, and (3) an ion channel that is specific for ions such as chloride (Fig. 6–1).[11,16,18] GABA

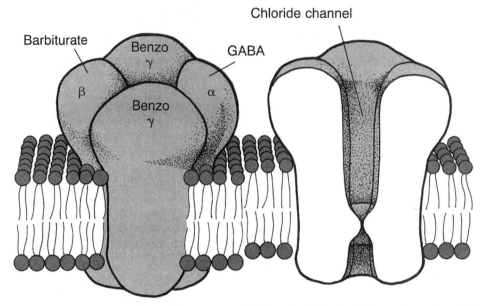

FIGURE 6–1. Putative structure of the gamma aminobutyric acid (GABA)–benzodiazepine–chloride ion channel complex. The centrally located chloride ion channel is modulated by the binding of GABA to the alpha subunit of the receptor. The binding and effects of GABA are enhanced by the binding of benzodiazepines to the gamma subunits or barbiturates to the beta subunit. (From Kandel, ER: Disorders of mood: Depression, mania, and anxiety disorders. In Kandel, ER, Schwartz, JH, and Jessell, TM (eds): Principles of Neural Science, ed 3. Appleton & Lange, Norwalk, CT, 1991, p 882, with permission.)

typically exerts its inhibitory effects by binding to its receptor site on this complex and by initiating an increase in chloride conductance through the channel. Increased chloride conductance facilitates chloride entry into the neuron and results in hyperpolarization or a decreased ability to raise the neuron to its firing threshold. By binding to their own respective site on the complex, benzodiazepines potentiate the effects of GABA and increase the inhibition at these synapses.

Consequently, the presence of the GABA–benzodiazepine–chloride ion channel complex accounts for the specific mechanism of action of this class of sedative-hypnotics. By increasing the inhibitory effects at GABA-ergic synapses located in the reticular formation, benzodiazepines can decrease the level of arousal of the individual. In other words, the general excitation level in the reticular activating system decreases, and relaxation and sleep are enhanced.

Research has also indicated that there are at least three primary types of GABA receptors, and these receptors are classified as $GABA_a$, $GABA_b$, and $GABA_c$ receptors, according to their structural and functional characteristics.[4] $GABA_a$ and $GABA_c$ receptors, for example, cause inhibition by increasing chloride entry, whereas $GABA_b$ receptors may cause inhibition by increasing potassium *exit* (efflux) from CNS neurons.[4] At the present time, it appears that most of GABA's inhibitory effects in the CNS are mediated through the $GABA_a$ receptors and that this receptor subtype tends to predominate in the brain.[18] Nonetheless, the fact that several subtypes of GABA receptors exist has enabled development of drugs that are more selective to certain GABA receptors than to others. The muscle relaxant baclofen, for example, may be more selective for $GABA_b$ receptors in the spinal cord than other GABA receptors (see Chap. 13). Future drug development may continue to exploit the differences between GABA receptor subtypes so that drugs are more selective and produce more specific beneficial effects, with fewer side effects.

Finally, the discovery of a CNS receptor that is specific for benzodiazepines has led to some interesting speculation as to the possible existence of some type of endogenous sedative-like agent. The presence of a certain type of receptor to indicate that the body produces an appropriate agonist for that receptor makes sense. For instance, the discovery of opiate receptors initiated the search for endogenous opiate-like substances, which culminated in the discovery of the enkephalins. However, no endogenous substances that bind specifically to the benzodiazepine receptor have yet been identified. Continued research in this area may someday reveal such a substance, and the focus of pharmacologic treatment can then be directed toward stimulating the release of endogenous sedative-hypnotic agents.

Barbiturates

Despite their extensive use in the past, the exact mechanism of the barbiturates remains somewhat unclear. When used in sedative-hypnotic doses, barbiturates may function in a somewhat similar fashion to the benzodiazepines in that they also potentiate the inhibitory effects of GABA.[11,18] This idea suggests that the barbiturates may affect the benzodiazepine–GABA–chloride ion channel complex described previously. Indeed, some evidence exists that barbiturates bind directly to this complex at a site that is different from the binding site for GABA or the benzodiazepines (see Fig. 6–1).[12,16] Barbiturates may, however, also exert effects that are not mediated through an effect on the GABA–benzodiazepine–chloride ion channel. For instance, barbiturates may also directly inhibit transmitter release from presynaptic terminals (i.e., independent of their GABA-enhancing effect), and barbiturates have been shown to have an antagonist-like effect on certain postsynaptic receptors that are excited by glutamate.[12,30] Regardless of their exact mechanism, barbiturates are effective sedative-hypnotics because of their specificity for neurons in the midbrain portion of the reticular formation as well as some limbic system structures. At higher doses, the barbiturates also depress neuronal excitability in other areas of the brain and spinal cord. Their role in producing general anesthesia by this more extensive CNS depression is discussed in Chapter 11.

Other Mechanisms

Alcohol (ethanol) and other sedative-hypnotics, which are neither benzodiazepine nor barbiturate in nature, work via poorly understood mechanisms. In the past, it was thought that alcohols exerted their depressant effects directly on neuronal membrane composition and fluidity. These and other highly lipid-soluble substances could simply dissolve in the lipid bilayer and inhibit neuronal excitability by temporarily disrupting membrane structure in the presynaptic and postsynaptic regions of CNS neurons.[7] Recent evidence, however, suggests that alcohol may act on protein receptors much as the barbiturates do; that is, alcohol may increase GABA-mediated inhibition by activating GABA receptors and decrease glutamate excitation by blocking certain glutamate receptors.[11,12] In any event, alcohol and similar agents bring about a decrease in neuronal transmission that causes fairly widespread CNS depression, which accounts for the subsequent sedative effects of such compounds.

PROBLEMS AND ADVERSE EFFECTS

Tolerance and Physical Dependence

The primary problem with many sedative-hypnotics is that prolonged use may cause tolerance and physical dependence. *Drug tolerance* is the need for more drug to be taken to exert the same effect. *Dependence* is described as the onset of withdrawal symptoms if the drug ceases to be taken. Although these problems were originally thought to be limited to the barbiturates, benzodiazepine sedative-hypnotics are now recognized as also causing tolerance and dependence when these drugs are taken continually for several weeks.

The manner and severity of withdrawal symptoms vary according to the type of drug and extent of the physical dependence.[13,37,38] Withdrawal after short-term benzodiazepine use may be associated with problems such as sleep disturbances (i.e., so-called rebound insomnia).[25,48] Long-term use and abuse may result in more severe problems such as psychosis and seizures if the drug is abruptly stopped.[10] When severe enough, seizures have been fatal in some cases of benzodiazepine withdrawal. Consequently, the long-term use of these drugs should be avoided, and other nonpharmacologic methods of reducing stress and promoting relaxation (e.g., mental imagery, biofeedback) should be instituted before tolerance and physical dependence become problems.[22] If the sedative-hypnotic has been used for an extended period, tapering off the dosage rather than abruptly stopping the drug has been recommended as a safer way to terminate administration.[37]

Residual Effects

Another problem associated with sedative-hypnotic use is the residual effects the day after administration. Individuals who take a sedative-hypnotic to get to sleep at night sometimes complain of drowsiness and decreased motor performance the next day.[8,14,49] These hangover-like effects may be caused by the drug's redistribution to the CNS from peripheral storage sites or may occur simply because the drug has not been fully metabolized. This problem may be resolved somewhat by using a smaller dose or by using a drug with a shorter half-life (see Table 6–2).[48,49] Anterograde amnesia is another problem sometimes associated with sedative-hypnotic use.[14,40] The patient may have trouble recalling details of events that occurred for a certain period of time before the drug was taken. Although usually a minor problem, this can become serious if the drug-induced amnesia exacerbates an already existing memory problem, as might occur in some elderly patients.

Other Side Effects

Other **side effects** such as gastrointestinal discomfort (nausea and vomiting), dry mouth, sore throat, and muscular incoordination have been reported, but these occur fairly infrequently. Cardiovascular and respiratory depression may also occur, but these problems are dose-related and are usually not significant except in cases of overdose.

ANTIANXIETY DRUGS

Anxiety can be described as a fear or apprehension over some situation or event that the individual feels is threatening. Such events can range from a change in employment or family life to somewhat irrational phobias concerning everyday occurrences. Anxiety disorders can also be classified in several clinical categories including generalized anxiety disorder, panic disorder, obsessive-compulsive disorder, and posttraumatic stress syndrome.[1,26] Antianxiety drugs can help decrease the tension and nervousness associated with many of these syndromes until the situation is resolved or the individual is counseled effectively in other methods of dealing with his or her anxiety.

Many drugs, including the sedative-hypnotics, have the ability to decrease anxiety levels, but this is usually at the expense of an increase in sedation. Frequently, alleviating anxiety without producing excessive sedation is desirable so that the individual can function in his or her home, on the job, and so on. Consequently, certain drugs are available that have significant anxiolytic properties at doses that produce minimal sedation. Benzodiazepine drugs and other nonbenzodiazepine strategies for dealing with anxiety are discussed here.

Benzodiazepines

As discussed previously, because of their relative safety, the benzodiazepines have replaced the barbiturates in the treatment of nervousness and anxiety. In terms of anxiolytic properties, diazepam (Valium) is the prototypical antianxiety benzodiazepine (Fig. 6–2). The extensive use of this drug in treating nervousness and apprehension has made the trade name of this compound virtually synonymous with a decrease in tension and anxiety. When prescribed in anxiolytic dosages, diazepam and certain other benzodiazepines (Table 6–3) are associated with a decrease in anxiety without major sedative effects. The mechanism of action of the benzodiazepines has been discussed previously in this chapter. The antianxiety properties of these drugs probably involve a mechanism similar or identical to their sedative-hypnotic effects (i.e., potentiating GABA-ergic transmission). However, the relative lack of sedation suggests that appropriate doses of these particular benzodiazepines may preferentially influence limbic structures with a lesser influence on the reticular activating system. Benzodiazepines also seem to increase presynaptic inhibition in the spinal cord, which produces some degree of skeletal muscle relaxation; this action may contribute to their antianxiety effects by making the individual feel more relaxed. The use of these drugs as skeletal muscle relaxants is further discussed in Chapter 13.

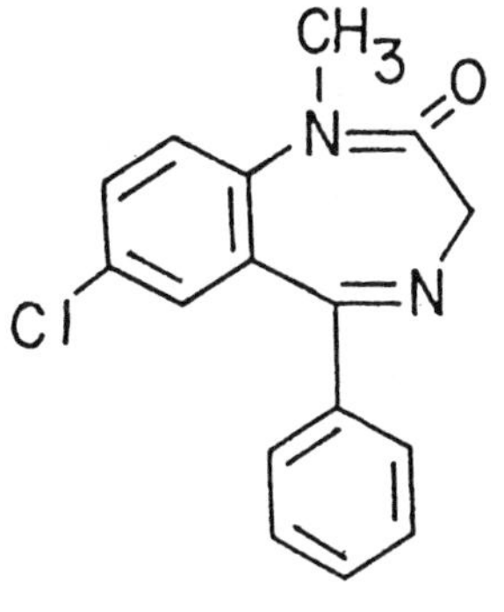

FIGURE 6–2. Diazepam (Valium).   Diazepam

TABLE 6–3 Benzodiazepine Antianxiety Drugs

Generic Name	Trade Name	Antianxiety Dose (mg)*	Relative Half-Life
Alprazolam	Xanax	0.25–0.5 TID	Short–intermediate
Chlordiazepoxide	Librium, others	5–25 TID or QID	Long
Clonazepam	Klonopin	0.25–0.50 BID	Intermediate
Clorazepate	Tranxene, others	7.5–15 BID to QID	Long
Diazepam	Valium, others	2–10 BID to QID	Long
Halazepam	Paxipam	20–40 TID or QID	Long
Lorazepam	Ativan	1–3 BID or TID	Short–intermediate
Oxazepam	Serax	10–30 TID or QID	Short–intermediate

*Doses refer to usual adult oral doses. Doses are often lower in elderly or debilitated patients.

Buspirone

Buspirone (BuSpar) is a relatively new antianxiety agent that was approved in 1986 for treating general anxiety disorder.[2] This agent is not a benzodiazepine but belongs instead to a drug class known as the azapirones.[3] Buspirone therefore does not act on the GABA receptor but exerts its antianxiety effects by increasing the effects of 5-hydroxy-tryptamine (serotonin) in certain areas of the brain.[46] Buspirone is basically a serotonin agonist that stimulates certain serotonin receptors, especially the 5-HT_{1A} serotonin receptor subtype.[19,46] This increase in serotoninergic influence is beneficial in treating general anxiety disorder and possibly other conditions, including panic disorder, obsessive-compulsive disorder, posttraumatic stress syndrome, and various other disorders that are influenced by CNS serotonin levels.[2] Buspirone also seems to be an effective treatment for patients who also have depression along with anxiety.[6,32]

More important, there is considerable evidence that buspirone has a much better side effect profile than traditional antianxiety drugs. Buspirone seems to produce less sedation and psychomotor impairment than benzodiazepine agents.[28,43] There is likewise a much smaller risk of developing tolerance and dependence to buspirone, and the potential for abuse is much lower with buspirone than with other anxiolytics.[32,34] Buspirone therefore offers an effective but safer alternative to traditional antianxiety drugs such as the benzodiazepines. Development of additional azapirones and other drugs that influence serotonin activity may continue to provide better and safer antianxiety agents in the future.

Other Antianxiety Drugs

The ideal antianxiety agent is nonaddictive, safe (i.e., relatively free from harmful side effects and potential for lethal overdose), and not associated with any sedative properties. Drugs such as meprobamate (Miltown) and the barbiturates are not currently used to any great extent because they do not meet any of these criteria and are no more effective in reducing anxiety than the benzodiazepines. As indicated earlier, buspirone currently offers an effective and somewhat safer method of treating anxiety, and use of this agent has increased dramatically since it was approved for clinical use. Another option is the beta-adrenergic antagonists (beta blockers, see Chap. 20) because these drugs can decrease situational anxiety without producing sedation.[9,20] In particular, beta blockers such as propranolol have been used by musicians and other performing artists to decrease cardiac palpitations, muscle tremors, hyperventilation, and other manifestations of anxiety that tend to occur before an important performance.[31] Beta blockers probably exert their antianxiety effects through their ability to decrease activity in the sympathetic nervous system, that is, through their sympatholytic effects. These drugs may exert both peripheral sympatholytic effects (e.g., blockade of myocardial beta-1 receptors) as well as by decreasing central sympathetic tone. In any event, beta blockers may offer a suitable alternative to decrease the effects of nervousness without a concomitant decrease in levels of alertness or motivation.[31] Hence, these drugs have gained a certain popularity with performing artists as a way to blunt the symptoms of performance anxiety without actually diminishing the anticipation and excitement that is requisite for a strong performance.

Problems and Adverse Effects

Most of the problems that occur with benzodiazepine anxiolytic drugs are similar to those mentioned regarding the use of these agents as sedative-hypnotics. Sedation is still the most common side effect of the anxiolytic benzodiazepines, even though this effect is not as pronounced as with their sedative-hypnotic counterparts.[41] Addiction and abuse are problems with chronic benzodiazepine use, and withdrawal from these drugs can be a serious problem. Also, rebound anxiety has been described when drugs such as diazepam are stopped.[15,17] Increased anxiety levels and other symptoms were noticed in one group of patients after diazepam was discontinued following a relatively short therapeutic trial of 6 weeks.[35] This observation again reinforces the idea that these drugs are not curative but should be used only for limited periods of time and as an adjunct to other nonpharmacologic procedures such as psychologic counseling.

Problems and side effects associated with buspirone include dizziness, headache, nausea, and restlessness. As indicated earlier, however, the side effect profile of buspirone is generally more acceptable than that of the benzodiazepines because buspirone produces only slight sedation (about one third of what occurs with benzodiazepines) and buspirone does not appear to cause addiction.

SPECIAL CONSIDERATIONS OF SEDATIVE-HYPNOTIC AND ANTIANXIETY AGENTS IN REHABILITATION

Although these drugs are not used to directly influence the rehabilitation of musculoskeletal or other somatic disorders, the prevalence of their use in patient populations is high. Any time a patient is hospitalized for treatment of a disorder, a substantial amount of apprehension and concern exists. The foreign environment of the institution as well as a change in the individual's daily routine can understandably result in sleep disturbances. Predictably, surveys reveal more than 50 percent of patients hospitalized for medical procedures receive some type of sedative-hypnotic drug.[33] Likewise, older adults often have trouble sleeping, and the use of sedative-hypnotic agents is common, especially in elderly people living in nursing homes or other facilities.[27,29] Individuals who are involved in rehabilitation programs, both as inpatients and as outpatients, may also have a fairly high anxiety level because of concern about their health and their ability to resume normal function.[44] Acute and chronic illness can create uncertainty about a patient's future family and job obligations, as well as doubts about his or her self-image. The tension and anxiety produced may necessitate pharmacologic management.

The administration of sedative-hypnotic and antianxiety drugs has several direct implications for the rehabilitation session. Obviously, the patient will be much calmer and more relaxed after taking an antianxiety drug, thus offering the potential benefit of gaining the patient's full cooperation during a physical therapy or occupational therapy treatment. Anxiolytic benzodiazepines, for example, reach peak blood levels 2 to 4 hours after oral administration, so scheduling the rehabilitation session during that time may improve the patient's participation in the treatment. Of course, this rationale will back-fire completely if the drug produces significant hypnotic effects. Therapy sessions that require the patient to actively participate in activities such as gait training or therapeutic exercise will be essentially useless and even hazardous if the patient is extremely drowsy. Consequently, scheduling patients for certain types of rehabilitation within several hours after administration of sedative-hypnotics or sedative-like anxiolytics is counterproductive and should be avoided.

Finally, sedative-hypnotic use is associated with falls and subsequent trauma, including hip fractures, especially in older adults.[21,24,50] The risk of falls is understandably greater in people who have a history of falls or who have other problems that would predispose them to falling (vestibular disorders, impaired vision, and so forth). Therapists can identify such people and intervene to help prevent a fall through balance training, environmental modifications (removing cluttered furniture, throw rugs, and so forth), and similar activities. Therapists can likewise help plan and implement nonpharmacologic interventions to decrease anxiety and improve sleep. Interventions such as regular physical activity, massage, and various relaxation techniques may reduce stress levels and promote normal sleep.[23,42] Therapists can therefore help substitute nonpharmacologic methods for traditional sedative-hypnotic and antianxiety drugs, thus improving the patient's quality of life by avoiding drug-related side effects.

CASE STUDY

SEDATIVE-HYPNOTIC DRUGS

Brief History. R.S. is a 34-year-old construction worker who sustained a fracture-dislocation of the vertebral column in an automobile accident. He was admitted to an acute care facility where a diagnosis was made of complete paraplegia at the T-12 spinal level. Surgery was performed to stabilize the vertebral column. During the next 3 weeks, his medical condition improved. At the end of 1 month, he was transferred to a rehabilitation facility to begin an intensive program of physical and occupational therapy. Rehabilitation included strengthening and range-of-motion (ROM) exercises, as well as training in wheelchair mobility, transfers, and activities of daily living (ADLs). However, upon arriving at the new institution, R.S. complained of difficulty sleeping. Flurazepam (Dalmane) was prescribed at a dosage of 20 mg administered orally each night at bedtime.

Problem/Influence of Medication. During his daily rehabilitation regimen, the therapists noted that R.S.'s performance and level of attentiveness were markedly poor during the morning sessions. He was excessively lethargic and drowsy, and his speech was slurred. These symptoms were present to a much greater extent than the normal slow starting that occurs in some patients on wakening in the morning. The therapists also found that when ADL or mobility training was taught during the morning sessions, there was poor carryover from day to day regarding these activities.

Decision/Solution. The benzodiazepine drug appeared to be producing a hangover effect, which limited the patient's cognitive skills during the early daily activities. Initially this problem was dealt with by reserving the early part of the morning session for stretching and ROM activities, and then gradually moving into upper-body strengthening. Activities that required more patient learning and comprehension were done later in the morning or in the afternoon. Also, this hangover problem was brought to the attention of the physician, and the hypnotic drug was ultimately switched to triazolam (Halcion) because this drug is a short-acting benzodiazepine with a half-life of 2.9 ± 1.0 hours (compared with flurazepam, which has a half-life of 74 ± 24 hours).

SUMMARY

Sedative-hypnotic and antianxiety drugs play a prominent role in today's society. The normal pressures of daily life often result in tension and stress, which affect an individual's ability to relax or cope. These problems are compounded when there is some type of illness or injury present. As would be expected, a number of patients seen in a rehabilitation setting are taking these drugs. The benzodiazepines (flurazepam, triazolam) are currently the drugs of choice in promoting sleep. Although these drugs are generally safer than their forerunners, they are not without their problems. Benzodiazepines are also used frequently to reduce anxiety, but the introduction of newer drugs such as buspirone have provided an effective but somewhat safer alternative for treating anxiety. Because of the potential for physical and psychologic dependence, sedative-hypnotic and antianxiety drugs should not be used indefinitely. These drugs should be prescribed judiciously as an adjunct to helping patients deal with the source of their problems.

REFERENCES

1. American Psychiatric Association: Diagnostic and Statistical Manual of Mental Disorders, ed 4. American Psychiatric Association, Washington, DC, 1994.
2. Apter, JT and Allen, LA: Buspirone: Future directions. J Clin Psychopharmacol 19:86, 1999.
3. Cadieux, RJ: Azapirones: An alternative to benzodiazepines for anxiety. Am Fam Physician 53:2349, 1996.
4. Costa, E: From GABA-A receptor diversity emerges a unified vision of GABAergic inhibition. Annu Rev Pharmacol Toxicol 38:321, 1998.
5. Fraser, AD: Use and abuse of the benzodiazepines. Ther Drug Monit 20:481, 1998.
6. Gammans, RE: Use of buspirone in patients with generalized anxiety disorder and coexisting depressive symptoms. A meta-analysis of eight randomized, controlled studies. Neuropsychobiology 25:193, 1992.
7. Goldstein, DB: The effects of drugs on membrane fluidity. Annu Rev Pharmacol Toxicol 24:43, 1984.
8. Gorenstein, C and Gentil, V: Residual and acute effects of flurazepam and triazolam in normal subjects. Psychopharmacology (Berl) 80:376, 1983.
9. Gossard, D, Dennis, C, and DeBusk, RF: Use of beta-blocking agents to reduce the stress of presentation at an international cardiology meeting: Results of a survey. Am J Cardiol 54:240, 1984.
10. Harrison, M, et al: Diazepam tapering in detoxification for high-dose benzodiazepine abuse. Clin Pharmacol Ther 36:527, 1984.
11. Hevers, W and Luddens, H: The diversity of GABA-A receptors. Pharmacological and electrophysiological properties of GABA-A channel subtypes. Mol Neurobiol 18:35, 1998.
12. Hobbs, WR, Rall, TW, and Verdoorn, TA: Hypnotics and sedatives; ethanol. In Hardman, JG, et al (eds): The Pharmacological Basis of Therapeutics, ed 9. McGraw-Hill, New York, 1996.
13. Hutchinson, MA, Smith, PF, and Darlington, CL: The behavioural and neuronal effects of the chronic administration of benzodiazepine anxiolytic and hypnotic drugs. Prog Neurobiol 49:73, 1996.
14. Jermain, DM: Sleep disorders. In DiPiro, JT, et al (eds): Pharmacotherapy: A Pathophysiologic Approach, ed 4. Appleton & Lange, Stamford, CT, 1999.
15. Kales, A, et al: Rebound insomnia and rebound anxiety: A review. Pharmacology 26:121, 1983.

16. Kandel, ER: Disorders of mood: Depression, mania, and anxiety disorders. In Kandel, ER, Schwartz, JH, and Jessell, TM (eds): Principles of Neural Science, ed 4. McGraw-Hill, New York, 2000.
17. Kirkwood, CK: Anxiety disorders. In DiPiro, JT, et al (eds): Pharmacotherapy: A Pathophysiologic Approach, ed 4. Appleton & Lange, Stamford, CT, 1999.
18. Korpi, ER, et al: GABA(A)-receptor subtypes: Clinical efficacy and selectivity of benzodiazepine site ligands. Ann Med 29:275, 1997.
19. Kunovac, JL and Stahl, SM: Future directions in anxiolytic pharmacotherapy. Psychiatr Clin North Am 18:895, 1995.
20. Landauer, AA and Pocock, DA: Stress reduction by oxoprenolol and placebo: Controlled investigation of the pharmacological and nonspecific effects. BMJ 289:529, 1984.
21. Leipzig, RM, Cumming, RG, and Tinetti, ME: Drugs and falls in older people: A systematic review and meta-analysis: I. Psychotropic drugs. J Am Geriatr Soc 47:30, 1999.
22. McClusky, HY, et al: Efficacy of behavioral versus triazolam treatment in persistent sleep-onset insomnia. Am J Psychiatry 148:121, 1991.
23. McDowell, JA, et al: A nonpharmacologic sleep protocol for hospitalized older patients. J Am Geriatr Soc 46:700, 1998.
24. Mendelson, WB: The use of sedative/hypnotic medication and its correlation with falling down in the hospital. Sleep 19:698, 1996.
25. Merlotti, L, et al: Rebound insomnia: Duration of use and individual differences. J Clin Psychopharmacol 11:368, 1991.
26. Michels, R and Marzuk, PM: Medical progress: Progress in psychiatry. N Engl J Med 329:552 (Part I), 628 (Part 2), 1993.
27. Monane, M, Glynn, RJ, and Avorn, J: The impact of sedative-hypnotic use on sleep symptoms in elderly nursing home residents. Clin Pharmacol Ther 59:83, 1996.
28. Napoliello, MJ and Domantay, AG: Buspirone: A worldwide update. Br J Psychiatry Suppl 12:40, 1991.
29. Neubauer, DN: Sleep problems in the elderly. Am Fam Physician 59:2551, 1999.
30. Nicoll, R: Selective actions of barbiturates on synaptic transmission. In Lipton, MA, DiMascio, A, and Killam, KF (eds): Psychopharmacology: A Generation of Progress. Raven, New York, 1978.
31. Nies, AS: Clinical pharmacology of the beta-adrenergic blockers. Medical Problems of Performing Artists 1:25, 1986.
32. Pecknold, JC: A risk-benefit assessment of buspirone in the treatment of anxiety disorders. Drug Saf 16:118, 1997.
33. Perry, SW and Wu, A: Rationale for the use of hypnotic agents in a general hospital. Ann Intern Med 100:441, 1984.
34. Petracca, A, et al: Treatment of generalized anxiety disorder: Preliminary clinical experience with buspirone. J Clin Psychiatry 51(Suppl):31, 1990.
35. Power, KG, et al: Controlled study of withdrawal symptoms and rebound anxiety after 6 week course of diazepam for generalized anxiety. BMJ 290:1246, 1985.
36. Richards, JG, et al: Benzodiazepine receptors resolved. Experientia 42:121, 1986.
37. Rickels, K, et al: Long-term therapeutic use of benzodiazepines: I. Effects of abrupt discontinuation. Arch Gen Psychiatry 47:899, 1990.
38. Salzman, C: Addiction to benzodiazepines. Psychiatr Q 69:251, 1998.
39. Schweizer, E and Rickels, K: Benzodiazepine dependence and withdrawal: A review of the syndrome and its clinical management. Acta Psychiatr Scand Suppl 393:95, 1998.
40. Shader, RI, et al: Sedative effects and impaired learning and recall after single doses of lorazepam. Clin Pharmacol Ther 39:562, 1986.
41. Shader, RI and Greenblatt, DJ. Drug therapy: Use of benzodiazepines in anxiety disorders. N Engl J Med 328:1398, 1993.
42. Shephard, RJ: Exercise and relaxation in health promotion. Sports Med 23:211, 1997.
43. Steinberg, JR: Anxiety in elderly patients. A comparison of azapirones and benzodiazepines. Drugs Aging 5:335, 1994.
44. Stoudemire, A: Epidemiology and psychopharmacology of anxiety in medical patients. J Clin Psychiatry 57(Suppl 7):64, 1996.
45. Tallman, JF and Gallager, DW: The GABA-ergic system: A locus of benzodiazepine action. Annu Rev Neurosci 8:21, 1985.
46. Taylor, DP: Buspirone, a new approach to the treatment of anxiety. FASEB J 2:2445, 1988.
47. Trevor, AJ and Way, WL: Sedative-hypnotic drugs. In Katzung, BG (ed): Basic and Clinical Pharmacology, ed 7. Appleton & Lange, Stamford, CT, 1998.
48. Walsh, JK, Schweitzer, PK, and Parwatikar, S: Effects of lorazepam and its withdrawal on sleep, performance and subjective state. Clin Pharmacol Ther 34:496, 1983.
49. Woo, E, Proulx, SM, and Greenblatt, DJ: Differential side effect profile of triazolam versus flurazepam in elderly patients undergoing rehabilitation therapy. J Clin Pharmacol 31:168, 1991.
50. Wysowski, DK, et al: Sedative-hypnotic drugs and the risk of hip fracture. J Clin Epidemiol 49:111, 1996.

CHAPTER *7*

Drugs Used to Treat Affective Disorders: Depression and Manic-Depression

Affective disorders comprise the group of mental conditions that includes depression and manic-depression (bipolar disorder).[2] These disorders are characterized by a marked disturbance in a patient's mood. Patients with an affective disorder typically display an inappropriate disposition, which is unreasonably sad and discouraged (depression) or may fluctuate between periods of depression and excessive excitation and elation (manic-depression).

Because these forms of mental illness are relatively common, many rehabilitation specialists will work with patients who are receiving drug therapy for an affective disorder. Also, serious injury or illness may precipitate an episode of depression in the patient undergoing physical rehabilitation. Consequently, this chapter will discuss the pharmacologic management of affective disorders, as well as how antidepressant and antimanic drugs may influence the patient involved in physical therapy and occupational therapy.

DEPRESSION

Clinical Picture

Depression is considered to be the most prevalent form of mental illness in the United States, with approximately 17 percent of adults experiencing major depression at some point in their lives.[29] Likewise, as many as 10 percent of Americans may experience major depression over a 1-year period.[29] In this sense, depression is a form of mental illness characterized by intense feelings of sadness and despair. Of course, a certain amount of disappointment and sadness is part of everyday life. However, a diagnosis of clinical depression indicates that these feelings are increased in both intensity and duration to the extent that they begin to be incapacitating.

Depressive disorders are characterized by a general dysphoric mood (sadness, irritability, "down in the dumps"), as well as by a general lack of interest in previously pleasurable activities. Other symptoms including anorexia, sleep disorders (either too much or too little), fatigue, lack of self-esteem, somatic complaints, and irrational guilt. Recurrent thoughts of death and suicide may also help lead to a diagnosis of depression. To initiate effective treatment, a proper diagnosis must be made; depression must not be confused with other mental disorders that also may influence mood and behavior (e.g., schizophrenia). To standardize the terminology and aid in recognizing depression, specific criteria for the diagnosis of a major depressive episode have been outlined by the American Psychiatric Association.[2] Depressive disorders can also be subclassified according to the type, duration, and intensity of the patient's symptoms.[2,42] For the purpose of this chapter, the term *depression* will be used to indicate major depressive disorder, but readers should be aware that the exact type of depression may vary somewhat from person to person.

The causes of depression seem to be complex and somewhat unclear. Although a recent stressful incident, misfortune, or illness can certainly exacerbate an episode of depression, some patients may become depressed for no apparent reason. The role of genetic factors in depression has been explored but remains uncertain. A great deal of evidence that a CNS neurochemical imbalance may be the underlying feature in depression, as well as in other forms of mental illness, has been accumulated over the past several decades. The importance of these findings as they relate to pharmacologic treatment will be discussed. However, factors responsible for initiating these changes in CNS function are unclear. Depression is undoubtedly caused by the complex interaction of a number of genetic, environmental, and biochemical factors.[27]

Treatment of depression is essential in minimizing the disruptive influence that this disease has on the patient's overall well-being and on his or her relationship to family and job. Depending on the severity and type of depression, procedures ranging from psychotherapy to electroconvulsive treatment have been prescribed. Drug treatment plays a major role in alleviating and preventing the occurrence of major depression, and this form of therapy is presented here.

Pathophysiology of Depression

Over the past several years, a great deal of attention has been focused on the idea that a neuronal or neurotransmitter defect may be responsible for causing depression. The emergence of such ideas was exciting in light of the fact that depression could be treated much more effectively if it were caused by a specific problem in CNS synaptic transmission.

Originally, depression was considered to be caused by a decrease in neural transmission in CNS synapses that use amine neurotransmitters[5,45]; that is, synapses containing norepinephrine, serotonin, and possibly dopamine were thought to be underactive in areas associated with mood and behavior, such as the limbic system. This so-called amine hypothesis was based on the fact that most of the drugs used to treat depression increased synaptic transmission in amine synapses. However, additional research on the effects of these drugs has caused the original amine hypothesis to be modified. Depression may be caused by an increased sensitivity of the postsynaptic receptor for norepinephrine—that is, the beta-adrenoreceptor.[25,53] This modification of the original theory was based primarily on the finding that effective antidepressant drugs all seem to work by decreasing the sensitivity of the CNS postsynaptic beta-adrenoreceptors.

The idea that depression is associated with changes in postsynaptic receptor sensitivity is summarized in Figure 7–1. For reasons that are still unclear, depression may occur because of an increase in postsynaptic receptor sensitivity to amine neurotransmitters, particularly norepinephrine and serotonin (see Fig. 7–1). Antidepressant drugs increase amine transmission by a variety of methods, thus overstimulating the postsynaptic receptor. (The exact method by which these drugs increase amine stimulation is discussed later in this chapter.) Overstimulation of the postsynaptic receptor leads to a compensatory down-regulation and decreased sensitivity of the receptor. As discussed in Chapter 4, this down-regulation is a normal response to overstimulation by either endogenous or exogenous agonists. As receptor sensitivity decreases, the clinical symptoms of depression are resolved.

It must be emphasized that it is difficult to prove the neurochemical changes that underlie depression, and the way that antidepressant drugs help resolve depression remains theoretical at present. Still, certain aspects of drug therapy tend to support the amine hypothesis and the putative changes in receptor sensitivity induced by drug therapy. For instance, there is usually a time lag of approximately 2 to 4 weeks before antidepressant drugs begin to work.[1,38] This latency period would be necessary for a compensatory change in postsynaptic receptor sensitivity to take place after drug therapy is initiated.[28]

Consequently, many antidepressants are believed to exert their effects by bringing about a decrease in sensitivity of the beta-adrenoreceptor at central norepinephrine synapses. The function of other amine neurotransmitters in this response requires some clarification as well. Serotonin (5-hydroxytryptamine) may play a permissive role in beta-receptor down-regulation, meaning that serotonergic activity must also be present

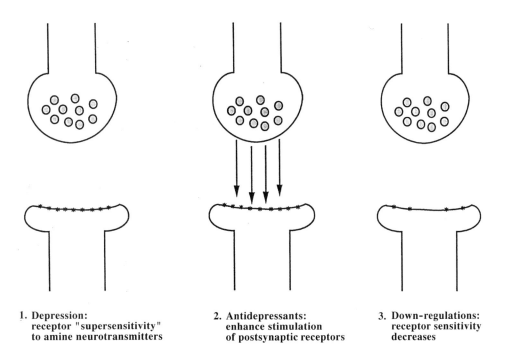

1. **Depression:**
   receptor "supersensitivity"
   to amine neurotransmitters

2. **Antidepressants:**
   enhance stimulation
   of postsynaptic receptors

3. **Down-regulations:**
   receptor sensitivity
   decreases

FIGURE 7–1. Theoretic basis for the mechanism and treatment of depression. Functionally active receptor sites are indicated by an "*." Depression is thought to be initiated by increased postsynaptic receptor sensitivity. Drugs that enhance stimulation of the receptors ultimately lead to receptor down-regulation, thus resolving the depression.

for the decrease in beta-receptor sensitivity to occur.[25,28] However, a defect in serotonin sensitivity may play a more central role in certain types of depression; that is, drugs that selectively influence serotonin activity (the so-called selective serotonin reuptake inhibitors, discussed later in this chapter) may be beneficial in certain types of depression. This fact suggests that selective regulation of serotonin receptors is an important factor in the pathogenesis and subsequent treatment of depression.[18,39] The role of dopamine in the cause and treatment of depression is even more speculative. Dopamine may not be directly involved in either the pathogenesis or the drug treatment of depression, but there is almost certainly some type of interaction between dopamine and the other two depression-related neurotransmitters (norepinephrine, serotonin).[8,28] By affecting dopamine synapses, many antidepressants also produce behavioral or motor side effects associated with antidepressant drug therapy.

Clearly, many factors contribute to the cause of depression, and the neurochemical changes underlying depression involve the complex interaction of several chemicals, including norepinephrine, serotonin, and dopamine. Future research will continue to clarify the exact cellular and subcellular events that occur during depression and how these events can be resolved pharmacologically. It is apparent, however, that current drug therapy is focused on modifying one or more receptor populations at brain synapses that use amine transmitters. These drugs are discussed here.

Antidepressant Drugs

The drugs that are currently used to treat depression are grouped into several categories according to chemical or functional criteria. These categories consist of the tricyclics, monoamine oxidase (MAO) inhibitors, and second-generation drugs (Table 7–1). All three groups attempt to increase aminergic transmission, but by different mechanisms (Fig. 7–2). Sympathomimetic stimulants such as the amphetamine drugs were also used on a limited basis to treat depression, but the powerful CNS excitation produced by amphetamine-like drugs and the potential for addiction and overdose have essentially eliminated their use as antidepressants. The pharmacologic effects of the primary antidepressant drug categories are discussed here.

Tricyclics. Drugs in this category share a common three-ring chemical structure (hence the name "tricyclic"). These drugs work by blocking the reuptake of amine neurotransmitters into the presynaptic terminal.[25,38] The active transport of amine neurotransmitters back into the presynaptic terminal is the method by which most (50 to 80 percent) of the released transmitter is removed from the synaptic cleft. By blocking reuptake, tricyclics allow the released amines to remain in the cleft and continue to exert their effects. The prolonged stimulation of these neurotransmitters (especially norepinephrine) leads to the compensatory decrease in receptor sensitivity, which ultimately leads to a decrease in depression.

In the past, tricyclic drugs were the most commonly used antidepressants, and these agents were the standard against which other antidepressants were measured.[1] Tricyclics are still widely used in various forms of depression, including melancholy depression.[38] Tricyclics, however, are associated with several adverse side effects that may limit their use in some patients (see Table 7–2 and "Problems and Adverse Effects"). The use of tricyclic drugs has therefore diminished somewhat in favor of some of the newer second-generation drugs that may have more favorable side effect profiles. Tricyclic agents, nonetheless, remain an important component in the management of depressive disorders.

TABLE 7–1 Common Antidepressant Drugs

Generic Name	Trade Name	Initial Adult Dose (mg/day)	Prescribing Limits* (mg/day)
Tricyclics			
Amitriptyline	Elavil, Endep, others	50–100	300
Amoxapine	Asendin	100–150	600
Clomipramine	Anafranil	75	300
Desipramine	Pertofrane, Norpramin	100–200	300
Doxepin	Sinequan, others	75	300
Imipramine	Tipramine, Tofranil, Norfranil	75–200	300
Nortriptyline	Aventyl, Pamelor	75–100	150
Protriptyline	Vivactil	15–40	60
Trimipramine	Surmontil	75	300
MAO inhibitors			
Isocarboxazid	Marplan	10–20	60
Phenelzine	Nardil	45	90
Tranylcypromine	Parnate	30	60
Second-generation agents			
Bupropion	Wellbutrin, Zyban	150	400
Citalopram	Celexa	20	60
Fluoxetine	Prozac	20	80
Fluvoxamine	Luvox	50	300
Maprotiline	Ludiomil	25–75	225
Mirtazapine	Remeron	15	45
Nefazodone	Serzone	200	600
Paroxetine	Paxil	20	50
Sertraline	Zoloft	50	200
Trazodone	Desyrel, Trazone, Trialodine	150	600
Venlafaxine	Effexor	75	375

*Upper limits reflect dosages administered to patients with severe depression who are being treated as inpatients.

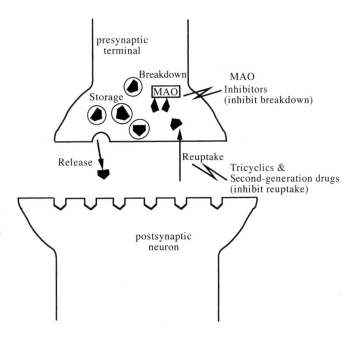

FIGURE 7–2. Effects of antidepressant drugs on amine synapses. All three types of drugs tend to increase the presence of amine transmitters (norepinephrine, dopamine, serotonin) in the synaptic cleft. Increased transmitter stimulation leads to postsynaptic receptor down-regulation and desensitization.

TABLE 7–2 Side Effects of Antidepressant Drugs*

Drug	Sedation	Anticholinergic Effects	Orthostatic Hypotension	Cardiac Arrhythmias	Seizures
Tricyclics					
Amitriptyline	++++	++++	+++	+++	+++
Amoxapine	++	+++	++	++	+++
Clomipramine	++++	++++	++	+++	++++
Desipramine	++	++	++	++	++
Doxepin	++++	+++	++	++	+++
Imipramine	+++	+++	++++	+++	+++
Nortriptyline	++	++	+	++	++
Protriptyline	+	++	++	+++	++
Trimipramine	++++	++++	+++	+++	+++
MAO inhibitors					
Phenelzine	++	+	++	+	+
Tranylcypromine	+	+	++	+	+
Second-generation agents					
Bupropion	0	+	0	+	++++
Citalopram	+	+	0	0	++
Fluoxetine	0	0	0	0	++
Fluvoxamine	0	0	0	0	++
Maprotiline	+++	+++	++	++	++++
Mirtazapine	++	+	++	+	+
Nefazodone	+++	0	+++	+	++
Paroxetine	+	+	0	0	++
Sertraline	0	0	0	0	++
Trazodone	++++	0	+++	+	++
Venlafaxine	+	+	0	+	++

*Zero denotes no side effect, + a very low incidence, ++ a low incidence, +++ a moderate incidence, and ++++ a high incidence.
Source: Adapted from Kando et al,[28] p 1148, with permission.

Monoamine Oxidase Inhibitors. Monoamine oxidase (MAO) is an enzyme that is located at amine synapses and helps remove the released transmitters through enzymatic destruction. Drugs that inhibit this enzyme allow more of the transmitter to remain in the synaptic cleft and continue to exert an effect.[54] As with the tricyclics, MAO inhibitors directly increase activity at amine synapses, which brings about a subsequent receptor down-regulation. MAO inhibitors are not usually the drugs of choice in depression, but these drugs may be helpful if patients do not respond to other agents (tricyclics, second-generation drugs) or if other antidepressants produce intolerable side effects.

The MAO enzyme exists in two primary forms or subtypes: MAO type A and MAO type B.[28] These two subtypes are differentiated according to their ability to degrade specific amines and according to the ability of various drugs to inhibit one or both subtypes of the MAO enzyme. Preliminary evidence suggests that selective inhibition of MAO type A may be desirable in treating depression,[28] whereas inhibition of MAO type B may be more important in prolonging the effects of dopamine in Parkinson disease (see Chapter 10). Regardless, the MAO inhibitors currently used as antidepressants are relatively nonselective, meaning that they inhibit MAO A and MAO B fairly equally. Development of new MAO inhibitors may produce agents that are more selective for the MAO A subtype and may therefore produce better antidepressant effects with fewer side effects.[28]

Second-Generation Antidepressants. Because of the limitations of first-generation drugs such as the tricyclics and MAO inhibitors, a number of diverse compounds have been developed and continue to be evaluated for their antidepressant effects. When compared with first-generation drugs, the goal of these newer drugs is threefold: (1) to have a more rapid onset in decreasing depression, (2) to have more tolerable side effects, and (3) to be safer—that is, to involve less chance of lethal overdose. In general, the second-generation drugs have been only partially successful in meeting these goals. None of the newer antidepressants appears to have a more rapid onset than their predecessors.[53] There is some evidence that certain second-generation drugs may be more effective in treating certain depressive symptoms, but the newer agents have not been proven to be categorically safer or more effective than their predecessors.[38] Some of the newer agents, however, have a lower incidence of certain side effects, such as cardiovascular problems and sedation (see Table 7–2). Hence, these newer drugs may be tolerated much better and may provide better long-term management of depression because of improved patient satisfaction and compliance with drug therapy.

The newer antidepressants are chemically diverse, but most work by mechanisms similar to tricyclic drugs; that is, they block reuptake of norepinephrine and other monoamines. Hence, these drugs appear to exert their beneficial effects by bringing about the decrease in receptor sensitivity that seems to be the common denominator of antidepressant drugs' action. The second-generation drugs and their proposed mechanisms of action are summarized in Table 7–3. In addition, certain second-generation drugs are distinguished by their ability to selectively influence specific monoamines rather than all the amine transmitters simultaneously. Subcategories of these selective drugs are discussed here.

Selective Serotonin Reuptake Inhibitors. Certain second-generation drugs have received attention because of their ability to selectively block the reuptake of 5-hydroxytryptamine (serotonin). Fluoxetine (Prozac) and similar agents (sertraline, paroxetine, fluvoxamine; see Table 7–3) are therefore grouped together functionally as selective serotonin reuptake inhibitors (SSRIs).[13,22] This action distinguishes them from the tricyclics, MAO inhibitors, and other second-generation drugs because these other drugs tend to be nonselective in their effect on amine neurotransmitters and block the reuptake of norepinephrine and dopamine as well as serotonin. The primary advantage of the SSRIs is that they produce fewer and less bothersome side effects than their nonselective counterparts (see Table 7–3). This improved side effect profile can be very helpful in the long-term management of depression because patients may tolerate these drugs better and be more willing to take these drugs on a regular basis.[23,48] SSRIs have therefore become the antidepressant drugs of choice for many patients, especially if side effects may limit compliance to drug therapy.[33,36]

Other Selective Drugs. Drugs that are relatively selective for other types of monoamines are also being considered as possible antidepressants. Reboxetine, for example, is a new agent that selectively inhibits transmitter reuptake at norepinephrine synapses.[11,44] There is likewise an emerging group of drugs such as venlafaxine that selectively decreases serotonin and norepinephrine reuptake without an appreciable effect on dopamine synapses.[24,43] These drugs are known as serotonin/norepinephrine reuptake inhibitors (SNRIs), and they may be effective in certain types of depression, including patients who are severely depressed.[43] The development of the SNRIs and various other selective drugs including SSRIs has opened new opportunities for the optimal management of depression. Future studies will undoubtedly shed light on how these more selective agents can be best used to treat specific depressive symptoms and types of depression.

TABLE 7–3 Second-Generation Antidepressant Drugs

Generic Name (Trade Name)	Mechanism (Amine Selectivity)	Advantages	Disadvantages
Selective serotonin reuptake inhibitors			
Citalopram (Celexa)	Strong, selective inhibition of serotonin reuptake	Low incidence of sedation and anticholinergic effects; does not cause orthostatic hypotension or cardiac arrhythmias	May cause sexual dysfunction (decreased libido, impotence)
Fluoxetine (Prozac)	Moderate, selective inhibition of serotonin reuptake	No sedative, anticholinergic, or cardiovascular side effects; helpful in obsessive-compulsive disorders	May cause anxiety, nausea, insomnia; long half-life can lead to accumulation
Fluvoxamine (Luvox)	Strong, selective inhibition of serotonin reuptake	Similar to fluoxetine	Similar to fluoxetine
Paroxetine (Paxil)	Strong, selective inhibition of serotonin reuptake	Similar to citalopram	Similar to citalopram
Sertraline (Zoloft)	Strong, selective inhibition of serotonin reuptake	Similar to fluoxetine	Similar to fluoxetine
Other second-generation agents			
Bupropion (Wellbutrin, Zyban)	Primarily inhibits dopamine reuptake; little effect on norepinephrine or serotonin	Low sedative, anticholinergic, and cardiovascular side effects	May cause overstimulation (insomnia, tremor) and induce psychotic symptoms
Maprotiline (Ludiomil)	Moderate inhibition of norepinephrine reuptake	Sedating: useful in agitation	Possibility of seizures; overdoses lethal; long half-life
Mirtazapine (Remeron)	Exact mechanism unclear; may increase norepinephrine and serotonin activity by blocking inhibitory presynaptic autoreceptors	Low incidence of sedative, anti-cholinergic, and cardiovascular side effects	May cause agitation, anxiety, other mood changes
Nefazodone (Serzone)	Slight inhibition of serotonin and norepinephrine reuptake; may also block CNS serotonin receptors	Sedating: useful in agitation	May cause orthostatic hypotension because of antagonistic effect on vascular alpha-1 receptors
Trazodone (Desyrel, others)	Slight inhibition of serotonin reuptake	Sedating: useful in agitation; lower relative risk of overdose	May cause orthostatic hypotension (similar to nefazodone); although rare, serious problems related to priapism may also occur in men
Venlafaxine (Effexor)	Strong inhibition of norepinephrine and serotonin reuptake	Low risk of ortho-static hypotension, sedation, and anti-cholinergic side effects	May cause hypertension

PHARMACOKINETICS

Antidepressants are usually administered orally. Dosages vary, depending not only on each drug but also on the individual patient. Initial doses generally start out relatively low and are increased slowly within the therapeutic range until beneficial effects are observed. Distribution within the body also varies with each type of antidepressant, but all eventually reach the brain to exert their effects. Metabolism takes place primarily in the liver, and metabolites of several drugs continue to show significant antidepressant activity. This fact may be responsible for prolonging the effects of the drug even after it has undergone hepatic biotransformation. Elimination takes place by biotransformation and renal excretion.

PROBLEMS AND ADVERSE EFFECTS

Tricyclics. A major problem with the tricyclic antidepressants is sedation (Table 7–2). Although a certain degree of sedation may be desirable in some agitated depressed patients, feelings of lethargy and sluggishness may impair patient adherence to drug therapy and result in a failure to take medication. A second major problem is that these drugs tend to have significant anticholinergic properties; that is, they act as if they are blocking certain central and peripheral acetylcholine receptors (see Table 7–2). Impairment of central acetylcholine transmission may cause confusion and del irium. The peripheral anticholinergic properties produce a variety of symptoms, including dry mouth, constipation, urinary retention, and tachycardia. Other cardiovascular problems include arrhythmias and orthostatic hypotension, with the latter particularly common in elderly patients. Because these drugs increase neurotransmitter activity in the brain, seizures may occur, especially in people with seizure disorders. Finally, tricyclics have the highest potential for fatal overdose from an antidepressant.[46] This fact leads to a serious problem, given the risk of suicide among depressed patients. These drugs should be dispensed in small quantities (i.e., giving the patient only a few days' worth of the drug) to diminish the risk of a fatal overdose.

MAO Inhibitors. In contrast to the tricyclics, MAO inhibitors tend to produce CNS excitation, which can result in restlessness, irritability, agitation, and sleep loss. These drugs also produce some central and peripheral anticholinergic effects (e.g., tremor, confusion, dry mouth, urinary retention), but these tend to occur to a lesser extent than with the tricyclics. Because of the systemic MAO inhibition, excess activity at peripheral sympathetic adrenergic terminals may cause a profound increase in blood pressure, leading to a hypertensive crisis. This situation is exacerbated if other drugs that increase sympathetic nervous activity are taken concurrently. Also, there is a distinct interaction between the MAO inhibitors and certain foods such as fermented cheese and wines.[54] These fermented foods contain tyramine, which stimulates the release of endogenous epinephrine and norepinephrine. The additive effect of increased catecholamine release (because of the ingested tyramine) and decreased catecholamine breakdown (because of MAO inhibition) can lead to excessive catecholamine levels and a hypertensive crisis.[54]

Another potential problem is the development of serotonin syndrome, which typically occurs when MAO inhibitors are administered concurrently with SSRIs or other drugs that increase serotonin activity.[4] Simultaneous use of two or more drugs that prolong the effects of serotonin can lead to excessive levels of this transmitter in the brain and other tissues, hence the term "serotonin syndrome." This syndrome is characterized by symptoms such as confusion, agitation, fever, sweating, shivering, tremor, ataxia, and diarrhea.[4] In severe cases, these symptoms can worsen and lead to seizures, coma, arrhythmias, renal failure, and death. Early recognition of serotonin syndrome is important so that the serotonin-potentiating drugs can be discontinued before this syndrome progresses to the more serious and potentially fatal stages.[4]

Second-Generation Drugs. The type and severity of side effects associated with the newer antidepressants vary according to the specific drug in use. SSRIs, for example, generally produce less sedation and fewer anticholinergic and cardiovascular effects than the tricyclics, MAO inhibitors, and other second-generation drugs. The SSRIs, however, are not devoid of side effects, and these agents often produce more gastrointestinal problems and insomnia than other antidepressants. SSRI agents may also produce movement disorders such as severe restlessness (akathisia), tardive dyskinesia, pseudoparkinsonism, and various dystonias and dyskinesias.[20,30]

Advantages and disadvantages of common second-generation drugs are listed in Table 7–3, and comparison of these drugs with the tricyclics and MAO inhibitors is summarized in Table 7–2. Various factors including potential side effects are considered in selecting one of these drugs, and selection of the best drug must be done on a patient-by-patient basis.

Use of Antidepressants in Chronic Pain

Many chronic pain syndromes (neuropathic pain, fibromyalgia, low back pain, and so forth) can be treated more effectively if antidepressants are included in the treatment regimen.[10,21,35] In particular, certain tricylic agents such as amitriptyline, nortriptyline, doxepin, and desipramine may help provide better pain relief when used along with traditional analgesic medications or, in some cases, when these tricyclic drugs are used alone.[37,55] Some studies attribute this effect to the fact that clinical depression is present in many patients with chronic pain; administering antidepressants will help provide optimal care by resolving the depressive symptoms.[41,51] There is considerable evidence, however, that antidepressants will help patients with chronic pain even if no symptoms of depression are present; that is, improvements in pain have been noted even when there has been no observed effect on the patient's mood. As indicated earlier, these drugs have the ability to modulate the influence of serotonin and other CNS monoamine neurotransmitters, and their effects on chronic pain may be related to the influence on monoamine transmission in critical pain pathways in the brain.[21] Many practitioners also feel that antidepressants may help resolve chronic pain by improving the patient's sleep patterns, but improvements in pain have been noted in patients even when no effect on sleep was seen.[34]

Hence, there is little doubt that antidepressants may be useful as an adjunct in the treatment of patients with chronic pain. However, the exact way that these drugs help diminish pain in these patients remains speculative.[10]

TREATMENT OF MANIC-DEPRESSION: ANTIMANIC DRUGS

Bipolar Syndrome

The form of depression discussed previously is often referred to as *unipolar depression*, in contrast to bipolar or "manic-depressive" syndrome. As these terms imply, **bipo-**

lar syndrome is associated with mood swings from one extreme (mania) to the other (depression). Manic episodes are characterized by euphoria, hyperactivity, and talkativeness, and depressive episodes are similar to those described previously. Approximately 10 percent of all depressed patients are considered to exhibit bipolar syndrome.[29]

As in unipolar depression, the exact causes of manic-depression are unknown. One theory is that genetic and environmental factors conspire to increase norepinephrine and possibly serotonin influence in the brain.[4,16] This increase in neurotransmitter activity appears to be responsible for the manic episodes of this disorder. The subsequent depression may simply be a rebound from the general excitement of the manic episode. The exact cause of manic-depression is not clear, however, and the manic episode of this condition may also be caused by neuroendocrine factors, an imbalance in cations such as sodium and calcium, or changes in the cellular and subcellular responses in specific brain neurons.[16] In any event, the treatment of bipolar syndrome focuses on preventing the start of these pendulum-like mood swings by preventing the manic episodes. Hence, drugs used to treat manic-depression are really "antimanic drugs." The primary form of drug treatment consists of lithium salts (i.e., lithium carbonate, lithium citrate). In addition, lithium is a useful adjunct to other antidepressant drugs in treating resistant cases of unipolar depression.[40]

Lithium

Lithium (Li^+) is a monovalent cation in the alkali metal group. Because of its small size (molecular weight 7) and single positive charge, lithium may influence neural excitability by competing with other cations, including sodium, potassium, and calcium.[4] The exact way that lithium helps stabilize mood, however, is not known.[31] Several theories have been proposed, and lithium has been shown to produce several neurochemical effects that could contribute to its antimanic properties. In particular, lithium may stabilize neuronal excitability by decreasing the sensitivity of certain postsynaptic receptors and by uncoupling these receptors from their subcellular second-messenger systems.[16] For example, studies have shown that lithium can diminish the function of cyclic adenosine monophosphate and other second-messenger systems that are normally stimulated by norepinephrine.[7,14] Lithium has also been shown to inhibit certain intracellular enzymes such protein kinase C and inositol monophosphatase, and this inhibition may help account for decreased neuronal excitation and desensitization.[31] Lithium has also been shown to directly decrease the release of certain amine neurotransmitters (norepinephrine and dopamine) and to increase the effects of other transmitters (serotonin, acetylcholine, and GABA).[16,49] Obviously, lithium has the potential to influence synaptic function and neural excitability in many ways. Exactly how this drug is able to stabilize mood and prevent the manic episode associated with bipolar syndrome remains to be determined.[4]

ABSORPTION AND DISTRIBUTION

Lithium is absorbed readily from the gastrointestinal tract and distributed completely throughout all the tissues in the body. During an acute manic episode, achieving blood serum concentrations between 1.0 and 1.4 mEq/L is desirable. Maintenance doses that are somewhat lower and serum concentrations that range from 0.5 to 1.3 mEq/L are optimal.

PROBLEMS AND ADVERSE EFFECTS OF LITHIUM

A major problem with lithium use is the danger of accumulation within the body.[3,9,16] Lithium is not metabolized, and drug elimination takes place almost exclusively through excretion in the urine. Consequently, lithium has a tendency to accumulate in the body, and toxic levels can frequently be reached during administration of this drug.

Side effects occur frequently with lithium, and the degree and type of side effects depend on the amount of lithium in the bloodstream. As Table 7–4 indicates, some side effects are present even when serum levels are within the therapeutic range.[15] However, toxic side effects become apparent when serum concentrations approach or exceed 2.5 mEq/L, and progressive accumulation of lithium can be fatal. Consequently, individuals dealing with a patient receiving lithium therapy should be aware of any changes in behavior that might indicate that this drug is reaching toxic levels. These changes can usually be resolved by adjusting the dosage or using a sustained-release form of lithium.[9] Also, serum titers of lithium should be monitored periodically to ensure that blood levels remain within the therapeutic range.[3,26]

Other Drugs Used in Manic-Depression

Although lithium remains the cornerstone of treatment for bipolar disorders, it is now recognized that other agents may be helpful, especially in the acute stages of the manic episode. In particular, antiseizure medications such as carbamazepine, valproic acid, gabapentin, and lamotrigine may help stabilize mood and limit the manic symptoms.[19,32,56] Antipsychotic medications including the newer agents such as clozapine and risperidone (see Chapter 8) may also be helpful as antimanic drugs.[32,50] Antiseizure and antipsychotic drugs are believed to be helpful because they act directly on CNS neurons to help prevent the neuronal excitation that seems to precipitate the manic symptoms. (Details about the pharmacology of antipsychotic and antiseizure drugs are addressed in Chapters 8 and 9, respectively.) Hence, these drugs can be used initially along with lithium to prevent or decrease the manic mood swing. These additional drugs are usually tapered off and discontinued, however, when mood is stabilized, and lithium treatment is often continued

TABLE 7–4 Side Effects and Toxicity of Lithium

Mild (Below 1.5 mEq/L)	Moderate (1.5–2.5 mEq/L)	Toxicity (2.5–7.0 mEq/L)
Metallic taste in mouth	Severe diarrhea	Nystagmus
Fine hand tremor (resting)	Nausea and vomiting	Coarse tremor
Nausea	Mild-to-moderate ataxia	Dysarthria
Polyuria	Incoordination	Fasciculations
Polydipsia	Dizziness, sluggishness, giddiness, vertigo	Visual or tactile hallucinations
Diarrhea or loose stools	Slurred speech	Oliguria, anuria
Muscular weakness or fatigue	Tinnitus	Confusion
	Blurred vision	Impaired consciousness
	Increasing tremor	Dyskinesia, chorea-athetoid movements
	Muscle irritability or twitching	Tonic-clonic convulsions
	Asymmetric deep tendon reflexes	Coma
	Increased muscle tone	Death

Source: Adapted from Harris, E: Lithium. Amer J Nurs 81(7):1312, 1981.

indefinitely to prevent relapses.[6,47,52] If lithium alone is not successful in preventing relapse, one of the alternative agents such as valproic acid or carbamazepine may be used along with or instead of lithium. Future research should help clarify how various types of drugs can be used most effectively to manage bipolar disorder, especially in people who are resistant to traditional treatment using lithium.

SPECIAL CONCERNS IN REHABILITATION PATIENTS

Some amount of depression is certain to be present as a result of a catastrophic injury or illness. Patients receiving physical therapy and occupational therapy for any number of acute or chronic illnesses may be taking antidepressant medications in order to improve their mood and general well-being. Of course, therapists working in a psychiatric facility will deal with many patients taking antidepressant drugs, and severe depression may be the primary reason the patient is institutionalized in the first place. However, these drugs are also frequently prescribed to patients suffering from spinal cord injury, stroke, severe burn, multiple sclerosis, amputation, and so on. Therapists must realize, however, that adequate treatment of depression is a very difficult clinical task. It is estimated that upwards of a third of the people with depression may not respond adequately, even with optimal pharmacologic and psychologic interventions.[17] Depression is a very serious and complex psychologic disorder, and the effects of drug treatment vary greatly from individual to individual. It is therefore imperative that the physician and other health-care professionals work closely with the patient and the patient's family to find the drug that produces optimal results with a minimum of side effects in each patient. Again, this task is complicated by many issues, including the complex interplay of the factors that cause depression in each patient and the rather unpredictable response of each patient to each type of antidepressant medication.

With regard to the impact of antidepressant and antimanic agents on the rehabilitation process, these drugs can be extremely beneficial in helping to improve the patient's outlook. The patient may become more optimistic regarding his or her future and may assume a more active role and interest in the rehabilitation process. This behavior can be invaluable in increasing patient cooperation and improving compliance with rehabilitation goals. However, certain side effects can be somewhat troublesome during physical therapy treatments. Sedation, lethargy, and muscle weakness can occur with the tricyclics and lithium, which can present a problem if the patient's active cooperation is required. Other unpleasant side effects such as nausea and vomiting can also be disturbing during treatment. A more common and potentially more serious problem is the orthostatic hypotension that occurs predominantly with the tricyclics. This hypotension can cause syncope and subsequent injury if patients fall during gait training. Blood pressure should also be monitored regularly, especially in patients taking MAO inhibitors. Care should be taken to avoid a hypertensive crisis, especially during therapy sessions that tend to increase blood pressure (e.g., certain forms of exercise).

Finally, rehabilitation specialists should remember that antidepressant treatment must often be administered for 1 month or more before an improvement in symptoms occurs.[1,38] During this period, drug therapy may actually precipitate an increase in depression, including increased thoughts of suicide in some patients.[12] Rehabilitation specialists should be alert for any signs that a patient is becoming more depressed and possibly suicidal, especially during the first few weeks after antidepressant drug therapy is initiated.

CASE STUDY

ANTIDEPRESSANT DRUGS

Brief History. J.G., a 71-year-old retired pharmacist, was admitted to the hospital with a chief complaint of an inability to move his right arm and leg. He was also unable to speak at the time of admission. The clinical impression was right hemiplegia caused by left middle cerebral artery thrombosis. The patient also had a history of hypertension and had been taking cardiac beta blockers for several years. J.G.'s medical condition stabilized, and the third day after admission he was seen for the first time by a physical therapist. Speech and occupational therapies were also soon initiated. The patient's condition improved rapidly, and motor function began to return in the right side. Balance and gross motor skills increased until he could transfer from his wheelchair to his bed with minimal assistance, and gait training activities were initiated. J.G. was able to comprehend verbal commands, but his speech remained markedly slurred and difficult to understand. During his first 2 weeks in the hospital, J.G. had shown signs of severe depression. Symptoms increased until cooperation with the rehabilitation and nursing staffs was compromised. Imipramine (Tofranil) was prescribed at a dosage of 150 mg/day.

Problem/Influence of Medication. Imipramine is a tricyclic antidepressant, and these drugs are known to produce orthostatic hypotension during the initial stages of drug therapy. Because the patient is expressively aphasic, he will have trouble telling the therapist that he feels dizzy or faint. Also, the cardiac beta blockers will blunt any compensatory increase in cardiac output if blood pressure drops during postural changes.

Decision/Solution. The therapist decided to place the patient on the tilt table for the first day after imipramine was started and to monitor blood pressure regularly. While the patient was on the tilt table, weight shifting and upper extremity facilitation activities were performed. The patient tolerated this well, so the therapist had him resume ambulation activities using the parallel bars on the following day. With the patient standing inside the bars, the therapist carefully watched for any subjective signs of dizziness or syncope in the patient (i.e., facial pallor, inability to follow instructions). Standing bouts were also limited in duration. By the third day, ambulation training continued with the patient outside the parallel bars, but the therapist made a point of having the patient's wheelchair close at hand in case the patient began to appear faint. These precautions of careful observation and short, controlled bouts of ambulation were continued throughout the remainder of the patient's hospital stay, and no incident of orthostatic hypotension was observed during physical therapy.

SUMMARY

Affective disorders such as depression and manic-depression are found frequently in the general population as well as in rehabilitation patients. Drugs commonly prescribed in the treatment of (unipolar) depression include the tricyclics and MAO inhibitors, as well as the newer second-generation antidepressants. Lithium is the drug of choice for treating bipolar syndrome, or manic-depression. All of these drugs seem to exert their effects by modifying CNS synaptic transmission and receptor sensitivity in amine pathways. The exact manner in which these drugs affect synaptic activity has shed some light on the possible neuronal changes that may underlie these forms of mental illness. Antidepressant and antimanic drugs can improve the patient's attitude and compliance during rehabilitation, but therapists should be aware that certain side effects may alter the patient's physical and mental behavior.

REFERENCES

1. Adams, J: Drug treatment of depression. N Z Med J 106:208, 1993.
2. American Psychiatric Association: Diagnostic and Statistical Manual of Mental Disorders, ed 4. American Psychiatric Association, Washington, DC, 1994.
3. Aronson, JK and Reynolds, DJM: ABC of monitoring drug therapy—lithium. BMJ 305:1273, 1992.
4. Baldessarini, RJ: Drugs and the treatment of psychiatric disorders: Depression and mania. In Hardman, JG, et al (eds): The Pharmacological Basis of Therapeutics, ed 9. McGraw-Hill, New York, 1996.
5. Baldessarini, RJ: The basis for amine hypothesis in affective disorders. Arch Gen Psychiatry 32:1087, 1975.
6. Baldessarini, RJ, Tondo, L, and Hennen, J: Effects of lithium treatment and its discontinuation on suicidal behavior in bipolar manic-depressive disorders. J Clin Psychiatry 60(Suppl 2):77, 1999.
7. Belmaker, RH: Receptors, adenylate cyclase, depression and lithium. Biol Psychiatry 16:333, 1981.
8. Bonhomme, N and Esposito, E: Involvement of serotonin and dopamine in the mechanism of action of novel antidepressant drugs: A review. J Clin Psychopharmacol 18:447, 1998.
9. Bowden, CL: Key treatment studies of lithium in manic-depressive illness: Efficacy and side effects. J Clin Psychiatry 59(Suppl 6):13, 1998.
10. Bryson, HM and Wilde, MI: Amitriptyline. A review of its pharmacological properties and therapeutic use in chronic pain states. Drugs Aging 8:459, 1996.
11. Burrows, GD, Maguire, KP, and Norman, TR: Antidepressant efficacy and tolerability of the selective norepinephrine reuptake inhibitor reboxetine: A review. J Clin Psychiatry 59(Suppl 14):4, 1998.
12. Damluji, NF and Ferguson, JM: Paradoxical worsening of depressive symptomatology caused by antidepressants. J Clin Psychopharmacol 8:347, 1988.
13. DeVane, CL: Differential pharmacology of newer antidepressants. J Clin Psychiatry 59(Suppl 20):85, 1998.
14. Ebstein, RP, Hermoni, M, and Belmaker, RH: The effect of lithium on noradrenaline-induced cyclic AMP accumulation in the rat: Inhibition after chronic treatment and absence of supersensitivity. J Pharmacol Exp Ther 213:161, 1980.
15. Emilien, G and Maloteaux, JM: Lithium neurotoxicity at low therapeutic doses. Hypotheses for causes and mechanism of action following a retrospective analysis of published case reports. Acta Neurol Belg 96:281, 1996.
16. Fankhauser, MP and Benefield, WH: Bipolar disorder. In DiPiro, JT, et al (eds): Pharmacotherapy: A Pathophysiologic Approach, ed 4. Appleton & Lange, Stamford, CT, 1999.
17. Fawcett, J and Barkin, RL: Efficacy issues with antidepressants. J Clin Psychiatry 58(Suppl 6):32, 1997.
18. Feighner, JP: Mechanism of action of antidepressant medications. J Clin Psychiatry 60(Suppl 4):4, 1999.
19. Ferrier, IN: Lamotrigine and gabapentin. Alternative in the treatment of bipolar disorder. Neuropsychobiology 38:192, 1998.
20. Gerber, PE and Lynd, LD: Selective serotonin-reuptake inhibitor-induced movement disorders. Ann Pharmacother 32:692, 1998.
21. Godfrey, RG: A guide to the understanding and use of tricyclic antidepressants in the overall management of fibromyalgia and other chronic pain syndromes. Arch Intern Med 156:1047, 1996.
22. Goodnick, PJ and Goldstein, BJ: Selective serotonin reuptake inhibitors in affective disorders: I. Basic pharmacology. J Psychopharmacol 12(3 Suppl B):S5, 1998.
23. Goodnick, PJ and Goldstein, BJ: Selective serotonin reuptake inhibitors in affective disorders: II. Efficacy and quality of life. J Psychopharmacol 12(3 Suppl B):S21, 1998.
24. Gorman, JM and Kent, JM: SSRIs and SNRIs: Broad spectrum of efficacy beyond major depression. J Clin Psychiatry 60(Supp l4):33, 1999.
25. Hollister, LE: Current antidepressants. Annu Rev Pharmacol Toxicol 26:23, 1986.
26. Johnson, G: Lithium: Early development, toxicity, and renal function. Neuropsychopharmacology 19:200, 1998.
27. Kandel, ER: Disorders of mood: Depression, mania, and anxiety disorders. In Kandel, ER, et al (eds): Principles of Neural Science, ed 4. McGraw-Hill, New York, 2000.
28. Kando, JC, Wells, BG, and Hayes, PE: Depressive disorders. In DiPiro, JT, et al (eds): Pharmacotherapy: A Pathophysiologic Approach, ed 4. Appleton & Lange, Stamford, CT, 1999.
29. Kessler, RC, et al: Lifetime and 12-month prevalence of DSM-III-R psychiatric disorders in the United States. Results from the national comorbidity survey. Arch Gen Psychiatry 51:8, 1994.

30. Lane, RM: SSRI-induced extrapyramidal side-effects and akathisia: Implications for treatment. J Psychopharmacol 12:192, 1998.
31. Lenox, RH, et al: Neurobiology of lithium: An update. J Clin Psychiatry 59(Suppl 6):37, 1998.
32. Licht, RW: Drug treatment of mania: A critical review. Acta Psychiatr Scand 97:387, 1998.
33. Majeroni, BA and Hess, A: The pharmacologic treatment of depression. J Am Board Fam Pract 11:127, 1998.
34. McQuay, HJ, Carroll, D, and Glynn, CJ: Low dose amitriptyline in the treatment of chronic pain. Anaesthesia 47:646, 1992.
35. McQuay, HJ, et al: A systematic review of antidepressants in neuropathic pain. Pain 68:217, 1996.
36. Mourilhe, P and Stokes, PE: Risks and benefits of selective serotonin reuptake inhibitors in the treatment of depression. Drug Saf 18:57, 1998.
37. Pettengill, CA and Reisner-Keller, L: The use of tricyclic antidepressants for the control of chronic orofacial pain. Cranio 15:53, 1997.
38. Potter, WZ, Rudorfer, MV, and Manji, H: Drug therapy: The pharmacologic treatment of depression. N Engl J Med 325:633, 1991.
39. Roth, BL, et al: Serotonin 5-HT2A receptors: Molecular biology and mechanisms of regulation. Crit Rev Neurobiol 12:319, 1998.
40. Rouillon, F and Gorwood, P: The use of lithium to augment antidepressant medication. J Clin Psychiatry 59(Suppl 5):32, 1998.
41. Ruoff, GE: Depression in the patient with chronic pain. J Fam Pract 43(Suppl):S25, 1996.
42. Rush, AJ and Thase, ME: Strategies and tactics in the treatment of chronic depression. J Clin Psychiatry 58(Suppl 13):14, 1997.
43. Schatzberg, AF: Antidepressant effectiveness in severe depression and melancholia. J Clin Psychiatry 60(Suppl 4):14, 1999.
44. Schatzberg, AF: Noradrenergic versus serotonergic antidepressants: Predictors of treatment response. J Clin Psychiatry 59(Suppl 14):15, 1998.
45. Schildkraut, JJ: Current status of the catecholamine hypothesis of affective disorders. In Lipton, MA, DiMascio, A, and Killam, KF (eds): Psychopharmacology: A Generation of Progress. Raven, New York, 1978.
46. Settle, EC: Antidepressant drugs: Disturbing and potentially dangerous adverse effects. J Clin Psychiatry 59(Suppl 16):25, 1998.
47. Sharma, V, et al: Continuation and prophylactic treatment of bipolar disorder. Can J Psychiatry 42(Suppl 2): 92S, 1997.
48. Shasha, M, et al: Serotonin reuptake inhibitors and the adequacy of antidepressant treatment. Int J Psychiatry Med 27:83, 1997.
49. Sheard, MH: The biological effects of lithium. Trends Neurosci 3:85, 1986.
50. Shelton, RC: Mood-stabilizing drugs in depression. J Clin Psychiatry 60(Suppl 5):37, 1999.
51. Sullivan, MJL, et al: The treatment of depression in chronic low back pain: Review and recommendations. Pain 50:5, 1992.
52. Tondo, L, et al: Lithium maintenance treatment of depression and mania in bipolar I and bipolar II disorders. Am J Psychiatry 155:638, 1998.
53. Tyrer, P and Marsden, C: New antidepressant drugs: Is there anything new they tell us about depression? Trends Neurosci 8:427, 1985.
54. Volz, HP and Gleiter, CH: Monoamine oxidase inhibitors. A perspective on their use in the elderly. Drugs Aging 13:341, 1998.
55. Watson, CP: Antidepressant drugs as adjuvant analgesics. J Pain Symptom Manage 9:392, 1994.
56. Xie, X and Hagan, RM: Cellular and molecular actions of lamotrigine: Possible mechanisms of efficacy in bipolar disorder. Neuropsychobiology 38:119, 1998.

CHAPTER **8**

Antipsychotic Drugs

Psychosis is the term used to describe the more severe forms of mental illness. Psychoses are a group of mental disorders characterized by a marked thought disturbance and an impaired perception of reality. By far the most common form of psychosis is schizophrenia, with an estimated 1.0 percent of the world population afflicted.[8,17] Other psychotic disorders include psychotic depression and severe paranoid disorders. In the past, strong, sedative-like drugs were the primary method of treating patients with psychosis. The goal was to pacify these patients so that they were no longer combative and abusive to themselves and others. Such drugs were commonly referred to as "major tranquilizers" and had the obvious disadvantage of producing so much sedation that the patient's cognitive and motor skills were compromised.

As more was learned about the neurologic changes involved in psychosis, drugs were developed to specifically treat psychosis rather than simply sedate the patient. These antipsychotic drugs, or **neuroleptics** as some clinicians refer to them, represent a major breakthrough in the treatment of schizophrenia and other psychotic disorders.

Physical therapists and occupational therapists frequently encounter patients taking antipsychotic drugs. Therapists employed in a psychiatric facility will routinely treat patients taking these medications. Therapists who practice in nonpsychiatric settings may still encounter these patients for various reasons. For instance, the patient on antipsychotic medication who sustains a fractured hip may be seen at an orthopedic facility. Consequently, knowledge of antipsychotic pharmacology will be useful to all rehabilitation specialists.

Because of the prevalence of schizophrenia, this chapter concentrates on the treatment of this psychotic disorder. Also, the pathogenesis and subsequent treatment of other forms of psychosis are similar to those of schizophrenia, and this specific condition will be used as an example of the broader range of psychotic conditions.

SCHIZOPHRENIA

The *Diagnostic and Statistical Manual of Mental Disorders* lists several distinct criteria necessary for a diagnosis of schizophrenia.[2] These criteria include a marked disturbance in the thought process, which may include bizarre delusions and auditory hallucinations (i.e., "hearing voices"). Also, a decreased level of function in work, social relations, and self-care may be present. The duration of these and other symptoms (at least 6 months) and a differential diagnosis from other forms of mental illness (such as affective disorders and organic brain syndrome) help round out these criteria.

The exact cause of schizophrenia is unknown. Extensive research has suggested that both genetic and environmental factors are important in bringing about changes in CNS dopamine pathways, but the precise role of these factors remains to be determined.[6,8]

The advent of antipsychotic drugs represents one of the most significant developments in the treatment of schizophrenia and similar disorders. These drugs are believed to be the single most important reason for the abrupt decrease in the number of mental patients admitted to public hospitals during the 1950s and 1960s.[13,18] This observation does not imply that these drugs cure schizophrenia. Schizophrenia and other psychoses are thought to be incurable, and psychotic episodes can recur throughout the lifetime of the patient. However, these drugs can normalize the patient's behavior and thinking during an acute psychotic episode, and maintenance doses are considered to help prevent the recurrence of psychosis. Consequently, these patients' ability to take care of themselves and cooperate with others is greatly improved.

NEUROTRANSMITTER CHANGES IN SCHIZOPHRENIA

Most of the current evidence indicates that schizophrenia may be caused by overactive dopaminergic pathways in certain parts of the brain.[8,17,20,22] Increased dopamine transmission in areas such as the limbic system may be responsible for the behavioral changes associated with this disorder. Increased dopamine influence could be caused by excessive dopamine synthesis and release by the presynaptic neuron, decreased dopamine breakdown at the synapse, increased postsynaptic dopamine receptor sensitivity, or a combination of these and other factors.

Consequently, the currently accepted theory is that schizophrenia is caused by overactivity in dopamine synapses.[18,20] This theory is based primarily on the fact that most antipsychotic drugs block dopamine receptors (see the next section of this chapter). However, given the complexity of central neurotransmitter interaction, this belief may ultimately prove to be an oversimplification. Future research in schizophrenia and other forms of psychosis will be needed to examine the contribution of additional factors such as changes in postsynaptic dopamine receptor sensitivity and imbalances in other transmitter pathways.[6,8]

ANTIPSYCHOTIC MECHANISM OF ACTION

The antipsychotic drugs that are used to successfully treat schizophrenia all block central dopamine receptors to some extent (Fig. 8–1).[3,8,17,20] These drugs share some structural similarity to dopamine, which allows them to bind to the postsynaptic receptor, but they do not activate it. This effectively blocks the receptor from the effects of the released endogenous neurotransmitter (see Fig. 8–1). Any increased activity at central dopamine synapses is therefore negated by postsynaptic receptor blockade.

It has become evident, however, that there are several subcategories of dopamine receptors, and these receptor subtypes are identified as D_1, D_2, D_3, and so on.[26] The clinical effects and side effects of specific antipsychotic medications are therefore related to their ability to affect certain dopamine receptor populations. The receptor that appears

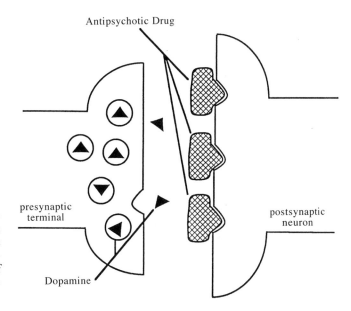

Antipsychotic Drug

presynaptic
terminal

postsynaptic
neuron

Dopamine

FIGURE 8–1. Effects of antipsychotic drugs on dopamine synapses. Antipsychotics act as postsynaptic receptor antagonists to block the effects of overactive dopamine transmission.

to be most important in mediating antipsychotic effects is the D_2 receptor subtype.[26] Most antipsychotic medications therefore have some ability to block the D_2 subtype. It is also clear, however, that other dopamine receptor subtypes play a role in the pathogenesis of psychosis and that certain antipsychotic drugs may produce specific effects because of their affinity for specific receptor subtypes. For example, newer antipsychotics such as clozapine also block D_4 receptors, and this action may help explain the differences in the effects and side effects of these drugs.[26]

Consequently, antipsychotic drugs all share a basic mechanism of action that involves dopamine receptor blockade. It is apparent, however, that they are not all equal in their ability to affect specific subtypes of dopamine receptors and that the effectiveness and side effects of specific drugs are related to their affinity and preference for certain receptors. As indicated earlier, other neurotransmitters may also be involved in the pathogenesis of psychosis, and differences in specific antipsychotic medications may be related to their ability to directly or indirectly affect these other transmitters as well as block dopamine influence. For example, some of the newer "atypical" antipsychotics (Tables 8–1 and 8–2) also block specific 5-hydroxytryptamine (serotonin) receptors such as the serotonin type 2 (5-HT$_2$) receptor.[8] Future studies will continue to clarify how current antipsychotics exert their beneficial effects and how new agents can be developed to be more selective in their effects on dopamine and other neurotransmitter pathways.

ANTIPSYCHOTIC MEDICATIONS

Antipsychotic medications are listed in Table 8–1. These agents comprise a somewhat diverse group in terms of their chemical background and potency—that is, the dosage range typically needed to achieve antipsychotic effects. As indicated earlier, these agents all block dopamine receptors to some extent, despite their chemical diversity. In addition to their chemical differences, antipsychotics can be classified as either traditional agents or newer "atypical" antipsychotics according to their efficacy and side effects. Differences between these two classes are described here.

TABLE 8–1 Common Antipsychotic Drugs

Generic Name	Trade Name	Usual Dosage Range (mg/day)*
Chlorpromazine	Thorazine	100–800
Chlorprothixene	Taractan	75–200
Clozapine†	Clozaril	50–500
Fluphenazine	Permitil, Prolixin	2–20
Haloperidol	Haldol	2–20
Loxapine	Loxitane	10–80
Molindone	Moban	10–100
Mesoridazine	Serentil	50–400
Olanzapine†	Zyprexa	10–20
Perphenazine	Trilafon	10–64
Prochlorperazine	Compazine	15–150
Quetiapine†	Seroquel	250–500
Risperidone†	Risperdal	2–8
Thioridazine	Mellaril	100–800
Thiothixene	Navane	4–40
Trifluoperazine	Stelazine	5–40
Triflupromazine	Vesprin	60–150

*Dosage range represents usual adult oral dose. Lower doses may be indicated in older or debilitated patients, and higher doses may be used for short periods to control severe psychotic episodes.
†Atypical antipsychotics. See text for details.

Traditional Antipsychotics

Traditional antipsychotics are associated with more side effects than their newer counterparts, including an increased incidence of extrapyramidal (motor) side effects. This increased risk may possibly be caused by the tendency of traditional agents to bind to several types of CNS dopamine receptors, including the receptors that influence motor function. This fact seems especially true for high-potency traditional agents such as haloperidol (Haldol) and fluphenazine (Prolixin). These high-potency agents have a fairly strong affinity for CNS dopamine receptors and can exert beneficial effects when used in fairly low doses (see Table 8–1). Other traditional agents such as chlorpromazine (Thorazine) and thioridazine (Mellaril) have lower potency and must be used in higher doses to exert an antipsychotic effect. These low-potency agents tend to cause fewer motor side effects but are associated with an increased incidence of other problems, such as sedative and anticholinergic side effects (e.g., dry mouth, constipation, urinary retention). These side effects and their possible long-term implications are discussed further in this chapter.

Traditional agents are also somewhat less predictable, and there tends to be more patient-to-patient variability in the beneficial (antipsychotic) effects of these medications.[8] Newer atypical drugs may be somewhat safer and more predictable, and these agents are described next.

Atypical Antipsychotics

Several newer antipsychotic medications have been developed that seem different or "atypical," compared with their predecessors. These agents include clozapine (Clozaril), risperidone (Risperdal), and several other atypical antipsychotics listed in Table 8–1. Although there is some debate about what exactly defines these drugs as

TABLE 8–2 Side Effects of Traditional and Atypical Antipsychotic Agents*

Drug	Extrapyramidal Symptoms	Sedative	Anticholinergic
Traditional antipsychotics			
Chlorpromazine	W–M	S	M–S
Chlorprothixene	S	W	W
Fluphenazine	S	W	W
Haloperidol	S	W	W
Loxapine	S	W	W
Molindone	S	W	W
Mesoridazine	W	M–S	M
Perphenazine	S	W–M	W–M
Prochlorperazine	S	M	W
Thioridazine	W	S	S
Thiothixene	S	W	W
Trifluoperazine	S	W	W
Triflupromazine	M–S	M–S	S
Atypical antipsychotics			
Clozapine	W	S	S
Olanzapine	W	W	M
Quetiapine	W	M	W
Risperidone	W	W	W

*Strengths of side effects are classified as follows: S = strong, M = moderate, W = weak.

"atypical," the most distinguishing feature of these drugs is that they have a much better side effect profile, including a decreased risk of producing extrapyramidal (motor) side effects.[5,9,10,24] There is also evidence that these atypical drugs are better at treating resistant forms of psychosis; that is, these newer agents may help resolve psychotic symptoms in patients who failed to respond to more traditional antipsychotic drugs.[7] It appears that these drugs may also be more successful in resolving some of the "negative" symptoms of psychosis, including lack of emotional expression (affective flattening), inability to speak (alogia), and lack of pleasure from acts that normally give pleasure (anhedonia).[8] It has likewise been suggested that early use of these atypical drugs (within the first 5 years of disease onset) may help prevent the progression and worsening of psychotic disease.[8]

Consequently, these atypical drugs are currently regarded as an important pharmacologic option and are often considered the drugs of first choice in treating psychosis.[8] These drugs are not devoid of side effects, however. As indicated in Table 8–2, clozapine has strong sedative and anticholinergic effects. Side effects of the other atypical drugs vary, but they can also cause specific problems, including orthostatic hypotension. Nonetheless, the newer atypical antipsychotics offer substantial advantages over the more traditional agents.

PHARMACOKINETICS

Antipsychotics are usually administered orally. During the acute stage of a psychotic episode, the daily dosage is often divided into three or four equal amounts. Maintenance doses are usually lower and can often be administered once each day. Under certain conditions, antipsychotics can be given intramuscularly. During acute episodes, intramuscular injections tend to reach the bloodstream faster than an orally administered drug and may be used if the patient is especially agitated. Conversely, certain forms of intramuscular antipsychotics that enter the bloodstream slowly have also been developed. Preparations such as fluphenazine decanoate and haloperidol decanoate can be injected every 2 to 4 weeks, respectively, and serve as a method of slow, continual release during the maintenance phase of psychosis. This method of administration may prove helpful if the patient has poor self-adherence to drug therapy and neglects to take his or her medication regularly.[16]

Metabolism of antipsychotics is through two mechanisms: conjugation with glucuronic acid and oxidation by hepatic microsomal enzymes. Both mechanisms of metabolism and subsequent inactivation take place in the liver. Some degree of enzyme induction may occur because of prolonged use of antipsychotics and may be responsible for increasing the rate of metabolism of these drugs.

OTHER USES OF ANTIPSYCHOTICS

Occasionally, these drugs are prescribed for conditions other than classic psychosis. As discussed in Chapter 7, an antipsychotic combined with lithium is often more effective than lithium alone during the acute manic phase of bipolar syndrome.[20] Low doses of antipsychotics may also be used in certain cases of organic brain syndrome to help control the patient's behavior.[14] These drugs are effective in decreasing the nausea and vomiting that often occur when dopamine agonists and precursors are administered to treat Parkinson disease. The antiemetic effect of the antipsychotics is probably caused by their ability to block dopamine receptors located on the brainstem that cause vomiting when stimulated by the exogenous dopamine.

PROBLEMS AND ADVERSE EFFECTS

Extrapyramidal Symptoms

Some of the more serious problems that occur with the use of antipsychotic drugs result in the production of abnormal movement patterns.[3,8] Many of these aberrant movements are similar to those seen in patients with lesions of the extrapyramidal system and are often referred to as extrapyramidal side effects. The basic reason that these motor problems occur is that dopamine is an important neurotransmitter in motor pathways, especially in the integration of motor function that takes place in the basal ganglia. Because antipsychotic drugs block CNS dopamine receptors, it makes sense that motor side effects are a potential complication of these drugs. The unintentional antagonism of dopamine receptors in areas of motor integration (as opposed to the beneficial blockade of behaviorally related receptors) results in a neurotransmitter imbalance that creates several distinct types of movement problems.

Thus, many antipsychotic drugs are associated with some type of motor side effect because these drugs are relatively nonselective in their ability to block CNS dopamine receptors. As noted earlier, the newer (atypical) agents such as clozapine and risperidone are not associated with as high an incidence of extrapyramidal side effects, possibly because these atypical agents are more selective for certain dopamine receptors that are located in the limbic system[4,6]; that is, these drugs may produce relatively fewer extrapyramidal side effects because of an apparent ability to bind more selectively to CNS receptors that affect behavior rather than receptors that influence motor function.

At present, however, extrapyramidal side effects continue to be one of the major drawbacks of antipsychotic medications. The primary types of extrapyramidal side effects, the manifestations of each type, and the relative time of their onset are shown in Figure 8–2. Some factors involved in patient susceptibility and possible treatment of these side effects are discussed here.

Tardive Dyskinesia. The disorder of **tardive dyskinesia** is characterized by a number of involuntary and fragmented movements. In particular, rhythmic movements of the mouth, tongue, and jaw are present, and the patient often produces involuntary sucking and smacking noises. Because this condition often involves the tongue and orofacial musculature, serious swallowing disorders (dysphagia) may also occur.[15] Other symptoms include choreoathetoid movements of the extremities and dystonias of the neck and trunk. As indicated in Table 8–2, certain traditional antipsychotics are associated with a greater incidence of tardive dyskinesia. Other risk factors include advanced patient age, affective mood disorders, diabetes mellitus, and continual use of the drug for 6 months or longer.[8,25] Tardive dyskinesia is also relatively common, with an estimated average prevalence between 15 and 30 percent of people with chronic psychosis.[3,8]

Tardive dyskinesia induced by antipsychotic drugs may be caused by "disuse supersensitivity" of the dopamine receptor.[3,8] Although the presynaptic neurons are still intact, drug blockade of the postsynaptic receptor induces the postsynaptic neuron to respond by "up-regulating" the number or sensitivity of the receptors. This increase in receptor sensitivity causes a functional increase in dopaminergic influence, leading to a

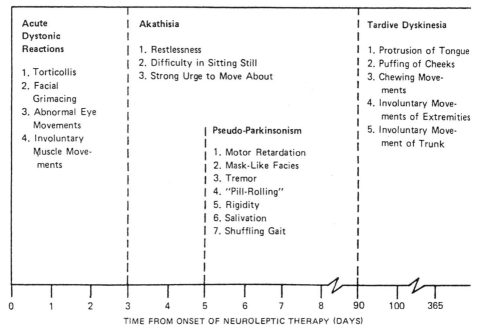

FIGURE 8–2. Extrapyramidal side effects and their relative onset after beginning antipsychotic drug therapy. (From Feigenbaum, JC and Schneider, F: Antipsychotic medications. In Mathewson, MK: Pharmacotherapeutics: A Nursing Approach. FA Davis, Philadelphia, 1986, p 404, with permission.)

neurotransmitter imbalance between dopamine and other central neurotransmitters such as acetylcholine and gamma-aminobutyric acid (GABA). This imbalance results in the symptoms of tardive dyskinesia.

Tardive dyskinesia is the most feared side effect of antipsychotic drugs.[6] In some patients, the symptoms will disappear if the drug is stopped or the dosage is decreased, but this can take from several weeks to several years to occur. In other individuals, drug-induced tardive dyskinesia appears irreversible.[3,8] To prevent the occurrence of tardive dyskinesia, the lowest effective dose of the antipsychotic should be used, especially during the maintenance phase of drug therapy. Also, patients taking these drugs for 3 months or more should undergo periodic reevaluation for any symptoms of tardive dyskinesia.[8] The motor symptoms of tardive dyskinesia can be dealt with by lowering drug dosage or by substituting an antipsychotic drug that tends to produce fewer extrapyramidal side effects (see Table 8–2). Early intervention is generally believed to be the most effective way of preventing the permanent changes associated with antipsychotic-induced tardive dyskinesia.[3]

Other drugs have been used to try to alleviate the symptoms of drug-induced tardive dyskinesia.[12] Agents such as anticholinergic drugs (e.g., atropine-like drugs) and GABA-enhancing drugs (e.g., benzodiazepines) have been used to attempt to rectify the transmitter imbalance created by the increased dopamine sensitivity. Reserpine has also been used in some patients because of its ability to deplete presynaptic stores of dopamine, thus limiting the influence of this neurotransmitter. However, these additional agents tend to be only marginally successful in reducing the dyskinesia symptoms, and their use tends to add complexity to the drug management of patients with psychoses. Thus, the best course of action continues to be judicious administration of these drugs, using the lowest effective dose, and early recognition and intervention if extrapyramidal symptoms appear.[3,8]

Pseudoparkinsonism. The motor symptoms seen in Parkinson disease (see Chap. 10) are caused by a deficiency in dopamine transmission in the basal ganglia. Because antipsychotic drugs block dopamine receptors, some patients may understandably experience symptoms similar to those seen in Parkinson disease. These symptoms include resting tremor, bradykinesia, and rigidity. Elderly patients are more susceptible to these drug-induced parkinsonian-like symptoms, probably because dopamine levels (and therefore dopaminergic influence) tend to be lower in older individuals.[23] The outcome of antipsychotic-induced parkinsonism is usually favorable, and these symptoms normally disappear when the dosage is adjusted or the drug is withdrawn. Drugs used as adjuncts in treating Parkinson disease (e.g., amantadine, benztropine mesylate) may also be administered to deal with the parkinsonian-like side effects. The primary antiparkinsonian drugs such as levodopa and dopamine agonists are not typically used to treat these parkinsonian-like side effects because they tend to exacerbate the psychotic symptoms.

Akathisia. Patients taking antipsychotics may experience sensations of motor restlessness and may complain of an inability to sit or lie still. This condition is known as **akathisia.**[19] Patients may also appear agitated, "pace the floor," and have problems with insomnia. Akathisia can usually be dealt with by altering the dosage or type of medication. If this is unsuccessful, beta-2–adrenergic receptor blockers (propranolol) may help decrease the restlessness associated with akathisia by a mechanism involving central adrenergic receptors.[1,11]

Dyskinesia and Dystonias. Patients may exhibit a broad range of bizarre movements of the arms, legs, neck, and face, including torticollis, oculogyric crisis, and opisthotonos.[3,8] These movements are involuntary and uncoordinated, and they may begin fairly soon after initiating antipsychotic therapy (i.e., even after a single dose).[21] If they persist during antipsychotic therapy, other drugs such as antiparkinsonian adjuncts or benzodiazepines (e.g., diazepam) may be used to try to combat the aberrant motor symptoms.

Neuroleptic Malignant Syndrome. Patients taking relatively high doses of the more potent antipsychotics may experience a serious disorder known as neuroleptic malignant syndrome (NMS).[8] Symptoms of NMS include catatonia, stupor, rigidity, tremors, and fever, and it can lead to death if untreated.[6] Treatment typically consists of stopping the antipsychotic drug and providing supportive care. The exact causes of NMS are unclear, but men younger than 40 and older patients with organic brain disease appear to be especially susceptible.

NONMOTOR EFFECTS

Sedation

Antipsychotics have varying degrees of sedative properties. Contrary to previous beliefs, sedative properties do not enhance the antipsychotic efficacy of these drugs. Consequently, sedative side effects offer no benefit and can be detrimental in withdrawn psychotic patients.

Anticholinergic Effects

Some antipsychotics also produce significant anticholinergic effects, manifested by symptoms such as blurred vision, dry mouth, constipation, and urinary retention. Fortunately, these problems are usually self-limiting, as many patients become tolerant to the anticholinergic side effects while remaining responsive to the antipsychotic properties.

Other Side Effects

Orthostatic hypotension is a frequent problem during the initial stages of antipsychotic therapy. This problem usually disappears after a few days. Certain antipsychotic drugs such as chlorpromazine are associated with photosensitivity, and care should be taken when exposing these patients to ultraviolet irradiation. Finally, abrupt withdrawal of antipsychotic drugs after prolonged use often results in nausea and vomiting, so it is advisable to decrease dosage gradually rather than stop administration suddenly.

SPECIAL CONCERNS IN REHABILITATION PATIENTS

Antipsychotic drugs have been a great benefit to patients seen in various rehabilitation facilities. Regardless of the reason these individuals are referred to physical therapy and occupational therapy, the improved behavior and reality perception usually provided by drug therapy will surely enhance the patient's cooperation during rehabilitation. Because these drugs tend to normalize patient behavior, the withdrawn patient often becomes more active and amiable, and the agitated patient becomes calmer and more relaxed. Also, remission of some of the confusion and impaired thinking will enable the patient to follow instructions more easily. Patients with paranoid symptoms may have fewer delusions of persecution and will feel less threatened by the entire therapy environment.

The benefits of antipsychotic drugs must be weighed against the risk of their side effects. The less serious side effects such as sedation and some of the anticholinergic effects (blurred vision, dry mouth, constipation) can be bothersome during the treatment session. Orthostatic hypotension should be guarded against, especially during the first few days after drug therapy is initiated. However, the major problems have to do with the extrapyramidal motor effects of these drugs. Therapists treating patients on antipsychotic medications should be continually on the alert for early signs of motor involvement. Chances are good that the therapist may be the first person to notice a change in posture, balance, or involuntary movements. Even subtle problems in motor function should be brought to the attention of the medical staff immediately. This early intervention may diminish the risk of long-term or even permanent motor dysfunction.

CASE STUDY

ANTIPSYCHOTIC DRUGS

Brief History. R.F., a 63-year-old woman, has been receiving treatment for schizophrenia intermittently for many years. She was last hospitalized for an acute episode 7 months ago and since then has been on a maintenance dose of haloperidol (Haldol), 25 mg/day. She is also being seen as an outpatient for treatment of rheumatoid arthritis in both hands. Her current treatment consists of gentle heat and active range-of-motion exercises, three times each week. She is being considered for possible metacarpophalangeal joint replacement.

Problem/Influence of Medication. During the course of physical therapy, the therapist noticed the onset and slow, progressive increase in writhing gestures of both upper extremities. Extraneous movements of her mouth and face were also observed, including chewinglike jaw movements and tongue protrusion.

Decision/Solution. These initial extrapyramidal symptoms suggested the onset of tardive dyskinesia. The therapist notified the patient's physician, and drug therapy was progressively shifted from haloperidol to the atypical agent clozapine (Clozaril), 450 mg/day. The extrapyramidal symptoms gradually diminished over the next 8 weeks and ultimately disappeared.

SUMMARY

Antipsychotic drugs represent one of the major advances in the management of mental illness. Drugs are currently available that diminish the symptoms of psychosis and improve the patient's ability to cooperate with others and to administer self-care. Despite their chemical diversity, antipsychotics all seem to exert their beneficial effects by blocking central dopamine receptors. Therefore, psychoses such as schizophrenia may be caused by an overactivity of CNS dopaminergic pathways. Because of the rather nonspecific blockade of dopaminergic receptors, antipsychotics are associated with several adverse side effects. The most serious of these are abnormal movement patterns that resemble tardive dyskinesia, Parkinson disease, and other lesions associated with the extrapyramidal system. In some cases, these aberrant motor activities may become irreversible and persist even after drug therapy is terminated. Rehabilitation specialists may play a critical role in recognizing the early onset of these motor abnormalities. When identified early, potentially serious motor problems can be dealt with by altering the dosage or type of antipsychotic agent.

REFERENCES

1. Adler, L, et al: Efficacy in propranolol in neuroleptic induced akathesia. J Clin Psychopharmacol 5:164, 1985.
2. American Psychiatric Association: Diagnostic and Statistical Manual of Mental Disorders, ed 4. American Psychiatric Association, Washington, DC, 1994.
3. Baldessarini, RJ: Drugs and the treatment of psychiatric disorders. In Hardman JG, et al (eds): The Pharmacological Basis of Therapeutics, ed 9. McGraw-Hill, New York, 1996.
4. Baldessarini, RJ and Frankenburg, FR: Drug therapy: Clozapine—a novel antipsychotic agent. N Engl J Med 324:746, 1991.
5. Beasley CM, et al: Randomized double-blind comparison of the incidence of tardive dyskinesia in patients with schizophrenia during long-term treatment with olanzapine or haloperidol. Br J Psychiatry 174:23, 1999.
6. Carpenter, WT and Buchanan, RW: Medical progress: Schizophrenia. N Engl J Med 330:681, 1994.
7. Conley, RR and Buchanan, RW: Evaluation of treatment-resistant schizophrenia. Schizophr Bull 23:663, 1997.
8. Crismon, ML and Dorson, PG: Schizophrenia. In DiPiro JT, et al (eds): Pharmacotherapy: A Pathophysiologic Approach, ed 4. Appleton & Lange, Stamford, CT, 1999.
9. Davies, A, et al: Risperidone versus haloperidol: I. Meta-analysis of efficacy and safety. Clin Ther 20:58, 1998.
10. De Oliveira, IR, et al: Risperidone versus haloperidol in the treatment of schizophrenia: A meta-analysis comparing their efficacy and safety. J Clin Pharm Ther 21:349, 1996.
11. Dorevitch, A, Durst, R, and Ginath, Y: Propranolol in the treatment of akathisia caused by antipsychotic drugs. South Med J 84:1505, 1991.
12. Egan, MF, Apud, J, and Wyatt, RJ: Treatment of tardive dyskinesia. Schizophr Bull 23:583, 1997.
13. Finkel, SI: Psychotherapeutic agents in older adults. Antipsychotics: Old and new. Clin Geriatr Med 14:87, 1998.
14. Gottlieb, GL and Kumar, A: Conventional pharmacological treatment for patients with Alzheimer's disease. Neurology 43(Suppl 4):S56, 1993.
15. Hayashi, T, et al: Life-threatening dysphagia following prolonged neuroleptic therapy. Clin Neuropharmacol 20:77, 1997.
16. Heyscue, BE, Levin, GM, and Merrick, JP: Compliance with depot antipsychotic medication by patients attending outpatient clinics. Psychiatr Serv 49:1232, 1998.
17. Kandel, ER: Disorders of thought and volition: Schizophrenia. In Kandel, ER, Schwartz, JH, and Jessell, TM (eds): Principles of Neural Science, ed 4. McGraw-Hill, New York, 2000.
18. Lasley, SM: Antipsychotic drugs. In Craig, CR and Stitzel, RE (eds): Modern Pharmacology with Clinical Applications, ed 5. Little Brown, Boston, 1997.
19. Miller, CH, et al: Risk factors for the development of neuroleptic induced akathisia. Eur Neuropsychopharmacol 7:51, 1997.
20. Potter, WZ and Hollister, LE: Antipsychotic agents and lithium. In Katzung, BG (ed): Basic and Clinical Pharmacology, ed 7. Appleton & Lange, Stamford, CT, 1998.
21. Rupniak, NMJ, Jenner, P, and Marsden, CD: Acute dystonia induced by neuroleptic drugs. Psychopharmacology (Berl) 88:403, 1986.
22. Seeman, P: Dopamine receptors and the dopamine hypothesis of schizophrenia. Synapse 1:133, 1987.
23. Stephen, PJ and Williamson, J: Drug induced parkinsonism in the elderly. Lancet 2:1082, 1984.
24. Tran, PV, et al: Extrapyramidal symptoms and tolerability of olanzapine versus haloperidol in acute treatment of schizophrenia. J Clin Psychiatry 58:205, 1997.
25. Van Os, J, et al: Tardive dyskinesia: Who is at risk? Acta Psychiatr Scand 96:206, 1997.
26. Wilson, JM, Sanyal, S, and Van Tol, HH: Dopamine D2 and D4 receptor ligands: Relation to antipsychotic action. Eur J Pharmacol 351:273, 1998.

CHAPTER 9

Antiepileptic Drugs

Epilepsy is a chronic neurologic disorder characterized by recurrent seizures.[28] **Seizures** are episodes of sudden, transient disturbances in cerebral excitation that occur when a sufficient number of cerebral neurons begin to fire rapidly and in synchronized bursts.[37] Depending on the type of seizure, the neuronal activity may remain localized in a specific area of the brain, or it may spread to other areas of the brain. In some seizures, neurons in the motor cortex are activated, leading to skeletal muscle contraction via descending neuronal pathways. These involuntary, paroxysmal skeletal muscle contractions seen during certain seizures are referred to as *convulsions*. However, convulsions are not associated with all types of epilepsy, and other types of seizures are characterized by a wide variety of sensory or behavioral symptoms.

Epilepsy is associated with the presence of a group or focus of cerebral neurons that are hyperexcitable, or "irritable." The spontaneous discharge of these irritable neurons initiates the epileptic seizure. The reason for the altered excitability of these focal neurons, and thus the cause of epilepsy, varies, depending on the patient.[8,13,21,35] In some patients, a specific incident such as a stroke, tumor, encephalopathy, head trauma, or other CNS injury probably caused damage to certain neurons, resulting in their altered threshold. In other patients, the reason for seizures may be less distinct or unknown, perhaps relating to a congenital abnormality, birth trauma, or genetic factor. A systemic metabolic disorder such as infection, hypoglycemia, hypoxia, or uremia may also precipitate seizure activity. In this last group of individuals, once the cause of the seizures is identified, the epilepsy is relatively easy to treat by resolving the metabolic disorder. Epilepsy resulting from these combined causes affects more than 2 million people in the United States and from 20 to 40 million worldwide, making it one of the most common neurologic disorders.[21,35]

Although some innovative approaches using surgery, neural stimulation, and dietary control have been reported,[14,15,17,33] drug therapy remains the primary method for treating epilepsy. Antiepileptic medications are successful in controlling seizures in 75 to 80 percent of the patient population.[3,10,24] Several types of drugs are currently available, and certain compounds work best in certain types of epilepsy. Consequently, the specific type of epilepsy must be determined by observing the patient and using diagnostic tests such as electroencephalography (EEG).[31,37] The classification system most commonly used in characterizing epilepsy is discussed here.

CLASSIFICATION OF EPILEPTIC SEIZURES

In an attempt to standardize the terminology used in describing various forms of epilepsy, the International League against Epilepsy[6] proposed the classification scheme outlined in Table 9–1. Seizures are divided into two major categories: partial and generalized. A third category of "unclassified" seizures is sometimes included to encompass additional seizure types that do not fit into the two major groupings.

In partial seizures, only part of the brain (i.e., one cerebral hemisphere) is involved, whereas in generalized seizures the whole cerebral brain is involved. Partial seizures that spread throughout the entire brain are referred to as "partial becoming generalized" or "secondarily generalized" seizures.

Partial and generalized seizures are subdivided depending on the specific symptoms that occur during the epileptic seizure (see Table 9–1). As a rule, the outward manifestations of the seizure depend on the specific area of the brain involved. Simple partial seizures that remain localized within the motor cortex for the right hand may cause involuntary, spasmlike movements of only the right hand. Other partial seizures produce motor and sensory symptoms, as well as affect consciousness and memory. These usually fall into the category of complex partial seizures. Generalized seizures are subclassified by the type and degree of motor involvement, as well as other factors such as

TABLE 9–1 Classification of Seizures

Seizure Type	Classification
I. Partial seizures	
A. Simple partial seizures	Limited (focal) motor or sensory signs (e.g., convulsions confined to one limb, specific sensory hallucinations); consciousness remains intact
B. Complex partial seizures	Consciousness impaired; bizarre behavior; wide variety of other manifestations; specific EEG abnormality (needed to differentiate this from absence seizures)
C. Partial becoming generalized	Symptoms progressively increase until seizure resembles a generalized (tonic-clonic) seizure
II. Generalized seizures	
A. Absence (petit mal) seizures	Sudden, brief loss of consciousness; motor signs may be absent or may range from rapid eye-blinking to symmetrical jerking movements of entire body
B. Myoclonic seizures	Sudden, brief, "shocklike" contractions of muscles in the face and trunk, or in one or more extremities; contractions may be single or multiple; consciousness may be impaired
C. Clonic seizures	Rhythmic, synchronized contractions throughout the body; loss of consciousness
D. Tonic seizures	Generalized sustained muscle contractions throughout body; loss of consciousness
E. Tonic-clonic (grand mal) seizures	Major convulsions of entire body; sustained contraction of all muscles (tonic phase) followed by powerful rhythmic contractions (clonic phase); loss of consciousness
F. Atonic seizures	Sudden loss of muscle tone in the head and neck, one limb, or thoughout the entire body; consciousness may be maintained or lost briefly
III. Unclassified seizures	
All other seizures that do not fit into one of the aforementioned categories	

Source: Modified from Commission on Classification and Terminology of the International League against Epilepsy,[6] pp 493–495, with permission.

the EEG recordings. The best-known and most dramatic of the generalized group is the tonic-clonic, or "grand mal," seizure. Absence, or "petit mal," seizures also fall into the category of generalized seizures. The drug therapy for generalized and partial seizures is discussed in "Drugs Used to Treat Epilepsy."

RATIONALE FOR DRUG TREATMENT

Even in the absence of drug therapy, individual seizures are usually self-limiting. Brain neurons are unable to sustain the high level of synaptic activity for more than a few minutes, and the seizure ends spontaneously. However, the uncontrolled recurrence of seizures is believed to cause further damage to the already injured neurons, as well as being potentially harmful to healthy cells. Certain types of seizures may be harmful if the patient loses consciousness or goes into convulsions and is injured during a fall. Certain types of convulsions are potentially fatal if cardiac irregularities result and the individual goes into cardiac arrest. Even relatively minor seizures may be embarrassing to a person, and social interaction may be compromised if the individual is afraid of having a seizure in public. Consequently, a strong effort is made to find an effective way to control or eliminate the incidence of seizures.

DRUGS USED TO TREAT EPILEPSY

Table 9–2 lists the primary drugs used to treat epilepsy according to their chemical classes and mechanisms of action. These drugs generally try to inhibit firing of certain cerebral neurons, usually by increasing the inhibitory effects of gamma-aminobutyric acid (GABA), by decreasing the effects of excitatory amino acids (glutamate, aspartate), or by altering the movement of ions (sodium, calcium) across the neuronal membrane.[11,13,23] In some cases, however, the exact way in which antiepileptic drugs exert their beneficial effects is obscure or unknown.[23] Specific details of each chemical class of drugs are discussed here. Because these drugs tend to have many adverse side effects, however, only the frequently occurring or more serious problems are listed for each category.

Barbiturates

Phenobarbital (various trade names) and other barbiturates such as mephobarbital (Mebaral) are prescribed in virtually all types of adult seizures but seem to be especially effective in generalized tonic-clonic and simple and complex partial seizures. These agents are considered to be very safe and effective in the treatment of seizures, but their use is often limited because of their strong tendency to produce sedation. Primidone (Mysoline) is another barbiturate-like drug that is recommended in several types of epilepsy but is particularly useful in generalized tonic-clonic seizures that have not responded to other drugs.

Mechanism of Action. Barbiturates are known to increase the inhibitory effects of GABA (see Chap. 6), and this effect is probably the primary way that these drugs decrease seizure activity. Barbiturates may also produce some of their antiseizure effects by inhibiting calcium entry into excitatory presynaptic nerve terminals and thereby decreasing the release of excitatory neurotransmitters such as glutamate.[21]

TABLE 9–2 Chemical Classification and Actions of Common Antiepileptic Agents

Chemical Class	Possible Mechanism of Action
Barbiturates Amobarbital (Amytal)* Mephobarbital (Mebaral) Pentobarbital (Nembutal)* Phenobarbital (Solfoton) Primidone (Mysoline) Secobarbital (Seconal)*	Potentiate inhibitory effects of GABA†; may also block excitatory effects of glutamate
Benzodiazepines Clonazepam (Klonopin) Clorazepate (Tranxene, others) Diazepam (Valium) Lorazepam (Ativan)	Potentiate inhibitory effects of GABA
Carboxylic acids Valproic acid (Depakene, others)	Unclear; may hyperpolarize membrane through an effect on potassium channels; higher concentrations increase CNS‡ GABA concentrations
Hydantoins Ethotoin (Peganone) Fosphenytoin (Cerebyx)* Mephenytoin (Mesantoin) Phenytoin (Dilantin)	Primary effect is to stabilize membrane by blocking sodium channels in repetitive-firing neurons; higher concentrations may also influence concentrations of other neurotransmitters (GABA, norepinephrine, others)
Iminostilbenes Carbamazepine (Tegretol, others)	Similar to hydantoins
Succinimides Ethosuximide (Zarontin) Methsuximide (Celontin) Phensuximide (Milontin)	Affect calcium channels; appear to inhibit spontaneous firing in thalamic neurons by limiting calcium entry

*Parenteral use only (IV injection).
†GABA = gamma-aminobutyric acid.
‡CNS = central nervous system.

Adverse Side Effects. Sedation (primary problem), nystagmus, ataxia, folate deficiency, vitamin K deficiency, and skin problems are typical side effects. A paradoxical increase in seizures and increased hyperactivity may occur in children.

Benzodiazepines

Several members of the benzodiazepine group are effective in treating epilepsy, but most are limited because of problems with sedation and tolerance. Some agents such as diazepam and lorazepam are used in the acute treatment of status epilepticus (see "Treatment of Status Epilepticus"), but only a few are used in the long-term treatment of epilepsy. Clonazepam (Klonopin) is recommended in specific forms of absence seizures (e.g., the Lennox-Gastaut variant) and may also be useful in minor generalized seizures such as akinetic spells and myoclonic jerks. Clorazepate (Tranxene) is another benzodiazepine that is occasionally used as an adjunct in certain partial seizures.

Mechanism of Action. These drugs are known to potentiate the inhibitory effects of GABA in the brain (see Chap. 6), and their antiepileptic properties are probably exerted through this mechanism.

Adverse Side Effects. Sedation, ataxia, and behavioral changes can be observed.

Hydantoins

This category includes phenytoin (Dilantin), mephenytoin (Mesantoin), ethotoin (Peganone), and fosphenytoin (Cerebyx). Phenytoin is often the first drug considered in treating many types of epilepsy, and it is especially effective in treating partial seizures and generalized tonic-clonic seizures. Mephenytoin has similar properties but is somewhat more toxic, and ethotoin has been effective in treating absence seizures. The latter two drugs are usually reserved for use if the patient has not responded to less toxic drugs. Finally, fosphenytoin can be administered intravenously in emergency situations to treat continuous, uncontrolled seizures (status epilepticus).

Mechanism of Action. Phenytoin stabilizes neural membranes and decreases neuronal excitability by decreasing sodium entry into rapidly firing neurons. This drug basically inhibits the ability of sodium channels to reset from an inactive to an active state after the neuron has fired an action potential. By inhibiting the reactivation of sodium channels, phenytoin prolongs the time between action potentials (absolute refractory period) so that neurons must slow their firing rate to a more normal level. Phenytoin may also decrease neuronal excitability by influencing the movement of potassium and calcium across the nerve membrane, but the effects on these other ions generally occur at drug concentrations that are higher than those used therapeutically to control seizures. Less is known about the molecular mechanisms of the other drugs in this category, but they probably work by a similar effect on the sodium channels.

Adverse Side Effects. Gastric irritation, confusion, sedation, dizziness, headache, cerebellar signs (nystagmus, ataxia, dysarthria), gingival hyperplasia, increased body and facial hair (hirsutism), and skin disorders are typical adverse effects.

Succinimides

Drugs in this category include ethosuximide (Zarontin), methsuximide (Celontin), and phensuximide (Milontin). All three drugs are primary agents in the treatment of absence (petit mal) seizures, but ethosuximide is the most commonly prescribed.

Mechanism of Action. These drugs are known to increase the seizure threshold and limit the spread of electrical activity in the brain, but their exact cellular mechanism is unknown. Some evidence suggests these drugs may exert their beneficial effects by decreasing calcium influx in certain thalamic neurons. The spontaneous, rhythmic entry of calcium into thalamic neurons may be responsible for initiating partial seizures, and the succinimides prevent the onset of these seizures by blunting calcium influx. Further research is needed to elaborate on this theory.

Adverse Side Effects. Gastrointestinal distress (nausea, vomiting), headache, dizziness, fatigue, lethargy, movement disorders (dyskinesia, bradykinesia), and skin rashes and itching are common side effects.

Carbamazepine

Carbamazepine (Tegretol) is classified chemically as an iminostilbene and is structurally similar to the tricyclic antidepressants. This drug has been shown to be effective in treating all types of epilepsy except absence seizures. Carbamazepine is regarded as equivalent to phenytoin in efficacy and side effects, and it may be substituted for that drug, depending on the individual patient response.

Mechanism of Action. Carbamazepine is believed to exert its primary antiepileptic effects in a manner similar to phenytoin—that is, stabilizing the neuronal membrane by slowing the recovery of sodium channels that are firing too rapidly. This drug may also inhibit the presynaptic uptake and release of norepinephrine, and this effect may contribute to its antiseizure activity.

Adverse Side Effects. Dizziness, drowsiness, ataxia, blurred vision, anemia, water retention (because of abnormal antidiuretic hormone [ADH] release), cardiac arrhythmias, and congestive heart failure can occur with use of this drug.

Valproic Acid

Valproic acid (Depakene, Depakote, other trade names) is classified as a carboxylic acid, and it is used primarily to treat absence seizures or as a secondary agent in generalized tonic-clonic forms of epilepsy. This drug is also used to treat bipolar syndrome (manic-depression), especially during the acute manic phase of bipolar disease (see Chap. 7).

Mechanism of Action. High concentrations of valproic acid are associated with increased levels of GABA in the brain, and this increase in GABA-ergic inhibition may be responsible for this drug's antiepileptic action. However, lower concentrations that are still effective in limiting seizures do not increase CNS GABA, indicating that some other mechanism must occur. Valproic acid also exerts some of its effects in a manner similar to phenytoin; that is, it limits sodium entry into rapidly firing neurons. Hence, the exact way in which this drug is effective against partial seizures remains to be determined, and valproic acid may actually work through a combination of several different molecular mechanisms.

Adverse Side Effects. Gastrointestinal distress, temporary hair loss, weight gain or loss, and impaired platelet function are documented adverse reactions.

Newer "Second-Generation" Agents

The medications described earlier have been on the market for many years and have been used routinely as the traditional drugs for decreasing seizure activity. Beginning with the introduction of felbamate in 1993, several new or "second-generation" drugs have also been approved by the FDA and are currently in use (Table 9–3). In most cases, these newer drugs are not more effective than their predecessors.[9,19] These newer agents, however, generally have favorable pharmacokinetic characteristics (absorption, distribution, metabolism, and so forth) and have relatively mild side effects that allow their use along with the more traditional antiseizure medications. Hence, these newer drugs are often used as adjuncts or "add-on" therapy to other drugs.[2,9,23] These drug combinations often allow adequate seizure control in patients who did not respond to a single traditional antiseizure agent. Likewise, as more is learned about these newer drugs, some are being used alone to treat certain types of seizures that are resistant to other drugs.

Second-generation antiseizure medications that are currently available are described here. There are likewise several other new agents including vigabatrin, zonisamide, oxcarbazepine, and levetiracetam that are undergoing clinical trials and may be available in the near future.[1] These newer agents should provide additional options for treating partial onset seizures and other seizure disorders, and future studies will be needed to determine how these drugs can be used most effectively.

TABLE 9–3 Second-Generation Antiepileptics

Generic Name	Trade Name	Primary Indication(s)
Felbamate	Felbatol	Used alone or as an adjunct in partial seizures in adults; treatment adjunct in partial and generalized seizures associated with Lennox-Gastaut syndrome in children
Gabapentin	Neurontin	Treatment adjunct in partial seizures in adults and children over age 12
Lamotrigine	Lamictal	Treatment adjunct in partial seizures in adults over age 16; treatment adjunct in generalized seizures associated with Lennox-Gastaut syndrome in adults and children over age 2
Tiagabine	Gabitril	Treatment adjunct in partial seizures in adults and children over age 12
Topiramate	Topamax	Treatment adjunct in partial onset seizures
Vigabatrine	Sabril	Used alone or as an adjunct to treat partial and generalized tonic-clonic seizures in adults and children

Felbamate (Felbatol). Felbamate is indicated for treatment of partial seizures in adults and children as well as generalized absence seizures (Lennox-Gastaut syndrome) in children. Felbamate appears to bind to specific receptors in the brain (the N-methyl-D-aspartate receptor) and block the effects of excitatory amino acids such as glutamate. Reduced influence of these excitatory amino acids results in decreased seizure activity. As indicated, this drug first appeared on the market in 1993 and represented the first "new-generation" antiseizure agent. It was soon recognized, however, that felbamate may cause severe toxic effects such as aplastic anemia and liver failure.[25] Felbamate is therefore not widely prescribed, and use is typically limited to patients with severe epilepsy who fail to respond to other antiseizure drugs. Other common side effects include insomnia, headache, dizziness, and gastrointestinal problems (anorexia, nausea, and vomiting).

Gabapentin (Neurontin). Gabapentin is used primarily to treat partial seizures in adults and partial seizures in children that have not responded to other treatments. As the name implies, gabapentin was designed to act as a GABA agonist. However, the exact antiseizure mechanism of this drug is unclear.[3,11] Gabapentin appears to work by increasing GABA release or by acting at some receptor that is different from the GABA receptor. The primary side effects of this drug are sedation, fatigue, dizziness, and ataxia.

Lamotrigine (Lamictal). Lamotrigine is used primarily as an adjunct to other medications in adults with partial seizures, although it has also been used alone to treat partial and generalized seizures in adults and children. This drug inhibits the release of excitatory amino acids by inhibiting sodium entry into presynaptic terminals of neurons that are firing too rapidly.[3,11] The primary side effects include dizziness, headache, ataxia, vision problems, and skin rashes.

Tiagabine (Gabitril). Tiagabine is used primarily as an adjunct to other drugs in adults with partial seizures that are poorly controlled by traditional drug therapy. This drug inhibits the reuptake of GABA after it is released from presynaptic terminals, thereby inhibiting seizure activity by enabling GABA to remain active in the synaptic cleft for longer periods.[23] The primary side effects of this drug are dizziness, weakness, and a slight tendency for psychiatric disturbances (anxiety, depression).

Topiramate (Topamax). Topiramate is used primarily as an adjunct to other medications in adults with partial seizures. This drug appears to limit seizure activity through several complementary mechanisms, including inhibition of sodium channel opening, blockade of excitatory amino acid receptors, and stimulation of GABA receptors. Primary side effects include sedation, dizziness, fatigue, and ataxia.

SELECTION OF A SPECIFIC ANTIEPILEPTIC AGENT

It is apparent from the preceding discussion that certain drugs are often preferred for treating specific types of seizures. Table 9–4 lists some of the more common types of seizures and the primary and alternative agents used to treat each seizure type. It is important to note, however, that Table 9–4 indicates general guidelines for drug selection, but selection of the best agent must be made on a patient-by-patient basis. Some patients exhibit a better response to agents that are not typically used as the first or second choice for a specific type of seizure. Hence, some trial and error may occur before the best drug is found for a given patient, and drug selection may need to be altered periodically throughout the patient's lifetime to achieve optimal results.[12]

Thus, a fairly large number of drugs can be used to treat epileptic seizures (see Tables 9–2 and 9–3), but certain agents are usually considered first to treat the most common seizures. These agents comprise a fairly small group of a dozen or so drugs that tend to be used most often. These commonly used drugs and their relevant pharmacologic parameters are listed in Table 9–5. Again, alternative antiseizure drugs can be used if these commonly used drugs are ineffective or poorly tolerated. As indicated earlier, one of the newer agents can also be added to these traditional drugs if patients do not respond to single-drug therapy with these traditional medications.

SINGLE-DRUG THERAPY VERSUS DRUG COMBINATIONS IN EPILEPSY

In the past, an effort was often made to use only one drug (primary agent), with an additional drug (secondary agent) added only if the epilepsy was especially resistant to management with the primary medication. The use of a single drug (monotherapy) offered several advantages, including fewer side effects, a lack of drug interactions, better

TABLE 9–4 Common Methods of Treating Specific Seizures*

Seizure Type	Primary Agents	Alternative Agents	Second-Generation Agents*
Partial seizures	Carbamazepine	Phenobarbital	Felbamate
	Phenytoin	Primidone	Gabapentin
	Valproic acid	Clonazepam	Lamotrigine
			Tiagabine
			Topiramate
Absence seizures	Ethosuximide	Clonazepam	Felbamate
	Valproic acid		Lamotrigine
Tonic-clonic seizures	Carbamazepine	Phenobarbital	Felbamate
	Phenytoin	Primidone	Lamotrigine
	Valproic acid	Clonazepam	Topiramate
Myoclonic seizures	Valproic acid	Clonazepam	Felbamate

*Therapy typically begins with one of the primary agents or one of the alternative agents. A second-generation drug can be added if the primary or alternative agent is not effective when used alone.

TABLE 9–5 Pharmacologic Parameters of Common Antiepileptic Drugs

Drug	Half-Life (hours)	Initial Target Dose (mg/day)*	Time to Reach Initial Target Dose*
Phenytoin	7–42	300	5–7 days
Carbamazepine	6–20	400–600	1 wk
Valproic acid	5–15	500–1000	3–7 days
Phenobarbital	65–110	60	2–4 wk
Primidone	8–15	750	4–6 wk
Ethosuximide	30–60	750	1–2 wk
Clonazepam	30–40	1–2	2–4 wk
Felbamate	18–24	2400–3600	2 wk
Gabapentin	5–8	900–1200	1–3 days
Lamotrigine	12–70	200	4 wk
Topiramate	20–30	200	4–8 wk
Tiagabine	2–9	24–32	5–7 wk

*Dosages are typically initiated at lower levels and increased progressively over several days to several weeks to reach initial target dose.

Source: Adapted from Abou-Kahil,[1] p 862, with permission.

ability of the patient to adhere to the drug regimen, lower cost, and better seizure control because the patient was able to tolerate a higher dose of a single agent.[12,29] Likewise, management of adverse side effects in single-drug therapy is easier because there is no question about which drug is producing the adverse effect.

As indicated earlier, the development of the newer antiseizure medications has advanced the strategy of using two drugs rather than a single agent. Because these newer drugs have relatively predictable pharmacokinetic and side effect profiles, they can be added to the traditional medications without excessive complications and risk to the patient.[16,24] Combination therapy is therefore a more common approach to treating seizure disorders than it was in the past.

PHARMACOKINETICS

When given for the long-term control of epilepsy, these drugs are normally administered orally. Daily oral doses are usually divided into three or four equal quantities, and the amount of each dose varies widely, depending on the specific drug and the severity of patient seizures. Distribution within the body is fairly extensive, with all antiepileptic drugs eventually reaching the brain to exert their beneficial effects. Drug biotransformation usually occurs via liver microsomal oxidases, and this is the primary method of drug termination.

SPECIAL PRECAUTIONS DURING PREGNANCY

Evidence exists that children of epileptic mothers have more birth defects than children of nonepileptic mothers.[7,27,34] Increases in the occurrence of problems such as stillbirth, microencephaly, mental retardation, infant seizures, and congenital malformations (cleft palate, cardiac defects) have been noted in children of women with seizure disorders. There is considerable debate as to whether this is a side effect of antiepileptic drug therapy or a sequela of the epilepsy itself. Because there is at least some concern that fetal malformations may be a drug side effect, some mothers may choose to discontinue drug therapy during their pregnancies.[22,27] This obviously places the mother at risk for uncontrolled seizures, which may be even more harmful to the mother and fetus. No consensus currently exists regarding this dilemma. Women taking antiepileptic drugs who wish to bear children should discuss the risks with their family members and physicians and try to arrive at a conclusion as to whether they will continue taking their medication.[4,22]

TREATMENT OF STATUS EPILEPTICUS

Status epilepticus is a series of seizures that occur without any appreciable period of recovery between individual seizures.[18,26] Essentially, the patient experiences one long, extended seizure. This may be brought on by a number of factors such as sudden withdrawal from antiepileptic drugs, cerebral infarct, systemic or intracranial infection, or withdrawal from addictive drugs including alcohol.[20,26] If untreated, status epilepticus will result in permanent damage or death, especially if the seizures are generalized tonic-clonic in nature.[18] Consequently, this event is regarded as a medical emergency that should be resolved as rapidly as possible.

Treatment begins with standard emergency procedures such as maintaining an airway and starting an IV line for blood sampling and drug administration.[26,36] The first drugs administered are usually benzodiazepines: either diazepam (Valium) or lorazepam (Ativan) given intravenously. This approach is followed by phenytoin, which is also administered intravenously. The phenytoin is given concurrently with or immediately after the benzodiazepine so that seizures are controlled when the relatively short-acting benzodiazepine is metabolized. If seizures continue despite these drugs, phenobarbital is given intravenously. If all other attempts fail, general anesthesia (e.g., halothane) may be used as a last resort. When the status epilepticus is eventually controlled, an attempt is made to begin or reinstitute chronic antiepileptic therapy.

WITHDRAWAL OF ANTISEIZURE MEDICATIONS

Many people with seizure disorders will need to adhere to a regimen of antiseizure medications throughout life. There appears, however, to be a certain percentage of patients who can discontinue their medications once their seizures are under control. It is estimated, for example, that as many as 60 to 70 percent of people who have epilepsy can remain seizure-free after their medication is withdrawn.[30,32] Factors associated with successful medication withdrawal include being free of seizures for at least 2 years while on medications, having a normal neurologic examination prior to withdrawal, and being young when the seizures started.[30,32]

Withdrawal of medications must, of course, be done under close medical supervision. Likewise, medications are usually tapered off over an extended period of time (6 months) rather than suddenly discontinued.[30] Nonetheless, it appears that a large proportion of people with epilepsy may be able to maintain seizure-free status once their seizures are controlled by the appropriate medications.

SPECIAL CONCERNS IN REHABILITATION PATIENTS

Rehabilitation specialists must always be cognizant of their patients who have a history of seizures and who are taking antiepileptic drugs. Patients being treated for conditions unrelated to epilepsy (e.g., the outpatient with low back pain) should be identified as potentially at risk for a seizure during the therapy session. This knowledge will better prepare the therapist to recognize and deal with such an episode. This approach emphasizes the need for a thorough medical history of all patients. Also, therapists may help determine the efficacy of antiepileptic drug therapy. The primary goal for any patient taking antiepileptic drugs is maintaining the drug dosage within a therapeutic window. Dosage must be high enough to adequately control seizure activity, but not so high as to invoke serious side effects. By constantly observing and monitoring patient progress, rehabilitation specialists may help determine if this goal is being met. By noting changes in either seizure frequency or side effects, physical therapists, occupational therapists, and other rehabilitation personnel may help the medical staff arrive at an effective dosing regimen. This information can be invaluable in helping achieve optimal patient care with a minimum of adverse side effects.[5]

Some of the more frequent side effects may affect physical therapy and other rehabilitation procedures. Headache, dizziness, sedation, and gastric disturbances (nausea, vomiting) may be bothersome during the therapy session. Often these reactions can be addressed by scheduling therapy at a time of day when these problems are relatively mild. The optimal treatment time will vary from patient to patient, depending on the particular drug, dosing schedule, and age of the patient. Cerebellar side effects such as ataxia also occur frequently and may impair the patient's ability to participate in various functional activities. If ataxia persists despite efforts to alter drug dosage or substitute another agent, coordination exercises may be instituted to help resolve this problem. Skin conditions (dermatitis, rashes) are another frequent problem in long-term antiepileptic therapy. Any therapeutic modalities that might exacerbate these conditions should be discontinued.

Finally, in some patients, seizures tend to be exacerbated by environmental stimuli such as lights and sound. In such patients, conducting the therapy session in a busy, noisy clinic may be sufficient to precipitate a seizure, especially if the epilepsy is poorly controlled by drug therapy. Also, certain patients may have a history of increased seizure activity at certain times of the day, which may be related to when the antiepileptic drug is administered. Consequently, certain patients may benefit if the therapy session is held in a relatively quiet setting at a time when the chance of a seizure for that individual is minimal.

CASE STUDY

ANTIEPILEPTIC DRUGS

Brief History. F.B. is a 43-year-old man who works in the mail room of a large company. He was diagnosed in childhood as having generalized tonic-clonic epilepsy, and his seizures have been managed successfully with various drugs over the years. Most recently, he has been taking carbamazepine (Tegretol), 800 mg/day (i.e., one 200-mg tablet, QID). One month ago, he began complaining of dizziness and blurred vision, so the dosage was reduced to 600 mg/day (one tablet TID). He usually took the medication after meals. Two weeks ago, he injured his back while lifting a large box at work. He was evaluated in physical therapy as having an acute lumbosacral strain. He began to attend physical therapy each day as an outpatient. Treatment included heat, ultrasound, and manual therapy, and the patient was also instructed in proper body mechanics and lifting technique. F.B. continued to work at his normal job, but he avoided heavy lifting. He would attend therapy on his way home from work, at about 5 PM.

Problem/Influence of Medication. F.B. arrived at physical therapy the first afternoon stating that he had had a particularly long day. He was positioned prone on a treatment table, and hot packs were placed over his low back. As the heat was applied, he began to drift off to sleep. Five minutes into the treatment, he had a seizure. Because of a thorough initial evaluation, the therapist was aware of his epileptic condition and protected him from injury during the seizure. The patient regained consciousness and rested quietly until he felt able to go home. No long-term effects were noted from the seizure.

Decision/Solution. The seizure may have been precipitated by a number of factors, including the recent decrease in drug dosage and the fact that he was nearing the end of a dosing interval. (He had taken his last dose at lunch and would take his next dose after he went home and had dinner.) The fact that he was tired and fell asleep during the treatment probably played a role. He reported later that when seizures do occur, they tend to be when he is asleep. To prevent the recurrence of seizures, the therapy session was rescheduled to earlier in the day, at 8 AM (his schedule was flexible enough that he could attend therapy before going to work). Also, he would have taken his first dose of the day approximately 1 hour before arriving at physical therapy. No further seizures occurred during the course of rehabilitation, and F.B.'s lumbosacral strain was resolved after 2 weeks of physical therapy.

SUMMARY

Epilepsy is a chronic condition characterized by recurrent seizures. Causes of this disorder range from a distinct traumatic episode to obscure or unknown origins. Seizures are categorized according to the clinical and electrophysiologic manifestations that occur during the seizure. Fortunately, most individuals with epilepsy (up to 80 percent) can be treated successfully with antiepileptic drugs. Although these drugs do not cure this disorder, reduction or elimination of seizures will prevent further CNS damage. Currently, a wide variety of drugs are used, with specific agents most successful in specific types of epilepsy. As in any area of pharmacotherapeutics, these drugs are not without adverse side effects. Some of these side effects may become a problem in rehabilitation patients, so therapists should be ready to alter the time and type of treatment as needed to accommodate these side effects. Physical therapists and other rehabilitation personnel should also be alert for any behavioral or functional changes in the patient that might indicate a problem in drug therapy. Insufficient drug therapy (as evidenced by increased seizures) or possible drug toxicity (as evidenced by increased side effects) should be brought to the physician's attention so that these problems can be rectified.

REFERENCES

1. Abou-Khalil, B: Seizures and epilepsy in adolescents and adults. In Rakel, RE (ed): Conn's Current Therapy. WB Saunders, Philadelphia, 2000.
2. Bazil, MK and Bazil, CW: Recent advances in the pharmacotherapy of epilepsy. Clin Ther 19:369, 1997.
3. Benetello, P: New antiepileptic drugs. Pharmacol Res 31:155, 1995.

4. Chang, SI and McAuley, JW: Pharmacotherapeutic issues for women of childbearing age with epilepsy. Ann Pharmacother 32:794, 1998.
5. Collaborative Group for Epidemiology of Epilepsy: Adverse reactions to antiepileptic drugs: A follow-up study of 355 patients with chronic antiepileptic drug treatment. Epilepsia 29:787, 1988.
6. Commission on Classification and Terminology of the International League against Epilepsy: Proposal for revised clinical and electroencephalographic classification of epileptic seizures. Epilepsia 30:389, 1989.
7. Dalessio, DJ: Current concepts: Seizure disorders and pregnancy. N Engl J Med 312:559, 1985.
8. Delanty, N, Vaughan, CJ, and French, JA: Medical causes of seizures. Lancet 352:383, 1998.
9. Elger, CE and Bauer, J: New antiepileptic drugs in epileptology. Neuropsychobiology 38:145, 1998.
10. Elwes, RDC, et al: The prognosis for seizure control in newly diagnosed epilepsy. N Engl J Med 311:944, 1984.
11. Emilien, G and Maloteaux, JM: Pharmacological management of epilepsy. Mechanism of action, pharmacokinetic drug interactions, and new drug discovery possibilities. Int J Clin Pharmacol Ther 36:181, 1998.
12. French, J: The long-term therapeutic management of epilepsy. Ann Intern Med 120:411, 1994.
13. Graves, NM and Garnett, WR: Epilepsy. In DiPiro, JT, et al (eds): Pharmacotherapy: A Pathophysiologic Approach, ed 4. Appleton & Lange, Stamford, CT, 1999.
14. Halloway, KL, et al: Epilepsy surgery: Removing the thorn from the lion's paw. South Med J 88:619, 1995.
15. Hornig, GW, et al: Left vagus nerve stimulation in children with refractory epilepsy: An update. South Med J 90:484, 1997.
16. Kalviainen, R, Keranen, T, and Reikkinen, PJ: Place of newer antiepileptic drugs in the treatment of epilepsy. Drugs 46:1009, 1993.
17. Keene, DL, Higgins, MJ, and Ventureyra, EC: Outcome and life prospects after surgical management of medically intractable epilepsy in patients under 18 years of age. Childs Nerv Syst 13:530, 1997.
18. Leppik, IE: Status epilepticus: The next decade. Neurology 40(Suppl 2):4, 1990.
19. Loscher, W: New visions in the pharmacology of anticonvulsion. Eur J Pharmacol 342:1, 1998.
20. Lothman, E: The biochemical basis and pathophysiology of status epilepticus. Neurology 40(Suppl 2):13, 1990.
21. McNamara, JO: Drugs effective in the therapy of the epilepsies. In Hardman, JG, et al (eds): The Pharmacological Basic of Therapeutics, ed 9. McGraw-Hill, New York, 1996.
22. Morrell, MJ: Guidelines for the care of women with epilepsy. Neurology 51(Suppl 4):S21, 1998.
23. Natsch, S, et al: Newer anticonvulsant drugs: Role of pharmacology, drug interactions, and adverse reactions in drug choice. Drug Saf 17:228, 1997.
24. Patsalos, PN and Sander, JW: Newer antiepileptic drugs. Towards an improved risk-benefit ratio. Drug Saf 11:37, 1994.
25. Perucca, E: The new generation of antiepileptic drugs: Advantages and disadvantages. Br J Clin Pharmacol 42:531, 1996.
26. Phelps, SJ, May, WN, and Rose, DF: Status epilepticus. In DiPiro, JT, et al (eds): Pharmacotherapy: A Pathophysiologic Approach, ed 4. Appleton & Lange, Stamford, CT, 1999.
27. Philbert, A and Pedersen, B: Treatment of epilepsy in women of child-bearing age: Patient's opinion of teratogenic potential of valproate. Acta Neurol Scand Suppl 94:35, 1983.
28. Scheuer, ML and Pedley, TA: Current concepts: The evaluation and treatment of seizures. N Engl J Med 323:1468, 1990.
29. Schmidt, D: Single drug therapy for intractable epilepsy. J Neurol 229:221, 1983.
30. Schmidt, D and Gram, L: A practical guide to when (and how) to withdraw antiepileptic drugs in seizure-free patients. Drugs 52:870, 1996.
31. Shorvon, SD: Medical assessment and treatment of chronic epilepsy. BMJ 302:363, 1991.
32. Sperling, MR, Bucurescu, G, and Kim, B: Epilepsy management. Issues in medical and surgical treatment. Postgrad Med 102:102, 1997.
33. Swink, TD, Vining, EP, and Freeman, JM: The ketogenic diet: 1997. Adv Pediatr 44:297, 1997.
34. Symposium (various authors): Pregnancy and teratogenesis in epilepsy. Neurology 42(Suppl 5):7, 1992.
35. Symposium (various authors): Basic mechanisms of the epilepsies: Molecular and cellular approaches. Adv Neurol 44:1, 1986.
36. Treiman, DM: The role of benzodiazepines in the management of status epilepticus. Neurology 40(Suppl 2):32, 1990
37. Westbrook, GL: Seizures and epilepsy. In Kandel, ER, Schwartz, JH, and Jessell, TM (eds): Principles of Neural Science, ed 4. McGraw-Hill, New York, 2000.

CHAPTER 10

Pharmacologic Management of Parkinson Disease

Parkinson disease is a movement disorder characterized by resting tremor, bradykinesia, rigidity, and postural instability.[12,26,86] In Parkinson disease, there is a slow, progressive degeneration of certain dopamine-secreting neurons in the basal ganglia.[14,40,64] Several theories have been proposed to explain this spontaneous neuronal degeneration, including the possibility that Parkinson disease may be related to some type of toxic substance (see "Etiology of Parkinson Disease: Potential Role of Toxic Substances").[8,59] However, the precise initiating factor in Parkinson disease is still largely unknown. The clinical syndrome of parkinsonism (i.e., rigidity, bradykinesia, and so on) may also be caused by other factors such as trauma, encephalitis, antipsychotic drugs, and various forms of cortical degeneration (including Alzheimer disease).[64] However, the most frequent cause of parkinsonism is the slow, selective neuronal degeneration characteristic of Parkinson disease itself.[86] Also, the drug management of parkinsonism caused by these other factors closely resembles the management of Parkinson disease.[64] Consequently, this chapter will address the idiopathic onset and pharmacologic treatment of Parkinson disease per se.

Parkinson disease usually begins in the fifth or sixth decade, and symptoms slowly but progressively worsen over a period of 10 to 20 years. It is estimated that more than 1 percent of the U.S. population older than age 60 is afflicted with this illness, making Parkinson disease one of the most prevalent neurologic disorders affecting elderly individuals.[12] In addition to the symptoms of bradykinesia and rigidity, the patient with advanced Parkinson disease maintains a flexed posture and speaks in a low, soft voice (microphonia). If left untreated, the motor problems associated with this illness eventually lead to total incapacitation of the patient. Because of the prevalence of Parkinson disease and the motor problems associated with this disorder, rehabilitation specialists are often involved in treating patients with this illness.

Fortunately, the pharmacologic management of Parkinson disease has evolved to the point that the symptoms associated with this disorder can be greatly diminished in many patients. The use of levodopa (L-dopa), alone or in combination with other drugs, can improve motor function and general mobility well into the advanced stages of this disease. Drugs used in treating Parkinson disease do not cure this condition, and motor function often tends to slowly deteriorate in these patients regardless of when drug therapy is initiated.[12,56,57] However, by alleviating the motor symptoms (i.e., bradykinesia and rigidity), drug therapy can allow patients with Parkinson disease to continue to lead relatively active lifestyles, thus improving their overall physiologic as well as psychologic well-being.

PATHOPHYSIOLOGY OF PARKINSON DISEASE

During the past 30 years, the specific neuronal changes associated with the onset and progression of Parkinson disease have been established. Specific alterations in neurotransmitter balance in the basal ganglia are responsible for the symptoms associated with this disorder.[12,14,86] The basal ganglia are groups of nuclei in the brain that are involved in the coordination and regulation of motor function. One such nucleus, the substantia nigra, contains the cell bodies of neurons that project to other areas, such as the putamen and caudate nucleus (known collectively as the "corpus striatum"). The neurotransmitter used in this nigrostriatal pathway is dopamine. The primary neural abnormality in Parkinson disease is that dopamine-producing cells in the substantia nigra begin to degenerate, resulting in the eventual loss of dopaminergic input into the corpus striatum.[12,14,64]

Consequently, the decrease in striatal dopamine seems to be the initiating factor in the onset of the symptoms associated with Parkinson disease. However, it also appears that the lack of dopamine results in an increase in activity in cholinergic pathways in the basal ganglia.[12,14,64] As illustrated in Figure 10–1, there is a balance between dopamin-

NORMAL

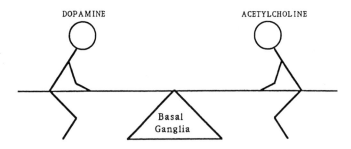

PARKINSON DISEASE

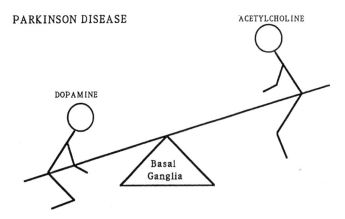

FIGURE 10–1. Schematic representation of the neurotransmitter imbalance in Parkinson disease. Normally, a balance exists between dopamine and acetylcholine in the basal ganglia. In Parkinson disease, decreased dopaminergic influence results in increased acetylcholine influence.

ergic and cholinergic influence in the basal ganglia under normal conditions. However, the loss of dopaminergic influence in Parkinson disease appears to allow cholinergic influence to dominate.

The relationship between these two neurotransmitters suggests that the role of striatal dopamine may be to modulate acetylcholine release; that is, the lack of inhibitory dopaminergic influence allows excitatory acetylcholine pathways to run wild. Thus, the symptoms associated with Parkinson disease may really be directly caused by increased cholinergic influence occurring secondary to the loss of dopamine. Current research also suggests that other imbalances involving transmitters such as gamma-aminobutyric acid (GABA), 5-hydroxytryptamine (serotonin), endogenous opioids, and excitatory amino acids (glutamate) may also be present in the basal ganglia subsequent to the loss of dopamine.[12,14,86] In any event, drug therapy focuses on resolving the dopamine-acetylcholine imbalance to restore normal motor function in Parkinson disease.

ETIOLOGY OF PARKINSON DISEASE: POTENTIAL ROLE OF TOXIC SUBSTANCES

As stated previously, the exact factors that initiate the loss of striatal dopamine are unknown in most patients with Parkinson disease. However, recent evidence suggests that some sort of environmental or endogenous toxin may be responsible for accelerating the destruction of dopaminergic neurons in the substantia nigra.[8,46,59,79] Much of this evidence is based on the finding that a compound known as 1-methyl-4-phenyl-1,2,3,6-tetrahydropyridine (MPTP) appears to be selectively toxic to these neurons and can invoke parkinsonism in primates.[6,50,51,55]

The theory that a toxin like MPTP might cause Parkinson disease was formulated in a rather interesting fashion. In 1982, several young adults in their 20s and 30s developed permanent, severe parkinsonism.[3] Because the onset of Parkinson disease before age 40 is extremely rare, these individuals aroused a great deal of interest. Upon close investigation, all of these individuals were found to have experimented with synthetic heroinlike drugs. These so-called designer drugs were manufactured by drug dealers in an attempt to create an illicit supply of narcotics for sale to heroin addicts. However, the illicit narcotics contained the toxin MPTP, which was discovered to cause selective destruction of substantia nigra neurons.[3]

The discovery of toxin-induced parkinsonism in drug addicts led to the idea that idiopathic Parkinson disease may be caused by previous exposure to some environmental toxin.[79] Exposure to such a toxin through industrial waste or certain herbicides may begin the neuronal changes that ultimately result in Parkinson disease. A specific environmental factor, however, has not been identified yet.

An alternative hypothesis to an environmental toxin is that the substantia nigra neurons may be damaged by some endogenously produced substance. Current research suggests that production of free radicals may be responsible for the selective degeneration of substantia nigra neurons in the brains of susceptible individuals.[8,45,85] A free radical is a chemical species that has an unpaired electron in its outer shell. In order to become more stable, the free radical steals an electron from some other cellular component such as a protein, DNA molecule, or membrane phospholipid. In this process, the free radical damages the cellular component, with subsequent damage to the cell. Cells subjected to this free radical–induced damage are said to undergo oxidative stress because loss of electrons (oxidation) of various cellular components leads to degeneration and possibly death of the cell.

Evidence therefore suggests that the degeneration of substantia nigra neurons in people with Parkinson disease may ultimately be caused by local production of free radicals.[8,40] Free radicals may be produced, for example, when dopamine is degraded enzymatically in the basal ganglia.[8,63] Although free radicals are often a normal by-product of cellular metabolism, it is possible that some defect in the production of and response to these chemicals may occur in people with Parkinson disease. Indeed, there is substantial evidence that people with Parkinson disease are susceptible to oxidative stress in the region of the substantia nigra.[45,85] The reason for this increased susceptibility is not clear, but there is reason to believe that Parkinson disease has a genetic basis.[33] Hence, it seems possible that a genetic defect may help account for the increased susceptibility of substantia nigra neurons to free radical–induced damage. Nonetheless, the exact cause of Parkinson disease remains unknown, and future research will hopefully clarify the link between genetic factors and the mechanism of cell death in the substantia nigra of people with this disease.

The idea that toxins such as free radicals may initiate Parkinson disease has also led to research in ways to delay or prevent the biochemical changes induced by such toxins. For example, it has been suggested that certain medications might have neuroprotective effects if they control the production and harmful effects of endogenous toxins such as free radicals. Such medications are often referred to as "antioxidants" because they may help control oxidative stress caused by free radicals. This idea has encouraged the development and use of agents that might delay the neurodegenerative changes seen in Parkinson disease. In particular, drugs used to decrease the symptoms of Parkinson disease (dopamine agonists, selegiline; see later), as well as antioxidants such as vitamin E, have been investigated for any possible neuroprotective effects.[62,68,71,89] To date, no agent has been identified that is overwhelmingly successful in delaying the neuronal changes that occur in Parkinson disease. Nonetheless, future research may continue to clarify the exact reason for the degeneration of substantia nigra neurons, and drugs that help prevent this degeneration could conceivably be developed to decrease or even eliminate the neuronal death that underlies Parkinson disease.

THERAPEUTIC AGENTS IN PARKINSONISM

An overview of the drugs used to treat Parkinson disease is shown in Table 10–1. The primary drug used to treat parkinsonism is levodopa. Other agents such as amantadine, anticholinergic drugs, and direct-acting dopamine agonists can be used alone or in conjunction with levodopa, depending on the needs of the patient. Each of these agents is discussed here.

Levodopa

Because the underlying problem in Parkinson disease is a deficiency of dopamine in the basal ganglia, simple substitution of this chemical would seem a logical course of action. However, dopamine does not cross the blood-brain barrier. Administration of dopamine, either orally or parenterally, will therefore be ineffective because it will be unable to cross from the systemic circulation into the brain where it is needed. Fortunately, the immediate precursor to dopamine, dihydroxyphenylalanine (dopa) (Fig. 10–2) does cross the blood-brain barrier quite readily. Dopa, or more specifically levodopa (the L-isomer of dopa), is able to cross the brain capillary endothelium through an

TABLE 10–1 Overview of Drug Therapy in Parkinson Disease

Drug	Mechanism of Action	Special Comments
Levodopa	Resolves dopamine deficiency by being converted to dopamine after crossing blood-brain barrier	Still the best drug for resolving parkinsonian symptoms; long-term use limited by side effects and decreased efficacy
Dopamine agonists Bromocriptine Pergolide Pramipexole Ropinirole	Directly stimulate dopamine receptors in basal ganglia	Often used in combination with levodopa to get optimal benefits with lower dose of each drug
Anticholinergics (see Table 10–2)	Inhibit excessive acetylcholine influence caused by dopamine deficiency	Use in Parkinson disease limited by frequent side effects
Amantadine	Unclear; may stimulate release of remaining dopamine or block effects of excitatory amino acids in brain	May be used alone during early/mild stages or added to drug regimen when levodopa loses effectiveness
Selegiline	Inhibits the enzyme that breaks down dopamine in the basal ganglia; enables dopamine to remain active for longer periods of time	May improve symptoms, especially in early stages of Parkinson disease; ability to produce long-term benefits unclear
COMT* inhibitors Tolcapone	Help prevent breakdown of levodopa in peripheral tissues; allow more levodopa to reach the brain	Useful as an adjunct to levodopa/ carbidopa administration; may improve and prolong effects of levodopa

*COMT = catechol-O-methyltransferase.

active transport process that is specific for this molecule and other large amino acids.[10,86] Upon entering the brain, levodopa is then transformed into dopamine by decarboxylation from the enzyme **dopa decarboxylase** (Fig. 10–3).

Administration of levodopa often dramatically improves all the symptoms of parkinsonism, especially bradykinesia and rigidity. In patients who respond well to this drug, the decrease in symptoms and increase in function are remarkable. As with any medication, some patients do not respond well or simply cannot tolerate the drug for unknown reasons. Also, prolonged use of levodopa is associated with some rather troublesome and frustrating side effects (see "Problems and Adverse Effects of Levodopa Therapy"). However, the use of levodopa has been the most significant advance in the management of Parkinson disease to date, and it remains the most effective single drug in the treatment of most patients with this disorder.[1,43,64]

LEVODOPA ADMINISTRATION AND METABOLISM: USE OF PERIPHERAL DECARBOXYLASE INHIBITORS

Levodopa is usually administered orally, beginning with dosages of 500 to 1000 mg/day. Dosages are progressively increased until a noticeable reduction in symptoms occurs, or until side effects begin to be a problem. Maximum doses can run as high as 8 g/day. Daily titers are usually divided into two to three doses per day, and individual doses are often given with meals to decrease gastrointestinal irritation.

Following absorption from the gastrointestinal tract, levodopa is rapidly converted to dopamine by the enzyme dopa decarboxylase. This enzyme is distributed extensively

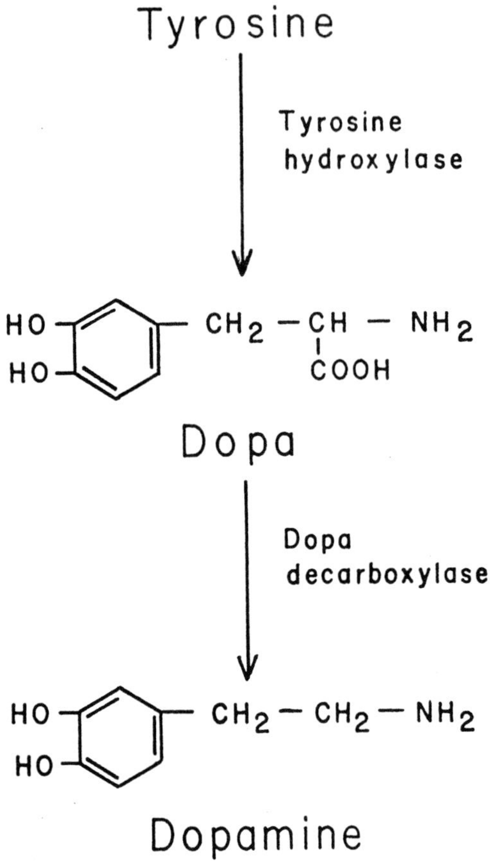

Tyrosine

Tyrosine
hydroxylase

HO—⬡— $CH_2 - \underset{\underset{COOH}{|}}{CH} - NH_2$

Dopa

Dopa
decarboxylase

HO—⬡— $CH_2 - CH_2 - NH_2$

Dopamine

FIGURE 10–2. Synthesis of dopamine.

throughout the body and can be found in such locations as the liver, intestinal mucosa, kidney, and skeletal muscle. Conversion of levodopa to dopamine in the periphery is rather extensive, such that only 1 to 3 percent of the administered levodopa reaches the brain in that form.[12,86] This fact is significant because only levodopa will be able to cross the blood-brain barrier to be subsequently transformed into dopamine. Any levodopa that is prematurely converted to dopamine in the periphery must remain in the periphery and is essentially useless in alleviating parkinsonism symptoms.

Consequently, when given alone, rather large quantities of levodopa must be administered to ensure that enough levodopa reaches the brain in that form. This is often undesirable because the majority of the levodopa ends up as dopamine in the peripheral circulation, and these high levels of circulating dopamine can cause some unpleasant gastrointestinal and cardiovascular side effects (see the next section). An alternative method is to give levodopa in conjunction with a peripheral decarboxylase inhibitor (Fig. 10–4). The simultaneous use of a drug that selectively inhibits the dopa decarboxylase enzyme outside the CNS enables more levodopa to reach the brain before being converted to dopamine. Carbidopa is such a drug and is given in conjunction with levodopa to prevent peripheral decarboxylation (see Fig. 10–4).[1,7,86] Use of carbidopa with levodopa dramatically decreases the amount of levodopa needed to achieve a desired effect, with the required levodopa dosage often being reduced by 75 to 80 percent.[4] Another decarboxylase inhibitor known as benserazide is available outside the United States, and this drug can also be used to prevent peripheral conversion of levodopa to dopamine.[7]

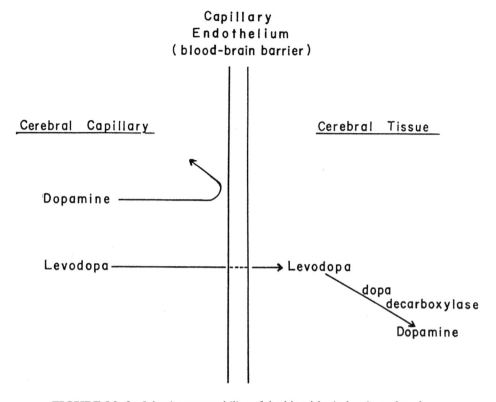

FIGURE 10–3. Selective permeability of the blood-brain barrier to levodopa.

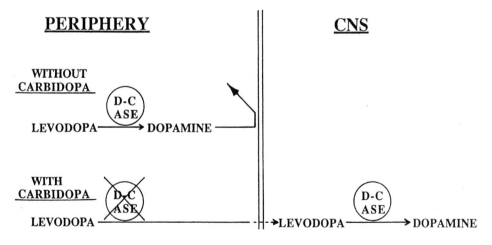

FIGURE 10–4. Use of a carbidopa, a peripheral decarboxylase inhibitor, on levodopa absorption. Without carbidopa, most of the levodopa is converted to dopamine in the periphery, rendering it unable to cross the blood-brain barrier. Carbidopa inhibits the peripheral decarboxylase (D-C ase) enzyme so that levodopa can cross the blood-brain barrier intact. Carbidopa does not cross the blood-brain barrier so that conversion of levodopa to dopamine still occurs within the CNS.

Hence, the effects of levodopa are accentuated by combining this drug with a decarboxylase inhibitor such as carbidopa; for this reason, these two drugs are often combined in the same pill and marketed under the trade name Sinemet. (Preparations of levodopa with benserazide are marketed as Madopar.) When prepared together as Sinemet, levodopa and carbidopa are combined in specific proportions, usually a fixed carbidopa-to-levodopa ratio of either 1:4 or 1:10.[7,64] The Sinemet preparation that is typically used to initiate therapy consists of tablets containing 25 mg of carbidopa and 100 mg of levodopa. This ratio is used to achieve a rapid and effective inhibition of the dopa decarboxylase enzyme. A 10:100- or 25:250-mg preparation of carbidopa to levodopa is usually instituted as the parkinsonism symptoms become more pronounced and there is a greater need for larger relative amounts of levodopa. The average maintenance dosage of levodopa is 600 to 700 mg/day, but this is highly variable according to the needs of the individual patient. Levodopa-carbidopa is also available in a controlled-release preparation (Sinemet CR) that is absorbed more slowly and is intended to provide more prolonged effects.[39,44,52] The use of this controlled-release preparation may be helpful to patients who respond well to levodopa initially but experience dyskinesias and fluctuations in response such as end-of-dose akinesia and the on-off phenomenon.[60] Problems related to levodopa therapy are described in the next section of this chapter.

PROBLEMS AND ADVERSE EFFECTS OF LEVODOPA THERAPY

Gastrointestinal Problems. Levodopa administration is often associated with nausea and vomiting. These symptoms can be severe, especially during the first few days of drug use. However, the incidence of this problem is greatly reduced if levodopa is given in conjunction with a peripheral decarboxylase inhibitor such as carbidopa. The reduction in nausea and vomiting when peripheral decarboxylation of levodopa to dopamine is inhibited suggests that these symptoms may in fact be caused by excessive levels of peripheral circulating dopamine.

Cardiovascular Problems. Some problems with cardiac arrhythmias may arise in the patient taking levodopa. However, these problems are usually fairly minor unless the patient has a history of cardiac irregularity. Caution should be used with cardiac patients undergoing levodopa therapy, especially during exercise.

Postural hypotension can also be an extremely troublesome problem for the patient taking levodopa. Again, this side effect is usually diminished when peripheral decarboxylation is inhibited and peripheral dopamine levels are not allowed to increase excessively. Still, patients undergoing physical therapy or similar regimens should be carefully observed during changes in posture and should be instructed to avoid sudden postural adjustments. This factor is especially true in patients beginning levodopa therapy or in those resuming taking levodopa after a period of time without this drug.

Dyskinesias. A more persistent and challenging problem is the appearance of various movement disorders in the patient taking levodopa for prolonged periods. Approximately 80 percent of patients receiving chronic levodopa therapy begin to exhibit various dyskinesias such as choreoathetoid movements, ballismus, dystonia, myoclonus, and various tics and tremors.[2] The specific type of movement disorder varies from patient to patient but seems to remain constant within a given patient. The onset of dyskinetic side effects is particularly frustrating in light of the ability of levodopa to ameliorate one form of movement disorder only to institute a different motor problem.

The onset of dyskinesias usually occurs after the patient has been receiving levodopa therapy for periods ranging from 3 months to several years. In some patients, these abnormal movements may simply be caused by drug-induced overstimulation of dopaminergic pathways in the basal ganglia, and decreasing the daily dosage of levodopa should help these patients. The reason for dyskinesias in other patients, however, may be far more complex. Certain patients, for example, may exhibit dyskinesias when plasma levodopa levels are rising or falling, or even when plasma levels are at a minimum.[10,64] There is evidently an intricate relationship between the basal ganglia neurons that continue to release or respond to dopamine and the pharmacologic replacement of dopamine through levopdopa therapy. Dyskinesias may actually be the result of functional and structural changes in these neurons due to a decline in normal endogenous dopaminergic influence combined with the periodic fluctuations in dopamine influence supplied from exogenous sources (levodopa).[86]

Regardless of the exact neural mechanism that underlies these dyskinesias, the goal of levodopa therapy is to find a regimen that diminishes the incapacitating parkinsonism symptoms without causing other movement disorders.[60] Strategies for minimizing dyskinesias include adjusting the dose of levodopa, using a controlled-release form of this drug, and incorporating other antiparkinson medications into the patient's drug regimen.[28,57] In some patients, dyskinesias may be somewhat difficult to control because the optimal dosage of levodopa may fall into a fairly narrow range, and some of the parkinsonism symptoms may appear quite similar to the dyskinetic side effects. The physician, physical therapist, patient, and other individuals who deal with the patient should make careful observations to determine if adjustments in levodopa therapy are resulting in the desired effect.

Behavioral Changes. A variety of mental side effects have been reported in patients taking levodopa. Psychotic symptoms seem especially prevalent, although depression, anxiety, and other changes in behavior have also been noted.[19,73] These problems are likely in older patients or in individuals who have some pre-existing psychologic disturbance.[7] Unlike the gastrointestinal and vascular problems described earlier, psychotic symptoms appear to be exacerbated if levodopa is used in conjunction with carbidopa. This event may be caused by the greater quantities of levodopa crossing the blood-brain barrier before being converted to dopamine, and thus generating higher quantities of dopamine within the brain. This idea seems logical, considering that increased activity in certain dopamine pathways seems to be the underlying cause of psychosis (see Chap. 8). Treatment of these symptoms is often difficult because traditional antipsychotic medications tend to increase the symptoms of Parkinson disease. However, some of the newer "atypical" antipsychotics such as clozapine (see Chap. 8) may help decrease psychotic symptoms without causing an increase in parkinsonism.[19,73]

Diminished Response to Levodopa. One of the most serious problems in levodopa therapy is that this drug seems to become less effective in many patients when it is administered for prolonged periods. When used continually for periods of 3 to 4 years, the ability of levodopa to relieve parkinsonism symptoms often progressively diminishes to the point where this drug is no longer effective in treating the patient.[2,57,91] One explanation for this occurrence is that the patient develops tolerance to the drug. A second theory is that the decreased effectiveness of levodopa may be caused by a progressive increase in the severity of the underlying disease rather than a decrease in drug efficacy. These two theories on the decreased effectiveness of levodopa have initiated a controversy as to whether levodopa therapy should be started early or late in the course of Parkinson disease (see "Clinical Course of Parkinson Disease: When to Use Specific Drugs"). Regardless of why this occurs, the loss of levodopa efficacy can be a devastating blow to the patient who had previously experienced excellent therapeutic results from this drug.

Fluctuations in Response to Levodopa. Several distinct fluctuations in the response to levodopa are fairly common in most patients.[2,7,57,78] **End-of-dose akinesia** describes the phenomenon in which the effectiveness of the drug simply seems to wear off prior to the next dose. This condition is usually resolved by adjusting the quantity and timing of levodopa administration (i.e., smaller doses may be given more frequently). A more bizarre and less understood fluctuation in response is the **on-off phenomenon.** Here the effectiveness of levodopa may suddenly and spontaneously decrease, resulting in the abrupt worsening of parkinsonism symptoms (off period). Remission of symptoms may then occur spontaneously or after taking a dose of levodopa (on period). This on-off pattern may repeat itself several times during the day. Although the exact reasons for this phenomenon are unclear, the off periods are directly related to diminishing plasma levels of levodopa.[65,77] These low levels may occur when the absorption of orally administered levodopa is delayed by poor gastrointestinal motility or when levodopa must compete with large amino acids for transport across the intestinal mucosa.[15,16,66] The off periods can be eliminated by administering levodopa continuously by intravenous infusion, thus preventing the fall in plasma levels. However, this is not a long-term solution, and alterations in the oral dosage schedule may have to be made in an attempt to maintain plasma levels at a relatively constant level. Specifically, the drug can be taken with smaller amounts of food and meals that are relatively low in protein so that levodopa absorption is not overwhelmed by dietary amino acid absorption. As indicated earlier, use of a controlled-release formulation such as Sinemet CR can also help alleviate various fluctuations by allowing a steadier, more controlled release of levodopa into the bloodstream, thus preventing the fluctuations in plasma levodopa that seem to be responsible for the on-off phenomenon and similar problems.

DRUG HOLIDAYS FROM LEVODOPA

Drug holidays are sometimes used in the patient who has become refractory to the beneficial effects of levodopa or has had a sudden increase in adverse side effects.[2,11] During this period, the patient is gradually removed from all antiparkinson medication for 3 days to 3 weeks while under close medical supervision. The purpose of the holiday is to allow the body to recover from any toxicity or tolerance that may have developed because of prolonged use of levodopa at relatively high dosages. Drug holidays are done with the hope that levodopa can eventually be resumed at a lower dosage and with better results. Drug holidays do appear to be successful in some patients with Parkinson disease. Beneficial effects may be achieved at only half the preholiday dosage, and the incidence of side effects (such as dyskinesias, confusion, and the on-off phenomenon) may be markedly reduced.[11,21,24,90] However, drug holidays are successful in only a limited number of patients with Parkinson disease, and there is no way of predicting which patients will benefit from such a holiday.[2,24,47] Also, there is no guarantee of how long the success will last, and the patient may return to the preholiday condition fairly quickly. Drug holidays have also been criticized lately because there is a certain amount of risk to the patient, and deaths have occurred when antiparkinson medications are suddenly discontinued.[7] Hence, drug holidays may still be used in some patients with Parkinson disease, but the continued use of this intervention remains controversial at the present time.

Other Drugs Used to Treat Parkinson Disease

DOPAMINE AGONISTS

Because the basic problem in Parkinson disease is a deficiency of striatal dopamine, it would seem logical that drugs similar in function to dopamine would be effective in treating this problem. However, many dopamine agonists have serious side effects that prevent their clinical use. A few dopamine agonists such as bromocriptine (Parlodel), pergolide (Permax), and several new agents such as pramipexole (Mirapex) and ropinirole (Requip) (see Table 10–1) have been developed to treat Parkinson disease without causing excessive adverse effects.[7,30,75,89] These dopamine agonists have traditionally been used in conjunction with levodopa, especially in patients who have begun to experience a decrease in levodopa effects, or in those who experience problems such as end-of-dose akinesia and the on-off effect.[41,75] Simultaneous administration of levodopa with a dopamine agonist permits optimal results with relatively smaller doses of each drug.

Dopamine agonists can also be used alone in the early stages of mild-to-moderate parkinsonism, thus providing an alternative if other antiparkinson drugs (including levodopa) are poorly tolerated.[25,89] For example, dopamine agonists when used alone do not usually cause the dyskinesias and fluctuations in motor responses that may occur with levodopa therapy.[89] There is also some preliminary evidence that dopamine agonists may help normalize endogenous dopamine activity and thus have a neuroprotective effect on substantia nigra neurons.[68,89] As indicated earlier, certain medications are being investigated for their potential to delay or prevent the degeneration of dopamine-producing neurons in the basal ganglia. Dopamine agonists could produce such a neuroprotective effect by preventing free radical–induced damage that is associated with abnormal dopamine synthesis and breakdown.[68,89] Future results from long-term studies should help clarify if early use of dopamine agonists is successful in slowing the progression of Parkinson disease.

Dopamine agonists may produce some adverse side effects such as nausea and vomiting. Postural hypotension is also a problem in some patients. With prolonged use, these drugs may cause CNS-related side effects such as confusion and hallucinations.

ANTICHOLINERGIC DRUGS

As mentioned previously, the deficiency of striatal dopamine results in excessive activity in certain cholinergic pathways in the basal ganglia. Consequently, drugs that limit acetylcholine transmission are used to help alleviate the symptoms of Parkinson disease, especially the tremor and rigidity associated with this disorder. Various **anticholinergic** agents are available for this purpose (Table 10–2), and these drugs work by blocking acetylcholine receptors in the basal ganglia.[86] These drugs are fairly nonselective, however, and they tend to produce a wide variety of side effects (see later) because they also block acetylcholine receptors in various other tissues throughout the body. When used alone, anticholinergics are usually only mildly to moderately successful in reducing symptoms, and they are typically used in conjunction with levodopa or other antiparkinson drugs to obtain optimal results.

TABLE 10–2 Anticholinergic Drugs Used in Treating Parkinsonism

Generic Name	Trade Name	Usual Daily Dose (mg)	Prescribing Limit (mg/day)
Benztropine	Cogentin	1.0–2.0	6
Biperiden	Akineton	6.0–8.0	16
Ethopropazine	Parsidol	50–100	600
Procyclidine	Kemadrin	7.5–15.0	20
Trihexyphenidyl	Artane	6.0–10.0	15
Diphenhydramine*	Benadryl, others	75–200	300

*Antihistamine drugs with anticholinergic properties.

Anticholinergics are associated with many troublesome side effects, including mood changes, confusion, hallucinations, drowsiness, and cardiac irregularities.[64] In addition, blurred vision, dryness of the mouth, nausea and vomiting, constipation, and urinary retention are fairly common. Antihistamine drugs with anticholinergic properties are also occasionally used (Table 10–2). These drugs tend to be somewhat less effective in treating parkinsonism but appear to have milder side effects than their anticholinergic counterparts.

AMANTADINE

Amantadine (Symmetrel) was originally developed as an antiviral drug, and its ability to reduce parkinsonian symptoms was discovered by chance.[23] Amantadine was being used to treat influenza in a patient with Parkinson disease, and a noticeable improvement in the patient's tremor and rigidity was observed. Since that time, amantadine has been approved for use in patients with Parkinson disease and is usually given along with levodopa or anticholinergic drugs. The exact mechanism of amantadine's antiparkinson activity remains unclear, although there is now evidence that this drug may inhibit the effects of excitatory amino acids (glutamate) by blocking the N-methyl-D-aspartate (NMDA) receptor in the brain.[13,31]

The primary adverse effects associated with amantadine are orthostatic hypotension, CNS disturbances (depression, confusion, hallucinations), and patches of skin discoloration on the lower extremities (livedo reticularis). However, these side effects are relatively mild compared with those of the other antiparkinson drugs and are usually reversed by altering the drug dosage.

SELEGILINE

Selegiline (deprenyl, Eldepryl) is a drug that potently and selectively inhibits the monoamine oxidase type B (MAO_B) enzyme. This enzyme is responsible for breaking down dopamine. By inhibiting this enzyme, selegiline prolongs the local effects of dopamine at CNS synapses. Thus, selegiline can be used alone in the early stages of Parkinson disease to prolong the effects of endogenous dopamine that is produced within the basal ganglia. Early administration of selegiline may alleviate motor symptoms so that patients do not need to begin taking levodopa until later in the course of this disease.[38,84] Selegiline may also be combined with levodopa therapy because selegiline prolongs the action of dopamine and allows parkinsonism symptoms to be reduced with a relatively lower dose of levodopa.[18,38,64,76]

It has also been suggested that selegiline may actually slow the progression of Parkinson disease.[71,72] Theoretically, selegiline could have neuroprotective effects because this drug inhibits dopamine oxidation, thus preventing excessive production of harmful free radicals during dopamine breakdown.[8,34] Preliminary clinical studies indicated that patients who started taking selegiline early in the course of Parkinson disease did not degenerate as quickly as patients who did not take this drug.[71] Additional research on these patients, however, indicated that the early benefits from selegiline were probably related to the symptomatic effects of this drug rather than to a protective effect on the substantia nigra neurons[67]; that is, patients appeared to have better motor function because selegiline prolonged the effects of endogenously produced dopamine. In fact, further research indicated that the progression of Parkinson disease in these patients was similar or possibly even accelerated compared with patients who did not receive selegiline.[70] Likewise, there was some preliminary evidence that administration of selegiline with levodopa may actually increase the mortality rate in patients with Parkinson disease,[69] but subsequent studies have not supported that finding.[37]

Selegiline is relatively safe in terms of short-term adverse side effects. With some MAO inhibitors, there is frequently a sudden, large increase in blood pressure if the patient ingests foods containing tyramine (see Chap. 7). However, selegiline does not appear to cause a hypertensive crisis even when such tyramine-containing foods are eaten.[37] Consequently, use of selegiline at the present time remains somewhat controversial. There is no doubt that this drug can be used alone or with levodopa to reduce the symptoms and improve motor function in people with Parkinson disease.[36,76] Additional research, however, is needed to clarify the long-term benefits and possible neuroprotective effects of selegiline.

CATECHOL-O-METHYLTRANSFERASE INHIBITORS

A relatively new drug group is being developed to enhance the effects of levodopa. These drugs inhibit an enzyme known as catechol-O-methyltransferase (COMT). This enzyme converts levodopa to an inactive metabolite known as 3-O-methyldopa; hence, these drugs are referred to as COMT inhibitors.[29,58] Because levodopa conversion is prevented in peripheral tissues, more levodopa is available to reach the brain and exert beneficial effects. Hence, these drugs are used as an adjunct to levodopa therapy to provide better therapeutic effects with smaller doses of levodopa.[5,32,81,82]

Tolcapone (Tasmar) is the drug in this category that is currently available. Other COMT inhibitors are currently being developed, and future clinical studies will determine how these agents can be used with traditional antiparkinson drugs to provide optimal treatment.

CLINICAL COURSE OF PARKINSON DISEASE: WHEN TO USE SPECIFIC DRUGS

Considerable controversy exists as to when specific antiparkinson drugs should be employed in treating this disease.[2,7,42,48] Much of the debate focuses on when levodopa therapy should be initiated. As mentioned previously, the effectiveness of this drug seems to diminish after several years of use. Consequently, some practitioners feel that levodopa therapy should be withheld until the parkinsonian symptoms become severe enough to truly impair motor function. In theory, this saves the levodopa for more advanced stages of this disease, when it would be needed the most.[20,80] In younger patients (under age 60) or in milder stages of Parkinson disease, other medications such as amantadine, anticholinergics, selegiline, or dopamine agonists could be prescribed.[83] Other physicians think that the decreased effectiveness of levodopa is simply the result of an increase in the severity of the disease itself. Consequently, there may be no advantage to delaying the start of levodopa, and it should be instituted as soon as the symptoms become obvious.[56,61] At present, the issue of when to begin levodopa remains largely unresolved, and the choice is ultimately left to the discretion of the physician.[7]

NEUROSURGICAL INTERVENTIONS IN PARKINSON DISEASE

Several innovative approaches have been studied to try to achieve a more permanent resolution to the dopamine imbalance in Parkinson disease. One approach is to surgically implant dopamine-producing cells into the substantia nigra to replace the cells that have been destroyed by the disease process.[7,35] This strategy, however, is limited by several issues, including how to get a supply of viable cells. A potential source of these cells has been from fetal mesenchymal tissues, but this approach has generated considerable concern about the ethical use of fetal tissues for medical research and treatment. An alternative source is the production of neuronlike cells from cultures of human chromaffin cells.[17] Such cell cultures could provide a viable source of dopamine-producing cells without the limitations inherent in using fetal tissues. Still, there are some practical limitations associated with implanting a sufficient number of these cells into a small area deep in the brain and then keeping these cells alive and producing dopamine. Patients who would benefit from such transplants are typically older and somewhat debilitated, with a possible reduction in blood flow and oxygenation of tissues deep in the brain. These facts, combined with the presence of the original pathologic process that caused Parkinson disease in the first place, may limit the chances for survival of the transplanted tissues.

Hence, tissue transplants have not shown overwhelming clinical success, and the future of this technique as an effective and widely used method of treating Parkinson disease remains doubtful at the present time. It may be possible that new developments, including the use of cell cultures as a source of dopamine-producing cells and the use of drugs to prolong the survival of transplanted tissues, may improve the clinical outcome of this technique. Still, it remains to be seen whether tissue transplants will ever be a practical and routine method of treating the rather large number of patients who are afflicted with Parkinson disease.

An alternative nonpharmacologic treatment is very specific surgery (pallidotomy) to interrupt specific neuronal pathways in people with advanced Parkinson disease.[49,53] There is likewise growing evidence that surgical implantation of electrodes and stimulation of deep brain structures, including the basal ganglia, may help control the motor symptoms of Parkinson disease.[27,54,88] It is beyond the scope of this chapter to review these newer surgical and electrical stimulation techniques. Nonetheless, these nonpharmacologic interventions continue to be developed and will hopefully provide an alternative treatment for patients who have become refractory to drug therapy during the advanced stages of Parkinson disease.[87]

SPECIAL CONSIDERATIONS FOR REHABILITATION

Therapists who are treating patients with Parkinson disease usually wish to coordinate the therapy session with the peak effects of drug therapy. In patients receiving levodopa, this usually occurs approximately 1 hour after a dose of the medication has been taken. If possible, scheduling the primary therapy session after the breakfast dose of levodopa often yields optimal effects from the standpoint of both maximal drug efficacy and low fatigue levels in these elderly patients.

Many therapists working in hospitals and other institutions are faced with the responsibility of treating patients who are on a drug holiday. As discussed previously, during those several days the patient is placed in the hospital and all antiparkinson medication is withdrawn so that the patient may recover from the adverse effects of prolonged levodopa administration. During the drug holiday, the goal of physical therapy is to maintain patient mobility as much as possible. Obviously, without antiparkinson drugs, this task is often quite difficult. Many patients are well into the advanced stages of this disease, and even a few days without medication can produce profound debilitating effects. Consequently, any efforts to maintain joint range of motion and cardio-vascular fitness during the drug holiday are crucial in helping the patient resume activity when medications are reinstated.

Therapists should also be aware of the need to monitor blood pressure in patients receiving antiparkinson drugs. Most of these drugs cause orthostatic hypotension, especially during the first few days of drug treatment. Dizziness and syncope often occur because of a sudden drop in blood pressure when the patient stands up. Because patients with Parkinson disease are susceptible to falls anyway, this problem is only enhanced by the chance of orthostatic hypotension. Consequently, therapists must be especially careful to guard against falls by the patient taking antiparkinson drugs.

Finally, rehabilitation specialists should recognize that they can have a direct and positive influence on the patient's health and need for drug treatment. There is consensus that an aggressive program of gait training, balance activities, and other appropriate exercises can be extremely helpful in promoting optimal health and function in patients with Parkinson disease.[9,22,74] Using physical therapy and occupational therapy to maintain motor function can diminish the patient's need for antiparkinson drugs. The synergistic effects of physical rehabilitation and the judicious use of antiparkinson drugs will ultimately provide better results than either intervention alone.

CASE STUDY

ANTIPARKINSON DRUGS

Brief History. M.M. is a 67-year-old woman who was diagnosed with Parkinson disease 6 years ago, at which time she was treated with anticholinergic drugs (i.e., benztropine, diphenhydramine). After approximately 2 years, the bradykinesia and rigidity associated with this disease began to be more pronounced, so she was started on a combination of levodopa-carbidopa. The initial levodopa dosage was 400 mg/day. She was successfully maintained on levodopa for the next 3 years, with minor adjustments in the dosage from time to time. During that time, M.M. had been living at home with her husband. During the past 12 months, her husband noted that her ability to get around seemed to be declining, so the levodopa dosage was progressively increased to 600 mg/day. The patient was also referred to physical therapy on an outpatient basis in an attempt to maintain her mobility and activities of daily living (ADL) skills. She began attending physical therapy three times per week, and a regimen designed to maintain musculoskeletal flexibility, posture, and balance was initiated.

Problem/Influence of Medication. The patient was seen by the therapist three mornings each week. After a few sessions, the therapist observed that there were certain days when the patient was able to actively and vigorously participate in the therapy program. On other days, the patient was essentially akinetic, and her active participation in exercise and gait activities was virtually impossible. There was no pattern to her good and bad days, and the beneficial effects of the rehabilitation program seemed limited by the rather random effects of her levodopa medication. The patient stated that these akinetic episodes sometimes occurred even on non-therapy days.

Decision/Solution. After discussions with the patient and her husband, the therapist realized that the morning dose of levodopa was sometimes taken with a rather large breakfast. On other days, the patient consumed only a light breakfast. In retrospect, the akinetic episodes usually occurred on days when a large morning meal was consumed. The therapist surmised that this probably occurred because the large breakfast was impairing absorption of levodopa from the gastrointestinal tract. The patient was probably exhibiting the on-off phenomenon sometimes seen in patients receiving long-term levodopa therapy, which was brought on by the impaired absorption of the drug. This problem was resolved by having the patient consistently take the morning dose with a light breakfast. On mornings when the patient was still hungry, she waited 1 hour before consuming additional food to allow complete absorption of the medication.

SUMMARY

The cause of Parkinson disease remains unknown. However, the neuronal changes that produce the symptoms associated with this movement disorder have been identified. Degeneration of dopaminergic neurons in the substantia nigra results in a deficiency of dopamine and subsequent overactivity of acetylcholine in the basal ganglia. Pharmacologic treatment attempts to rectify this dopamine-acetylcholine imbalance. Although no cure is currently available, drug therapy can dramatically improve the clinical picture in many patients by reducing the incapacitating symptoms of parkinsonism.

The use of levodopa and several other medications has allowed many patients with Parkinson disease to remain active despite the steadily degenerative nature of this disease. Levodopa, currently the drug of choice in treating parkinsonism, often produces remarkable improvements in motor function. However, levodopa is associated with several troublesome side effects, and the effectiveness of this drug tends to diminish with time. Other agents, such as dopamine agonists, amantadine, selegiline, and anticholinergic drugs, and COMT inhibitors can be used alone or in combination with levodopa or with each other to prolong the functional status of the patient. Physical therapists and other rehabilitation specialists can maximize the effectiveness of their treatments by coordinating therapy sessions with drug administration. Therapists also play a vital role in maintaining function in the patient with Parkinson disease when the efficacy of these drugs begins to diminish.

REFERENCES

1. Ahlskog, JE: Treatment of early Parkinson's disease: Are complicated strategies justified? Mayo Clin Proc 71:659, 1996.
2. Aminoff, MJ: Pharmacologic management of parkinsonism and other movement disorders. In Katzung, BG (ed): Basic and Clinical Pharmacology, ed 7. Appleton & Lange, Stamford, CT, 1998.
3. Ballard PA, Tetrud, JW, and Langston, JW: Permanent human parkinsonism due to 1-methyl-4-phenyl-1,2,3,6-tetrahydropyridine (MPTP): Seven cases. Neurology 35:949, 1985.
4. Bianchine, JR: Drug therapy of parkinsonism. N Engl J Med 295:814, 1976.
5. Bonifati, V and Meco, G: New, selective catechol-O-methyltransferase inhibitors as therapeutic agents in Parkinson's disease. Pharmacol Ther 81:1, 1999.
6. Burns, RS, et al: A primate model of parkinsonism: Selective destruction of dopaminergic neurons in pars compacta of the substantia nigra by N-methyl-4-phenyl-1,2,3,6-tetrahydropyridine. Proc Natl Acad Sci U S A 80:4546, 1983.
7. Calne, DB: Drug therapy: Treatment of Parkinson's disease. N Engl J Med 329:1021, 1993.
8. Ciccone, CD: Free-radical toxicity and antioxidant medications in Parkinson's disease. Phys Ther 78:313, 1998.
9. Comela, CL, et al: Physical therapy and Parkinson's disease: A controlled clinical trial. Neurology 44:376, 1994.

10. Contin, M, et al: Pharmacokinetic optimisation in the treatment of Parkinson's disease. Clin Pharmacokinet 30:463, 1996.
11. Corona, T, et al: A longitudinal study of the effects of an L-dopa drug holiday on the course of Parkinson's disease. Clin Neuropharmacol 18:325, 1995.
12. Cutson, TM, Laub, KC, and Schenkman, M: Pharmacological and nonpharmacological interventions in the treatment of Parkinson's disease. Phys Ther 75:363, 1995.
13. Danielczyk, W: Twenty-five years of amantadine therapy in Parkinson's disease. J Neural Transm Suppl 46:399, 1995.
14. DeLong, MR: The basal ganglia. In Kandel, ER, Schwartz, JH, and Jessell, TM (eds): Principles of Neural Science, ed 4. McGraw-Hill, New York, 2000.
15. Djaldetti, R and Melamed, E: Management of response fluctuations: Practical guidelines. Neurology 51(Suppl 2):S36, 1998.
16. Djaldetti, R, Ziv, I, and Melamed, E: Impaired absorption of oral levodopa: A major cause of response fluctuations in Parkinson's disease. Isr J Med Sci 32:1224, 1996.
17. Drucker-Colin, R, et al: Transplant of cultured neuron-like differentiated chromaffin cells in a Parkinson's disease patient. A preliminary report. Arch Med Res 30:33, 1999.
18. Elizan, TS, Moros, DA, and Yahr, MD: Early combination of selegiline and low-dose levodopa as initial symptomatic therapy in Parkinson's disease: Experience in 26 patients receiving combined therapy for 26 months. Arch Neurol 48:31, 1991.
19. Factor, SA, et al: Parkinson's disease: Drug-induced psychiatric states. Adv Neurol 65:115, 1995.
20. Fahn, S and Bressman, SB: Should levodopa therapy for parkinsonism be started early or late? Evidence against early treatment. Can J Neurol Sci 11(Suppl):200, 1984.
21. Feldman, RG, Kaye, JA, and Lannon, MC: Parkinson's disease: Follow-up after "drug holiday." J Clin Pharmacol 26:662, 1986.
22. Formisano, R, et al: Rehabilitation and Parkinson's disease. Scand J Rehabil Med 24:157, 1992.
23. Forssman, B, Kihlstrand, S, and Larsson, LE: Amantadine therapy in parkinsonism. Acta Neurol Scand 48:1, 1972.
24. Friedman, JH: Drug holidays in the treatment of Parkinson's disease. A brief review. Arch Intern Med 145:913, 1985.
25. Fukuyama, H, et al: Bromocriptine therapy in early-stage Parkinson's disease. Eur Neurol 36:164, 1996.
26. Gelb, DJ, Oliver, E, and Gilman, S: Diagnostic criteria for Parkinson disease. Arch Neurol 56:33, 1999.
27. Ghika, J, et al: Efficiency and safety of bilateral contemporaneous pallidal stimulation (deep brain stimulation) in levodopa-responsive patients with Parkinson's disease with severe motor fluctuations: A 2-year follow-up review. J Neurosurg 89:713, 1998.
28. Giron, LT and Koller, WC: Methods of managing levodopa-induced dyskinesias. Drug Saf 14:365, 1996.
29. Goetz, CG: Influence of COMT inhibition on levodopa pharmacology and therapy. Neurology 50(Suppl 5):S26, 1998.
30. Goetz, CG: New strategies with dopaminergic drugs: Modified formulations of levodopa and novel agonists. Exp Neurol 144:17, 1997.
31. Greulich, W and Fenger, E: Amantadine in Parkinson's disease: Pro and contra. J Neural Transm Suppl 46:415, 1995.
32. Guay, DR: Tolcapone, a selective catechol-O-methyltransferase inhibitor for treatment of Parkinson's disease. Pharmacotherapy 19:6, 1999.
33. Hagan, JJ, et al: Parkinson's disease: Prospects for improved drug therapy. Trends Pharmacol Sci 18:156, 1997.
34. Hao, R, Ebadi, M, and Pfeiffer, RF: Selegiline protects dopaminergic neurons in culture from toxic factors present in cerebrospinal fluid of patients with Parkinson's disease. Neurosci Lett 200:77, 1995.
35. Hauser, RA, et al: Long-term evaluation of bilateral fetal nigral transplantation in Parkinson's disease. Arch Neurol 56:179, 1999.
36. Hauser, RA and Zesiewicz, TA: Management of early Parkinson's disease. Med Clin North Am 83:393, 1999.
37. Heinonen, EH and Myllyla, V: Safety of selegiline (deprenyl) in the treatment of Parkinson's disease. Drug Saf 19:11, 1998.
38. Hely, MA and Morris, JG: Controversies in the treatment of Parkinson's disease. Curr Opin Neurol 9:308, 1996.
39. Hempel, AG, et al: Pharmacoeconomic analysis of using Sinemet CR over standard Sinemet in parkinsonian patients with motor fluctuations. Ann Pharmacother 32:878, 1998.
40. Hirsch, EC: Mechanism and consequences of nerve cell death in Parkinson's disease. J Neural Transm Suppl 56:127, 1999.
41. Hoehn, MMM and Elton, RL: Low doses of bromocriptine added to levodopa in Parkinson's disease. Neurology 35:199, 1985.
42. Hubble, JP: Novel drugs for Parkinson's disease. Med Clin North Am 83:525, 1999.
43. Hurtig, HI: Problems with current pharmacologic treatment of Parkinson's disease. Exp Neurol 144:10, 1997.
44. Hutton, JT and Morris, JL: Long-acting carbidopa-levodopa in the management of moderate and advanced Parkinson's disease. Neurology 42(Suppl 1):51, 1992.

45. Jenner, P and Olanow, CW: Oxidative stress and the pathogenesis of Parkinson's disease. Neurology 47(Suppl 3):S161, 1996.
46. Jenner, P, Schapira, AHV, and Marsden, CD: New insights into the cause of Parkinson's disease. Neurology 42:2241, 1992.
47. Kofman, OS: Are levodopa "drug holidays" justified? Can J Neurol Sci 11(Suppl):206, 1984.
48. Koller, WC: Initiating treatment of Parkinson's disease. Neurology 42(Suppl 1):33, 1992.
49. Kondziolka, D, et al: Outcomes after stereotactically guided pallidotomy for advanced Parkinson's disease. J Neurosurg 90:197, 1999.
50. Langston, JW: MPTP and Parkinson's disease. Trends Neurosci 8:79, 1985.
51. Langston, JW, et al: Selective nigral toxicity after systemic administration of 1-methyl-4-phenyl-1,2,5,6-tetrahydropyridine (MPTP) in the squirrel monkey. Brain Res 292:390, 1984.
52. LeWitt, PA: Clinical studies with and pharmacokinetic consideration of sustained-released levodopa. Neurology 42(Suppl 1):29, 1992.
53. Limousin, P, et al: The effects of posteroventral pallidotomy on the preparation and execution of voluntary hand and arm movements in Parkinson's disease. Brain 122:315, 1999.
54. Limousin, P, et al: Electrical stimulation of the subthalamic nucleus in advanced Parkinson's disease. N Engl J Med 339:1105, 1998.
55. Markey, SP, et al (eds): MPTP: A Neurotoxin Producing a Parkinsonian Syndrome. Academic Press, New York, 1986.
56. Markham, CH and Diamond, SG: Long-term follow up of early DOPA treatment in Parkinson's disease. Ann Neurol 19:365, 1986.
57. Marsden, CD: Problems with long-term levodopa therapy for Parkinson's disease. Clin Neuropharmacol 17(Suppl 2):S32, 1994.
58. Martinez-Martin, P and O'Brien, CF: Extending levodopa action: COMT inhibition. Neurology 50(Suppl 6): S27, 1998.
59. Maruyama, W, et al: An endogenous MPTP-like dopaminergic neurotoxin, N-methyl(R)salsolinol, in the cerebrospinal fluid decreases with progression of Parkinson's disease. Neurosci Lett 262:13, 1999.
60. Montgomery, EB: Pharmacokinetics and pharmacodynamics of levodopa. Neurology 42(Suppl 1):17, 1992.
61. Muenter, MD: Should levodopa therapy be started early or late? Can J Neurol Sci 11(Suppl):295, 1984.
62. Myllyla, VV, et al: Selegiline as initial treatment in de novo parkinsonian patients. Neurology 42:339, 1992.
63. Naoi, M and Maruyama, W: Type B monoamine oxidase and neurotoxins. Eur Neurol 33(Suppl 1):31, 1993.
64. Nelson, MV, Berchou, RC, and LeWitt, PA: Parkinson's disease. In: DiPiro, JT, et al (eds): Pharmacotherapy: A Pathophysiologic Approach, ed 4. Appleton & Lange, Stamford, CT, 1999.
65. Nutt, JG, et al: Effect of long-term therapy on the pharmacodynamics of levodopa: Relation to on-off phenomenon. Arch Neurol 49:1123, 1992.
66. Nutt, JG, et al: The "on-off" phenomenon in Parkinson's disease. N Engl J Med 310:483, 1984.
67. Olanow, CW: Selegiline: Current perspectives on issues related to neuroprotection and mortality. Neurology 47(Suppl 3):S210, 1996.
68. Olanow, CW, Jenner, P, and Brooks, D: Dopamine agonists and neuroprotection in Parkinson's disease. Ann Neurol 44(Suppl 1):S167, 1998.
69. Parkinson's Disease Research Group of the United Kingdom: Comparison of therapeutic effects and mortality data of levodopa and levodopa combined with selegiline in patients with early, mild Parkinson's disease. BMJ 311:1602, 1995.
70. Parkinson's Study Group: Impact of deprenyl and tocopherol treatment on Parkinson's disease in DATATOP subjects not requiring levodopa. Ann Neurol 39:29, 1996.
71. Parkinson's Study Group: Effects of tocopherol and deprenyl on the progression of disability in early Parkinson's disease. N Engl J Med 328:176, 1993.
72. Parkinson's Study Group: Effects of deprenyl on the progression of disability in early Parkinson's disease. N Engl J Med 321:1364, 1989.
73. Peyser, CE, et al: Psychoses in Parkinson's disease. Semin Clin Neuropsychiatry 3:41, 1998
74. Pfeiffer, R: Optimization of levodopa therapy. Neurology 42(Suppl 1):39, 1992.
75. Poewe, W: Adjuncts to levodopa therapy: Dopamine agonists. Neurology 50(Suppl 6):S23, 1998.
76. Przuntek, H, et al: SELEDO: A 5-year long-term trial on the effect of selegiline in early parkinsonian patients treated with levodopa. Eur J Neurol 6:141, 1999.
77. Quinn, N, Parkes, JD, and Marsden, CD: Control of on/off phenomenon by continuous infusion of levodopa. Neurology 34:1131, 1984.
78. Quinn, NP: Classification of fluctuations in patients with Parkinson's disease. Neurology 51(Suppl 2):S25, 1998.
79. Rajput, AH: Environmental causation of Parkinson's disease. Arch Neurol 50:651, 1993.
80. Rajput, AH, Stern, W, and Laverty, WH: Chronic low-dose levodopa therapy in Parkinson's disease: An argument for delaying levodopa therapy. Neurology 34:991, 1984.
81. Ruottinen, HM and Rinne, UK: COMT inhibition in the treatment of Parkinson's disease. J Neurol 245(Suppl 3):P25, 1998.
82. Siderowf, A and Kurlan, R: Monoamine oxidase and catechol-O-methyltransferase inhibitors. Med Clin North Am 83:445, 1999.
83. Silver, DE and Ruggieri, S: Initiating therapy for Parkinson's disease. Neurology 50(Suppl 6):S18, 1998.

84. Silverstein, PM: Moderate Parkinson's disease. Strategies for maximizing treatment. Postgrad Med 99:52, 1996.
85. Simonian, NA and Coyle, JT: Oxidative stress in neurodegenerative diseases. Annu Rev Pharmacol Toxicol 36:83, 1996.
86. Standaert, DG and Young, AB: Treatment of central nervous system degenerative disorders. In Hardman, JG, et al (eds): The Pharmacological Basis of Therapeutics, ed 9. McGraw-Hill, New York, 1996.
87. Starr, PA, Vitek, JL, and Bakay, RA: Ablative surgery and deep brain stimulation for Parkinson's disease. Neurosurgery 43:989, 1998.
88. Volkmann, J, et al: Bilateral high-frequency stimulation of the internal globus pallidus in advanced Parkinson's disease. Ann Neurol 44:953, 1998.
89. Watts, RL: The role of dopamine agonists in early Parkinson's disease. Neurology 49(Suppl 1):S34, 1997.
90. Weiner, WJ, et al: Drug holiday and the management of Parkinson's disease. Neurology 30:1257, 1980.
91. Yahr, MD: Limitations of long-term use of antiparkinson drugs. Can J Neurol Sci 11(Suppl):191, 1984.

CHAPTER 11

General Anesthetics

The discovery and development of anesthetic agents has been one of the most significant contributions to the advancement of surgical technique. Before the use of anesthesia, surgery was used only as a last resort and was often performed with the patient conscious but physically restrained by several large "assistants." During the past century, general and local anesthetic drugs have been used to allow surgery to be performed in a manner that is both safer and much less traumatic for the patient and that permits lengthier and more sophisticated surgical procedures.

Anesthetics are categorized as general or local, depending on whether the patient remains conscious when the anesthetic is administered. General anesthetics are usually administered during more extensive surgical procedures. Local anesthetics are given when analgesia is needed in a relatively small, well-defined area or when the patient should remain conscious during surgery. The use of general anesthesia and general anesthetic agents is presented in this chapter; local anesthetics are dealt with in Chapter 12.

Most physical therapists and other rehabilitation specialists are not usually involved in working with patients while general anesthesia is actually being administered. However, knowledge of how these agents work will help the therapist understand some of the residual effects that may occur when the patient is recovering from the anesthesia. This knowledge will help the therapist understand how these effects may directly influence the therapy sessions that take place during the first few days after procedures in which general anesthesia was used.

GENERAL ANESTHESIA: REQUIREMENTS

During major surgery (such as laparotomy, thoracotomy, joint replacement, amputation), the patient should be unconscious throughout the procedure and, upon awakening, have no recollection of what occurred during the surgery. An ideal anesthetic agent must be able to produce each of the following conditions:

1. Loss of consciousness and sensation.
2. Amnesia (i.e., no recollection of what occurred during the surgery).
3. Skeletal muscle relaxation (this requirement is currently met with the aid of skeletal muscle blockers used in conjunction with the anesthetic; see "Neuromuscular Blockers").

4. Inhibition of sensory and autonomic reflexes.
5. A minimum of toxic side effects (i.e., be relatively safe).
6. Rapid onset of anesthesia; easy adjustment of the anesthetic dosage during the procedure; and rapid, uneventful recovery after administration is terminated.

Current general anesthetics meet these criteria quite well, providing that the dosage is high enough to produce an adequate level of anesthesia but not so high that problems occur. The relationship between dosage and level or plane of anesthesia is discussed in the next section.

STAGES OF GENERAL ANESTHESIA

During general anesthesia, the patient goes through a series of stages as the anesthetic dosage and the amount of anesthesia reaching the brain progressively increase. Four stages of anesthesia are commonly identified[35]:

Stage I. Analgesia: The patient begins to lose somatic sensation but is still conscious and somewhat aware of what is happening.
Stage II. Excitement (Delirium):   The patient is unconscious and amnesiac but appears agitated and restless. This paradoxical increase in the level of excitation is highly undesirable because patients may injure themselves while thrashing about. Thus, an effort is made to move as quickly as possible through this stage and on to stage III.
Stage III. Surgical Anesthesia: As the name implies, this level is desirable for the surgical procedure and begins with the onset of regular, deep respiration. Some sources subdivide this stage according to respiration rate and reflex activity.[20]
Stage IV. Medullary Paralysis: This stage is marked by the cessation of spontaneous respiration because respiratory control centers located in the medulla oblongata are inhibited by excessive anesthesia. The ability of the medullary vasomotor center to regulate blood pressure is also affected, and cardiovascular collapse ensues. If this stage is inadvertently reached during anesthesia, respiratory and circulatory support must be provided or the patient will die.[35]

Consequently, the goal of the anesthetist is to bring the patient to stage III as rapidly as possible and to maintain the patient at that stage for the duration of the surgical procedure. This goal is often accomplished by using both an intravenous and an inhaled anesthetic agent (see "General Anesthetic Agents: Classification and Use According to Route of Administration"). Finally, the anesthetic should not be administered for any longer than necessary, or recovery will be delayed. This state is often accomplished by beginning to taper off the dosage toward the end of the surgical procedure, so that the patient is already recovering as the surgery is completed.

GENERAL ANESTHETIC AGENTS: CLASSIFICATION AND USE ACCORDING TO ROUTE OF ADMINISTRATION

Specific agents are classified according to the two primary routes of administration: intravenous or inhaled.[22,35] Intravenously injected anesthetics offer the advantage of a rapid onset, thus allowing the patient to pass through the first two stages of anesthesia very quickly. The primary disadvantage is that there is a relative lack of control over the level of anesthesia if too much of the drug is injected. Inhaled anesthetics provide an easier method of making adjustments in the dosage during the procedure, but it takes a relatively long time for the onset of the appropriate level of anesthesia when administered through inhalation. Consequently, a combination of injected and inhaled agents is often used sequentially during the lengthier surgical procedures. The intravenous drug is injected first to quickly get the patient to stage III, and an inhaled agent is then administered to maintain the patient in a stage of surgical anesthesia. Ultimately, the selection of exactly which agents will be used depends on the type and length of the surgical procedure and any possible interactions with other anesthetics or the medical problems of the patient. Specific injected and inhaled anesthetics are presented here.

GENERAL ANESTHETICS: SPECIFIC AGENTS

Inhalation Anesthetics

Anesthetics administered by this route exist either as gases or as volatile liquids that can be easily mixed with air or oxygen and then inhaled by the patient. A system of tubing and valves is usually employed to deliver the anesthetic drug directly to the patient through an endotracheal tube or a mask over the patient's face (Fig. 11–1). This delivery system offers the obvious benefit of focusing the drug on the patient without anesthetizing everyone else in the room. These systems also allow for easy adjustment of the rate of delivery and concentration of the inhaled drug.

Inhaled anesthetics currently in use include halogenated volatile liquids such as halothane, enflurane, desflurane, isoflurane, and methoxyflurane (Table 11–1). These volatile liquids are all chemically similar, but newer agents such as desflurane and sevoflurane are often used preferentially because they permit a more rapid onset, faster recovery, and better control during anesthesia compared with older agents such as halothane.[10,12] These volatile liquids likewise represent the primary form of inhaled anesthetics. The only gaseous anesthetic currently in widespread use is nitrous oxide,

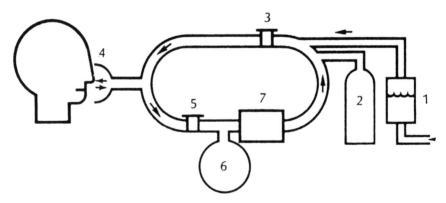

FIGURE 11–1. Schematic diagram of a closed anesthesia system. (*1*) Vaporizer for volatile liquid anesthetics. (*2*) Compressed gas source. (*3*) Inhalation unidirectional valve. (*4*) Mask. (*5*) Unidirectional exhalation valve. (*6*) Rebreathing bag. (*7*) Carbon dioxide absorption chamber. (From Brown, BR: Pharmacology of general anesthesia. In Clark, WG, Brater, DC, and Johnson, AR: Goth's Medical Pharmacology, ed 13. CV Mosby, St. Louis, 1992, p 385, with permission.)

TABLE 11–1 General Anesthetics

Anesthetic	Representative Structure
Inhaled Anesthetics	

Volatile liquids
  Enflurane (Ethrane)
  Halothane (Fluothane)
  Isoflurane (Forane)
  Methoxyflurane (Penthrane)
	Halothane

Gas Nitrous oxide	Nitrous oxide
Intravenous Anesthetics	

Barbiturates
  Methohexital (Brevital)
  Thiopental (Pentothal)
	Thiopental

Benzodiazepines
  Diazepam (Valium)
  Lorazepam (Ativan)
  Midazolam (Versed)
	Diazepam

Opioids
  Fentanyl derivatives (Sublimaze, others)
  Meperidine (Demerol)
  Morphine
	Meperidine

Ketamine (Ketalar)	Ketamine

which is usually reserved for relatively short-term procedures (e.g., tooth extractions). Earlier inhaled anesthetics, such as ether, chloroform, and cyclopropane, are not currently used because they are explosive in nature or they produce toxic effects that do not occur with the more modern anesthetic agents.

Intravenous Anesthetics

When given in appropriate doses, several categories of CNS depressants can serve as general anesthetics (see Table 11–1).[22,33] The most widely used are the barbiturate drugs such as thiopental and methohexital. Barbiturates are noted for their fast onset (when administered intravenously) and relative safety when used appropriately. Several other types of drugs, including benzodiazepines (diazepam, lorazepam, midazolam) and opioid analgesics (fentanyl, morphine, meperidine, others), have also been used to induce or help maintain general anesthesia. These other agents are often used as preoperative sedatives, but larger doses can be used alone or in combination with other general anesthetics to produce anesthesia in short surgical or diagnostic procedures or when other general anesthetics may be contraindicated (e.g., cardiovascular disease).

Another intravenous general anesthetic is ketamine (Ketalar). This agent produces a somewhat different type of condition known as *dissociative anesthesia*.[22,35] This term is used because of the clinical observation that the patient appears detached or dissociated from the surrounding environment. The patient appears awake but is sedated and usually unable to recall events that occurred when the ketamine was in effect. Dissociative anesthesia is useful during relatively short diagnostic or surgical procedures (e.g., endoscopy) or during invasive procedures in children.[34,35] A similar type of anesthesia is produced by combining the opioid fentanyl with the antipsychotic drug droperidol. The combination of these two agents produces a condition known as *neuroleptanalgesia*, which is also characterized by dissociation of the patient from what is happening around him or her with or without loss of consciousness.[4] An inhaled anesthetic such as nitrous oxide can also be added to convert neuroleptanalgesia to a deeper level of dissociation known as neuroleptanesthesia.[22] Neuroleptanalgesia and neuroleptanesthesia are typically used for short surgical procedures, including endoscopy or burn dressings, or for patients who are seriously ill and may not tolerate general anesthesia by more conventional methods.

Finally, newer intravenous anesthetics such as etomidate (Amidate) and propofol (Diprivan) are available. Etomidate is a hypnotic-like drug that causes a rapid onset of general anesthesia with a minimum of cardiopulmonary side effects. Hence, this drug may be useful in patients with compromised cardiovascular or respiratory function. Propofol is a short-acting hypnotic that is useful as a general anesthetic in some short invasive procedures, and it can be used as an adjunct to other general anesthetics in longer procedures. Recovery from propofol may also be more rapid than with other anesthetics, making this drug useful when early mobilization of the patient is desirable.

PHARMACOKINETICS

Following either injection or inhalation administration, general anesthetics become widely and uniformly distributed throughout the body, largely because of their high degree of lipid solubility. As a result, a great deal of the anesthetic may be temporarily stored in adipose tissues and slowly wash out of these tissues when the patient is recovering from surgery. If the person was anesthetized for an extended period of time and has large deposits of fat, this washout may take quite some time.[9] During this period, symptoms such as confusion, disorientation, and lethargy may occur, presumably because the drug is being redistributed to the CNS. The patient's age also influences anesthetic requirements and distribution, with older individuals usually requiring less anesthetic for a given procedure.[19] Because older people need smaller concentrations of anesthetic, the chance that, during surgery, more anesthetic may be administered than is needed is increased, and recovery will be somewhat delayed.

Depending on the individual drug, elimination occurs through excretion of the drug from the lungs, biotransformation in the liver, or a combination of these two methods.[8,11] If the patient has any pulmonary or hepatic dysfunction, elimination of the anesthetic will be further delayed.

MECHANISM OF ACTION

A great deal of debate still exists as to how general anesthetics work. Clearly, these drugs are able to inhibit the neuronal activity within all levels of the CNS, and generally they decrease the level of consciousness in the brain through an effect on neurons in the reticular activating system. However, the exact way in which these drugs affect these neurons remains speculative. In the past, it was believed that general anesthetics primarily affected the lipid bilayer of CNS neurons. This so-called general perturbation theory was based on the premise that general anesthetic molecules become dissolved directly in the lipid bilayer of the nerve membrane and temporarily disrupt membrane function by increasing membrane fluidity and disturbing the phospholipid environment that surrounds the protein channel.[16,17,21] Membrane excitability would be decreased because ion channels, including the sodium channels, are unable to open and allow the influx of sodium needed to initiate an action potential (Fig. 11–2). The primary support for the membrane perturbation theory was the direct correlation between anesthetic potency and lipid solubility,[21] meaning that the more easily the drug can become dissolved in the bilayer, the less drug is needed to achieve a given level of anesthesia. This theory was further supported by the fact that general anesthetics all produce a similar effect, even though they have quite diverse chemical structures (see Table 11–1). Presumably, if drugs bind to some type of receptor, they should share some structural similarities.

More recent evidence, however, suggests that general anesthetics primarily affect CNS synaptic transmission by binding directly to protein channels.[14,15,30] This idea is certainly logical for the injected anesthetics such as the barbiturates, benzodiazepines, and opioids. As discussed in Chapter 6, the barbiturates and the benzodiazepines work by binding to CNS chloride ion channels and thereby enhancing the inhibitory effects of gamma-aminobutyric acid (GABA). Opioids decrease transmission in nociceptive pathways by binding to specific presynaptic and postsynaptic receptors in the brain and spinal cord (see Chap. 14). Other injected anesthetics also appear to affect synaptic transmission by binding to protein receptors. Etomidate and propofol, for example, appear to bind to GABA receptors and enhance the inhibitory effects of GABA when these drugs are used at lower dosages yet exerting a direct GABA-like effect at higher doses.[24,28] Ketamine seems to work by binding to

No Drug
(Na⁺ channel shown open)

Anesthetized
(Na⁺ channel closed)

A. General Perturbation Theory

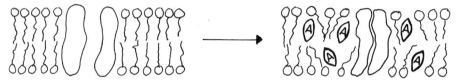

B. Specific Receptor Theory

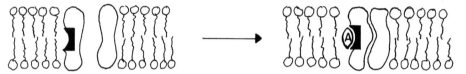

FIGURE 11–2. Schematic illustration of two possible ways in which general anesthetics may act on the nerve membrane. In the general perturbation theory, anesthetic molecules lodge in the lipid bilayer and inhibit sodium channel function by disrupting membrane structure. In the specific receptor theory, anesthetics inhibit opening of the sodium channel by binding directly to the channel protein.

N-methyl-D-aspartate (NMDA) receptors in the brain, thus inhibiting the excitatory effects of glutamate.[35]

Injected anesthetics therefore act on specific protein channels and exert their effects by either increasing the effects at inhibitory synapses or decreasing the effects at excitatory synapses in the CNS. It appears that many of the inhaled anesthetics also bind to protein receptors and modify synaptic transmission. For example, the classic inhaled agents (halothane, enflurane, and similar drugs) appear to act primarily at GABA receptors and enhance the inhibitory effects of GABA in the CNS.[18,27] This idea is a departure from the general perturbation theory described earlier—that is, that the inhaled anesthetics affected the lipid bilayer rather than a specific protein. The details of how inhaled anesthetics affect GABA receptors remain somewhat unclear. It is not known, for example, if these agents bind to the outer portion of the GABA receptor, within the central pore of the receptor, or at some other site such as the interface between the receptor and adjacent phospholipids (see Fig. 11–2). The preponderance of evidence, however, suggests that these drugs bind to a site somewhere on or near the GABA receptor protein rather than via a general effect on the lipid bilayer.

Other proteins, including the receptors for acetylcholine, glycine, and serotonin may also be affected by various general anesthetics, and specific agents may exert their anesthetic effects by binding to certain types of receptors in certain synaptic pathways in the CNS.[3,13] Research will continue to clarify the mechanism of these drugs, and future studies may lead to newer agents that produce more selective anesthetic effects by acting at specific receptor sites in the brain and spinal cord.

ADJUVANTS IN GENERAL ANESTHESIA

Preoperative Medications

Frequently, a preoperative sedative is given to the patient 1 to 2 hours before the administration of general anesthesia.[20,23,25,36] Sedatives are usually administered via intramuscular injection and are given while the patient is still in his or her room. This approach serves to relax the patient and reduce anxiety when the patient arrives at the operating room. Frequently used preoperative sedatives include barbiturates (secobarbital, pentobarbital), opioids (morphine, meperidine), and benzodiazepines (diazepam, lorazepam) (Table 11–2). Different sedatives are used, depending on the patient, the type of general anesthesia used, and the preference of the physician.

A number of other medications may be used preoperatively to achieve various goals (see Table 11–2).[20,25,36] Antihistamines (promethazine, hydroxyzine) offer the dual advantages of producing sedation and reducing vomiting (antiemesis). Antacids and other drugs that increase gastric pH are sometimes used to decrease stomach acidity and thus reduce the risk of serious lung damage if gastric fluid is aspirated during general surgery. In the past, anticholinergics (atropine, scopolamine) were often administered to help reduce bronchial secretions and aid in airway intubation. However, anesthetics currently in use do not produce excessive airway secretions (as did prior agents), so the preoperative use of anticholinergics is no longer critical.[23,25]

Neuromuscular Blockers

Skeletal muscle paralysis is essential during surgical procedures. The patient must be relaxed to allow proper positioning on the operating table and to prevent spontaneous muscle contractions from hampering the surgery.[7,32] Imagine the disastrous effects that a muscular spasm in the arm would have on a delicate procedure such as

TABLE 11–2 Drugs and Doses Used for Preoperative Premedication

Classification	Drug	Typical Adult Dose (mg)	Route of Administration (Oral, IM*)
Barbiturates	Secobarbital	50–150	Oral, IM
	Pentobarbital	50–150	Oral, IM
Opioids	Morphine	5–15	IM
	Meperidine	50–100	IM
Benzodiazepines	Diazepam	5–10	Oral
	Lorazepam	2–4	Oral, IM
Antihistamines	Diphenhydramine	25–75	Oral, IM
	Promethazine	25–50	IM
	Hydroxyzine	50–100	IM
Anticholinergics	Atropine	0.3–0.6	IM
	Scopolamine	0.3–0.6	IM
	Glycopyrrolate	0.1–0.3	IM
Antacids	Particulate	15–30 mL	Oral
	Nonparticulate	15–30 mL	Oral

*IM = intramuscular.
Source: Modified from Stoelting, RK: Psychological preparation and preoperative medication. In Stoelting, RK and Miller, RD (eds): Basics of Anesthesia. Churchill Livingstone, New York, 1984, p 381, with permission.

nerve repair or limb reattachment. Most currently used general anesthetics produce skeletal muscle relaxation, but it takes a larger dose of the anesthetic to produce adequate muscular relaxation than is needed to produce unconsciousness and amnesia; that is, the patient must be well into stage III and almost into stage IV before muscle paralysis is complete. Consequently, a drug that blocks the skeletal neuromuscular junction is given in conjunction with the general anesthetic to allow a lower dose of anesthetic to be used while still ensuring skeletal muscle paralysis. These drugs work by blocking the postsynaptic acetylcholine receptor located at the skeletal neuromuscular junction.

Several different neuromuscular blockers are currently available, and the choice of a specific agent depends primarily on the desired length of action and the potential side effects of each agent (Table 11–3).[6,29] Possible side effects include cardiovascular problems (tachycardia), increased histamine release, and immunologic reactions (anaphylaxis).[1,6,26] Selection of a specific agent is therefore designed to minimize the risk of a specific side effect in a specific patient; for example, a drug that produces relatively few cardiovascular effects would be selected for the patient with cardiovascular disease. Efforts are also made to use small doses of relatively short-acting agents so that the length of muscle paralysis is kept to a minimum.[31] The paralytic effects of these agents should therefore disappear by the end of the surgical procedure. However, complications such as prolonged paralysis, hyperkalemia, and muscle rigidity may occur, especially if the patient has a concurrent neuromuscular condition such as a spinal cord injury, peripheral neuropathies, intracranial lesions, or muscle pathologies.[2] It should be realized, however, that neuromuscular junction blockers are an adjunct to general anesthesia but that these blockers do not cause anesthesia or analgesia when used alone.[31] The patient must therefore receive an adequate amount of the general anesthetic throughout the surgery when a neuromuscular junction blocker is used. This idea is critical in that the patient will be paralyzed by the neuromuscular junction blocker and unable to respond to painful stimuli if the anesthesia is inadequate. Failure to provide adequate anesthesia has resulted in some harrowing reports from patients who were apparently fully awake during surgery but unable to move or cry out.[31]

Discussed here are the two general types of neuromuscular blockers, which are clas-

TABLE 11–3 Neuromuscular Junction Blockers

Drug	Onset of Initial Action* (min)	Time to Peak Effect (min)	Duration of Peak Effect (min)
Nondepolarizing blockers			
Atracurium	Within 2	3–5	20–35
Gallamine	1–2	3–5	15–30
Pancuronium	Within 0.75	4.5	35–45
Tubocurarine	Within 1	2–5	20–40
Vecuronium	1	3–5	25–30
Depolarizing blockers			
Succinylcholine	0.5–1	1–2	4–10

*Reflects usual adult intravenous dosage.

Source: Copied from *USP DI®, 20th Edition* Copyright 2000. The USP Convention, Inc. Permission granted. The USP is not responsible for any inaccuracy of quotation nor for any false or misleading implication that may arise due to the text used or due to the quotation of information subsequently changed in later editions.

sified according to whether they depolarize the skeletal muscle cell when binding to the cholinergic receptor.[5,6]

Nondepolarizing Blockers. These drugs act as competitive antagonists of the post-synaptic receptor; that is, they bind to the receptor but do not activate it (see Chap. 4). This binding prevents the agonist (acetylcholine) from binding to the receptor, and paralysis of the muscle cell results. These drugs all share a structural similarity, which apparently explains their affinity and relative selectivity for the cholinergic receptor at the skeletal neuromuscular junction. Specific agents and their onset and duration of action are listed in Table 11–3.

Depolarizing Blockers. Although these drugs also inhibit transmission at the skeletal neuromuscular junction, their mechanism is different from that of the nondepolarizing agents. These drugs initially act like acetylcholine by binding to and stimulating the receptor, resulting in depolarization of the muscle cell. However, the enzymatic degradation of the drug is not as rapid as the destruction of acetylcholine, so the muscle cell remains depolarized for a prolonged period of time. While depolarized, the muscle is unresponsive to further stimulation. The cell must become repolarized or reprimed before the cell will respond to a second stimulus. This event is often referred to as phase I blockade.[29] If the depolarizing blocker remains at the synapse, the muscle cell does eventually repolarize but remains unresponsive to stimulation by acetylcholine. This occurrence is referred to as phase II blockade and is believed to occur because the drug exerts some sort of modification on the receptor. This modification could be in the form of a temporary conformational change on the receptor. Clinically, when these drugs are first administered, they are often associated with a variable amount of muscle tremor and fasciculation (because of the initial depolarization), but this is followed by a period of flaccid paralysis. Although several drugs that act as depolarizing blockers are available, the only agent currently in clinical use is succinylcholine (see Table 11–3).[5]

SPECIAL CONCERNS IN REHABILITATION

The major problems that a rehabilitation specialist may encounter occur when the patient is not quite over the effects of the anesthesia. Dealing with a patient the day after surgery or possibly even the same day as surgery may be difficult because the patient is woozy. Some anesthetics may produce confusion or psychotic-like behavior during the recovery period. Muscle weakness may also be present for a variable amount of time, especially if a neuromuscular blocker was used during the surgical procedure. Of course, patients who are in relatively good general health and who have had relatively short or minor surgeries will have minimal residual effects. However, patients who are debilitated or who have other medical problems that impair drug elimination may continue to show some anesthesia aftereffects for several days. These problems should disappear with time, so the therapist must plan activities accordingly until recovery from the anesthetic effects is complete.

Another problem that therapists frequently deal with is the tendency for bronchial secretions to accumulate in the lungs of patients recovering from general anesthesia. General anesthetics depress mucociliary clearance in the airway, leading to pooling of mucus, which may produce respiratory infections and atelectasis. Therapists play an important role in preventing this accumulation by encouraging early mobilization of the patient and by implementing respiratory hygiene protocols (i.e., breathing exercises and postural drainage).

CASE STUDY

GENERAL ANESTHETICS

Brief History. B.W., a 75-year-old woman, fell at home and experienced a sudden sharp pain in her left hip. She was unable to walk and was taken to a nearby hospital, where x-ray examination showed an impacted fracture of the left hip. The patient was alert and oriented at the time of admission. She had a history of arteriosclerotic cardiovascular disease and diabetes mellitus, but her medical condition was stable. The patient was relatively obese, and a considerable amount of osteoarthritis was present in both hips. Two days after admission, a total hip arthroplasty was performed under general anesthesia. Meperidine (Demerol) was given intramuscularly as a preoperative sedative. General anesthesia was induced by intravenous administration of thiopental (Pentothal) and sustained by inhalation of halothane (Fluothane). The surgery was completed successfully, and physical therapy was initiated at the patient's bedside on the subsequent day.

Problem/Influence of Medication. At the initial therapy session, the therapist found the patient to be extremely lethargic and disoriented. She appeared confused about recent events and was unable to follow most commands. Apparently, she was experiencing some residual effects of the general anesthesia.

Decision/Solution. The patient's confusion and disorientation precluded any activities that required her cooperation, including any initial attempts at weight-bearing activities. The therapist limited the initial session to passive and active-assisted exercises of both lower extremities. Active upper-extremity exercises were encouraged within the limitations of the patient's ability to follow instructions. These upper-extremity exercises were instituted to help increase metabolism and excretion of the remaining anesthesia. The patient was also placed on a program of breathing exercises in an effort to facilitate excretion of the anesthetic, as well as to maintain respiratory function and prevent the accumulation of mucus in the airways. As the patient's mental disposition gradually improved, partial weight bearing in the parallel bars was initiated. From there, the patient progressed to a walker and was soon able to ambulate independently with that device. Within 1 week after the surgery, no overt residual effects of the anesthesia were noted, and the remainder of the hospital stay was uneventful.

SUMMARY

General anesthesia has been used for some time to permit surgical procedures of various types and durations to be performed. Several different effective agents are currently available and relatively safe in producing a suitable anesthetic condition in the patient. General anesthetics are classified according to their two primary routes of administration: by inhalation and by intravenous infusion. Specific anesthetic agents and anesthetic adjuvants (preoperative sedatives, neuromuscular blockers, etc.) are selected primarily according to the type of surgical procedure being performed and the overall condition of the patient. Health professionals should be cognizant of the fact that their patients may take some time to fully recover from the effects of general anesthesia and should adjust their postoperative care of the patient accordingly.

REFERENCES

1. Abel, M, Book, WJ, and Eisenkraft, JB: Adverse effects of nondepolarizing neuromuscular blocking agents. Incidence, prevention and management. Drug Saf 10:420, 1994.
2. Azar, I: Complications of neuromuscular blockers. Interaction with concurrent diseases. Anesthesiol Clin North Am 11:409, 1993.
3. Barann, M, Wenningmann, I, and Dilger, JP: Interaction of general anesthetics within the pore of an ion channel. Toxicol Lett 100:155, 1998.
4. Bissonnette, B, et al: Neuroleptanesthesia: Current status. Can J Anaesth 46:154, 1999.
5. Booij, LH: Neuromuscular transmission and its pharmacological blockade. Part 2: Pharmacology of neuromuscular blocking agents. Pharm World Sci 19:13, 1997.
6. Book, WJ, Abel, M, and Eisenkraft, JB: Adverse effects of depolarizing neuromuscular blocking agents. Incidence, prevention and management. Drug Saf 10:331, 1994.
7. Brull, SJ and Silverman, DG: Intraoperative use of muscle relaxants. Anesthesiol Clin North Am 11:325, 1993.
8. Carpenter, RL, Eger, EI, and Johnson, BH: Pharmacokinetics of inhaled anesthetics in humans: Measurements during and after the simultaneous administration of enflurane, halothane, isoflurane, methoxyflurane and nitrous oxide. Anesth Analg 65:572, 1986.
9. Carpenter, RL, et al: The extent of metabolism of inhaled anesthetics in humans. Anesthesiology 65:201, 1986.
10. Clark, KW: Desflurane and sevoflurane. New volatile anesthetic agents. Vet Clin North Am Small Anim Pract 29:793, 1999.
11. Davis, PJ and Cook, DR: Clinical pharmacokinetics of the newer intravenous anesthetic agents. Clin Pharmacokinet 11:18, 1986.
12. Eger, EI: New drugs in anesthesia. Int Anesthesiol Clin 33:61, 1995.
13. Flood, P and Role, LW: Neuronal nicotinic acetylcholine receptor modulation by general anesthetics. Toxicol Lett 100:149, 1998.
14. Forman, SA, Miller, KW, and Yellen, G: A discrete site for general anesthetics on a postsynaptic receptor. Mol Pharmacol 48:574, 1995.
15. Franks, NP and Lieb, WR: Molecular and cellular mechanisms of general anaesthesia. Nature 367:607, 1994.
16. Godin, DV and McGinn, P: Perturbational actions of barbiturate analogs on erythrocyte and synaptosomal membranes. Can J Physiol Pharmacol 63:937, 1985.
17. Goldstein, DB: The effects of drugs on membrane fluidity. Annu Rev Pharmacol Toxicol 24:43, 1984.
18. Hirota, K, et al: GABAergic mechanisms in the action of general anesthetics. Toxicol Lett 100:203, 1998.
19. Homer, TD and Stanski, DR: The effect of increasing age on thiopental disposition and anesthetic requirement. Anesthesiology 62:714, 1985.
20. Kennedy, SK and Longnecker, DE: History and principles of anesthesiology. In Hardman, JG, et al (eds): The Pharmacological Basis of Therapeutics, ed 9. McGraw-Hill, New York, 1996.
21. Koblin, DD: Mechanisms of action. In Miller, RD (ed): Anesthesia, Vol 1, ed 5. Churchill Livingstone, Philadelphia, 2000.
22. Marshall, BE and Longnecker, DE: General anesthetics. In Hardman, JG, et al (eds): The Pharmacological Basis of Therapeutics, ed 9. McGraw-Hill, New York, 1996.
23. Mirakhur, RK: Preanesthetic medication: A survey of current usage. J R Soc Med 84:481, 1991.
24. Moody, EJ, et al: Distinct structural requirements for the direct and indirect actions of the anaesthetic etomidate at $GABA_A$ receptors. Toxicol Lett 100:209, 1998.
25. Moyers, JR: Preoperative medication. In Barash, PG, Cullen, BF, and Stoelting, RK (eds): Clinical Anesthesia. JB Lippincott, Philadelphia, 1989.
26. Naguib, M and Magboul, MM: Adverse effects of neuromuscular blockers and their antagonists. Middle East J Anesthesiol 14:341, 1998.
27. Narahashi, T, et al: Ion channel modulation as the basis for general anesthesia. Toxicol Lett 100:185, 1998.
28. Orser, BA, et al: General anesthetics and their effects on $GABA_A$ receptor desensitization. Toxicol Lett 100:217, 1998.
29. Ramsey, FM: Basic pharmacology of the neuromuscular blocking agents. Anesthesiol Clin North Am 11:219, 1993.
30. Richards, CD: The synaptic basis of general anaesthesia. Eur J Anaesthesiol 12:5, 1995.
31. Savarese, JJ, et al: Pharmacology of muscle relaxants and their antagonists. In Miller, RD (ed): Anesthesia, Vol 1, ed 5. Churchill Livingstone, Philadelphia, 2000.
32. Shanks, CA: Pharmacokinetics of the nondepolarizing neuromuscular relaxants applied to calculation of bolus and infusion dosage regimens. Anesthesiology 64:72, 1986.
33. Stoelting, RK: Pharmacology and Physiology in Anesthetic Practice, ed 3. Lippincott-Raven, Philadelphia, 1999.
34. Tobias, JD, et al: Oral ketamine premedication to alleviate the distress of invasive procedures in pediatric oncology patients. Pediatrics 90:537, 1992.
35. Trevor, AJ and Miller, RD: General anesthetics. In Katzung, BG (ed): Basic and Clinical Pharmacology, ed 7. Appleton & Lange, Stamford, CT, 1998.
36. White, SE: The preoperative visit and premedication. In Kirby, RR and Gravenstein, N (eds): Clinical Anesthesia Practice. WB Saunders, Philadelphia, 1994.

CHAPTER 12

Local Anesthetics

Local anesthesia is used to produce loss of sensation in a specific body part or region. Frequently, this application occurs when a relatively minor surgical procedure is to be performed. This approach involves introducing an anesthetic drug near the peripheral nerve that innervates the area in question. The basic goal is to block afferent neural transmission along the peripheral nerve so that the procedure can be performed painlessly. When the local anesthetic is introduced in the vicinity of the spinal cord, transmission of impulses may be effectively blocked at a specific level of the cord to allow more extensive surgical procedures to be performed (e.g., caesarean delivery) because a larger region of the body is being anesthetized. This approach, however, is still considered a form of local anesthesia because the drug acts locally at the spinal cord and the patient remains conscious during the surgical procedure.

Using a local anesthetic during a surgical procedure offers several advantages over the use of general anesthesia, including the relatively rapid recovery and lack of residual effects from the local anesthetic.[7,9,47] There is a virtual absence of the postoperative confusion and lethargy often seen after general anesthesia. In most cases of minor surgery, patients are able to leave the practitioner's office or the hospital almost as soon as the procedure is completed. In more extensive procedures, local anesthesia offers the advantage of not interfering with cardiovascular, respiratory, and renal function. This fact can be important in patients with problems in these physiologic systems. During childbirth, local (spinal) anesthesia imposes less of a risk to the neonate than general anesthesia.[52] The primary disadvantages of local anesthesia are the length of time required to establish an anesthetic effect and the risk that analgesia will be incomplete or insufficient for the procedure.[7] The latter problem can usually be resolved by administering additional local anesthesia if the procedure is relatively minor or by switching to a general anesthetic during a major procedure in the event of an emergency arising during surgery.

Local anesthetics are sometimes used to provide analgesia in nonsurgical situations. These drugs may be used for short-term pain relief in conditions such as musculoskeletal and joint pain (e.g., bursitis, tendinitis), or in longer-term situations such as pain relief in cancer. Also, local anesthetics may be used to block efferent sympathetic activity in conditions such as complex regional pain syndrome. During these nonsurgical applications, physical therapists and other rehabilitation personnel often will be directly involved in treating the patient while the local anesthetic is in effect. If prescribed by the physician, the local anesthetic may actually be administered by the physical therapist via iontophoresis or phonophoresis. Consequently, these individuals should have an adequate knowledge of the pharmacology of local anesthetic agents.

TYPES OF LOCAL ANESTHETICS

Commonly used local anesthetics are listed in Table 12–1. These drugs share a common chemical strategy consisting of both a lipophilic and hydrophilic group, connected

TABLE 12–1 Common Local Anesthetics

Generic Name	Trade Name(s)	Relative Onset* of Action	Relative Duration* of Action	Principal Use(s)
Benzocaine	Americaine, others	—	—	Topical
Bupivacaine	Marcaine, Sensorcaine	Slow to intermediate	Long	Infiltration Peripheral nerve block Epidural Spinal Sympathetic block
Butamben	Butesin	—	—	Topical
Chloroprocaine	Nesacaine	Rapid	Short	Infiltration Peripheral nerve block Epidural Intravenous regional block
Dibucaine	Nupercainal	—	—	Topical
Etidocaine	Duranest	Rapid	Long	Infiltration Peripheral nerve block Epidural
Lidocaine	Xylocaine	Rapid	Intermediate	Infiltration Peripheral nerve block Epidural Spinal Transdermal Topical Sympathetic block Intravenous regional block
Mepivacaine	Carbocaine, Polocaine	Intermediate to rapid	Intermediate	Infiltration Peripheral nerve block Epidural Intravenous regional block
Pramoxine	Prax, Tronothane	—	—	Topical
Prilocaine	Citanest	Rapid	Intermediate	Infiltration Peripheral nerve block
Procaine	Novocain	Intermediate	Short	Infiltration Peripheral nerve block Spinal
Tetracaine	Pontocaine	Rapid	Intermediate to long	Topical Spinal

*Values for onset and duration of action refer to use during injection. Relative durations of action are as follows: short = 30–60 min; intermediate = 1–3 hr; and long = 3–10 hr of action.

Source: Copied from *USP DI®, 20th Edition* Copyright 2000. The USP Convention, Inc. Permission granted. The USP is not responsible for any inaccuracy of quotation nor for any false or misleading implication that may arise due to the text or due to the quotation of information subsequently changed in later editions.

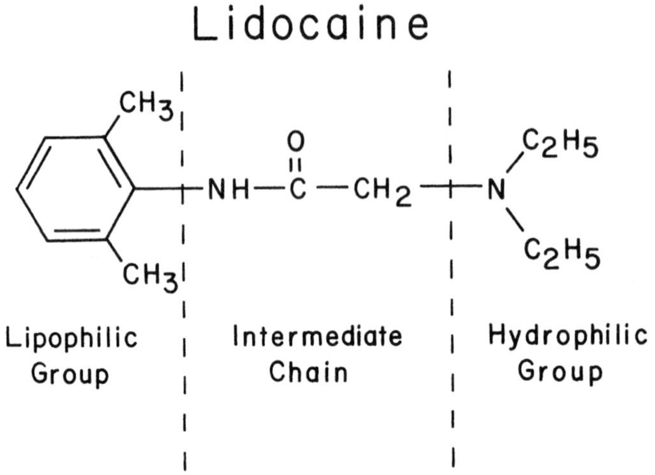

Lidocaine

Lipophilic Group | Intermediate Chain | Hydrophilic Group

FIGURE 12-1. Structure of lidocaine. The basic structure of a lipophilic and hydrophilic group connected by an intermediate chain is common to the local anesthetics.

by an intermediate chain (Fig. 12–1). The choice of a specific local anesthetic is made depending on factors such as (1) the operative site and nature of the procedure, (2) the type of regional anesthesia desired (such as single peripheral nerve block or spinal anesthesia), (3) the patient's size and general health, and (4) the duration of action of the anesthetic.[3]

Local anesthetics can usually be identified by their "-caine" suffix (lidocaine, procaine, and so on). Cocaine was identified as the first clinically useful local anesthetic in 1884. However, its tendency for abuse and its high incidence of addiction and systemic toxicity initiated the search for safer local anesthetics such as those in Table 12–1. One should note that cocaine abuse is based on its effects on the brain, not for its local anesthetic effects. Cocaine is believed to produce intense feelings of euphoria and excitement through increased synaptic transmission in the brain. This fact explains why cocaine abusers inject this drug or apply it to the nasal mucous membranes (i.e., "snorting," so that it is absorbed through those membranes and into the systemic circulation, where it ultimately reaches the brain).

PHARMACOKINETICS

Local anesthetics are administered through a variety of routes and techniques depending on the specific clinical situation (see "Clinical Use of Local Anesthetics"). In local anesthesia, the drug should remain at the site of administration. For instance, procaine (Novocain) injected into the area of the trigeminal nerve during a dental procedure will be more effective if it is not washed away from the site of administration by the blood flow through that region. Likewise, injection of a local anesthetic into the area surrounding the spinal cord (e.g., epidural or spinal injection; see "Clinical Use of Local Anesthetics") will be more effective if the drug remains near the administration site.[2] Consequently, a vasoconstricting agent (e.g., epinephrine) is often administered simultaneously to help prevent washout from the desired site.[9] Preventing the anesthetic from reaching the bloodstream is also beneficial because local anesthetics can cause toxic side effects when sufficient amounts reach the systemic circulation (see "Systemic Effects of Local Anesthetics"). This occurrence is usually not a problem in most cases of a single dose of regional anesthesia, but the build-up of the local anesthetic in the bloodstream should be monitored if these drugs are administered repeatedly or if the drug is administered continuously to treat chronic pain.[22]

Local anesthetics are usually eliminated by hydrolyzing or breaking apart the drug molecule. This metabolic hydrolysis is catalyzed by hepatic enzymes or enzymes circulating in the plasma (e.g., the plasma cholinesterase). Once metabolized, the polar drug metabolites are excreted by the kidney.

CLINICAL USE OF LOCAL ANESTHETICS

The primary clinical uses of local anesthetics, according to their method of administration and specific indications, are presented here.

1. *Topical administration.* Local anesthetics can be applied directly to the surface of the skin, mucous membranes, cornea, and other regions to produce analgesia, and this is usually done for the symptomatic relief of minor surface irritation and injury (minor burns, abrasions, inflammation). Local anesthetics can also be applied topically to reduce pain prior to minor surgical procedures such as wound cleansing, myringotomy, and circumcision.[20,27,28,49] Topical anesthesia can be produced in these situations by applying a single agent or by applying a mixture of two or more local anesthetics (e.g, lidocaine and prilocaine).[6,25,30,45]

    Topical anesthesia has also been used to improve motor function in some patients with skeletal muscle hypertonicity that resulted from a cerebrovascular accident or head trauma.[40] In this situation, a local anesthetic (e.g., 20 percent benzocaine) can be sprayed on the skin that overlies hypertonic muscles, and then various exercises and facilitation techniques can be performed to increase and improve mobility in the affected limbs. The rationale of this treatment is to temporarily decrease abnormal or excessive excitatory feedback of cutaneous receptors on efferent motor pathways so that normal integration and control of motor function can be re-established. Preliminary evidence has suggested that repeated applications of this technique may produce fairly long-lasting improvements in joint mobility and gait characteristics in patients with hypertonicity caused by various CNS disorders.[40]

2. *Transdermal administration.* The drug is applied to the surface of the skin or other tissues with the intention that the drug will be absorbed into underlying tissues. Transdermal administration of some local anesthetics may be enhanced by the use of electrical current (iontophoresis) or ultrasound (phonophoresis) (see Appendix A).[10,24,44] These approaches offer the advantage of treating painful subcutaneous structures (bursae, tendons, other soft tissues) without breaking the skin. Physical therapists can therefore use iontophoresis and phonophoresis to administer local anesthetics such as lidocaine for treating certain musculoskeletal injuries. However, a comprehensive discussion of the efficacy of these techniques in physical therapy practice is beyond the scope of this chapter. Readers are directed to several references at the end of this chapter that address this topic in more detail.[8,10,13,54]

    Administration of local anesthetics via iontophoresis can also be used to produce topical anesthesia prior to certain dermatologic procedures. For example, lidocaine iontophoresis can adequately anesthetize a small patch of skin so that a minor surgical procedure (placement of an intravenous catheter, laser treatment of port-wine stains, and so forth) can be performed.[1,26,36,53] Iontophoretic application of local anesthetics offers a noninvasive alternative to subcutaneous injection of these drugs, and use of iontophoresis seems to be gaining popularity as a method for producing local anesthesia before specific dermatologic surgeries.

3. *Infiltration anesthesia.* The drug is injected directly into the selected tissue and allowed

to diffuse to sensory nerve endings within that tissue. This technique is used to saturate an area such as a skin laceration so that surgical repair (suturing) can be performed.

4. *Peripheral nerve block.*   The anesthetic is injected close to the nerve trunk so that transmission along the peripheral nerve is interrupted.[50] This type of local anesthesia is common in dental procedures (restorations, tooth extractions, and so on) and can also be used to block other peripheral nerves to allow certain surgical procedures or to reduce pain and improve function in chronic conditions such as rheumatoid arthritis.[16] Injection near larger nerves (sciatic) or around a nerve plexus (brachial plexus) can also be used to anesthetize larger areas of an upper or lower extremity.[32,46,50] Nerve blocks can be classified as minor, when only one distinct nerve (e.g., ulnar, median) is blocked, or major, when several peripheral nerves or a nerve plexus (brachial, lumbosacral) is involved.

5. *Central neural blockade.*   The anesthetic is injected within the spaces surrounding the spinal cord[5] (Fig.12–2). Specifically, the term **epidural nerve blockade** refers to injection of the drug into the epidural space—that is, the space between the bony vertebral column and the dura mater. A variation of epidural administration known as

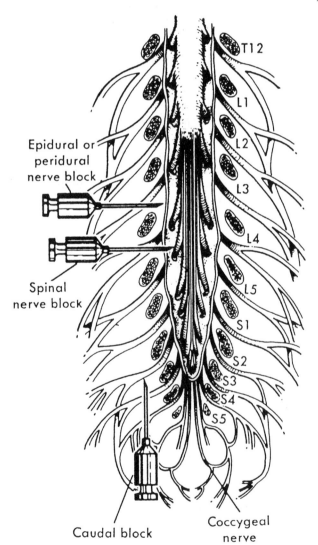

Epidural or peridural nerve block

Spinal nerve block

Caudal block

Coccygeal nerve

T12
L1
L2
L3
L4
L5
S1
S2
S3
S4
S5

FIGURE 12–2. Sites of epidural and spinal administration of local anesthetics. Caudal block represents epidural administration via the sacral hiatus. (From Clark, JB, Queener, SF, and Karb, VB: Pharmacological Basis of Nursing Practice, ed 4. CV Mosby, St. Louis, 1993, p 688, with permission.)

a "caudal block" is sometimes performed by injecting the local anesthetic into the lumbar epidural space via the sacral hiatus (see Fig. 12–2). **Spinal nerve blockade** refers to injection within the subarachnoid space—that is, the space between the arachnoid membrane and the pia mater. Spinal blockade is also referred to as "intrathecal anesthesia" because the drug is injected within the tissue sheaths that surround the spinal cord (*intrathecal* means within a sheath; see Chapter 2).

In theory, epidural and spinal blocks can be done at any level of the cord, but they are usually administered at the L3-4 or L4-5 vertebral interspace (i.e., caudal to the L-2 vertebral body, which is the point where the spinal cord ends). Epidural anesthesia is somewhat easier to perform than spinal blockade because the epidural space is larger and more accessible than the subarachnoid space. However, spinal anesthesia usually creates a more effective or solid block using a smaller amount of the local anesthetic.[5] The drawback, of course, is that higher concentrations of the drug are administered in close proximity to neural structures during spinal anesthesia. Local anesthetics are neurotoxic when administered in high concentrations.[21] Spinal anesthesia therefore carries a somewhat higher risk for neurotoxicity because a relatively large amount of the local anesthetic is being introduced fairly close to the spinal cord and related neural structures (cauda equina). Any physical damage from the injection technique or neurotoxicity from the local anesthetic drugs will therefore be more problematic during spinal administration than during use of the epidural route.

Central neural blockade is used whenever analgesia is needed in a large region, and epidural and spinal routes are used frequently to administer local anesthetics during obstetric procedures, including caesarean delivery. These routes can also be used as an alternative to general anesthesia for various other surgical procedures, including lumbar spine surgery and hip and knee arthroplasty.[5,47] The epidural and intrathecal routes have also been used to administer anesthetics and narcotic analgesics for relief of acute and chronic pain.[31,33] In these instances, an indwelling catheter is often left implanted in the epidural or subarachnoid space to allow repeated or continuous delivery of the anesthetic to the patient. The use of implanted drug delivery systems in managing chronic and severe pain is discussed further in Chapters 14 and 17.

6. *Sympathetic block.* Although blockade of sympathetic function usually occurs during peripheral and central nerve blocks, sometimes the selective interruption of sympathetic efferent discharge is desirable. This intervention is especially useful in cases of complex regional pain syndrome (CRPS). This syndrome, known also as reflex sympathetic dystrophy syndrome (RSDS) and causalgia, involves increased sympathetic discharge to an upper or lower extremity, often causing severe pain and dysfunction in the distal part of the extremity. As part of the treatment, a local anesthetic can be administered to interrupt sympathetic discharge to the affected extremity.[37,48] One approach is to inject the local anesthetic into the area surrounding the sympathetic chain ganglion that innervates the affected limb. For example, injection near the stellate ganglion is performed when the upper extremity is involved, and injections around the sympathetic ganglion at the L-2 vertebral level are used for lower-extremity CRPS.[23,38] Usually, a series of five injections on alternate days is necessary to attenuate the sympathetic discharge and provide remission from the CRPS episode. Alternatively, the local anesthetic can be administered subcutaneously to an affected area[29] or injected intravenously into the affected limb by using regional intravenous block techniques (see next section).[12,55] Hence, several techniques are currently being used to promote sympathetic blockade with local anesthetic drugs. With these techniques, the anesthetic is not to provide analgesia but rather to impair efferent sympathetic outflow to the affected extremity.

7. *Intravenous Regional Anesthesia (Bier block).* During intravenous regional anesthesia

(also known as Bier block), the anesthetic is injected into a peripheral vein located in a selected limb (arm or leg).[9] The local vasculature can then carry the anesthetic to the nerves in that extremity, thereby producing anesthesia in the limb. A tourniquet is also applied proximally on the limb to temporarily localize the drug within the extremity and to prevent the anesthetic from reaching the systemic circulation, where it would cause toxic effects on the heart and CNS. This technique is somewhat difficult to use because the tourniquet can cause pain, and diminished blood flow to the extremity can cause nerve damage (ischemic neuropathy) if it is left in place for more than 2 hours.[9] Intravenous regional block, however, can be used to anesthetize the forearm-hand or distal leg-ankle-foot for short periods to allow certain surgical procedures or to treat conditions such as CRPS.

MECHANISM OF ACTION

Local anesthetics work by blocking action potential propagation along neuronal axons, which is thought to occur from the anesthetic molecule inhibiting the opening of membrane sodium channels.[9,15,43] The sudden influx of sodium into the neuron through open (activated) ion channels depolarizes the neuron during impulse propagation. If the sodium ion channels are inhibited from opening along a portion of the axon, the action potential will not be propagated past that point. If the neuron is sensory in nature, this information will not reach the brain, and anesthesia of the area innervated by that neuron will result.

Exactly how the local anesthetic inhibits sodium channel opening has been the subject of much debate. Although several theories exist, the current consensus is that local anesthetics temporarily attach to a binding site or receptor located on or within the sodium channel.[9,15,43] These receptors probably control the opening of the channel, and when bound by the anesthetic molecule, the sodium channel is maintained in a closed, inactivated position. Several sites have been proposed to explain exactly where the local anesthetic binds on the sodium channel protein (Fig. 12–3).[9,43] The most likely binding

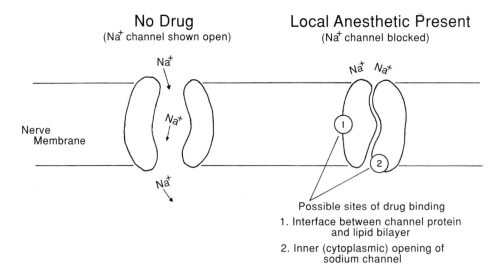

FIGURE 12–3. Schematic diagram showing mechanism of action of local anesthetics on the nerve membrane. Local anesthetics appear to inhibit channel opening by binding to one of the sites indicated.

site is within the lumen or pore of the channel itself, possibly at the inner, cytoplasmic opening of the channel.[9,15] When bound by the anesthetic molecule, this site may effectively lock the sodium channel shut (much in the same way that the appropriate key fitting into a door keyhole is able to lock a door).

Consequently, local anesthetics appear to bind directly to sodium channels on the nerve axon. By keeping these channels in a closed, inactivated state, the anesthetic prevents action potential propagation along the affected portion of the axon. Any sensory or motor information transported by that neuron cannot be transmitted past the point of the blockade.

DIFFERENTIAL NERVE BLOCK

Differential nerve block refers to the ability of a given local anesthetic dose to block specific nerve fiber groups and not others, depending on the size (diameter) of the nerve fibers.[9,39,43] In general, smaller diameter fibers seem to be the most sensitive to anesthetic effects, with progressively larger fibers affected as anesthetic concentration increases.[14,18,35] This point is significant because different diameter fibers transmit different types of information (Table 12–2). Thus, information transmitted by the smallest fibers will be lost first, with other types of transmission successively lost as the local anesthetic effect increases. The smallest diameter (type C) fibers that transmit pain are usually the first sensory information blocked as the anesthetic takes effect. Type C fibers also transmit postganglionic autonomic information, including the sympathetic vasomotor control of the peripheral vasculature, and are also most susceptible to block by local anesthetics. Other sensory information such as temperature, touch, and position sense (proprioception) is successively lost as the concentration and effect of the anesthetic increase. Finally, skeletal motor function is usually last to disappear, because efferent impulses to the skeletal muscle are transmitted over the large, type A–alpha fibers.

The exact reason for the differential susceptibility of nerve fibers based on their axonal diameter is not known. One possible suggestion is that the anesthetic is simply able to diffuse more rapidly and completely around the thinner fibers, thus inactivating them first.[51] In fact, some evidence suggests that it is actually the largest (type A) fibers that are the most susceptible to various types of stress, including that of local anesthetic drugs.[19] However, the larger fibers are the last ones affected because of the relatively poor ability

TABLE 12–2 Relative Size and Susceptibility to Block of Types of Nerve Fibers

Fiber Type*	Function	Diameter (μm)	Myelination	Conduction Velocity (m/s)	Sensitivity to Block
Type A					
Alpha	Proprioception, motor	12–20	Heavy	70–120	+
Beta	Touch, pressure	5–12	Heavy	30–70	++
Gamma	Muscle spindles	3–6	Heavy	15–30	++
Delta	Pain, temperature	2–5	Heavy	12–30	+++
Type B	Preganglionic autonomic	<3	Light	3–15	++++
Type C					
Dorsal root	Pain	0.4–1.2	None	0.5–2.3	++++
Sympathetic	Postganglionic	0.3–1.3	None	0.7–2.3	++++

*Fiber types are classified according to the system established by Gasser and Erlanger.[18]
Source: Katzung, BG (ed): Basic and Clinical Pharmacology, ed 7. Appleton & Lange, Stamford, CT, 1998, p 429, with permission.

of the drug to reach them. Myelination, which is found more extensively in larger-diameter fibers, may also play a role in differential nerve block, although exactly how myelination affects anesthetic efficacy is complex and somewhat unclear. In any event, from a clinical perspective the smaller-diameter fibers are the ones that appear to be affected first, although the exact reasons for this phenomenon remain to be determined.

The clinical importance of a differential nerve block is that certain sensory modalities may be blocked without the loss of motor function. Fortuitously, the most susceptible modality is pain because analgesia is usually the desired effect. If the dosage and administration of the anesthetic are optimal, analgesia will be produced without any significant loss of skeletal muscle function. This fact may be advantageous if motor function is required, such as during labor and delivery.[52] If local anesthetics are used to produce sympathetic blockade, postganglionic type C fibers are fortunately the first to be blocked, thus producing the desired effect at the lowest anesthetic concentration.

SYSTEMIC EFFECTS OF LOCAL ANESTHETICS

The intent of administering a local anesthetic is to produce a regional effect on specific neurons. However, these drugs may occasionally be absorbed into the general circulation and exert various effects on other organs and tissues. The most important systemic effects involve the central nervous system and the cardiovascular system.[34,41,42] Virtually all local anesthetics stimulate the brain initially, and symptoms such as somnolence, confusion, agitation, excitation, and seizures can occur if sufficient amounts of local anesthetic reach the brain via the bloodstream.[17,34,41] Central excitation is usually followed by a period of CNS depression. This depression may result in impaired respiratory function, and death may occur because of respiratory depression.[34] The primary cardiovascular effects associated with local anesthetics include decreased cardiac excitation, decreased heart rate, and decreased force of contraction.[34] Again, this general inhibitory effect on the myocardium may produce serious consequences if sufficient amounts of the local anesthetic reach the general circulation.[41]

Systemic effects are more likely to occur if an excessive dose is used, if absorption into the bloodstream is accelerated for some reason, or if the drug is accidentally injected into the systemic circulation rather than into extravascular tissues.[34] Other factors that can predispose a patient to systemic effects include the type of local anesthetic administered and the route and method of administration.[3] Therapists and other health-care professionals should always be alert for signs of the systemic effects of local anesthetics in patients receiving these drugs. Early recognition of symptoms listed in the preceding paragraph (confusion, restlessness, bradycardia, and so forth) may help avert fatalities due to the systemic effects of these drugs.

SIGNIFICANCE IN REHABILITATION

Because of the various clinical applications of local anesthetics, physical therapists may encounter the use of these agents in several patient situations. Therapists may be directly involved in the topical or transdermal administration of local anesthetics. As discussed earlier, repeated topical application of local anesthetics may help produce long-term improvements in motor function in patients with skeletal muscle hypertonicity, so therapists may want to consider incorporating topical anesthetics into the treatment of certain patients with CNS dysfunction. Therapists may also administer local anesthetics transdermally, using the techniques of iontophoresis and phonophoresis. Agents such as lidocaine can be administered through these methods for the treatment of acute inflammation in bursitis, tendinitis, and so on.

Therapists may also be working with patients who are receiving local anesthetic injections for the treatment of CRPS/RSDS. These patients often receive a series of anesthetic injections, so therapists may want to schedule the rehabilitation session immediately after each injection so that exercises and other rehabilitation techniques are performed while the anesthetic is still in effect. This strategy may help re-establish normal sympathetic function and blood flow to the affected extremity so that optimal results are obtained from the sympathetic blockade.

Finally, therapists may work with patients who are receiving central neural blockade in the form of an epidural or spinal injection. These procedures are common during natural and caesarean childbirth and in some other surgical procedures. Administration of local anesthetics into the spaces around the spinal cord may also be used to treat individuals with severe and chronic pain—that is, patients recovering from extensive surgery, patients who have cancer, or patients with other types of intractable pain. In these situations, therapists may notice that an indwelling catheter has been placed in the patient's epidural or subarachnoid space to allow repeated or sustained administration of the spinal anesthesia.

In situations when central neural blockade is used, therapists should be especially aware that sensation may be diminished below the level of epidural or spinal administration. Decreased sensation to thermal agents and electrical stimulation can occur when the central block is in effect.[4] Likewise, motor function may be affected in the lower extremities when local anesthetics are administered spinally or epidurally.[11] Hence, therapists should test sensation and motor strength before applying any physical agents or attempting ambulation with patients who have received some type of central neural blockade with a local anesthetic.

CASE STUDY

LOCAL ANESTHETICS

Brief History. R.D. is a 35-year-old man who developed pain in his right shoulder after spending the weekend chopping firewood. He was examined by a physical therapist and evaluated as having supraspinatus tendinitis. Apparently, this tendinitis recurred intermittently, usually after extensive use of the right shoulder. During past episodes, the tendinitis was resistant to treatment and usually took several months to resolve.

Decision/Solution. The therapist began an aggressive rehabilitation program of daily heat, ultrasound, soft-tissue massage, and exercise. Soft-tissue massage consisted of transverse-friction techniques applied to the supraspinatus tendon. In order to improve the patient's tolerance to this technique, 5 percent lidocaine (Xylocaine) solution was administered via iontophoresis prior to the transverse-friction massage. This approach allowed both the massage technique and subsequent exercises to be performed more aggressively by the therapist and patient, respectively. Under this regimen, the supraspinatus tendinitis was resolved and the patient had full, pain-free use of the right shoulder within 3 weeks.

SUMMARY

Local anesthetics are frequently used when a limited, well-defined area of anesthesia is required, as is the case for most minor surgical procedures. Depending on the method of administration, local anesthetics can be used to temporarily block transmission in the area of peripheral nerve endings, along the trunk of a single peripheral nerve, along several peripheral nerves or plexuses, or at the level of the spinal cord. Local anesthetics may also be used to block efferent sympathetic activity. These drugs appear to block transmission along nerve axons by binding to membrane sodium channels and preventing the channels from opening during neuronal excitation. Physical therapists may frequently encounter the use of these agents in their patients for both short-term and long-term control of pain, as well as in the management of sympathetic hyperactivity.

REFERENCES

1. Ashburn, MA, et al: Iontophoretic administration of 2% lidocaine HCl and 1:100,000 epinephrine in humans. Clin J Pain 13:22, 1997.
2. Batra, MS: Adjuvants in epidural and spinal anesthesia. Anesthesiol Clin North Am 10:13, 1992.
3. Berde, CB and Strichartz, GR: Local anesthetics. In Miller, RD (ed): Anesthesia, Vol 1, ed 5. Churchill Livingstone, Philadelphia, 2000.
4. Brennum, J, et al: Quantitative sensory examination in human epidural anaesthesia and analgesia: Effects of lidocaine. Pain 51:27, 1992.
5. Brown, DL: Spinal, epidural, and caudal anesthesia. In In Miller, RD (ed): Anesthesia, Vol 1, ed. 5. Churchill Livingstone, Philadelphia, 2000.
6. Buckley, MM and Benfield, P: Eutectic lidocaine/prilocaine cream: A review of the topical anaesthetic analgesic efficacy of a eutectic mixture of local anaesthetics (EMLA). Drugs 46:126, 1993.
7. Buist, RJ: A survey of the practice of regional anesthesia. J R Soc Med 83:709, 1990.
8. Byl, NN: The use of ultrasound as an enhancer for transcutaneous drug delivery: Phonophoresis. Phys Ther 75:539, 1995.
9. Catterall, WA and Mackie, K: Local anesthetics. In Hardman, JG, et al (eds): The Pharmacological Basis of Therapeutics, ed 9. McGraw-Hill, New York, 1996.
10. Ciccone, CD. Iontophoresis. In Robinson, AJ, and Snyder-Mackler, L (eds): Clinical Electrophysiology, ed 2. Williams & Wilkins, Baltimore, 1994.
11. Cohen, S, et al: Adverse effects of epidural 0.03 percent bupivacaine during analgesia after cesarean section. Anesth Analg 75:753, 1992.
12. Connelly, NR, Reuben, S, and Brull, SJ: Intravenous regional anesthesia with ketorolac-lidocaine for the management of sympathetically-mediated pain. Yale J Biol Med 68:95, 1995.
13. Costello, CT and Jeske, AH: Iontophoresis: Applications in transdermal medication delivery. Phys Ther 75:554, 1995.
14. Franz, DN and Perry, RS: Mechanisms for differential nerve block among similar myelinated and non-myelinated axons by procaine. J Physiol 236:193, 1974.
15. French, RJ, Zamponi, GW, and Sierralta, IE: Molecular and kinetic determinants of local anaesthetic action on sodium channels. Toxicol Lett 100–101:247, 1998.
16. Gado, K and Emery, P: Modified suprascapular nerve block with bupivacaine alone effectively controls chronic shoulder pain in patients with rheumatoid arthritis. Ann Rheum Dis 52:215, 1993.
17. Garfield, JM and Gugino, L: Central effects of local anesthetic agents. In Strichartz, GR (ed): Handbook of Experimental Pharmacology, Vol. 81, Local Anesthetics. Springer-Verlag, New York, 1987.
18. Gasser, HS and Erlanger, J: Role of fiber size in the establishment of nerve block by pressure or cocaine. Am J Physiol 88:581, 1929.
19. Gissen, AJ, Covino, BG, and Gregus, J: Differential sensitivities of mammalian nerve fibers to local anesthetic agents. Anesthesiology 53:467, 1980.
20. Hansson, C, et al: Repeated treatment with lidocaine prilocaine cream (EMLA) as a topical anaesthetic for the cleansing of venous leg ulcers—a controlled study. Acta Derm Venereol (Stockh) 73:231, 1993.
21. Hodgson, PS, et al: The neurotoxicity of drugs given intrathecally (spinal). Anesth Analg 88:797, 1999.
22. Inoue, R, et al: Plasma concentrations of lidocaine and its principal metabolites during intermittent epidural anesthesia. Anesthesiology 63:304, 1985.
23. Kapral, S, et al: Ultrasound imaging for stellate ganglion block: Direct visualization of puncture site and local anesthetic spread. Reg Anesth 20:323, 1995.
24. Kassan, DG, Lynch, AM, and Stiller, MJ: Physical enhancement of dermatologic drug delivery: Iontophoresis and phonophoresis. J Am Acad Dermatol 34:657, 1996.

25. Keyes, PD, Tallon, JM, and Rizos, J: Topical anesthesia. Can Fam Physician 44:2152, 1998.
26. Kim, MK, et al: A randomized clinical trial of dermal anesthesia by iontophoresis for peripheral intravenous catheter placement in children. Ann Emerg Med 33:395, 1999.
27. Koren, G: Use of the eutectic mixture of local anesthetics in young children for procedure-related pain. J Pediatr 122(Suppl 5, part 2):S30, 1993.
28. Lener, EV, et al: Topical anesthetic agents in dermatologic surgery: A review. Dermatol Surg 23:673, 1997.
29. Linchitz, RM and Raheb, JC: Subcutaneous infusion of lidocaine provides effective pain relief for CRPS patients. Clin J Pain 15:67, 1999.
30. Lycka, BAS: EMLA: A new and effective topical anesthetic. J Dermatol Surg Oncol 18:859, 1992.
31. Mandabach, MG: Intrathecal and epidural analgesia. Crit Care Clin 15:105, 1999.
32. Mehrkens, HH and Geiger, PK: Continuous brachial plexus blockade via the vertical infraclavicular approach. Anaesthesia 53(Suppl 2):19, 1998.
33. Mercadante, S: Neuraxial techniques for cancer pain: An opinion about unresolved therapeutic dilemmas. Reg Anesth Pain Med 24:74, 1999.
34. Naguib, M, et al: Adverse effects and drug interactions associated with local and regional anesthesia. Drug Saf 18:221, 1998.
35. Nathan, PW and Sears, TA: Some factors concerned in differential nerve block by local anesthetics. J Physiol 157:565, 1961.
36. Nunez, M, et al: Iontophoresis for anesthesia during pulsed dye laser treatment of port-wine stains. Pediatr Dermatol 14:397, 1997.
37. Owenfalkenberg, A and Olsen, KS: Continuous stellate ganglion blockade for reflex sympathetic dystrophy. Anesth Analg 75:1041, 1992.
38. Price, DD, et al: Analysis of peak magnitude and duration of analgesia produced by local anesthetics injected into sympathetic ganglia of complex regional pain syndrome patients. Clin J Pain 14:216, 1998.
39. Raymond, SA and Gissen, AJ: Mechanisms of differential nerve block. In Strichartz, GR (ed): Handbook of Experimental Pharmacology, Vol 81, Local Anesthetics. Springer-Verlag, New York, 1987.
40. Sabbahi, MA and De Luca, CJ: Topical anesthetic-induced improvements in the mobility of patients with muscular hypertonicity: Preliminary results. J Electromyogr Kinesiol 1:41, 1991.
41. Scott, DB: Toxicity caused by local anesthetic drugs. Br J Anaesth 53:553, 1981.
42. Singh, R and Erwin, D: Local anaesthetics: An overview of current drugs. Hosp Med 59:880, 1998.
43. Strichartz, GR and Ritchie, JM: The action of local anesthetics on ion channels in excitable tissues. In Strichartz, GR (ed): Handbook of Experimental Pharmacology, Vol 81, Local Anesthetics. Springer-Verlag, New York, 1987.
44. Tachibana, K and Tachibana, S: Use of ultrasound to enhance the local anesthetic effect of topically applied aqueous lidocaine. Anesthesiology 78:1091, 1993.
45. Taddio, A, et al: A systematic review of lidocaine-prilocaine cream (EMLA) in the treatment of acute pain in neonates. Pediatrics 101:E1, 1998.
46. Tagariello, V: Sciatic nerve blocks: Approaches, techniques, local anaesthetics and manipulations. Anaesthesia 53(Suppl 2):15, 1998.
47. Tetzlaff, JE, et al: Spinal anesthesia for elective lumbar spine surgery. J Clin Anesth 10:666, 1998.
48. Van Wyngarden, TM and Bleyaert, AL: Reflex sympathetic dystrophy: Objective clinical signs in diagnosis and treatment. J Am Podiatr Assoc 81:580, 1991.
49. Weatherstone, KB, et al: Safety and efficacy of topical anesthetic for neonate circumcision. Pediatrics 92:710, 1993.
50. Wedel, DJ: Nerve blocks. In Miller, RD (ed): Anesthesia, Vol 1, ed 5. Churchill Livingstone, Philadelphia, 2000.
51. Wildsmith, JAW: Peripheral nerve and local anesthetic drugs. Br J Anaesth 58:692, 1986.
52. Writer, D: Epidural anesthesia for labor. Anesthesiol Clin North Am 10:59, 1992.
53. Zempsky, WT, et al: Lidocaine iontophoresis for topical anesthesia before intravenous line placement in children. J Pediatr 132:1061, 1998.
54. Zempsky, WT and Ashburn, MA: Iontophoresis: Noninvasive drug delivery. Am J Anesthesiol 25:158, 1998.
55. Zyluk, A: Results of the treatment of posttraumatic reflex sympathetic dystrophy of the upper extremity with regional intravenous blocks of methylprednisolone and lidocaine. Acta Orthop Belg 64:452, 1998.

SECTION III

Drugs Affecting Skeletal Muscle

CHAPTER 13

Skeletal Muscle Relaxants

Skeletal muscle relaxants are used to treat conditions associated with hyperexcitable skeletal muscle—specifically, spasticity and muscle spasms. Although these two terms are often used interchangeably, spasticity and muscle spasms represent two distinct abnormalities. The use of relaxant drugs, however, is similar in each condition because the ultimate goal is to normalize muscle excitability without a profound decrease in muscle function. Considering the number of rehabilitation patients with muscle hyperexcitability associated with either spasm or spasticity, skeletal muscle relaxants represent an important class of drugs to the rehabilitation specialist.

Drugs discussed in this chapter are used to decrease muscle excitability and contraction via an effect at the spinal cord level, at the neuromuscular junction, or within the muscle cell itself. Some texts also classify neuromuscular junction blockers such as curare and succinylcholine as skeletal muscle relaxants. These drugs are more appropriately classified as skeletal muscle *paralytics* because they eliminate muscle contraction by blocking transmission at the myoneural synapse. This type of skeletal muscle paralysis is used primarily during general anesthesia; using neuromuscular blockers as an adjunct in surgery was discussed in Chapter 11. Skeletal muscle relaxants do not prevent muscle contraction; they attempt only to normalize muscle excitability to decrease pain and improve motor function.

INCREASED MUSCLE TONE: SPASTICITY VERSUS MUSCLE SPASMS

Much confusion and consternation often arise from the erroneous use of the terms "spasticity" and "spasm." For the purpose of this chapter, these terms will be used to describe two different types of increased excitability, which result from different underlying pathologies. *Spasticity* is characterized primarily by an exaggerated muscle stretch reflex (Fig. 13–1).[18,46,71,93] This abnormal reflex activity is velocity dependent, with a rapid lengthening of the muscle invoking a strong contraction in the stretched muscle. The neurophysiologic mechanisms underlying spasticity are complex, but this phenomenon occurs when supraspinal inhibition or control is lost because of some lesion in the spinal cord or brain.[14,47,93] Presumably, specific upper motor neuron lesions interrupt

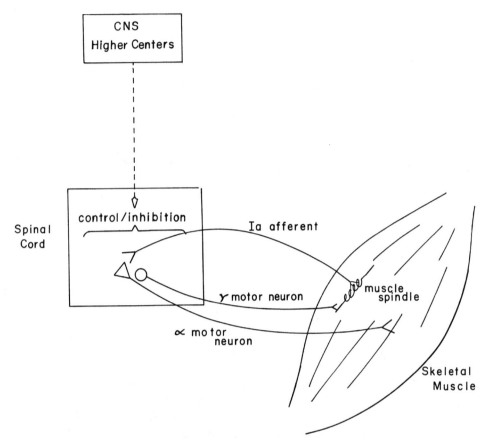

FIGURE 13–1. Schematic illustration of the basic components of the stretch reflex. Normally, higher CNS centers control the sensitivity of this reflex by inhibiting synaptic connections within the spinal cord. Spasticity is thought to occur when this higher center influence is lost because of cerebral trauma or damage to descending pathways in the spinal cord.

the cortical control of stretch reflex and alpha motor neuron excitability. Spasticity, therefore, is not in itself a disease but rather the motor sequela to such pathologies as cerebrovascular accident (CVA), cerebral palsy, multiple sclerosis (MS), and traumatic lesions to the brain and spinal cord (including quadriplegia and paraplegia).

Skeletal muscle *spasms* are used to describe the increased tension often seen in skeletal muscle after certain musculoskeletal injuries and inflammation (e.g., muscle strains, nerve root impingements).[12,83] This tension is involuntary, so the patient is unable to relax the muscle. Spasms are different from spasticity because spasms involve the afferent nociceptive input from the damaged tissue, which excites the outflow of alpha motor neuron to the muscle. This results in a tonic contraction of the affected muscle, which is quite painful because of the build-up of pain-mediating metabolites (e.g., lactate). In effect, a vicious cycle is created, with the increased pain caused by the spasm causing more nociceptive input, which further excites the alpha motor neuron to cause more spasms, and so on.[81,83]

Consequently, various skeletal muscle relaxants attempt to decrease skeletal muscle excitation and contraction in cases of spasticity and spasm. Specific drugs and their mechanisms of action are discussed here.

SPECIFIC AGENTS USED TO PRODUCE SKELETAL MUSCLE RELAXATION

Skeletal muscle relaxants are categorized here according to their primary clinical application: agents used to decrease spasms and agents used to decrease spasticity. One agent, diazepam, is indicated for both conditions and will appear in both categories. Finally, the use of botulinum toxin as an alternative strategy for reducing focal spasms or spasticity will be addressed.

AGENTS USED TO TREAT MUSCLE SPASMS

Two primary pharmacologic strategies are used to treat muscle spasms: diazepam and polysynaptic inhibitors. Diazepam (Valium) is a drug traditionally used to decrease anxiety, but this drug can also be used as a muscle relaxant. Polysynaptic inhibitors are a group of agents that are often used to treat spasms associated with musculoskeletal injuries. These two strategies are described here.

Diazepam

The effect of diazepam (Valium) on the CNS and its use as an antianxiety drug are discussed in Chapter 6. Basically, diazepam and other benzodiazepines work by increasing the central inhibitory effects of GABA; that is, diazepam binds to receptors located at GABA-ergic synapses and increases the GABA-induced inhibition at that synapse. Diazepam appears to work as a muscle relaxant through this mechanism, potentiating the inhibitory effect of GABA on alpha motor neuron activity in the spinal cord.[53,94] Diazepam also exerts some supraspinal sedative effects; in fact, some of its muscle relaxant properties may derive from the drug's ability to produce a more generalized state of sedation.[23,61,69]

Uses. Diazepam has been used extensively in treating muscle spasms associated with musculoskeletal injuries such as acute low-back strains.

Adverse Effects. The primary problem with diazepam is that dosages successful in relaxing skeletal muscle also produce sedation and a general reduction in psychomotor ability.[53,61] This effect may not be a problem and may actually be advantageous for the patient recovering from an acute musculoskeletal injury. A patient with an acute lumbosacral strain, for example, may benefit from the sedative properties because he or she will remain fairly inactive, thereby allowing better healing during the first few days after the injury. Continued use, however, may be problematic because of diazepam's sedative effects. Diazepam can produce tolerance and physical dependence, and long-term use in the treatment of muscle spasms should be discouraged.

Polysynaptic Inhibitors

A variety of centrally acting compounds have been used in an attempt to enhance muscle relaxation and decrease muscle spasms (Table 13–1). Some examples are carisoprodol (Soma, Vanadom), chlorphenesin carbamate (Maolate), chlorzoxazone (Paraflex, Parafon Forte, other trade names), cyclobenzaprine (Flexeril), metaxalone

TABLE 13–1 Drugs Commonly Used to Treat Skeletal Muscle Spasms

Generic Name (Trade Name)	Usual Adult Oral Dosage (mg)	Onset of Action (min)	Duration of Action (hr)
Carisoprodol (Soma, Vanadom)	350 TID and bedtime	30	4–6
Chlorphenesin carbamate (Maolate)	400 QID	—	—
Chlorzoxazone (Paraflex, Parafon Forte, others)	250–750 TID or QID	Within 60	3–4
Cyclobenzaprine (Flexeril)	10 TID	Within 60	12–24
Diazepam (Valium)	2–10 TID or QID	15–45	Variable
Metaxalone (Skelaxin)	800 TID or QID	60	4–6
Methocarbamol (Carbacot, Robaxin, Skelex)	1000 QID	Within 30	24
Orphenadrine citrate (Antiflex, Norflex, others)	100 BID	Within 60	12

(Skelaxin), methocarbamol (Carbacot, Robaxin, Skelex), and orphenadrine citrate (Antiflex, Norflex, other trade names). The mechanism of action of these drugs is not well defined.[81] Research in animals has suggested that some of these drugs may decrease polysynaptic reflex activity in the spinal cord, hence the term "polysynaptic inhibitors." By decreasing activity in polysynaptic pathways that lead to the alpha motor neuron, these drugs could decrease alpha motor neuron excitability, with subsequent relaxation of skeletal muscle. These compounds, however, also have a general depressant effect on the CNS; that is, they cause a global decrease in CNS excitability that results in generalized sedation.

The consensus, therefore, is that any muscle relaxant effect of these drugs stems from their sedative effects rather than a selective effect on specific neuronal reflex pathways.[23] This observation is not to say that they are ineffective, because clinical research has shown these drugs to be superior to a **placebo** in producing subjective muscle relaxation.[23,81] However, the specific ability of these drugs to relax skeletal muscle remains doubtful, and it is generally believed that their muscle relaxant properties are secondary to a nonspecific CNS sedation.

Uses. These drugs are typically used as adjuncts to rest and physical therapy for the relief of muscle spasms associated with acute, painful musculoskeletal injuries.[81] When used to treat spasms, these compounds are sometimes incorporated into the same tablet with an analgesic such as acetaminophen or aspirin. For instance, Norgesic is one of the trade names for orphenadrine combined with aspirin (and caffeine). Such combinations have been reported to be more effective than the individual components given separately.[5,38]

Adverse Effects. Because of their sedative properties, the primary side effects of these drugs are drowsiness and dizziness (Table 13–2). A variety of additional adverse effects, including nausea, light-headedness, vertigo, ataxia, and headache, may occur, depending on the patient and the specific drug administered (see Table 13–2). These medications may also cause tolerance and physical dependence, and the long-term use of these drugs should be discouraged. In particular, carisoprodol should be used cautiously because this drug is metabolized in the body to form meprobamate, which is a controlled substance that has sedative and anxiolytic properties but is not used exten-

TABLE 13–2 Relative Side Effects of Polysynaptic Inhibitors Used
as Antispasmodic Agents

Drug	Drowsiness	Dizziness or light-headedness	Headache	Nausea and Vomiting
Carisoprodol	M	L	L	L
Chlorphenesin carbamate	L	L	R	R
Chlorzoxazone	M	M	L	L
Cyclobenzaprine	M	M	L	L
Metaxalone	M	M	M	M
Methocarbamol	M	M	L	L
Orphenadrine citrate	L	L	L	L

Relative incidence of side effects: M = more frequent; L = less frequent; R = rare.
Source: Copied from *USP DI®, 20th Edition* Copyright 2000. The USP Convention, Inc. Permission granted. The USP is not responsible for any inaccuracy of quotation nor for any false or misleading implication that may arise due to the text or due to the quotation of information subsequently changed in later editions.

sively because it has strong potential for abuse.[52,76,77] Hence, use of carisoprodol represents an uncommon situation in which the metabolic byproduct (meprobamate) can produce effects and side effects that lead to addiction and abuse.[77]

AGENTS USED TO TREAT SPASTICITY

The three agents traditionally used in the treatment of spasticity are baclofen, dantrolene sodium, and diazepam (Table 13–3; Fig. 13–2). Two newer agents, gabapentin and tizanidine, are also available for treating spasticity in various conditions. These agents are addressed here.

Baclofen

The chemical name of baclofen is beta-(*p*-chlorophenyl)-GABA. As this name suggests, baclofen is a derivative of the central inhibitory neurotransmitter gamma-aminobutyric acid (GABA). There appear to be some differences between baclofen and GABA. Baclofen seems to bind only to certain GABA receptors, which have been classified as $GABA_b$ receptors (as opposed to $GABA_a$ receptors).[8,66] Preferential binding to $GABA_b$ receptors enables baclofen to act as a GABA agonist in that it inhibits transmission within the spinal cord at specific synapses.[27,72] To put this in the context of its use as a muscle relaxant, baclofen appears to have an inhibitory effect on alpha motor neuron activity within the spinal cord. Whether this inhibition is by an effect on the alpha motor neuron itself (postsynaptic inhibition), through inhibition of other excitatory neurons that synapse with the alpha motor neuron (presynaptic inhibition), or through a combination of presynaptic and postsynaptic inhibition is unclear.[94] In any event, the result is decreased firing of the alpha motor neuron, with a subsequent relaxation of the skeletal muscle.

Uses. Baclofen is administered orally to treat spasticity associated with lesions of the spinal cord, including traumatic injuries resulting in paraplegia or quadriplegia and spinal cord demyelination resulting in multiple sclerosis (MS).[42] Baclofen is often the drug of choice in reducing muscle spasticity associated with MS because it produces beneficial effects with a remarkable lack of adverse side effects when used in patients with MS.[24,29] Baclofen likewise does not cause as much generalized muscle weakness as direct-acting relaxants such as dantrolene, which can be a major advantage of baclofen treatment in many

TABLE 13–3 Antispasticity Drugs

Drug	Oral Dosage	Comments
Baclofen (Lioresal)	*Adults:* 5 mg TID initially; increase by 15 mg/day at 3-day intervals as required; maximum recommended dosage is 80 mg/day. *Children:* No specific pediatric dosage is listed; the adult dose must be decreased according to the size and age of the child.	More effective in treating spasticity resulting from spinal cord lesions (versus cerebral lesions).
Dantrolene sodium (Dantrium)	*Adults:* 25 mg/day initially; increase up to 100 mg 2, 3, or 4 times per day as needed; maximum recommended dose is 400 mg/day. *Children* (older than 5 yr): Initially, 0.5 mg/kg body weight BID; increase total daily dosage by 0.5 mg/kg every 4–7 days as needed, and give total daily amount in 4 divided doses; maximum recommended dose is 400 mg/day.	Exerts an effect directly on the muscle cell; may cause generalized weakness in all skeletal musculature.
Diazepam (Valium)	*Adults:* 2–10 mg TID or QID. *Children* (older than 6 mo): 1.0–2.5 mg TID or QID (in both adults and children, begin at lower end of dosage range and increase gradually as tolerated and needed).	Produces sedation at dosages that decrease spasticity.
Gabapentin (Neurontin)	*Adults**: Initially, 300 mg TID can be gradually increased up to 3600 mg/day based on desired response. *Children:* The safety and efficacy of this drug in treating spasticity in children has not been established.	Developed originally as an anti-convulsant; may also be helpful as an adjunct to other drugs in treating spasticity associated with spinal cord injury and multiple sclerosis.
Tizanidine (Zanaflex)	*Adults:* Initially, 4 mg TID can be gradually increased in 2- to 4-mg steps until spasticity is adequately reduced or a total daily dosage of 36 mg (12 mg TID) is reached. *Children:* The safety and efficacy of this drug in treating spasticity in children have not been established.	May reduce spasticity in spinal cord disorders while producing fewer side effects and less generalized muscle weakness than other agents (oral baclofen, diazepam).

*Anticonvulsant dose.

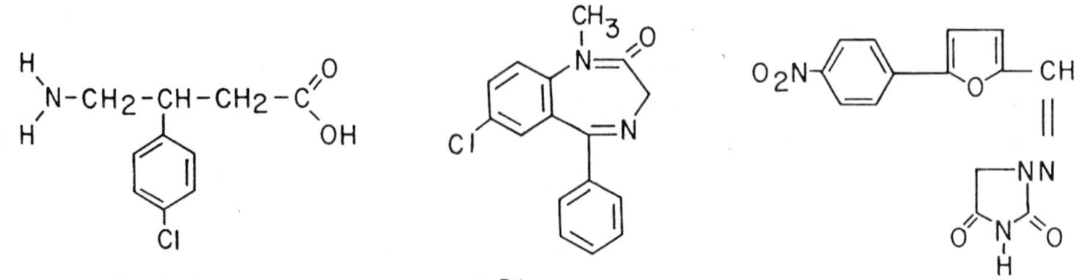

FIGURE 13–2. Structure of three primary antispasticity drugs.

patients with MS.[61] Baclofen also appears to produce few side effects when used appropriately to reduce spasticity secondary to traumatic spinal cord lesions, thus providing a relatively safe and effective form of treatment.[94] When administered systemically, baclofen is less effective in treating spasticity associated with supraspinal lesions (stroke, cerebral palsy), because these patients are more prone to the adverse side effects of this drug.

Adverse Effects. When baclofen therapy is initiated, the most common side effect is transient drowsiness, which usually disappears within a few days. When it is given to patients with spinal cord lesions, there are usually few other adverse effects. For patients who have had a CVA or for elderly individuals, there is sometimes a problem with confusion and hallucinations. Other side effects, occurring on an individual basis, include fatigue, nausea, dizziness, muscle weakness, and headache.

Intrathecal Baclofen

Baclofen is administered orally in most patients (see Table 13–2). Baclofen can, however, be administered intrathecally in patients with severe, intractable spasticity.[13,41] Intrathecal administration is the delivery of a drug directly into the subarachnoid space surrounding a specific level of the spinal cord. This places the drug very close to the spinal cord, thus allowing increased drug effectiveness with much smaller doses of the drug. Likewise, fewer systemic side effects occur because the drug tends to remain in the area of the cord rather than circulating in the bloodstream and causing adverse effects on other tissues.

When baclofen is administered intrathecally for the long-term treatment of spasticity, a small catheter is usually implanted surgically so that the open end of the catheter is located in the subarachnoid space and the other end of the catheter is attached to some type of programmable pump. The pump is implanted subcutaneously in the abdominal wall and is adjusted to deliver the drug at a slow, continuous rate. The rate of infusion is titrated over time to achieve the best clinical reduction in spasticity.

Uses. Intrathecal baclofen delivery using implantable pumps has been used in a variety of patients with spasticity of spinal origin. Studies involving these patients have typically noted a substantial decrease in rigidity with an increase in ability to perform functional activities, including activities of daily living (ADLs).[15,58,60,74] Muscle function also increased in some patients whose voluntary motor control was being masked by spasticity.[13,48,57,74] Similar beneficial effects have been noted when intrathecal baclofen was administered to patients with spasticity resulting from supraspinal (cerebral) injury, including cerebral palsy, CVA, and traumatic brain injury. In these patients, long-term continuous infusion of intrathecal baclofen has generally resulted in decreased spasticity (as indicated by decreased Ashworth scores, decreased reflex activity, and so forth) and improvement in various other impairments and functional limitations.[4,13,28,56,59,89]

Adverse Effects. Despite these benefits, intrathecal baclofen is associated with a number of potential complications. Primary among these is the possibility of a disruption in the delivery system; that is, a pump malfunction or a problem with the delivery catheter can occur.[4,58,74] Increased drug delivery because of a pump malfunction could cause overdose and lead to respiratory depression, decreased cardiac function, and coma.[73] Conversely, abrupt stoppage of the drug because of pump failure or displacement or blockage of the delivery catheter may cause a withdrawal syndrome that includes fever, confusion, delirium, and seizures.[73,76] A second major concern is the possibility that tolerance could develop with long-term, continuous baclofen administration. Tolerance is the need for more drug to achieve a beneficial effect when the drug is used for prolonged periods. Several studies have reported that doses must indeed be increased progressively when intrathecal baclofen systems are used for periods of several months to several years.[15,58,74] Tolerance to intrathecal baclofen, however, can usually be dealt with by periodic adjustments in dosage, and tolerance does not usually develop to such an extent that intrathecal baclofen must be discontinued.

Hence, intrathecal baclofen offers a means of treating certain patients with severe spasticity who have not responded to more conventional means of treatment, including oral baclofen. Additional research will help determine optimal ways that this intervention can be used to decrease spasticity in various types of patients. Further improvements in the technologic and mechanical aspects of intrathecal delivery, including better pumps and catheter systems, will also make this a safer and more practical method of treating these patients.

Dantrolene Sodium

The only available muscle relaxant that exerts its effect directly on the skeletal muscle cell is dantrolene sodium (Dantrium).[42] This drug works by impairing the release of calcium from the sarcoplasmic reticulum within the muscle cell during excitation (Fig. 13–3).[18,85,94] In response to an action potential, the release of calcium from sarcoplasmic storage sites initiates myofilament cross-bridging and subsequent muscle contraction. By inhibiting this release, dantrolene attenuates muscle contraction and therefore enhances relaxation.

Uses. Dantrolene is often effective in treating severe spasticity, regardless of the underlying pathology.[62,94] Patients with traumatic cord lesions, advanced MS, cerebral palsy, or CVAs will probably experience a reduction in spasticity with this drug. Dantrolene is not prescribed to treat muscle spasms caused by musculoskeletal injury.

Adverse Effects. The most common side effect of dantrolene is generalized muscle weakness; this makes sense, considering that dantrolene impairs sarcoplasmic calcium re-

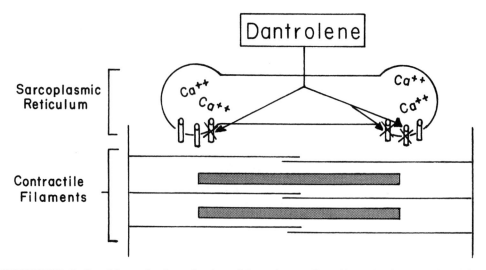

FIGURE 13–3. Possible mechanism of action of dantrolene sodium (Dantrium). Dantrolene blocks channels in the sarcoplasmic reticulum, thus interfering with calcium release onto the contractile (actin, myosin) filaments. Muscle contraction is reduced because less calcium is available to initiate cross-bridge formation between actin and myosin filaments.

lease in skeletal muscles throughout the body, not just in the hyperexcitable tissues. Thus, the use of dantrolene is sometimes counterproductive because the increased motor function that occurs when spasticity is reduced may be offset by the generalized motor weakness. This drug may also cause severe hepatotoxicity, and cases of fatal hepatitis have been reported.[51] The risk of toxic effects on the liver seems to be greater in women, in patients older than 35, and in individuals receiving drugs such as estrogen.[94] Less serious side effects that sometimes occur during the first few days of dantrolene therapy include drowsiness, dizziness, nausea, and diarrhea, but these problems are usually transient.

Diazepam

As indicated earlier, diazepam is effective in reducing spasticity as well as muscle spasms because this drug increases the inhibitory effects of GABA in the CNS.

Uses. Diazepam is used in patients with spasticity resulting from cord lesions and is sometimes effective in patients with cerebral palsy.

Adverse effects. Use of diazepam as an antispasticity agent is limited by the sedative effects of this medication; that is, patients with spasticity who do not want a decrease in mental alertness will not tolerate diazepam therapy very well. Extended use of diazepam can cause tolerance and physical dependence, and use of diazepam for the long-term treatment of spasticity should be avoided whenever possible.[10]

Gabapentin

Developed originally an antiseizure drug (see Chap. 9), gabapentin (Neurontin) has also shown some promise in treating spasticity. This drug appears to enhance the inhibitory effects of GABA in the spinal cord by either increasing GABA release or by stimulating GABA-like receptors on spinal neurons. Gabapentin may therefore decrease spasticity by increasing GABA-mediated inhibition of the alpha motor neuron, but the exact way that this drug exerts its antispasticity effects remains to be determined.

Uses. Preliminary studies suggest that gabapentin is effective in decreasing spasticity associated with spinal cord injury[33,75] and multiple sclerosis.[21,63] The primary benefit of this drug may be its ability to be used in conjunction with more traditional antispasticity agents. Combining gabapentin with baclofen, for example, may provide better effects than either drug used alone. In addition, gabapentin does not affect the liver's ability to metabolize other drugs, thus reducing the risk of an interaction between gabapentin and other antispasticity agents. Gabapentin may likewise be helpful in reducing certain types of chronic pain, an effect that may be especially beneficial in people with spasticity that is accompanied by painful sensations. Additional research should clarify how this drug can be used alone or with other agents to provide optimal benefits in spasticity resulting from various spinal and possibly cerebral injuries.

Adverse effects. The primary side effects of this drug are sedation, fatigue, dizziness, and ataxia.

Tizanidine

Tizanidine (Zanaflex) is classified as an alpha-2 adrenergic agonist, meaning that this drug binds selectively to the alpha-2 receptors in the CNS and stimulates these receptors. Alpha-2 receptors are found at various locations in the brain and spinal cord, including the presynaptic and postsynaptic membranes of spinal interneurons that control alpha motor neuron excitability. Stimulation of these alpha-2 receptors inhibits firing of the interneurons that relay information to the alpha motor neuron—that is, interneurons that comprise polysynaptic reflex arcs within the spinal cord.[17] Tizanidine appears to bind to receptors on these spinal interneurons, decrease the release of excitatory neurotransmitters from their presynaptic terminals (presynaptic inhibition), and also decrease excitability of the postsynaptic neuron (postsynaptic inhibition).[20] Inhibition of spinal interneurons results in decreased excitatory input onto the alpha motor neuron, with a subsequent decrease in spasticity of the skeletal muscle supplied by that neuron.

Hence, tizanidine is the primary alpha-2 agonist used to treat spasticity. Another type of alpha-2 agonist known as clonidine (Catapres) is also available. Clonidine exerts antispasticity as well as antihypertensive effects because this drug stimulates alpha-2 receptors in the cord and brainstem, respectively.[88,92] Use of clonidine in treating spasticity, however, is limited because of the cardiovascular side effects, and clonidine is used primarily for treating hypertension (see Chap. 21).

Uses. Tizanidine has been used successfully to control spasticity resulting from spinal lesions (multiple sclerosis, spinal cord injury)[64,65,80,84] and from cerebral lesions (CVA).[6,55,68] This drug appears to be as effective in reducing spasticity as orally administered baclofen or diazepam, but tizanidine generally has milder side effects and produces less generalized muscle weakness than these other agents.[32,49,50,54] Tizanidine is also superior to other alpha-2 agonists such as clonidine because tizanidine does not cause as much hypotension and other cardiovascular side effects.

Adverse Effects. The most common side effects associated with tizanidine include sedation, dizziness, and dry mouth.[86,87] As indicated, however, tizanidine tends to have a more favorable side effect profile than other alpha-2 agonists, and this drug produces less generalized weakness than oral baclofen or diazepam. Tizanidine may therefore be a better alternative to these other agents in patients who need to reduce spasticity while maintaining adequate muscle strength for ambulation, transfers, and so forth.

USE OF BOTULINUM TOXIN AS A MUSCLE RELAXANT

Injection of botulinum toxin is a rather innovative way to control localized muscle hyperexcitability. Botulinum toxin is a purified version of the toxin that causes botulism. This toxin enters the presynaptic terminal at the skeletal neuromuscular junction and binds strongly to presynaptic acetylcholine vesicles (Fig. 13–4). Once bound by the toxin, these vesicles are unable to release acetylcholine into the synaptic cleft.[40,44] Local injection of botulinum toxin into specific muscles will therefore decrease muscle excitation by disrupting synaptic transmission at the neuromuscular junction. The affected muscle will invariably undergo some degree of paresis and subsequent relaxation because the toxin blocks the release of acetylcholine.

Several types of botulinum toxin are currently available (botulinum toxin types A, B, and F), and these types differ somewhat in their chemistry, duration of action, and so forth. The type most commonly used therapeutically is botulinum toxin type A, and this agent is marketed commercially under such trade names as Botox and Dysport. Botulinum toxin type A has been used for some time to control localized muscle dystonias, including conditions such as spasmodic torticollis, blepharospasm, laryngeal dystonia,

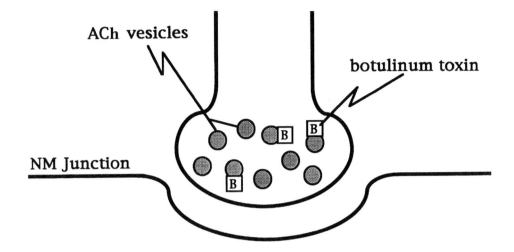

Skeletal Muscle Cell

FIGURE 13–4. Mechanism of action of botulinum toxin. Botulinum toxin (B) enters the presynaptic terminal at the skeletal neuromuscular (NM) junction and prevents release of acetylcholine (ACh) from the presynaptic vesicles.

strabismus, and several other types of focal dystonias.[19,31,37,40,43,82] When used therapeutically, small amounts of this toxin are injected directly into the dystonic muscles, and relaxation of these muscles typically occurs within a few days to 1 week. This technique appears to be fairly safe and effective in many patients, but relief may be only temporary. Symptoms often return within 3 months after each injection, necessitating additional treatments.[37,40,82] Still, this technique represents a method for treating patients with severe, incapacitating conditions marked by focal dystonias and spasms.

Uses. In addition to treating certain spasms and focal dystonias, there has been considerable interest in using botulinum toxin to reduce spasticity in specific muscles or muscle groups. This treatment has been used to treat spasticity resulting from various disorders including cerebral palsy,[3,30,45,91,95] traumatic brain injury,[70,90] CVA,[11,35] and spinal cord injury.[2] As with treatment of focal dystonias, the toxin is injected directly into selected muscles. If necessary, electromyography can be used to identify specific muscles and guide the injection to the desired site within the muscle belly (e.g, the motor point of the muscle).[25,67] There is also some evidence that electrical stimulation of the nerve supplying the muscle for the first few days following injection may help increase the efficacy of the toxin, presumably by enhancing the uptake of the toxin by the presynaptic nerve terminals.[34,36]

Botulinum toxin injection has therefore provided a means to control severe spasticity in certain situations. This intervention can help remove spastic dominance in certain patients so that volitional motor function can be facilitated. For example, judicious administration of botulinum toxin can result in improved gait and other functional activities in selected patients with cerebral palsy or traumatic brain injury.[3,30,91,95] Even if voluntary motor function is not improved dramatically by these injections, reducing spasticity in severely affected muscles may produce other musculoskeletal benefits. Injection of botulinum toxin, for example, can reduce spasticity so that muscles can be stretched more effectively, thus helping to prevent joint contractures and decrease the need for surgical procedures such as heel-cord lengthening and adductor release.[16,22,26,45]

These injections can likewise enable patients to wear and use orthotic devices more effectively. Injection into the triceps surae musculature, for example, can improve the fit and function of an ankle-foot orthosis by preventing excessive plantar flexor spasticity from "pistoning" the foot out of the orthosis.[93] Finally, botulinum toxin injections into severely spastic muscles can increase patient comfort and ability to perform ADLs and hygiene activities. Consider, for example, the patient with severe upper-extremity flexor spasticity following a CVA. Local injection of botulinum toxin into the affected muscles may enable the patient to extend his or her elbow, wrist, and fingers, thereby allowing better hand cleansing, ability to dress, decreased pain, and so forth.[7,78]

Adverse Effects and Limitations. Despite the potential benefits of using botulinum toxin, one must realize that this drug does not cure spasticity and that there are a number of limitations to the use of this intervention. In particular, only a limited number of muscles can be injected during a given treatment because only a limited amount of botulinum toxin can be administered during each set of injections. For example, the total amount of Botox injected during each treatment session is typically between 200 and 300 units in adults, with proportionally smaller amounts used in children, depending on the size and age of the child.[7] Exceeding this dosage will cause an immune response whereby antibodies are synthesized against the toxin, making subsequent treatments ineffective because the patient's immune system will recognize and inactivate the toxin. The number of muscles that can be injected is therefore often limited to one or two muscle groups—for example, the elbow and wrist flexors in one upper extremity of an adult, or the bilateral triceps surae musculature of a child.

As indicated earlier, the relaxant effects of the toxin are likewise temporary, and these effects typically disappear within 3 to 6 months after injection.[9,39] The effects apparently wear off because a new presynaptic terminal "sprouts" from the axon that contains the presynaptic terminal originally affected by the toxin. This new terminal grows downward and reattaches to the skeletal muscle, thus creating a new motor end plate with a new source of acetylcholine. The effects of the previous injection are therefore overcome when this new presynaptic terminal begins to function. Another injection will be needed to block the release from this new presynaptic terminal, thus allowing another 3 to 6 months of antispasticity effects.

Consequently, botulinum toxin represents a strategy for dealing with spasticity that is especially problematic in specific muscles or groups of muscles. Despite the rather ominous prospect of injecting a potentially lethal toxin into skeletal muscles, this intervention has a remarkably small incidence of severe adverse effects when administered at therapeutic doses.[79] Botulinum toxin can therefore be used as part of a comprehensive rehabilitation program to provide optimal benefits for certain patients with severe spasticity.

PHARMACOKINETICS

Most muscle relaxants are absorbed fairly easily from the gastrointestinal tract, and the oral route is the most frequent method of drug administration. In cases of severe spasms, certain drugs such as methocarbamol and orphenadrine can be injected intramuscularly or intravenously to permit a more rapid effect. Likewise, diazepam and dantrolene can be injected to treat spasticity if the situation warrants a faster onset. As discussed earlier, continuous intrathecal baclofen administration may be used in certain patients with severe spasticity, and local injection of botulinum toxin is a possible strategy for treating focal dystonias and spasticity. Metabolism of muscle relaxants is usually accomplished by hepatic microsomal enzymes, and excretion of the metabolite or the intact drug is through the kidneys.

SPECIAL CONCERNS IN REHABILITATION PATIENTS

Because of the very nature of their use, skeletal muscle relaxants are prescribed for many patients involved in rehabilitation programs. Physical therapists and other rehabilitation professionals will encounter these drugs applied as both antispasm and antispasticity agents. When used to reduce muscle spasms following nerve root impingements, muscle strains, and the like, these drugs will complement the physical therapy interventions. Concomitant use of muscle relaxants with thermal, electrotherapeutic, and manual techniques can produce optimal benefits during the acute phase of musculoskeletal injuries that cause spasms. Of course, the long-term use of antispasmodic agents is not practical because these drugs often cause sedation, and they can have addictive properties that lead to tolerance and physical dependence. This fact further emphasizes the need for aggressive physical therapy so that these drugs can be discontinued as soon as possible. Physical therapists and occupational therapists can also help prevent reinjury and recurrence of spasms by improving the patient's muscle strength, flexibility, and posture and by teaching proper body mechanics and lifting techniques. These interventions may help decrease the incidence of spasms and the need for drugs used to treat these spasms.

The pharmacologic reduction of spasticity is also an important goal in patients receiving physical therapy and occupational therapy. As indicated earlier, decreased spasticity can result in increased motor function, easier self-care or nursing care, and decreased painful and harmful effects of strong spastic contractions. Drug treatment is likewise synergistic with rehabilitation; that is, antispasticity agents can allow more effective passive range-of-motion and stretching activities, as well as permit more effective use of neuromuscular facilitation techniques, orthotic devices, and other interventions designed to reduce spasticity and improve function.

Rehabilitation specialists also play a critical role in helping patients adapt to sudden changes in muscle excitability caused by antispasticity drugs. Reducing spasticity may, in fact, adversely affect the individual who has come to rely on increased muscle tone to assist in functional activities such as ambulation. For example, patients who have had a CVA and who use extensor spasticity in the lower extremity to support themselves when walking may begin to have episodes of falling if this spasticity is reduced suddenly by drugs. This loss of support from the hypertonic muscles will hopefully be replaced by a more normal form of motor function.

Physical therapists and occupational therapists can therefore play a vital role in facilitating the substitution of normal physiologic motor control for the previously used spastic tone. Therapists need to be involved especially when one of the parenteral antispasticity techniques is used, such as intrathecal baclofen or botulinum toxin injections. For example, patients who receive intrathecal baclofen through programmable pump systems often require a period of intensive rehabilitation to enable them to benefit from the decreased spasticity and increased voluntary motor function that can occur when this form of drug therapy is initiated.[58] Therapists must therefore be ready to use aggressive rehabilitation techniques to help patients adapt to the relatively rapid and dramatic decrease in muscle tone that is often associated with antispasticity drug therapy.

Rehabilitation specialists can also play a critical role in using certain antispasticity drugs effectively. In particular, therapists can help identify patients who are suitable candidates for botulinum toxin injections and help evaluate these patients preinjection and postinjection to determine if these injections are achieving the desired outcomes.[1] Rehabilitation specialists are, in fact, often in the best position to evaluate the effects of all antispasticity drugs. By working closely with the patient, the patient's family, and the physician, therapists can provide valuable feedback about the efficacy of antispasticity drugs and whether these drugs are helping to produce improvements in the patient's function and well-being.

Finally, therapists may have to deal with the side effects of these drugs. Depending on the drug in question, problems with sedation, generalized muscle weakness, and hepatotoxicity can negate any beneficial effects from a reduction in muscle tone. Sedation, which may occur to a variable degree with all skeletal muscle relaxants, must sometimes be accommodated in the rehabilitation program. If the patient needs to be awake and alert, treatments may have to be scheduled at a time of the day when the sedative effects are minimal.

In situations of generalized muscle weakness (i.e., during the use of dantrolene sodium or oral baclofen), there is often little the physical therapist can do to resolve this problem. For instance, the patient with paraplegia who requires adequate upper-extremity strength to perform transfers, wheelchair mobility, and ambulation with crutches and braces may find his or her ability to perform these activities compromised by the antispasticity drug. The role of the therapist in this situation may simply be to advise the patient that voluntary muscular power is limited and that some upper-extremity strength deficits can be expected. The therapist may also work closely with the physician in trying to find the minimum acceptable dose for that patient or in attempting to find a better drug (e.g., switching from dantrolene to tizanidine).

CASE STUDY

MUSCLE RELAXANTS

Brief History. F.D. is a 28-year-old man who sustained complete paraplegia below the L-2 spinal level during an automobile accident. Through the course of rehabilitation, he was becoming independent in self-care, and he had begun to ambulate in the parallel bars and with crutches while wearing temporary long leg braces. He was highly motivated to continue this progress and was eventually fitted with permanent leg orthoses. During this period, spasticity had increased in his lower extremities to the point where dressing and self-care were often difficult. Also, his ability to put on his leg braces was often compromised by the lower-extremity spasticity. The patient was started on oral baclofen (Lioresal) at an initial oral dosage of 15 mg/day. The daily dosage of baclofen was gradually increased until he was receiving 60 mg/day.

Problem/Influence of Medication. Although the baclofen was effective in controlling his spasticity, F.D. began to notice weakness in his arms and upper torso when he attempted to ambulate and transfer. This decrease in voluntary power in his upper extremities was caused by the generalized muscle weakness sometimes seen when this drug is used.

Decision/Solution. The therapist conferred with the patient's physician, and the decreased voluntary muscle power was noted. As an alternative, the patient was switched to tizanidine (Zanaflex). The dosage was adjusted until the spasticity was adequately reduced, and no further problems were noted.

SUMMARY

Skeletal muscle relaxants are used to treat muscle spasms that result from musculoskeletal injuries or spasticity that occurs following lesions in the CNS. Depending on the specific agent, these drugs reduce muscle excitability by acting on the spinal cord, at the neuromuscular junction, or directly within the skeletal muscle fiber. Diazepam and polysynaptic inhibitors are used in the treatment of muscle spasms, but their effectiveness as muscle relaxants may be because of their nonspecific sedative properties. Agents used to treat spasticity include baclofen, dantrolene, diazepam, gabapentin, and tizanidine. Each drug works by a somewhat different mechanism, and the selection of a specific antispasticity agent depends on the patient and the underlying CNS lesion (e.g., stroke, MS). Local injection of botulinum toxin can also be used to treat focal dystonias and spasticity, and this technique may help control spasms and spasticity in specific muscles or muscle groups. Physical therapists and other rehabilitation personnel will frequently work with patients taking these drugs for the treatment of either spasticity or spasms. Although there are some side effects that may be troublesome, these drugs generally facilitate the rehabilitation program by directly providing benefits (muscle relaxation) that are congruent with the major rehabilitation goals.

REFERENCES

1. Albany, K: Physical and occupational therapy considerations in adult patients receiving botulinum toxin injections for spasticity. Muscle Nerve Suppl 6:S221, 1997.
2. Al-Khodairy, AT, Gobelet, C, and Rossier, AB: Has botulinum toxin type A a place in the treatment of spasticity in spinal cord injury patients? Spinal Cord 36:854, 1998.
3. Arens, LJ, Leary, PM, and Goldschmidt, RB: Experience with botulinum toxin in the treatment of cerebral palsy. S Afr Med J 87:1001, 1997.
4. Armstrong, RW, et al: Intrathecally administered baclofen for treatment of children with spasticity of cerebral origin. J Neurosurg 87:409, 1997.
5. Basmajian, JV: Acute back pain and spasm. A controlled multicenter trial of combined analgesic and antispasm agents. Spine 14:438, 1989.
6. Bes, A, et al: A multi-centre, double-blind trial of tizanidine, a new antispastic agent, in spasticity associated with hemiplegia. Curr Med Res Opin 10:709, 1988.
7. Bhakta, BB, et al: Use of botulinum toxin in stroke patients with severe upper limb spasticity. J Neurol Neurosurg Psychiatry 61:30, 1996.
8. Bowery, NG, Hill, DR, and Hudson, AL: Characteristics of GABA$_b$ receptor binding sites on rat whole brain synaptic membranes. Br J Pharmacol 78:191, 1983.
9. Brin, MF: Dosing, administration, and a treatment algorithm for use of botulinum toxin A for adult-onset spasticity. Spasticity study group. Muscle Nerve Suppl 6:S208, 1997.
10. Broderick, CP, Radnitz, CL, and Bauman, WA: Diazepam usage in veterans with spinal cord injury. J Spinal Cord Med 20:406, 1997.
11. Burbaud, P, et al: A randomized, double blind, placebo controlled trial of botulinum toxin in the treatment of spastic foot in hemiparetic patients. J Neurol Neurosurg Psychiatry 61:265, 1996.
12. Calliet, R: Low Back Pain Syndrome, ed 4. FA Davis, Philadelphia, 1988.
13. Campbell, SK, et al: The effects of intrathecally administered baclofen on function in patients with spasticity. Phys Ther 75:352, 1995.
14. Clemente, CD: Neurophysiological mechanisms and neuroanatomic substrates related to spasticity. Neurology 28:40, 1978.
15. Coffey, RJ, et al: Intrathecal baclofen for intractable spasticity of spinal origin: Results of a long-term multicenter study. J Neurosurg 78:226, 1993.
16. Cosgrove, AP and Graham, HK: Botulinum toxin A prevents the development of contractures in the hereditary spastic mouse. Dev Med Child Neurol 36:379, 1994.

17. Coward, DM: Tizanidine: Neuropharmacology and mechanism of action. Neurology 44(Suppl 9):S6, 1994.
18. Davidoff, RA: Pharmacology of spasticity. Neurology 28:46, 1978.
19. Davidson, BJ and Ludlow, CL: Long-term effects of botulinum toxin injections in spasmodic dysphonia. Ann Otol Rhinol Laryngol 105:33, 1996.
20. Delwaide, PJ and Pennisi, G: Tizanidine and electrophysiologic analysis of spinal control mechanisms in humans with spasticity. Neurology 44(Suppl 9):S21, 1994.
21. Dunevsky, A and Perel, AB: Gabapentin for relief of spasticity associated with multiple sclerosis. Am J Phys Med Rehabil 77:451, 1998.
22. Eames, NW, et al: The effect of botulinum toxin A on gastrocnemius length: Magnitude and duration of response. Dev Med Child Neurol 41:226, 1999.
23. Elenbaas, JK: Centrally acting oral skeletal muscle relaxants. Am J Hosp Pharm 37:1313, 1980.
24. Feldman, RG, et al: Baclofen for spasticity in multiple sclerosis: Double blind cross-over and three year study. Neurology 28:1094, 1978.
25. Finsterer, J, Fuchs, I, and Mamoli, B: Automatic EMG-guided botulinum toxin treatment of spasticity. Clin Neuropharmacol 20:195, 1997.
26. Flett, PJ, et al: Botulinum toxin A versus fixed cast stretching for dynamic calf tightness in cerebral palsy. J Paediatr Child Health 35:71, 1999.
27. Fukuda, T, Kudo, Y, and Ono, H: Effects of beta-(p-chlorophenyl)-GABA (baclofen) on spinal synaptic activity. Eur J Pharmacol 44:17, 1977.
28. Gerszten, PC, Albright, AL, and Barry, MJ: Effect on ambulation of continuous intrathecal baclofen infusion. Pediatr Neurosurg 27:40, 1997.
29. Gidal, BE, Fleming, JO, and Dalmady-Israel, C: Multiple sclerosis. In DiPiro, JT, et al (eds): Pharmacotherapy: A Pathophysiologic Approach, ed 4. Appleton & Lange, Stamford, CT, 1999.
30. Gooch, JL and Sandell, TV: Botulinum toxin for spasticity and athetosis in children with cerebral palsy. Arch Phys Med Rehabil 77:508, 1996.
31. Greene, P, et al: Double-blind, placebo-controlled trial of botulinum toxin injections for the treatment of spasmodic torticollis. Neurology 40:1213, 1990.
32. Groves, L, Shellenberger, MK, and Davis, CS: Tizanidine treatment of spasticity: A meta-analysis of controlled, double-blind, comparative studies with baclofen and diazepam. Adv Ther 15:241, 1998.
33. Gruenthal, M, et al: Gabapentin for the treatment of spasticity in patients with spinal cord injury. Spinal Cord 35:686, 1997.
34. Hesse, S, et al: Botulinum toxin type A and short-term electrical stimulation in the treatment of upper limb flexor spasticity after stroke: A randomized, double-blind, placebo-controlled trial. Clin Rehabil 12:381, 1998.
35. Hesse, S, et al: Ankle muscle activity before and after botulinum toxin therapy for lower limb extensor spasticity in chronic hemiparetic patients. Stroke 27:455, 1996.
36. Hesse, S, et al: Short-term electrical stimulation enhances the effectiveness of botulinum toxin in the treatment of lower limb spasticity in hemiparetic patients. Neurosci Lett 201:37, 1995.
37. Hughes, AJ: Botulinum toxin in clinical practice. Drugs 48:888, 1994.
38. Hunskaar, S and Donnell, D: Clinical and pharmacological review of the efficacy of orphenadrine and its combination with paracetamol in painful conditions. J Int Med Res 19:71, 1991.
39. Jankovic, J and Brin, MF: Botulinum toxin: Historical perspective and potential new indications. Muscle Nerve Suppl 6:S129, 1997.
40. Jankovic, J and Brin, MF: Therapeutic uses of botulinum toxin. N Engl J Med 324:1186, 1991.
41. Kamensek, J: Continuous intrathecal baclofen infusions. An introduction and overview. Axone 20:67, 1999.
42. Katz, RT: Management of spasticity. Am J Phys Med Rehabil 67:108, 1988.
43. Kaufman, DM: Use of botulinum toxin injections for spasmodic torticollis of tardive dystonia. J Neuropsychiatry Clin Neurosci 6:50, 1994.
44. Kessler, KR and Benecke, R: Botulinum toxin: From poison to remedy. Neurotoxicology 18:761, 1997.
45. Koman, LA, et al: Management of cerebral palsy with botulinum-A toxin: Preliminary investigation. J Pediatr Orthop 13:489, 1993.
46. Lance, JW: Symposium synopsis. In Feldman, RG, Young, RR, and Koella, WP (eds): Spasticity: Disordered Motor Control. Year Book, Chicago, 1980.
47. Lance, JW and Burke, D: Mechanisms of spasticity. Arch Phys Med Rehabil 55:332, 1974.
48. Latash, ML, et al: Effects of intrathecal baclofen on voluntary motor control in spastic paresis. J Neurosurg 72:388, 1990.
49. Lataste, X, et al: Comparative profile of tizanidine in the management of spasticity. Neurology 44(Suppl 9):S53, 1994.
50. Lawson, K: Tizanidine: A therapeutic weapon for spasticity? Physiotherapy 84:418, 1998.
51. Lee, WM: Drug-induced hepatotoxicity. N Engl J Med 333:1118, 1995.
52. Littrell, RA, Hayes, LR, and Stillner, V: Carisoprodol (Soma): A new and cautious perspective on an old agent. South Med J 86:753, 1993.
53. Lossius, R, Dietrichson, P, and Lunde, PKM: Effects of diazepam and desmethyl-diazepam in spasticity and rigidity: A quantitative study of reflexes and plasma concentrations. Acta Neurol Scand 61:378, 1980.
54. Mathias, CJ, et al: Pharmacodynamics and pharmacokinetics of the oral antispastic agent tizanidine in patients with spinal cord injury. J Rehabil Res Dev 26:9, 1989.

55. Medici, M, Pebet, M, and Ciblis, D: A double-blind, long-term study of tizanidine (Sirdalud) in spasticity due to cerebrovascular lesions. Curr Med Res Opin 11:398, 1989.
56. Meythaler, JM, et al: Long-term continuously infused intrathecal baclofen for spastic-dystonic hypertonia in traumatic brain injury: 1-year experience. Arch Phys Med Rehabil 80:13, 1999.
57. Meythaler, JM, et al: Intrathecal baclofen in hereditary spastic paraparesis. Arch Phys Med Rehabil 73:794, 1992.
58. Meythaler, JM, et al: Continuous intrathecal baclofen in spinal cord spasticity: A prospective study. Arch Phys Med Rehabil 71:321, 1990.
59. Meythaler, JM, Guin-Renfroe, S, and Hadley, MN: Continuously infused intrathecal baclofen for spastic/dystonic hemiplegia: A preliminary report. Am J Phys Med Rehabil 78:247, 1999.
60. Meythaler, JM, McCary, A, and Hadley, MN: Prospective assessment of continuous intrathecal infusion of baclofen for spasticity caused by acquired brain injury: A preliminary report. J Neurosurg 87:415, 1997.
61. Miller, RD: Skeletal muscle relaxants. In Katzung, BG (ed): Basic and Clinical Pharmacology, ed 7. Appleton & Lange, Stamford, CT, 1998.
62. Monster, AW: Spasticity and the effect of dantrolene sodium. Arch Phys Med Rehabil 55:373, 1974.
63. Mueller, ME, et al: Gabapentin for relief of upper motor neuron symptoms in multiple sclerosis. Arch Phys Med Rehabil 78:521, 1997.
64. Nance, PW, et al: Relationship of the antispasticity effect of tizanidine to plasma concentration in patients with multiple sclerosis. Arch Neurol 54:731, 1997.
65. Nance, PW, et al: Efficacy and safety of tizanidine in the treatment of spasticity in patients with spinal cord injury. North American Tizanidine Study Group. Neurology 44(Suppl 9):S44, 1994.
66. Newberry, NR and Nicoll, RA: Direct hyperpolarizing action of baclofen on hippocampal pyramidal cells. Nature 308:450, 1984.
67. O'Brien, CF: Injection techniques for botulinum toxin using electromyography and electrical stimulation. Muscle Nerve Suppl 6:S176, 1997.
68. Ogawa, N, et al: Development of a simple spasticity quantification method: Effects of tizanidine on spasticity in patients with sequelae of cerebrovascular disease. J Int Med Res 20:78, 1992.
69. Ollinger, H, Gruber, J, and Singer, F: Outcomes of electromyographic investigations with muscle relaxant drugs acting primarily at a supraspinal or spinal level: Considerations on assessment, reproducibility and clinical significance. EEG EMG 16:104, 1985.
70. Pavesi, G, et al: Botulinum toxin type A in the treatment of upper limb spasticity among patients with traumatic brain injury. J Neurol Neurosurg Psychiatry 64:419, 1998.
71. Pearson, K and Gordon, J: Spinal reflexes. In Kandel, ER, Schwartz, JH, and Jessell, TM (eds): Principles of Neural Science, ed 4. McGraw-Hill, New York, 2000.
72. Pedersen, E, Alien-Soborg, P, and Mai, J: The mode of action of the GABA derivative baclofen in human spasticity. Acta Neurol Scand 50:665, 1974.
73. Peng, CT, et al: Prolonged severe withdrawal symptoms after acute-on-chronic baclofen overdose. J Toxicol Clin Toxicol 36:359, 1998.
74. Penn, RD and Kroin, JS: Long-term intrathecal baclofen infusion for treatment of spasticity. J Neurosurg 66:181, 1987.
75. Priebe, MM, et al: Effectiveness of gabapentin in controlling spasticity: A quantitative study. Spinal Cord 35:171, 1997.
76. Reeves, RK, et al: Hyperthermia, rhabdomyolysis, and disseminated intravascular coagulation associated with baclofen pump failure. Arch Phys Med Rehabil 79:353, 1998.
77. Reeves, RR, et al: Carisoprodol (Soma): Abuse potential and physician awareness. J Addict Dis 18:51, 1999.
78. Sampaio, C, et al: Botulinum toxin type A for the treatment of arm and hand spasticity in stroke patients. Clin Rehabil 11:3, 1997.
79. Simpson, DM: Clinical trials of botulinum toxin in the treatment of spasticity. Muscle Nerve Suppl 6:S169, 1997.
80. Smith, C, et al: Tizanidine treatment of spasticity caused by multiple sclerosis: Results of a double-blind, placebo-controlled trial. US tizanidine study group. Neurology 44(Suppl 9):S34, 1994.
81. Stanko, JR: Review of oral skeletal muscle relaxants for the craniomandibular disorder (CMD) practitioner. Cranio 8:234, 1990.
82. Stell, R, Thompson, PD, and Marsden, CD: Botulinum toxin in spasmodic torticollis. J Neurol Neurosurg Psychiatry 51:920, 1988.
83. Travell, JG and Simons, DG: Myofascial Pain and Dysfunction: The Trigger Point Method, Vol 2. Williams & Wilkins, Baltimore, 1992.
84. United Kingdom Tizanidine Trial Group: A double-blind, placebo-controlled trial of tizanidine in the treatment of spasticity caused by multiple sclerosis. Neurology 44(Suppl 9):S70, 1994.
85. VanWinkle, WB: Calcium release from skeletal muscle sarcoplasmic reticulum: Site of action of dantrolene sodium? Science 193:1130, 1976.
86. Wagstaff, AJ and Bryson, HM: Tizanidine. A reivew of its pharmacology, clinical efficacy and tolerability in the management of spasticity associated with cerebral and spinal disorders. Drugs 53:435, 1997.
87. Wallace, JD: Summary of combined clinical analysis of controlled clinical trials with tizanidine. Neurology 44(Suppl 9):S60, 1994.
88. Weingarden, SI and Belen, JG: Clonidine transdermal system for treatment of spasticity in spinal cord injury. Arch Phys Med Rehabil 73:876, 1992.

89. Wiens, HD: Spasticity in children with cerebral palsy: A retrospective review of the effects of intrathecal baclofen. Issues Compr Pediatr Nurs 21:49, 1998.
90. Wilson, DJ, et al: Kinematic changes following botulinum toxin injection after traumatic brain injury. Brain Inj 11:157, 1997.
91. Wong, V: Use of botulinum toxin injection in 17 children with spastic cerebral palsy. Pediatr Neurol 18:124, 1998.
92. Yablon, SA and Sipski, ML: Effect of transdermal clonidine on spinal spasticity: A case series. Am J Phys Med Rehabil 72:154, 1993.
93. Young, RR: Spasticity: A review. Neurology 44(Suppl 9):S12, 1994.
94. Young, RR and Delwaide, PJ: Drug therapy: Spasticity (parts 1 and 2). N Engl J Med 304:28, 96, 1981.
95. Zelnik, N, et al: The role of botulinum toxin in the treatment of lower limb spasticity in children with cerebral palsy: A pilot study. Isr J Med Sci 33:129, 1997.

SECTION IV

Drugs Used to Treat Pain and Inflammation

CHAPTER 14

Opioid Analgesics

Analgesic drug therapy and certain rehabilitation interventions share a common goal: pain relief. Consequently, analgesics are among the most frequently taken drugs by patients in a rehabilitation setting. The vast array of drugs that are used to treat pain can be roughly divided into two categories: opioid and nonopioid **analgesics**. Nonopioid analgesics are composed of drugs such as acetaminophen, aspirin, and similar agents. These drugs are discussed in Chapter 15. **Opioid** analgesics are a group of naturally occurring, semisynthetic, and synthetic agents that are characterized by their ability to relieve moderate-to-severe pain. These drugs exert their effects by binding to specific neuronal receptors that are located primarily in the CNS. Opioid analgesics are also characterized by their potential ability to produce physical dependence, and these agents are classified as controlled substances in the United States because of their potential for abuse (see Chapter 1 for a description of controlled substance classification). Morphine (Fig. 14–1) is considered the prototypical opioid analgesic, and other drugs of this type are often compared with morphine in terms of efficacy and potency.[5,43]

In the past, the term "narcotic" was often applied to these compounds because they tend to have sedative or sleep-inducing side effects and high doses can produce a state of unresponsiveness and stupor. Narcotic is a misleading name, however, because it describes a side effect of these agents rather than their principal therapeutic effect. Likewise, these drugs are sometimes referred to as "opiate" analgesics because some of these compounds are derived from opium (see the next section, "Source of Opioid Analgesics"). More recently, the term "opioid" has been instituted to represent all types of narcotic analgesic-like agents, regardless of their origin.[61,79] Hence, most sources preferentially use the term "opioid" to describe these drugs, and clinicians should recognize that this term represents all of the morphinelike medications.

SOURCE OF OPIOID ANALGESICS

As mentioned previously, opioid analgesics can be obtained from natural, synthetic, or semisynthetic sources. Synthetic agents, as the designation implies, are simply formulated from basic chemical components in the laboratory. The source of the naturally occurring and the semisynthetic narcotic analgesics is the opium poppy.[79] When the extract from the seeds of this flower is allowed to dry and harden, the resulting sub-

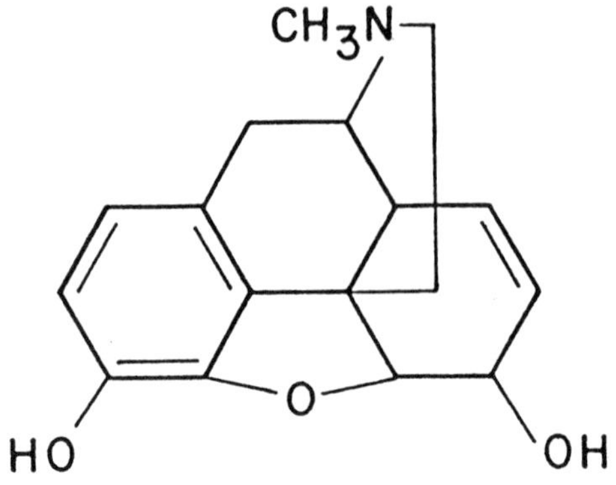

Morphine

FIGURE 14–1. Structure of morphine.

stance is opium. Opium contains about 20 biologically active compounds, including morphine and codeine. Other derivatives from opium can also directly produce analgesia in varying degrees or can serve as precursors for analgesic drugs. The most notable of these precursors is thebaine, which can be modified chemically to yield compounds such as heroin. Hence, the semisynthetic narcotic analgesics are derived from these precursors. Semisynthetic opioids can also be formulated by modifying one of the other naturally occurring narcotic drugs, such as morphine.

In addition to analgesic drugs and their precursors, opium also contains compounds that do not have any analgesic properties. These compounds can actually antagonize the analgesic effects of opioid agonists such as morphine. (As defined in Chapter 4, an *agonist* stimulates its respective receptor and exerts a physiologic response, whereas an *antagonist* blocks the receptor, thus preventing the response.) The role of these opioid antagonists is discussed in "Classification of Specific Agents."

ENDOGENOUS OPIOID PEPTIDES AND OPIOID RECEPTORS

Endogenous Opioids

Neurons at specific locations within the brain and spinal cord have been identified as having receptors that serve as binding sites for morphine and similar exogenous substances. Exogenous opioids exert their effects by binding to these receptors; the proposed mechanisms of these drug-receptor interactions are discussed in "Mechanism of Action." The discovery of these opioid receptors also suggested the existence of an endogenous opioidlike substance. Rather than isolating one such compound, the search for an "endogenous morphine" has actually revealed several groups of peptides with analgesic and other pharmacologic properties. It is now recognized that three distinct families of endogenous opioids exist: the endorphins, enkephalins, and dynorphins.[61] These peptides are manufactured and released within the body to control pain under specific conditions.[3,6,10,55,77] This chapter is not intended to elucidate all the known details of the endogenous opioid peptide system or how these endogenous compounds can be influenced by opioid drugs. These endogenous compounds do exert their effects, however, via the same receptors as the exogenous opioid drugs. There is obviously the possibility for a great deal of interaction between the endogenous and exogenous opioids, and research continues to investigate how exogenous drugs influence the function of the endogenous peptides, and vice versa.[1]

Opioid Receptors

Since their discovery, the opioid receptors have been examined in considerable detail. Studies in animals have suggested that rather than one homogeneous opioid receptor, there are at least three primary classes known as mu, kappa, and delta receptors[20,23,37,48,65] (Table 14–1). Furthermore, some of the primary classes may have subclassifications (e.g., there are believed to be two types of mu receptors, usually referred to as mu_1 and mu_2).[40,61,67] At the moment, we do not know if all of these subpopulations are present in humans, or if all are important in the response to exogenous opioids.[65] However, some specialization regarding both the location and the response of specific types of opioid receptors does appear to exist (see Table 14–1).

Stimulation of all three classes of opioid receptors causes analgesia. The mu receptor, however, seems to be the most important in mediating the analgesic effects of many opioids, including morphine.[17,56] Mu receptors are located in specific locations in the brain and spinal cord, and the analgesic effects of these receptors are mediated at the supraspinal and spinal levels by the mu_1 and mu_2 receptors, respectively.[61] Unfortunately, some of the more problematic side effects of opioid drugs may also be mediated by stimulation of mu receptors. For example, stimulation of mu_2 receptors may also cause respiratory depression, constipation, and an increase in the chance of addiction and opioid abuse in certain people.[58,79]

The existence of several classes of opioid receptors has therefore led to the development of drugs that are somewhat more selective in the receptor class or subclass that they stimulate. In particular, drugs that selectively stimulate kappa or delta receptors may still provide sufficient analgesia but will be less likely to provoke problems like res-

TABLE 14–1 Opioid Receptors

Primary Receptor	Subtypes	Site of Analgesic Action	Other Effects
Mu (μ)	μ_1	Supraspinal	Sedation* Inhibit acetylcholine release
	μ_2	Spinal	Respiratory depression Constipation Inhibit dopamine release
Kappa (κ)	κ_1	Spinal	Sedation* Psychotic effects* Constipation*
	κ_3	Supraspinal	
Delta (δ)	δ_1	Supraspinal	Inhibit dopamine release*
	δ_2	Spinal, supraspinal	

*Effect is associated with the primary receptor type (μ, κ, or δ), but the effect has not yet been attributed to a specific subtype within the primary receptor type.

Source: Adapted from Reisine, T and Pasternak, G: Opioid analgesics and antagonists. In Hardman, JG, et al (eds): The Pharmacological Basis of Therapeutics, ed 9. McGraw-Hill, New York, 1996, pp 523–525.

piratory depression and opioid abuse if they avoid or even block (antagonize) the mu receptors. Certain opioid drugs, for example, stimulate kappa receptors while avoiding or blocking the mu receptors. These agents are known as mixed agonist-antagonist opioids, and their clinical significance is addressed in the next section, "Classification of Specific Agents."

The discovery of several classes of opioid receptors that cause different effects and side effects has important pharmacologic implications. Research in this area continues to expand our knowledge about the structural and functional aspects of these receptor classes. Drug developers will hopefully capitalize on the unique aspects of opioid receptor classes, and new agents will be produced that are even more specific in relieving pain without provoking excessive side effects.

CLASSIFICATION OF SPECIFIC AGENTS

Opioid analgesics are classified as strong agonists, mild-to-moderate agonists, mixed agonist-antagonists, and antagonists according to their interaction with opioid receptors. Some opioids in these categories are listed in Table 14–2. The basic characteristics of each category and clinically relevant examples are also discussed here.

Strong Agonists. These agents are used to treat severe pain. As the name implies, these drugs have a high affinity for certain receptors and are believed to interact primarily with mu opioid receptors in the CNS. The best-known member of this group is morphine, and the other strong agonists are similar pharmacologically. Examples of strong opioid agonists include the following:

- fentanyl (Sublimaze)
- hydromorphone (Hydrostat, Dilaudid)
- levorphanol (Levo-Dromoran)
- meperidine (Demerol)
- methadone (Dolophine, Methadose)
- morphine (Duramorph, Epimorph, Roxanol, Statex, others)
- oxymorphone (Numorphan)

Mild-to-Moderate Agonists. These drugs are still considered agonists that stimulate opioid receptors, but they do not have as high an affinity or efficacy as the drugs listed previously. These drugs are more appropriate for treating pain of moderate intensity. Examples include the following:

- codeine
- hydrocodone (Hycodan)
- oxycodone (OxyContin, Roxicodone)
- propoxyphene (Darvon)

Mixed Agonist-Antagonists. These drugs exhibit some agonist and antagonist-like activity at the same time because of the ability of the drug to act differently at specific classes of opioid receptors. For instance, drugs in this category cause analgesia because they bind to and activate kappa receptors; that is, they are kappa-receptor agonists. At the same time, these drugs block or only partially activate mu receptors, thus acting as mu-receptor antagonists or partial agonists, respectively.[14,56] (The effects of partial agonists are described in more detail in Chapter 4.) Mixed agonist-antagonist opioids ap-

TABLE 14–2 Opioid Analgesics

Drug	Route of Administration*	Onset of Action (min)	Time to Peak Effect (min)	Duration of Action (hr)
Strong Agonists				
Fentanyl	IM	7–15	20–30	1–2
(Sublimaze)	IV	1–2	3–5	0.5–1
Hydromorphone	Oral	30	90–120	4
(Hydrostat, Dilaudid)	IM	15	30–60	4–5
	IV	10–15	15–30	2–3
	Sub-Q	15	30–90	4
Levorphanol	Oral	10–60	90–120	4–5
(Levo-Dromoran)	IM	—	60	4–5
	IV	—	Within 20	4–5
	Sub-Q	—	60–90	4–5
Meperidine	Oral	15	60–90	2–4
(Demerol)	IM	10–15	30–50	2–4
	IV	1	5–7	2–4
	Sub-Q	10–15	30–50	2–4
Methadone	Oral	30–60	90–120	4–6
(Dolophine, Methadose)	IM	10–20	60–120	4–5
	IV	—	15–30	3–4
Morphine	Oral	—	60–120	4–5
(many trade names)	IM	10–30	30–60	4–5
	IV	—	20	4–5
	Sub-Q	10–30	50–90	4–5
	Epidural	15–60	—	Up to 24
	Intrathecal	15–60	—	Up to 24
Oxymorphone	IM	10–15	30–90	3–6
(Numorphan)	IV	5–10	15–30	3–4
	Sub-Q	10–20	—	3–6
	Rectal	15–30	120	3–6
Mild-to-Moderate Agonists				
Codeine	Oral	30–40	60–120	4
(generic)	IM	10–30	30–60	4
	Sub-Q	10–30	—	4
Hydrocodone (Hycodan)	Oral	10–30	30–60	4–6
Oxycodone (OxyContin, Roxicodone)	Oral	—	60	3–4
Propoxyphene (Darvon)	Oral	15–60	120	4–6
Mixed Agonist-Antagonist				
Butorphanol	IM	10–30	30–60	3–4
(Stadol)	IV	2–3	30	2–4
Nalbuphine	IM	Within 15	60	3–6
(Nubain)	IV	2–3	30	3–4
	Sub-Q	Within 15	—	3–6
Pentazocine	Oral	15–30	60–90	3
(Talwin)	IM	15–20	30–60	2–3
	IV	2–3	15–30	2–3
	Sub-Q	15–20	30–60	2–3

*IM = intramuscular; IV = intravenous; sub-Q = subcutaneous.

pear to have the advantage of producing adequate analgesia with less risk of the side effects associated with mu receptors, including respiratory depression. These drugs are therefore safer in terms of a reduced risk of fatal overdose.[12,46,56] These drugs may also have fewer addictive qualities than strong mu receptor agonists such as morphine.[43,46] Mixed agonist-antagonists, however, may produce more psychotropic effects (hallucinations, vivid dreams), and their maximal analgesic effect may not be as great as strong mu agonists.[7] Consequently, these drugs are not used extensively, but they offer an alternative to strong-moderate opioid agonists in certain patients. Examples include the following:

- butorphanol (Stadol)
- nalbuphine (Nubain)
- pentazocine (Talwin)

Antagonists. These drugs block all opioid receptors, with a particular affinity for the mu variety. Because of their antagonistic properties, these agents will not produce analgesia but will displace opioid agonists from the opioid receptors and block any further effects of the agonist molecules. Consequently, these drugs are used primarily in the treatment of opioid overdose and addiction. Certain opioid antagonists (e.g., naloxone) can rapidly (within 1 to 2 minutes) and dramatically reverse the respiratory depression that is usually the cause of death in excessive opioid ingestion. Other antagonists (e.g., naltrexone) are used in conjunction with behavioral therapy to maintain an opioid-free state in individuals recovering from opioid addiction. Hence, the primary agents used clinically as opioid antagonists are the following:

- naloxone (Narcan)
- naltrexone (ReVia)

PHARMACOKINETICS

Some opioid analgesics can be given orally, a preferred route of administration in terms of convenience and safety. Several of these enteral drugs also come in suppository form, permitting rectal administration if nausea and vomiting prohibit the oral route. Some opioids including morphine are now available in sustained-release enteral preparations, thus allowing more prolonged effects and wider intervals between doses.[28] Because of poor intestinal absorption or significant first-pass inactivation, other agents must be administered parenterally, usually through subcutaneous or intramuscular injection. Intravenous administration is also sometimes used but must be done slowly and with caution. When the intravenous route is used, the narcotic is frequently diluted, and infusion pumps are used to allow the slow, controlled administration of the drug. The intravenous route or other parenteral routes (epidural and intrathecal infusion) can also be used to administer opioids during patient-controlled analgesia; this concept is addressed in Chapter 17.

The feasibility of using other relatively new methods for administering opioids has also been investigated. For instance, the intranasal route may be a suitable means of administering fentanyl, a potent and fast-acting opioid.[74,75] Other agents including morphine can be given through the transdermal route by using skin patches or iontophoresis techniques.[2,4] It will be interesting to see if these newer methods of administration will gain widespread acceptance in the future.

Because of different degrees of solubility, the distribution and subsequent onset of action of specific agents vary (see Table 14–2). Opioids are ultimately distributed throughout all tissues, and these agents probably exert their principal analgesic effects after they reach the CNS. Some opioid effects may also be mediated by peripheral receptors located at the site of painful inflammation (see "Mechanism of Action"). Metabolic inactivation of these drugs takes place primarily in the liver, although some degree of metabolism also occurs in other tissues, such as the kidneys, lungs, and CNS. The kidneys excrete the drug metabolite and, to a lesser extent, the intact drug in the urine.

MECHANISM OF ACTION

Effect of Opioids on the Central Nervous System

As discussed earlier, opioid receptors exist at specific locations throughout the CNS and possibly in peripheral nerve tissues as well. In the spinal cord, these receptors are concentrated on neurons responsible for transmitting nociceptive input to higher (supraspinal) levels.[82] Opioid receptors have likewise been identified in several locations of the brain that are associated with pain transmission and interpretation. These areas include the periaqueductal gray region of the spinoreticular tract, medial thalamic nuclei, hypothalamus, limbic system, and several other areas.[27,68]

Opioids basically exert their analgesic effects by inhibiting synaptic transmission in key pain pathways in the spinal cord and brain. This inhibitory effect is mediated by opioid receptors that are located on both presynaptic and postsynaptic membranes of pain-mediating synapses (Fig. 14–2). In the spinal cord, for example, receptors are located on the presynaptic terminals of primary (first-order) nociceptive afferents, and when bound by opioids, they directly decrease the release of pain-mediating transmitters such as sub-

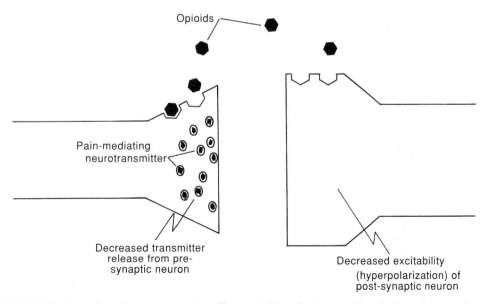

FIGURE 14–2. Schematic representation of how opioid analgesics may impair synaptic transmission in pain-mediating pathways. The drug binds to specific opioid receptors on the presynaptic and postsynaptic membranes.

stance P.[8,24,82] Opioid drug-receptor interactions also take place on the postsynaptic membrane of the secondary afferent neuron—that is, the second-order nociceptive afferent neuron in the spinal cord.[8,82] When stimulated, these receptors also inhibit pain transmission by hyperpolarizing the postsynaptic neuron.

Opioids therefore inhibit synaptic transmission by decreasing neurotransmitter release from the presynaptic terminal and by decreasing the excitability of (hyperpolarizing) the postsynaptic neuron within key pain pathways in the spinal cord and brain. These effects are mediated through opioid receptors that are located on the membrane of these neurons but are linked to the internal chemistry on the presynaptic and postsynaptic neurons through regulatory G proteins.[9,20,69] As described in Chapter 4, regulatory G proteins act as an intermediate link between receptor activation and the intracellular effector mechanism that ultimately causes a change in cellular activity. In the case of opioid receptors, these G proteins interact with three primary cellular effectors: calcium channels, potassium channels, and the adenyl cyclase enzyme.[9,11,23,29] At the presynaptic terminal, stimulation of opioid receptors activates G proteins that in turn inhibit the opening of calcium channels on the nerve membrane.[9,11] Decreased calcium entry into the presynaptic terminal causes decreased neurotransmitter release because calcium influx mediates transmitter release at a chemical synapse. At the postsynaptic neuron, opioid receptors are linked via G proteins to potassium channels, and activation of the receptor leads to opening of these channels and loss of potassium from the postsynaptic neuron.[9,11] A relative loss of potassium from the postsynaptic neuron causes hyperpolarization because efflux of potassium (a cation) results in a relative increase in the negative intracellular electric potential. The postsynaptic neuron is therefore more difficult to excite because the interior of the cell is more negative.

Finally, opioid receptors are linked via G proteins to the adenyl cyclase enzyme, and stimulation of the receptor leads to inhibition of this enzyme and decreased synthesis of cyclic adenosine monophosphate (cAMP). Cyclic AMP is an important second messenger that regulates neurotransmitter release from the presynaptic terminal and may also regulate the firing threshold of the postsynaptic neuron.[23,29] Opioid-mediated inhibition of this second messenger therefore helps explain how these drugs alter pain transmission. Hence, opioid drugs exert their analgesic effects by interacting with receptors that are linked to several intracellular effector mechanisms that ultimately lead to decreased synaptic transmission in specific pain pathways.

Peripheral Effects of Opioids

Opioid receptors may exist outside the CNS, and some of the analgesic effects of opioid drugs may be mediated at peripheral sites.[70,71] Opioid receptors have been identified on the distal (peripheral) ends of primary afferent (sensory) neurons.[70–72] Binding of opioid agents to these peripheral receptors will provide an analgesic effect by decreasing the excitability of these sensory neurons (Fig. 14–3). This idea is supported by the fact that endogenous opioids (endorphins, enkephalins) are often produced in peripheral tissues during certain types of painful inflammation and that these endogenous substances seem to act locally on the peripheral sensory nerve terminals.[71,72] Likewise, results from some studies in animals and humans suggest that exogenous opioids can be administered directly into peripheral tissues (e.g., injected into an inflamed joint) and that these agents exert analgesic effects even though the drug never reaches the CNS.[31,70]

Hence, some evidence suggests that opioid receptors exist outside the CNS and that opioid drugs may help produce analgesia at these peripheral sites. However, the clinical

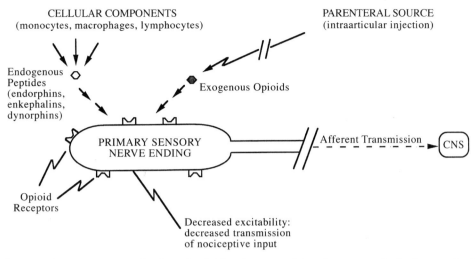

FIGURE 14–3. Putative mechanism of opioid action on peripheral nerve terminals. See text for discussion.

significance of these peripheral opioid effects remains to be fully determined. For instance, these receptors may play a role in mediating only certain types of pain, such as the pain associated with inflammation.[70] Nonetheless, the fact that certain types of pain might be controlled by peripherally acting opioids has important pharmacologic implications. For instance, opioids that work exclusively in the periphery would not cause CNS-mediated side effects such as sedation, respiratory depression, and tolerance. Peripheral-acting opioids could be developed by creating lipophobic compounds that are unable to cross the blood-brain barrier.[70–72] The use of these peripheral-acting drugs remains fairly experimental at the present time, and additional clinical trials will be needed to determine whether this becomes a viable means of treating certain types of pain.

CLINICAL APPLICATIONS

Treatment of Pain

Opioid analgesics are most effective in treating moderate-to-severe pain that is more or less constant in duration. These drugs are not as effective in treating sharp, intermittent pain, although higher doses can relieve this type of pain as well. Some examples of the clinical use of opioid analgesics include the treatment of acute pain following surgery, trauma, and myocardial infarction, as well as the treatment of chronic pain in patients with conditions such as cancer. Because of the potential for serious side effects (see "Problems and Adverse Effects"), these drugs should be used only when necessary, and the dose should be titrated according to the patient's pain. Generally, oral administration of a mild-to-moderate opioid agonist should be used first, with stronger agonists being instituted orally and then parenterally if needed. In cases of chronic pain, pain control by nonopioid drugs should be attempted first. However, opioid analgesics should be instituted when the improved quality of life offered to the patient with chronic pain clearly outweighs the potential risks of these drugs.[26,41,62]

Opioid analgesics often produce a unique form of analgesia as compared with the nonopioid agents. Opioids frequently alter the perception of pain rather than eliminating the painful sensation entirely. The patient may still be aware of the pain, but it is no longer the primary focus of his or her attention. In a sense, the patient is no longer preoccupied by the pain. This type of analgesia is also often associated with euphoria and a sensation of floating. These sensations may be caused by the stimulation of specific types of opiate receptors within the limbic system (i.e., delta receptors).

The route of opioid administration appears to be important in providing effective pain relief.[43] Although the oral route is the easiest and most convenient, parenteral routes may be more effective in chronic or severe, intractable pain. In particular, administration directly into the epidural or intrathecal space has been suggested as optimal in relieving pain following certain types of surgery or in terminal cancer.[16,21,33,45,54,60,78,80] Because reinsertion of a needle every time the drug is needed is impractical, indwelling catheters are often implanted surgically so that the tip of the catheter lies in the epidural or intrathecal space. The free end of the catheter can be brought out through the patient's skin and used to administer the opioid directly into the area surrounding the spinal cord. Alternatively, the catheter can be connected to some sort of a drug reservoir or pump that contains the opioid drug. Such devices can be located outside the patient's body or implanted surgically beneath the patient's skin (e.g., in the abdominal wall), and these pumps are programmed to deliver the drug at a fixed rate into the indwelling catheter.[44] Programmable drug delivery systems may have some risks, such as errors in programming the pump, displacement or obstruction of the catheter, and pump malfunction that leads to overdose or underdose. Nonetheless, these systems appear to be an effective way of treating severe, chronic pain in selected patients, such as those with terminal cancer.[21,33,44,54,63,78]

The effectiveness of opioid analgesics also appears to be influenced by the dosing schedule. The current consensus is that orally administered opioids are more effective when given at regularly scheduled intervals rather than when the patient feels the need for the drug.[66] This may be because with regularly scheduled dosages, plasma concentrations may be maintained within a therapeutic range, rather than allowing the large plasma fluctuations that may occur if the drugs are given at sporadic intervals. Consistent with this hypothesis is the finding that continuous infusion of the opioid (either intravenously or spinally) provides optimal pain relief postoperatively or in chronic, intractable pain.[21,33,44,54,78] Continuous infusion is associated with certain side effects, especially nausea and constipation, as well as the potential for disruption of the drug delivery system.[22,44,54,78,80] Problems with tolerance have also been reported during continuous administration,[39,47] but it is somewhat controversial whether tolerance really develops when these drugs are used appropriately in the clinical management of pain (see "Concepts of Addiction, Tolerance, and Physical Dependence"). Hence, the benefit-to-risk ratio for continuous infusion is often acceptable in patients with severe pain. This method of opioid administration continues to gain acceptance.[60,78]

Use of Opioids in Patient-Controlled Analgesia

Finally, some rather innovative techniques have allowed the patient to control the delivery of the analgesic.[25,35,53] These techniques are collectively known as patient-controlled analgesia (PCA) because the patient is able to periodically administer a specific dose of the drug (by pushing a button or some other device). PCA systems have some distinct advantages over conventional administration, and PCAs are often used in the treatment of severe, chronic pain, as well as following various types of surgery.[25,35,53] The use of opioids and other drugs in PCA systems is discussed in Chapter 17.

Other Opioid Uses

Opioids have several other clinical applications. These agents can be used as an anesthetic premedication or as an adjunct in general anesthesia. Opioids are effective in cough suppression, and the short-term use of codeine in this regard is quite common. Opioid agonists decrease gastrointestinal motility and can be used to control cases of severe diarrhea. This effect is probably mediated indirectly through an effect on the CNS, as well as through a direct effect on the intestine. Finally, opioid agonists are used as an adjunct in cases of acute pulmonary edema. These drugs probably do not directly improve ventilatory capacity, but they do serve to reduce feelings of intense panic and anxiety associated with the dyspnea of this disorder. Patients feel they can breathe more easily following opioid administration.

PROBLEMS AND ADVERSE EFFECTS

Opioid analgesics produce a number of central and peripheral side effects. Virtually all of these drugs have sedative properties and induce some degree of mental slowing and drowsiness. Patients taking opioids for the relief of pain may also become somewhat euphoric, although the manner and degree of such mood changes vary from individual to individual. One of the more potentially serious side effects is the respiratory depression often seen after narcotic administration.[12] Within a few minutes after administration, these drugs cause the breathing rate to slow down, which can last for several hours. Although not usually a major problem when therapeutic doses are given to relatively healthy individuals, respiratory depression can be severe or even fatal in seriously ill patients, in patients with pre-existing pulmonary problems, or in cases of overdose. Some cardiovascular problems such as orthostatic hypotension may also occur immediately after opioids are administered, especially when parenteral routes are used. Finally, gastrointestinal distress in the form of nausea and vomiting is quite common with many of the narcotic analgesics. Because of their antiperistaltic action, these drugs can also cause constipation.[38]

CONCEPTS OF ADDICTION, TOLERANCE, AND PHYSICAL DEPENDENCE

When used inappropriately, opioid drugs can produce addiction. The term *addiction* typically refers to situations in which certain individuals repeatedly seek out and ingest certain substances for mood-altering and pleasurable experiences, such as the heroin addict who takes this drug illicitly to achieve an opioid "high." In this sense, addiction is a very complex phenomenon that has strong psychologic implications regarding why certain chemicals cause this behavior in certain people. This concept of addiction is often separated from the physiologic changes that can accompany prolonged opioid use—namely, tolerance and physical dependence.

Tolerance is the need for more drug to achieve a given effect, and **physical dependence** is the onset of withdrawal symptoms if a drug is suddenly discontinued. Tolerance and physical dependence are also rather complex phenomena, and a complete discussion of the factors involved in producing them is beyond the scope of this chapter. The primary characteristics of tolerance and physical dependence will be briefly discussed here as they relate to opioid usage.

Tolerance

Tolerance is defined as the need for more drug to achieve the same effect when the drug is used for prolonged periods. When used for the treatment of pain in some patients, the dosage of the opioid may need to be increased periodically to continue to provide adequate relief. The physiologic reasons for tolerance are complex and probably involve changes in the intracellular response to repeated stimulation of opioid receptors. Prolonged exposure to opioids can also cause a decrease in the number and sensitivity of the opioid receptors, a phenomenon known as receptor down-regulation and desensitization[18,34] (see Chap. 4). However, these changes in the quantity and sensitivity of opioid receptors do not seem to be the primary reasons for opioid tolerance.[30] It seems more likely that tolerance is caused by changes in the intracellular effectors that are coupled to the opioid receptor—namely, the G proteins and intracellular effector mechanisms.[51,52] As described earlier, opioid receptors mediate their effects through regulatory G proteins that are linked to intracellular effectors, including the adenyl cyclase enzyme. Tolerance to opioid drugs therefore seems to be caused by long-term changes in G protein function and adenyl cyclase–induced synthesis of second messengers like cAMP.[51,52] In a sense, tolerance occurs because the internal biochemistry of the cell has been blunted by repeated stimulation of the G protein–effector mechanisms.

The physiologic changes that cause opioid tolerance typically follow a predictable time course. Tolerance begins after the first dose of the narcotic, but the need for increased amounts of the drug usually becomes obvious after 2 to 3 weeks of administration. Tolerance seems to last approximately 1 to 2 weeks after the drug is removed. This does not mean that the patient no longer has any desire for the drug, but that the patient will again respond to the initial dosage after 14 days or so. Other factors may influence the individual's desire for the drug long after any physiologic effects have disappeared (see "Physical Dependence").

Physical Dependence

Physical dependence is usually defined as the onset of withdrawal symptoms when the drug is abruptly removed. **Withdrawal syndrome** from opioid dependence is associated with a number of obvious and unpleasant symptoms (Table 14–3). In severe dependence, withdrawal symptoms become evident within 6 to 10 hours after the last dose of the drug and reach their peak in the second or third day after the drug has been stopped. Withdrawal symptoms last approximately 5 days. This does not necessarily mean that the individual no longer desires the drug, only that the physical symptoms of withdrawal have ceased. Indeed, an addict may continue to crave the drug after months or years of abstinence.

TABLE 14–3 Abstinence Syndromes: Symptoms of Narcotic Withdrawal

Body aches	Runny nose
Diarrhea	Shivering
Fever	Sneezing
Gooseflesh	Stomach cramps
Insomnia	Sweating
Irritability	Tachycardia
Loss of appetite	Uncontrollable yawning
Nausea/vomiting	Weakness/fatigue

Physical dependence must therefore be differentiated from the more intangible concepts of addiction and psychologic dependence. Psychologic dependence seems to be related to pleasurable changes in mood and behavior evoked by the drug. The individual is motivated to continually reproduce these pleasurable sensations because of the feelings of well-being, relaxation, and so on. Psychologic dependence seems to create the drug-seeking behavior that causes the addict to relapse into use of the drug long after the physiologic effects have disappeared.

Tolerance and Dependence during Therapeutic Opioid Use

Although tolerance and dependence can occur whenever opioid drugs are used indiscriminately for prolonged periods, there is some debate as to whether these phenomena must always accompany the therapeutic use of opioid drugs for the treatment of chronic pain. There is growing evidence that the risk of tolerance and dependence is actually very low when opioid drugs are used appropriately to treat chronic pain.[59,64] For example, there appear to be relatively few problems with long-term opioid use when these drugs are administered to treat pain in patients who do not have a history of substance abuse, who adhere to the prescribed opioid regimen, and who have pain from physiologic rather than psychologic causes.[57,59,76]

Some experts also feel that tolerance and physical dependence will not occur if the dosage is carefully adjusted to meet the patient's needs.[43,63] It is thought that when the opioid dose exactly matches the patient's need for pain control, there is no excess drug that will stimulate the drug-seeking behavior commonly associated with opioid addiction. The opioid is essentially absorbed by the patient's pain. Of course, patients with chronic pain may still need to have the dosage increased periodically. This observation would be explained by the fact that the pain has increased because the patient's condition has worsened (e.g., the cancer has increased) rather than the idea that the patient developed pharmacologic tolerance to the drug.[19,59,63]

Thus, many practitioners think that problems with addiction, tolerance, and dependence are minimized when opioid drugs are used therapeutically. These agents are essentially being used for a specific reason, treatment of pain, rather than for the pleasure-seeking purpose associated with the recreational use of these drugs. These drugs must, of course, be used carefully and with strict regard to using the lowest effective dose. Hence, there is consensus that opioids are very effective and important analgesic agents and should be used under appropriate therapeutic conditions without excessive fear that the patient will develop addiction or become especially tolerant to the drug's effects.[26,42,62]

Use of Methadone to Treat Opioid Addiction

The illegal use and abuse of narcotics such as heroin is a major problem in many countries, and many therapists will work with patients who are undergoing pharmacologic and nonpharmacologic treatment of opioid addiction. With regard to pharmacologic management, methadone is often used to treat people who are addicted to heroin. Methadone is a strong narcotic agonist, similar in potency and efficacy to morphine. Although giving an opioid to treat opioid addiction may at first appear odd, methadone offers several advantages, such as milder withdrawal symptoms. Methadone is essentially substituted for the heroin and then slowly withdrawn as various methods of counseling are employed to discourage further drug abuse.[49] Use of methadone, however, remains controversial because of the rather low success rate of this intervention and the tendency for many subjects to relapse and return to heroin abuse.[13] Hence, efforts continue to provide more effective programs that use methadone and related interventions to treat heroin addiction.[36,50,81] For a detailed discussion on the use of methadone in heroin addiction, the reader is referred to several sources listed at the end of this chapter.[24,36,50,73]

SPECIAL CONCERNS IN REHABILITATION PATIENTS

Physical therapists will encounter the use of opioid analgesics in patients requiring acute pain relief (e.g., following surgery, trauma) and chronic analgesia (for patients with terminal cancer and other types of severe chronic pain). The usual side effects of sedation and gastrointestinal discomfort may be bothersome during some of the therapy sessions. However, the relief of pain afforded by these drugs may be helpful in allowing a relatively more vigorous and comprehensive rehabilitation regimen. The benefits of pain relief usually outweigh side effects such as sedation. Scheduling therapy when these drugs reach their peak effects may be advantageous (see Table 14–2). One side effect that should be taken into account during therapy is the tendency of these drugs to produce respiratory depression. Opioids tend to make the medullary chemoreceptors less responsive to carbon dioxide, thus slowing down the respiratory rate and inducing a relative hypoxia and hypercapnia.[15] This fact should be considered if any exercise is instituted as part of the rehabilitation program. The respiratory response to this exercise may be blunted.

The tendency for these drugs to produce constipation is another side effect that could have important implications for patients receiving physical rehabilitation. Opioid-induced constipation is especially problematic in patients with spinal cord injury or other conditions that decrease gastrointestinal motility. In such patients, opioids are often administered along with laxatives and GI stimulants (see Chap. 27) to minimize the constipating effects and risk of fecal impaction. Therapists should therefore be aware of these constipating effects and help educate patients and their families so that these effects do not result in serious problems.

Therapists may also be working with patients who are experiencing withdrawal symptoms from opioid drugs. Such patients may be in the process of being weaned off the therapeutic use of these agents, or they may be heroin addicts who have been hospitalized for other reasons (e.g., trauma, surgery). If not on some type of methadone maintenance, the addict may be experiencing a wide variety of physical symptoms, including diffuse muscle aches. The therapist should be aware that these aches and pains may be caused by opioid withdrawal rather than by an actual somatic disorder. Therapists may, however, help the patient cope with opioid withdrawal by using various physical agents (heat, electrotherapy) and manual (massage, relaxation) techniques to alleviate these somatic symptoms.

CASE STUDY

OPIOID ANALGESICS

Brief History. N.P., a 45-year-old woman, was involved in an automobile accident approximately 6 months ago. She received multiple contusions from the accident, but no major injuries were sustained. Two months later, she began to develop pain in the right shoulder. This pain progressively increased, and she was treated for bursitis using anti-inflammatory drugs. Her shoulder motion became progressively more limited, however; any movement of her glenohumeral joint caused rather severe pain. She was reevaluated, and a diagnosis of adhesive capsulitis was made. The patient was admitted to the hospital, and while she was under general anesthesia, a closed manipulation of the shoulder was performed. When the patient recovered from the anesthesia, meperidine (Demerol) was prescribed for pain relief. This drug was given orally at a dosage of 75 mg every 4 hours. Physical therapy was also initiated the afternoon following the closed manipulation. Passive range-of-motion exercises were used to maintain the increased joint mobility achieved during the manipulative procedure.

Relevance to Therapy/Clinical Decision. The therapist arranged the treatment schedule so that the meperidine was reaching peak effects during the therapy session. The patient was seen approximately 1 hour following the oral administration of the drug. The initial session was scheduled at the patient's bedside because the patient was still woozy from the anesthesia. On the following day, therapy was continued in the physical therapy department. However, the patient was brought to the department on a stretcher to prevent an episode of dizziness brought on by orthostatic hypotension. On the third day, the patient's medication was changed to hydrocodone (Hycodan), a mild-to-moderate opioid agonist. By this time, the patient was being transported to physical therapy in a wheelchair, and the therapy session also included active exercise. The patient was discharged on the fourth day after the manipulative procedure. She continued to attend therapy as an outpatient, and full function of her right shoulder was ultimately restored.

SUMMARY

Opioid analgesics represent some of the most effective methods of treating moderate-to-severe pain. When used properly, these agents can alleviate acute and chronic pain in a variety of situations. The use of these drugs is sometimes tempered by their tendency to produce tolerance and physical dependence, but their potential for abuse seems relatively low when these drugs are used appropriately to treat pain. Opioid drugs therefore represent the most effective pharmacologic means of helping patients deal with acute and chronic pain. The analgesic properties of these drugs often provide a substantial benefit in patients involved in rehabilitation. Physical therapists should be aware of some of the side effects such as sedation and respiratory depression and should be cognizant of the impact of these effects during the rehabilitation session.

REFERENCES

1. Adams, ML, et al: The role of endogenous peptides in the action of opioid analgesics. Ann Emerg Med 15:1030, 1986.
2. Ahmedzai, S: Current strategies for pain control. Ann Oncol 8(Suppl 3):S21, 1997.
3. Akil, H, et al: Endogenous opioids: Biology and function. Annu Rev Neurosci 7:223, 1984.
4. Ashburn, MA, et al: Iontophoretic delivery of morphine for postoperative analgesia. J Pain Symptom Manage 7:27, 1992.
5. Austrup, ML and Korean, G: Analgesic agents for the postoperative period: Opioids. Surg Clin North Am 79:253, 1999.

6. Basbaum, AI and Fields, HL: Endogenous pain control systems: Brainstem spinal pathways and endorphin circuitry. Annu Rev Neurosci 7:309, 1984.
7. Baumann, TJ: Pain management. In DiPiro, JT, et al (eds): Pharmacotherapy: A Pathophysiologic Approach, ed 4. Appleton & Lange, Stamford, CT, 1999.
8. Besson, JM: The neurobiology of pain. Lancet 353:1610, 1999.
9. Blake, AD, et al: Molecular regulation of opioid receptors. Receptors Channels 5:231, 1997.
10. Bloom, FE: The endorphins: A growing family of pharmacologically pertinent peptides. Annu Rev Pharmacol Toxicol 23:151, 1983.
11. Bovill, JG: Mechanisms of actions of opioids and non-steroidal anti-inflammatory drugs. Eur J Anaesthesiol Suppl 15:9, 1997.
12. Bowdle, TA: Adverse effects of opioid agonists and agonist-antagonists in anaesthesia. Drug Saf 19:173, 1998.
13. Brewer, DD, et al: A meta-analysis of predictors of continued drug use during and after treatment for opiate addiction. Addiction 93:73, 1998.
14. Burkey, TH, et al: The efficacy of delta-opioid receptor-selective drugs. Life Sci 62:1531, 1998.
15. Camporesi, EM, et al: Ventilatory CO_2 sensitivity after intravenous and epidural morphine in volunteers. Anesth Analg 62:633, 1983.
16. Chaplan, SR, et al: Morphine and hydromorphone epidural analgesia: A prospective, randomized comparison. Anesthesiology 77:1090, 1992.
17. Childers, SR: Opioid receptors: Pinning down the opiate targets. Curr Biol 7:R695, 1997.
18. Collin, E and Cesselin, F: Neurobiological mechanisms of opioid tolerance and dependence. Clin Neuropharmacol 14:465, 1991.
19. Collin, E, et al: Is disease progression the major factor in morphine tolerance in cancer pain treatment. Pain 55:319, 1993.
20. Connor, M and Christie, MD: Opioid receptor signaling mechanisms. Clin Exp Pharmacol Physiol 26:493, 1999.
21. Coombs, DW, et al: Relief of continuous chronic pain by intraspinal narcotics infusion via an implanted reservoir. JAMA 250:2336, 1983.
22. Dahm, P, et al: Efficacy and technical complications of long-term continuous intraspinal infusions of opioid and/or bupivacaine in refractory nonmalignant pain: A comparison between the epidural and the intrathecal approach with externalized or implanted catheters and infusion pumps. Clin J Pain 14:4, 1998.
23. Dickenson, AH: Mechanisms of the analgesic actions of opiates and opioids. BMJ 47:690, 1991.
24. Dole, VP: Implications of methadone maintenance for theories of narcotic addiction. JAMA 260:3025, 1988.
25. Etches, RC: Patient-controlled analgesia. Surg Clin North Am 79:297, 1999.
26. Gardner, JR and Sandhu, G: The stigma and enigma of chronic non-malignant back pain (CNMBP) treated with long-term opioids (LTO). Contemp Nurse 6:61, 1997.
27. Goodman, RR and Pasternak, GW: Visualization of mu_1 opiate receptors in the rat brain by using a computerized autoradiographic subtraction technique. Proc Natl Acad Sci U S A 82:6667, 1985.
28. Gourlay, GK: Sustained relief of chronic pain. Pharmacokinetics of sustained release morphine. Clin Pharmacokinet 35:173, 1998.
29. Grudt, TJ and Williams, JT: Opioid receptors and the regulation of ion conductances. Rev Neurosci 6:279, 1995.
30. Harrison, LM, Kastin, AJ, and Zadina, JE: Opiate tolerance and dependence: Receptors, G-proteins, and antiopiates. Peptides 19:1603, 1998.
31. Joshi, GP, et al: Intra-articular morphine for pain relief after knee arthroscopy. J Bone Joint Surg Br 74:749, 1992.
32. Keats, AS: The effect of drugs on respiration in man. Annu Rev Pharmacol Toxicol 25:41, 1985.
33. Krames, ES, et al: Continuous infusion of spinally administered narcotics for the relief of pain due to malignant disorders. Cancer 56:696, 1986.
34. Law, PY and Loh, HH: Regulation of opioid receptor activities. J Pharmacol Exp Ther 289:607, 1999.
35. Lehmann, KA: Patient-controlled analgesia: An efficient therapeutic tool in the postoperative setting. Eur Surg Res 31:112, 1999.
36. Lewis, DC: Access to narcotic addiction treatment and medical care: Prospects for the expansion of methadone maintenance treatment. J Addict Dis 18:5, 1999.
37. Lutz, RA and Pfister, HP: Opioid receptors and their pharmacological profiles. J Recept Res 12:267, 1992.
38. Mancini, I and Bruera, E: Constipation in advanced cancer patients. Support Care Cancer 6:356, 1998.
39. Marshall, HUW, et al: Relief of pain by infusion of morphine after operation: Does tolerance develop? BMJ 291:19, 1985.
40. Martin, WR: Pharmacology of opioids. Pharmacol Rev 35:283, 1983.
41. McGivney, WT and Crooks, GM: The care of patients with severe chronic pain in terminal illness. JAMA 251:1182, 1984.
42. McQuay, H: Opioids in pain management. Lancet 353:2229, 1999.
43. McQuay, HJ: Opioid clinical pharmacology and routes of administration. Br Med Bull 47:703, 1991.
44. Mercadante, S: Problems of long-term spinal opioid treatment in advanced cancer patients. Pain 79:1, 1999.
45. Mercadante, S: Controversies over spinal treatment in advanced cancer patients. Support Care Cancer 6:495, 1998.

46. Millan, MJ: K-opioid receptors and analgesia. Trends Pharmacol Sci 11:70, 1990.
47. Milne, B, et al: Analgesia and tolerance to intrathecal morphine and norepinephrine infusion via implanted miniosmotic pumps in the rat. Pain 22:165, 1985.
48. Minami, M and Satoh, M: Molecular biology of the opioid receptors: Structures, functions and distributions. Neurosci Res 23:121, 1995.
49. Murray, JB: Effectiveness of methadone maintenance for heroin addiction. Psychol Rep 83:295, 1998.
50. National Consensus Development Panel: Effective medical treatment of opiate addiction. JAMA 280:1936, 1998.
51. Nestler, EJ: Molecular mechanisms of opiate and cocaine addiction. Curr Opin Neurobiol 7:713, 1997.
52. Nestler, EJ, Berhow, MT, and Brodkin, ES: Molecular mechanisms of drug addiction: Adaptations in signal transduction pathways. Mol Psychiatry 1:190, 1996.
53. Nolan, MF and Wilson, M-C: Patient-controlled analgesia: A method for the controlled self-administration of opioid pain medications. Phys Ther 75:374, 1995.
54. Ohlsson, L, et al: Cancer pain relief by continuous administration of epidural morphine in a hospital setting and at home. Pain 48:349, 1992.
55. Olson, GA, et al: Endogenous opiates: 1997. Peptides 19:1791, 1998.
56. Pan, ZZ: mu-Opposing actions of the kappa-opioid receptor. Trends Pharmacol Sci 19:94, 1998.
57. Pappagallo, M and Heinberg, LJ: Ethical issues in the management of chronic nonmalignant pain. Semin Neurol 17:203, 1997.
58. Pasternak, GW: Pharmacological mechanisms of opioid analgesics. Neuropharmacology 16:1, 1993.
59. Portenoy, RK and Savage, SR: Clinical realities and economic considerations: Special therapeutic issues in intrathecal therapy—tolerance and addiction. J Pain Symptom Manage 14(Suppl):S27, 1997.
60. Rawal, N: Epidural and spinal agents for postoperative analgesia. Surg Clin North Am 79:313, 1999.
61. Reisine, T and Pasternak, G: Opioid analgesics and antagonists. In Hardman, JG, et al (eds): The Pharmacological Basis of Therapeutics, ed 9. McGraw-Hill, New York, 1996.
62. Savage, SR: Opioid use in the management of chronic pain. Med Clin North Am 83:761, 1999.
63. Schultheiss, R, et al: Dose changes in long-term and medium-term intrathecal morphine therapy of cancer pain. Neurosurgery 31:664, 1992.
64. Shannon, CN and Baranowski, AP: Use of opioids in non-cancer pain. Br J Hosp Med 58:459, 1997.
65. Singh, VK, et al: Molecular biology of opioid receptors: Recent advances. Neuroimmunomodulation 4:285, 1997.
66. Slattery, PJ and Boas, RA: Newer methods of delivery of opiates for relief of pain. Drugs 30:539, 1985.
67. Snyder, SH: Neuronal receptors. Annu Rev Physiol 48:461, 1986.
68. Snyder, SH: Drug and neurotransmitter receptors in the brain. Science 224:22, 1984.
69. Standifer, KM and Pasternak, GW: G proteins and opioid receptor-mediated signalling. Cell Signal 9:237, 1997.
70. Stein, C: Peripheral mechanisms of opioid analgesia. Anesth Analg 76:182, 1993.
71. Stein, C, et al: Peripheral opioid receptors. Ann Med 27:219, 1995.
72. Stein, C, et al: Local anesthetic effect of endogenous opioid peptides. Lancet 342:321, 1993.
73. Strain, EC, et al: Dose-response effects of methadone in the treatment of opioid dependence. Ann Intern Med 119:23, 1993.
74. Streibel, HW, Koenigs, D, and Kramer, J: Postoperative pain management by intranasal demand-adapted fentanyl titration. Anesthesiology 77:281, 1992.
75. Streibel, HW, Pommerening, J, and Rieger, A: Intranasal fentanyl titration for postoperative pain management in an unselected population. Anaesthesia 48:753, 1993.
76. Swift, JQ and Roszkowski, MT: The use of opioid drugs in management of chronic orofacial pain. J Oral Maxillofac Surg 56:1081, 1998.
77. Terenius, L: Endogenous peptides and analgesia. Annu Rev Pharmacol Toxicol 18:189, 1978.
78. Vandongen, RTM, Crul, BJP, and Debock, M: Long-term intrathecal infusion of morphine and morphine bupivacaine mixtures in the treatment of cancer pain: A retrospective analysis of 51 cases. Pain 55:119, 1993.
79. Way, WL, Fields, HL, and Way, EL: Opioid analgesics and antagonists. In Katzung, BG (ed): Basic and Clinical Pharmacology, ed 7. Appleton & Lange, Stamford, CT, 1998.
80. White, MJ, et al: Side effects during continuous epidural infusion of morphine and fentanyl. Can J Anaesth 39:576, 1992.
81. Wolff, K and Strang, J: Therapeutic drug monitoring for methadone: Scanning the horizon. Eur Addict Res 5:36, 1999.
82. Yaksh, TL and Noueihed, R: The physiology and pharmacology of spinal opiates. Annu Rev Pharmacol Toxicol 25:433, 1985.

CHAPTER **15**

Nonsteroidal Anti-Inflammatory Drugs

This chapter discusses a chemically diverse group of substances that exert several distinct pharmacologic properties. These properties include (1) the ability to decrease inflammation, (2) the ability to relieve mild-to-moderate pain (**analgesia**), (3) the ability to decrease the elevated body temperature associated with fever (**antipyresis**), and (4) the ability to decrease blood clotting by inhibiting platelet aggregation (**anticoagulation**). These drugs are commonly referred to as nonsteroidal anti-inflammatory drugs (NSAIDs) to distinguish them from the glucocorticoids (i.e., the other main group of drugs used to treat inflammation). Obviously, the term NSAIDs does not fully describe the pharmacologic actions of these agents, and a more inclusive terminology should also mention the analgesic, antipyretic, and anticoagulant effects of these drugs. However, these drugs are typically referred to as NSAIDs, and this terminology is used throughout this chapter.

Because of their analgesic and anti-inflammatory effects, NSAIDs are often taken by patients receiving physical therapy for any number of problems. These drugs are a mainstay in the treatment of many types of mild-to-moderate pain, and NSAIDs are especially useful in treating pain and inflammation that occur in acute and chronic musculoskeletal disorders. Other patients are given NSAIDs to treat fever or to prevent excessive blood clotting. Consequently, physical therapists and other rehabilitation specialists will see these drugs used quite frequently in their patient population, with the specific therapeutic goal related to the individual needs of each patient.

ASPIRIN AND OTHER NSAIDS: GENERAL ASPECTS

The best representative of the NSAIDs is aspirin (acetylsalicylic acid) (Fig. 15–1). Newer NSAIDs are usually compared to aspirin in terms of efficacy and safety. Acetaminophen is another agent that is similar to aspirin and other NSAIDs in its ability to decrease pain and fever. Acetaminophen, however, is not considered one of the NSAIDs because it lacks anti-inflammatory and anticoagulant properties. For a discussion of the comparative effects of aspirin, newer NSAIDs, and acetaminophen, see "Comparison of Aspirin with Other NSAIDs."

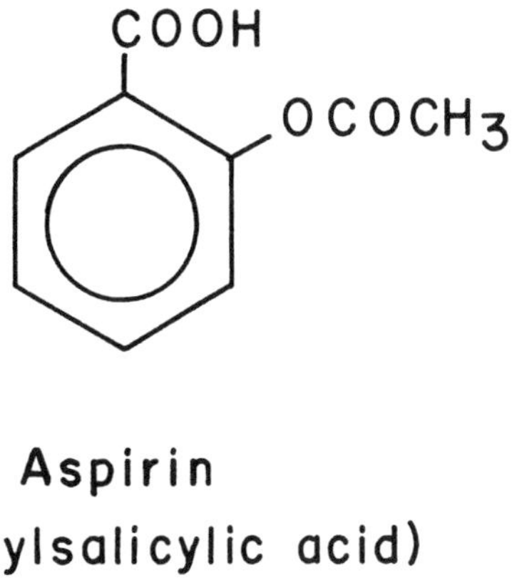

$$COOH$$
$$OCOCH_3$$

Aspirin
(acetylsalicylic acid)

FIGURE 15–1. Structure of aspirin.

For years, it was a mystery how a drug like aspirin could exert such a diverse range of therapeutic effects; that is, how could one drug influence so many different systems to effectively alleviate pain and inflammation, decrease fever, and even affect blood clotting? This issue was essentially resolved in the early 1970s, when aspirin was found to inhibit the synthesis of a group of endogenous compounds known collectively as the "prostaglandins." We now know that aspirin and the other NSAIDs exert most, if not all, of their therapeutic effects by interfering with the biosynthesis of prostaglandins and other related compounds.[10,67,118,119] To understand the way in which these drugs work, a brief discussion of prostaglandins and similar endogenously produced substances is presented here.

PROSTAGLANDINS, THROMBOXANES, AND LEUKOTRIENES

Prostaglandins are a group of lipidlike compounds that exhibit a wide range of pharmacologic activities.[15,43,49,95,99] With the exception of the red blood cell, virtually every type of living cell in the human body has been identified as being able to produce prostaglandins. These compounds appear to be hormones that act locally to help regulate cell function under normal and pathologic conditions. Other biologically active compounds known as the "thromboxanes" and "**leukotrienes**" are derived from the same precursor as the prostaglandins.[41,43,69,88,95] Together, the prostaglandins, thromboxanes, and leukotrienes are often referred to as **eicosanoids** because they all are derived from 20-carbon fatty acids that contain several double bonds.[41,43,49,107] (The term *eicosanoid* is derived from *eicosa*, meaning "20-carbon," and *enoic*, meaning "containing double bonds.")

Eicosanoid Biosynthesis

The biosynthetic pathway of prostaglandins and other eicosanoids is outlined in Figure 15–2. Basically, these compounds are derived from a 20-carbon essential fatty acid. In humans, this fatty acid is usually arachidonic acid.[15,94,99] Arachidonic acid is ingested in the diet and stored as a phospholipid in the cell membrane. Thus, the cell has an abundant and easily accessible supply of this precursor. When needed, arachidonic acid is cleaved from the cell membrane by a phospholipase enzyme (i.e., phospholipase

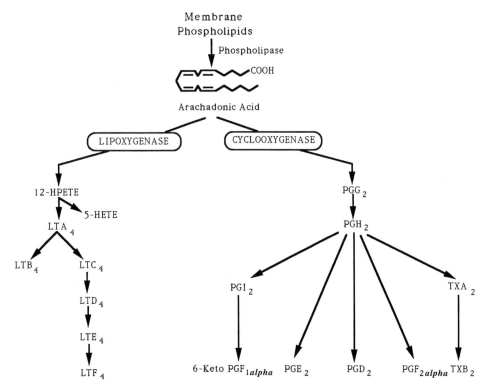

FIGURE 15–2. Eicosanoid biosynthesis. PG = prostaglandin; TX = thromboxane; LT = leukotriene.

A_2). The 20-carbon fatty acid can then be metabolized by several enzyme systems to generate a variety of biologically active compounds. One of the primary enzyme systems involves the **cyclooxygenase (COX)** enzyme, and a second system involves the **lipoxygenase (LOX)** enzyme. The prostaglandins and thromboxanes are ultimately synthesized from the cyclooxygenase pathway, and the leukotrienes come from the lipoxygenase system (see Fig. 15–2).[15,33,90,94,99,107]

Exactly which pathway is used in any particular cell depends on the type and quantity of enzymes in that cell, as well as the physiologic status of the cell. The end products within a given pathway (i.e., exactly which prostaglandins, thromboxanes, or leukotrienes will be formed) also depend on the individual cell. Any drug that inhibits one of these enzymes will also inhibit the formation of all of the subsequent products of that particular pathway. A drug that blocks the cyclooxygenase will essentially eliminate all prostaglandin and thromboxane synthesis in that cell. As this chapter will later discuss, aspirin and the other NSAIDs are cyclooxygenase inhibitors, and this is the way that these drugs exert their therapeutic effects (see "Mechanism of NSAID Action: Inhibition of Prostaglandin and Thromboxane Synthesis").

Aspirin and other NSAIDs do not inhibit the lipoxygenase enzyme and thus do not appreciably decrease leukotriene synthesis.[54,90,99] Like the prostaglandins, leukotrienes are pro-inflammatory, but leukotrienes seem to be more important in mediating airway inflammation in conditions such as asthma and allergic rhinitis (see Chap. 26).[69,78,80,100,124] Drugs have therefore been developed to reduce leukotriene-mediated inflammation by either inhibiting the lipoxygenase enzyme (e.g., zileuton) or by blocking leukotriene receptors on respiratory tissues (e.g., montelukast and zafirlukast).[80,113,124] These antileukotriene drugs will be discussed in more detail in Chapter 26. The remainder of this chapter will focus on drugs that inhibit prostaglandin and thromboxane production by selectively inhibiting the cyclooxygenase enzyme.

Role of Eicosanoids in Health and Disease

The prostaglandins, thromboxanes, and leukotrienes have been shown to have a variety of effects on virtually every major physiologic system. Studies have indicated that these compounds can influence cardiovascular, respiratory, renal, gastrointestinal, nervous, and reproductive function.[15,33,41,43,49] The biologic effects of the various eicosanoids cannot be generalized. Different classes of eicosanoids and even different members within the same class may exert different effects on the same system. For instance, certain prostaglandins such as the PGAs and PGEs tend to produce vasodilation in most vascular beds, whereas other prostaglandins (e.g., PGF_{2a}) and the thromboxanes are often vasoconstrictors.[15] Some of the major effects of the eicosanoids are summarized in Table 15–1.

All of the effects of different prostaglandins, thromboxanes, and leukotrienes on various systems in the body cannot be reviewed in this chapter. Besides, this issue has been reviewed extensively elsewhere.[15,33,41,43,49,99,117] Of greater interest in this chapter is the role of prostaglandins and related substances in pathologic conditions. In general, cells that are subjected to various types of trauma or disturbances in homeostasis tend to increase the production of prostaglandins.[15,107] This finding suggests that prostaglandins and other eicosanoids may be important in the protective response to cellular injury. In addition, prostaglandins are important in mediating some of the painful effects of injury and inflammation, as well as the symptoms of other pathologic conditions. Some of the better documented conditions associated with excessive prostaglandin synthesis are listed here.

Inflammation. Increased prostaglandin synthesis is usually detected at the site of local inflammation.[48,95,107] Certain prostaglandins, such as PGE_2, are thought to help mediate the local erythema and edema associated with inflammation by increasing local blood flow, increasing capillary permeability, and potentiating the permeability effects of histamine and bradykinin.[65,118] Leukotrienes, particularly LTB_4, also contribute to the inflammatory response by increasing vascular permeability, and LTB_4 has a potent chemotactic effect on polymorphonuclear leukocytes.[5,65,69,88,100]

Pain. Prostaglandins appear to help mediate painful stimuli in a variety of conditions (including inflammation). The compounds do not usually produce pain directly but are believed to increase the sensitivity of pain receptors to the effects of other pain-producing substances such as bradykinin.[15]

Fever. Prostaglandins appear to be pyretogenic; that is, they help produce the elevated body temperature during fever.[23] Although the details are somewhat unclear, increased prostaglandin production may help alter the thermoregulatory set-point within the hypothalamus so that body temperature is maintained at a higher level.[23]

Dysmenorrhea. The painful cramps that accompany menstruation in some women have been attributed at least in part to increased prostaglandin production in the endometrium of the uterus.[19,82]

Thrombus Formation. The thromboxanes, especially TXA_2, cause platelet aggregation, resulting in blood clot formation.[18,77,102] Whether excessive thrombus formation (as in deep vein thrombosis) is initiated by abnormal thromboxane production is unclear. Certainly, inhibition of thromboxane synthesis will help prevent platelet-induced thrombus formation in individuals who are prone to specific types of excessive blood clotting.[14,32,37,102,126]

TABLE 15-1 Primary Physiologic Effects of the Major Classes of Prostaglandins (PGs), Thromboxanes (TX), and Leukotrienes (LT)

Class	Vascular Smooth Muscle	Airway Smooth Muscle	Gastrointestinal Smooth Muscle	Gastrointestinal Secretions	Uterine Muscle (Nonpregnant)	Platelet Aggregation
PGAs	Vasodilation	—	—	Decrease	Relaxation	—
PGEs	Vasodilation	Bronchodilation	Contraction	Decrease	Relaxation	Variable
PGIs	Vasodilation	—	Relaxation	Decrease	—	Decrease
PGFs	Variable	Bronchoconstriction	Contraction	—	Contraction	—
TXA$_2$	Vasoconstriction	Bronchoconstriction	—	—	—	Increase
LTs	Vasoconstriction	Bronchoconstriction	Contraction	—	—	—

Other Pathologies. Because of their many varied physiologic effects, the eicosanoids are involved in a number of other pathologic conditions. Prostaglandins have been implicated in cardiovascular disorders (hypertension), neoplasms (colon cancer), respiratory dysfunction (asthma), neurologic disorders (multiple sclerosis, allergic encephalomyelitis), endocrine dysfunction (Bartter syndrome, diabetes mellitus), and a variety of other problems.[15,33,40,41,46,49] The exact role of prostaglandins and the other eicosanoids in various diseases continues to be evaluated, and the role of these compounds in health and disease has become clearer with ongoing research.

MECHANISM OF NSAID ACTION: INHIBITION OF PROSTAGLANDIN AND THROMBOXANE SYNTHESIS

Aspirin and the other NSAIDs are all potent inhibitors of the cyclooxygenase enzyme.[27,33,58,67] Because cyclooxygenase represents the first step in the synthesis of prostaglandins and thromboxanes, drugs that inhibit this enzyme in any given cell will block the production of all prostaglandins and thromboxanes in that cell. Considering that prostaglandins and thromboxanes are implicated in producing pain, inflammation, fever, and excessive blood clotting, virtually all of the therapeutic effects of aspirin and similar drugs can be explained by their ability to inhibit the synthesis of these two eicosanoid classes.[58]

The cyclooxygenase or COX enzyme system is therefore the key site of NSAID action within the cell. It is now realized, however, that there are at least two primary subtypes (isozymes) of the COX enzyme, known as COX-1 and COX-2.[10,33,94,95,117,119] The COX-1 enzyme is a normal constituent in certain cells, and prostaglandins synthesized by COX-1 are typically responsible for mediating normal cell activity and maintaining homeostasis. For example, COX-1 enzymes located in the stomach mucosa synthesize prostaglandins that help protect the stomach lining from gastric acid, and COX-1 enzymes in the kidney produce beneficial prostaglandins that help maintain renal function, especially when kidney function is compromised.[33,44,117,118] COX-1 is also the enzyme responsible for synthesizing prostaglandins and thromboxanes that regulate normal platelet activity.[44] The COX-2 enzyme, however, seems to be produced primarily in cells when they are injured in some way; that is, other chemical mediators (**cytokines**) induce the injured cell to synthesize the COX-2 enzyme, and this enzyme then produces prostaglandins that mediate pain and other aspects of the inflammatory response.[10,48,105,119]

The roles of COX-1 and COX-2 enzymes therefore seem quite different. The COX-1 enzyme is a "normal" cell component that synthesizes prostaglandins to help regulate and maintain cell activity. COX-2 represents an "emergency" enzyme that often synthesizes prostaglandins in response to cell injury (i.e., pain and inflammation). This difference has important implications for how NSAIDs exert their therapeutic effects and side effects. Aspirin and most of the traditional NSAIDs are nonselective, and they inhibit both the COX-1 and COX-2 enzymes. These nonselective NSAIDs therefore cause their primary beneficial effects (decreased pain and inflammation) by inhibiting the COX-2 enzyme. Because these drugs also inhibit the COX-1 enzyme, they also decrease the production of the beneficial and protective prostaglandins. It is the loss of these beneficial prostaglandins that accounts for the primary side effects of the NSAIDs; that is, loss of protective prostaglandins in the stomach and kidney result in gastric damage and decreased renal function, respectively.

It follows that drugs that selectively inhibit the COX-2 enzyme would offer certain advantages over aspirin and the nonselective NSAIDs. Selective COX-2 inhibitors should decrease the production of prostaglandins that mediate pain and inflammation while sparing the synthesis of protective prostaglandins that are synthesized by COX-1. Such COX-2 selective drugs are currently available, and the pharmacology of these drugs is addressed later in this chapter.

ASPIRIN: PROTOTYPICAL NSAID

Acetylsalicylic acid, or aspirin, as it is commonly known (see Fig. 15–1), represents the major form of a group of drugs known as the **salicylates**. Other salicylates (sodium salicylate, choline salicylate) are also used clinically, but aspirin is the most frequently used and appears to have the widest range of therapeutic effects of the salicylate drugs. Because aspirin has been used clinically for more than 100 years, is inexpensive, and is readily available without prescription, many individuals may be under the impression that this drug is only a marginally effective therapeutic agent. On the contrary, aspirin is a very powerful and effective drug that should be considered a major medicine.[58,66] As discussed previously, aspirin is a potent inhibitor of all cyclooxygenase activity (COX-1 and COX-2), and thus it has the potential to affect a number of conditions that involve excessive prostaglandin and thromboxane production.

As indicated previously, aspirin is the oldest and most widely used NSAID, and other NSAIDs are compared with aspirin in terms of efficacy and safety. Hence, this discussion focuses primarily on the clinical applications of aspirin and the problems typically associated with aspirin. For the most part, these clinical uses and problems can also be applied to most of the nonaspirin NSAIDs. The major similarities and differences between aspirin and the other NSAIDs are discussed in "Comparison of Aspirin with Other NSAIDs."

CLINICAL APPLICATIONS OF ASPIRIN-LIKE DRUGS

Treatment of Pain and Inflammation

Aspirin and other NSAIDs are effective in treating mild-to-moderate pain of various origins, including headache, toothache, and diffuse muscular aches and soreness. Aspirin appears to be especially useful in treating pain and inflammation in musculo-skeletal and joint disorders.[7,123] The safe and effective use of aspirin in both rheumatoid arthritis and osteoarthritis is well documented (see Chap. 16).[11,26,56,87,108] Aspirin is also recommended for treating pain and cramping associated with primary dysmenorrhea.[11,19,82]

Aspirin and aspirin-like drugs are also used to manage pain following certain types of surgery, including arthroscopic surgery.[84,92] These drugs can serve as the primary analgesic following other types of minor or intermediate surgery, and they can also be used after extensive surgery to decrease the need for high doses of other drugs such as the opioids.[16,17,79,93] Ketorolac tromethamine (Toradol) is a relatively new NSAID that has shown exceptional promise in treating postoperative pain. This drug can be given orally or by intramuscular injection, and it has been reported to provide analgesic effects similar to opioid drugs (morphine) but without the side effects and risks associated with opioid analgesics.[31,39,81,93] Hence, ketorolac tromethamine provides a reasonable alternative for nonopioid management of postoperative pain and may be especially valuable when opioid side effects (sedation, respiratory depression) are harmful or undesirable.[72,75,93]

Treatment of Fever

Although the use of aspirin in treating fever in children is contraindicated (because of the association with Reye syndrome; see "Problems and Adverse Effects of Aspirin-like Drugs"), aspirin remains the primary NSAID used in treating fever in adults.[58] Ibuprofen is also used frequently as a nonprescription antipyretic NSAID.

Treatment of Vascular Disorders

As discussed previously, aspirin inhibits platelet-induced thrombus formation through its ability to inhibit thromboxane biosynthesis. Aspirin has therefore been used to help prevent the onset or recurrence of heart attacks in some individuals by inhibiting thrombus formation in the coronary arteries.[3,68,83,110] Similarly, daily aspirin use may help prevent transient ischemic attacks and stroke by preventing cerebral infarction in certain patients.[3,32,36,37] The role of aspirin in treating coagulation disorders is discussed in more detail in Chapter 25.

Prevention of Cancer

There is now considerable evidence that regular aspirin use decreases the risk of colon cancer and possibly other types of gastrointestinal cancer.[1,71,111,112,116] It has been estimated, for example, that people who use aspirin on a regular basis have a 40 to 50 percent lower risk of fatal colon cancer as compared with people who do not use aspirin.[73,114] It appears that certain prostaglandins help promote tumor growth and that aspirin and similar NSAIDs exert anticancer effects by inhibiting the synthesis of these prostaglandins.[40,73,111] Hence, aspirin continues to gain acceptance as an anticancer drug, especially in individuals who are at an increased risk for developing colon cancer.

PROBLEMS AND ADVERSE EFFECTS OF ASPIRIN-LIKE DRUGS

Gastrointestinal Problems

The primary problem with all of the NSAIDs, including aspirin, is gastrointestinal damage. Problems ranging from minor stomach discomfort to variable amounts of upper gastrointestinal hemorrhage and ulceration are fairly common.[2,9,28,55,62–64] These effects may be caused by aspirin directly irritating the gastric mucosa or by the loss of protective prostaglandins from the mucosal lining (i.e., aspirin may locally inhibit the formation of prostaglandins that protect the stomach from the acidic gastric juices).[59,74,85] Certain patients are more susceptible to gastrointestinal injury from aspirin-like drugs, and factors such as increased age and a history of ulcers appear to increase the risk of serious gastrointestinal damage.[30,63,97,101]

Several pharmacologic and nonpharmacologic strategies have been employed to manage the gastrointestinal problems associated with the aspirin-like drugs. One strategy has been to coat the aspirin tablet so that dissolution and release of the drug is delayed until it reaches the small intestine. These so-called enteric-coated forms of aspirin spare the stomach from irritation, but the duodenum and upper small intestine may still be subjected to damage.[2] Enteric-coated aspirin also has the disadvantage of delaying the onset of analgesic effects, so that relief from acute pain may also be delayed. Other methods such as buffering the aspirin tablet have also been used to help decrease stomach irritation. The rationale here is that including a chemical buffer helps blunt the acidic effects of the aspirin molecule on the stomach mucosa. It is questionable, however, whether sufficient buffer is added to commercial aspirin preparations to actually make a difference in stomach irritation. During chronic aspirin therapy (e.g., treatment of arthritis), taking aspirin with meals may help decrease gastrointestinal irritation because the food in the stomach will offer some direct protection of the gastric mucosa. The presence of food, however, will also delay drug absorption, which may decrease the peak levels of drug that reach the bloodstream.

A great deal of attention has been focused recently on other drugs that can prevent or treat the gastrointestinal side effects associated with aspirin and the other NSAIDs. Misoprostol (Cytotec) is a prostaglandin E_1 analog that inhibits gastric acid secretion and prevents gastric damage.[91,103,109,121] This drug has been beneficial in decreasing aspirin-induced irritation, but the clinical use of misoprostol is limited somewhat by side effects such as diarrhea.[121] Omeprazole (Prilosec) is a drug that inhibits the "proton pump" that is ultimately responsible for secreting gastric acid from mucosal cells into the lumen of the stomach (see Chap. 27). Omeprazole has therefore been used successfully to decrease NSAID-induced ulcers and increase the healing of these ulcers.[61,91,103,104] Drugs that antagonize certain histamine receptors—that is, the H_2 receptor blockers—have also been used to decrease gastrointestinal damage.[13,109] As indicated in Chapter 27, histamine receptor (H_2) blockers such as cimetidine (Tagamet) and ranitidine (Zantac) inhibit gastric acid secretion by antagonizing histamine receptors in the gastric mucosa. These drugs are tolerated quite well but are generally not as effective in controlling NSAID-induced ulceration as other drugs such as misoprostol and omeprazole.[103]

Hence, currently available drugs such as misoprostol, omeprazole, and the H_2 receptor blockers can be used to prevent or treat gastrointestinal damage in patients taking aspirin and other NSAIDs. These protective agents are not usually prescribed on a routine basis to every person taking aspirin-like drugs but are typically reserved for people who exhibit symptoms of gastrointestinal irritation or who are at risk for developing ulceration while undergoing NSAID therapy.[13,30,62,109,121]

Other Side Effects

Aspirin and similar NSAIDs can cause other toxic side effects if used improperly or if taken by patients who have pre-existing diseases. For instance, serious hepatotoxicity is rare with normal therapeutic use, but high doses of aspirin-like drugs can produce adverse changes in hepatic function in patients with liver disease.[9,45,89] Likewise, aspirin does not seem to cause renal disease in an individual with normal kidneys,[125] but problems such as nephrotic syndrome, acute interstitial nephritis, and even acute renal failure have been observed when aspirin is given to patients with impaired renal function.[22,35,52,60,120] Aspirin causes these problems by inhibiting the synthesis of renal prostaglandins, which serve a protective role in maintaining renal blood flow and glomerular filtration rate during various forms of renal dysfunction.[34,35,38,125] These protective renal prostaglandins appear to be important in sustaining adequate renal function when renal blood flow and perfusion pressure become compromised. Consequently, aspirin and aspirin-like drugs may create problems in other conditions such as hypovolemia, shock, hepatic cirrhosis, congestive heart failure, and hypertension.[21,35,38,52,120]

In cases of aspirin overdose, a condition known as aspirin intoxication or poisoning may occur. This event is usually identified by a number of symptoms, including headache, tinnitus, difficulty in hearing, confusion, and gastrointestinal distress. More severe cases also result in metabolic acidosis and dehydration, which are the life-threatening aspects of aspirin overdose. In adults, a dose of 10 to 30 g of aspirin is sometimes fatal, although much higher doses (130 g in one documented case) have been ingested without causing death.[58] Of course, much smaller doses can produce fatalities in children.

Evidence has suggested that aspirin may also be associated with a relatively rare condition known as Reye syndrome.[25,122] This condition occurs in children and teenagers, usually following a bout of influenza or chickenpox. Reye syndrome is marked by a high fever, vomiting, liver dysfunction, and increasing unresponsiveness, often progressing rapidly and leading to delirium, convulsions, coma, and possibly death. Because aspirin is one factor that may contribute to Reye syndrome, it is recommended that aspirin and other aspirin-like drugs should not be used to treat fever in children and teenagers.[122] Nonaspirin antipyretics such as acetaminophen and ibuprofen are not associated with Reye syndrome, so products containing these drugs are preferred for treating fever in children and teenagers.[122]

A small number of individuals (approximately 1 percent of the general population) exhibit aspirin intolerance or supersensitivity.[4,58] These patients will display allergic-like reactions, including acute bronchospasm, urticaria, and severe rhinitis, within a few hours after taking aspirin and aspirin-like NSAIDs.[58,106] These reactions may be quite severe in some individuals, and cardiovascular shock may occur. Consequently, the use of all NSAIDs is contraindicated in these individuals.

Finally, there is preliminary evidence from animal and in vitro studies that aspirin-like drugs may actually delay certain types of tissue healing. Aspirin and some of the other commonly used NSAIDs have been shown to inhibit the synthesis and transport of connective tissue components such as proteoglycans.[6,24,29,53,57] This finding has implications concerning the healing of cartilage, tendons, ligaments, and bone. It is unclear at the present time, however, whether aspirin-like drugs will cause a meaningful decrease in tissue healing when these drugs are used clinically in humans. Additional research will be needed to determine the extent to which aspirin and other NSAIDs can affect the healing process of articular cartilage and other tissues.

COMPARISON OF ASPIRIN WITH OTHER NSAIDS

A number of drugs that bear a functional similarity to aspirin have been developed during the past several decades, and a comprehensive list of currently available NSAIDs is shown in Table 15–2. Other NSAIDs are like aspirin in that they exert their therapeutic effects by inhibiting prostaglandin and thromboxane synthesis. Although specific approved uses of individual members of this group vary, NSAIDs are used in much the same way as aspirin; that is, they are administered primarily for their analgesic and anti-inflammatory effects, with some members also used as antipyretic and anticoagulant agents. Dosages commonly used to achieve analgesic or anti-inflammatory effects with some of the more common NSAIDs are listed in Table 15–3.

TABLE 15–2 Common Nonsteroidal Anti-Inflammatory Drugs

Generic Name	Trade Name(s)	Specific Comments—Comparison with Other NSAIDs
Aspirin	Many trade names	Most widely used NSAID for analgesic and anti-inflammatory effects; also used frequently for antipyretic and anticoagulant effects.
Diclofenac	Voltaren	Substantially more potent than naproxen and several other NSAIDs; adverse side effects occur in 20% of patients.
Diflunisal	Dolobid	Has potency 3–4 times greater than aspirin in terms of analgesic and anti-inflammatory effects but lacks antipyretic activity.
Etodolac	Lodine	Effective as analgesic/anti-inflammatory agent with fewer side effects than most NSAIDs; may have gastric-sparing properties.
Fenoprofen	Nalfon	GI side effects fairly common but usually less intense than those occurring with similar doses of aspirin.
Flurbiprofen	Ansaid	Similar to aspirin's benefits and side effects; also available as topical ophthalmic preparation (Ocufen).
Ibuprofen	Motrin, many others	First nonaspirin NSAID also available in nonprescription form; fewer GI side effects than aspirin but GI effects still occur in 5–15% of patients.
Indomethacin	Indocin	Relative high incidence of dose-related side effects; problems occur in 25–50% of patients.
Ketoprofen	Orudis, Oruvail, others	Similar to aspirin's benefits and side effects but has relatively short half-life (1–2 hr).
Ketorolac	Toradol	Can be administered orally or by intramuscular injection; parenteral doses provide postoperative analgesia equivalent to opioids.
Meclofenamate	Meclomen	No apparent advantages or disadvantages compared with aspirin and other NSAIDs.
Mefenamic acid	Ponstel	No advantages; often less effective and more toxic than aspirin and other NSAIDs.
Nabumetone	Relafen	Effective as analgesic/anti-inflammatory agent with fewer side effects than most NSAIDs.
Naproxen	Anaprox, Naprosyn, others	Similar to ibuprofen in terms of benefits and adverse effects.
Oxaprozin	Daypro	Analgesic and anti-inflammatory effects similar to aspirin; may produce fewer side effects than other NSAIDs.
Phenylbutazone	Cotylbutazone	Potent anti-inflammatory effects but long-term use limited by high incidence of side effects (10–45% of patients).
Piroxicam	Feldene	Long half-life (45 hr) allows once-daily dosing; may be somewhat better tolerated than aspirin.
Sulindac	Clinoril	Relatively little effect on kidneys (renal-sparing) but may produce more GI side effects than aspirin.
Tolmetin	Tolectin	Similar to aspirin's benefits and side effects but must be given frequently (QID) because of short half-life (1 hr).

With respect to therapeutic effects, there is no clear evidence that any of the commonly used NSAIDs are markedly better than aspirin as anti-inflammatory analgesics.[12,127] The primary differences between aspirin and other NSAIDs are related to the side effects and safety profile of each agent (see Table 15–2).[127] As a group, the nonaspirin NSAIDs tend to be associated with less gastrointestinal discomfort than plain aspirin, but most of these NSAIDs (with the exception of the COX-2 drugs; see later) are

TABLE 15–3 Dosages of Common Oral NSAIDs

Drug	Dosages (According to Desired Effect)	
	Analgesia	Anti-Inflammation
Aspirin (many trade names)	325–650 mg every 4 hr	3.6–5.4 g/day in divided doses
Diclofenac (Voltaren)	Up to 100 mg for the first dose; then up to 50 mg TID thereafter	Initially: 150–200 mg/day in 3–4 divided doses; try to reduce to 75–100 mg/d in 3 divided doses
Diflunisal (Dolobid)	1 g initially; 500 mg every 8–12 hr as needed	250–500 mg BID
Etodolac (Lodine)	400 mg initially; 200–400 mg every 6–8 hr as needed	400 mg BID or TID or 300 mg TID or QID; total daily dose is typically 600–1200 mg/day
Fenoprofen (Nalfon)	200 mg every 4–6 hr	300–600 mg TID or QID
Flurbiprofen (Ansaid)	—	200–300 mg/day in 2–4 divided doses
Ibuprofen (Advil, Motrin, Nuprin, others)	200–400 mg every 4–6 hr as needed	1.2–3.2 g/day in 3–4 divided doses
Indomethacin (Indocin)	—	25–50 mg 2–4 times each day initially; can be increased up to 200 mg/day as tolerated
Ketoprofen (Orudis)	25–50 mg every 6–8 hr	150–300 mg/day in 3–4 divided doses
Meclofenamate (Meclomen)	50 mg every 4–6 hr	200–400 mg/day in 3–4 divided doses
Mefenamic acid (Ponstel)	500 mg initially; 250 mg every 6 hr as needed	—
Nabumetone (Ponstel)	—	Initially: 1000 mg/day in a single dose or 2 divided doses; can be increased to 1500–2000 mg/day in 2 divided doses if needed
Naproxen (Naprosyn)	500 mg initially; 250 mg every 6–8 hr	250, 375, or 500 mg BID
Naproxen sodium (Aleve, Anaprox, others)	500–650 mg initially; 275 mg every 6–8 hr	275 or 550 mg BID
Oxaprozin (Daypro)	—	Initially: 1200 mg/day, then adjust to patient tolerance
Phenylbutazone (Butazolidin, Cotylbutazone)	—	300–600 mg/day in 3–4 divided doses initially; reduce as tolerated to lowest effective dose
Piroxicam (Feldene)	—	20 mg/day single dose; or 10 mg BID
Sulindac (Clinoril)	—	150 or 200 mg BID
Tolmetin (Tolectin)	—	400 mg TID initially; 600 mg–1.8 g/day in 3–4 divided doses

still associated with some degree of stomach irritation[76] (Table 15–4). Likewise, certain NSAIDs may offer an advantage because they are less toxic to certain organs. Ibuprofen, for instance, does not affect liver function as much as aspirin,[45] and sulindac (Clinoril) is described as a renal-sparing NSAID because it does not have any appreciable effect on kidney function.[20,38] Some of the other NSAIDs, however, may produce more serious

TABLE 15–4 Cyclooxygenase Type 2 (COX-2) Inhibitors

Generic Name	Trade Name	Indications and Dosages
Celecoxib	Celebrex	*Rheumatoid arthritis:* 200 mg OD, or 100 mg BID
		Osteoarthritis: 100–200 mg BID
Rofecoxib	Vioxx	*Pain (including dysmenorrhea):* 50 mg on day 1 and 50 mg OD as needed for no more than 5 days
		Osteoarthritis: 12.5–25.0 mg OD

toxic renal and hepatic effects than aspirin.[127] Hence, it cannot be generalized that the newer NSAIDs are significantly better or worse than plain aspirin in terms of either therapeutic or adverse effects.

The primary difference between aspirin and the newer NSAIDs is cost. Most of the NSAIDs still require a physician's prescription for their use. The cost of these prescription NSAIDs can be anywhere between 10 and 20 times more expensive than an equivalent supply of plain aspirin. NSAIDs that are available in nonprescription form (e.g., ibuprofen) can still cost up to five times as much as aspirin.

Consequently, the newer NSAIDs have not always been shown to be clinically superior to aspirin, but some agents may provide better effects in some patients. Considering the interpatient variability in the response to drugs, there are surely cases in which one of the other NSAIDs will produce better therapeutic effects than aspirin with fewer side effects.[12,127] If a patient responds equally well to a variety of NSAIDs, however, efforts should be made to use the NSAID that will produce adequate therapeutic effects at a minimal cost.[51]

COX-2 SELECTIVE DRUGS

As discussed earlier, the cyclooxygenase enzyme that synthesizes prostaglandins exists in at least two forms: COX-1 and COX-2.[47,48] Aspirin and most other NSAIDs are nonselective cyclooxygenase inhibitors; that is, they inhibit both the COX-1 and COX-2 forms of the cyclooxygenase. This nonselective inhibition results in decreased synthesis of prostaglandins that cause pain and inflammation (COX-2 prostaglandins), as well as loss of prostaglandins that are protective and beneficial to tissues such as the stomach lining and kidneys (COX-1 prostaglandins). Recently, drugs have been developed that are selective for the COX-2 enzyme, hence the name COX-2 inhibitors (see Table 15–4). These COX-2 selective drugs offer the obvious advantage of inhibiting synthesis of the inflammatory prostaglandins while sparing synthesis of the prostaglandins that are beneficial and help regulate normal physiologic function.[47,96]

It follows that use of COX-2 selective drugs should decrease pain and inflammation with minimal or no adverse effects on the stomach and other tissues. Preliminary results indicate that this is indeed true; that is, the COX-2 drugs have analgesic and anti-inflammatory efficacy similar to other NSAIDs but have a negligible incidence of gastric ulcers.[44,48,67] Likewise, COX-2 drugs do not inhibit platelet function because prostaglandins that influence platelet activity are under the control of the COX-1 isozyme.[8,44,48,70] Use of COX-2 drugs should therefore be beneficial in people who are at risk for prolonged bleeding and hemorrhage.

COX-2 drugs therefore represent an important addition to the NSAID armamentarium. Although these drugs are not necessarily more effective in reducing pain and inflammation, they may avoid some of the most common side effects associated with aspirin and the other NSAIDs. The COX-2 drugs are not devoid of side effects, of course, and they may increase the risk of upper respiratory tract infections. Even though these drugs are purportedly easier on the stomach than traditional NSAIDs, certain patients may still experience gastrointestinal problems such as diarrhea, heartburn, stomach cramps, and upper GI bleeding. Nonetheless, COX-2 drugs offer an alternative to more traditional NSAIDs, and COX-2 agents may be especially useful to patients who cannot tolerate other NSAIDs because of gastric irritation or other side effects typically associated with aspirin and the more traditional NSAIDs.[50]

ACETAMINOPHEN

Acetaminophen has several distinct differences from aspirin and the other NSAIDs. Acetaminophen does appear to be equal to aspirin and the other NSAIDs in terms of analgesic and antipyretic effects, but it does not have any appreciable anti-inflammatory or anticoagulant effects.[58,86] One major advantage of acetaminophen is that this drug is not associated with upper gastrointestinal tract irritation.[58] Consequently, acetaminophen has been used widely in the treatment of noninflammatory conditions associated with mild-to-moderate pain and in patients who have a history of gastric damage (such as ulcers). In addition, Reye syndrome has not been implicated with acetaminophen use, so this drug is often preferentially used in treating fever in children and teenagers.[122] Acetaminophen is not a totally innocuous drug devoid of any adverse effects, however. High doses of acetaminophen (e.g., 15 g) can be especially toxic to the liver and may be fatal because of hepatic necrosis.[98,115] People with pre-existing liver disease or individuals who are chronic alcohol abusers may be particularly susceptible to liver damage caused by high doses of acetaminophen.[98]

The mechanism of action of acetaminophen is not fully understood. Acetaminophen does inhibit the cyclooxygenase enzyme, and its analgesic and antipyretic effects are probably mediated through prostaglandin inhibition. Why acetaminophen fails to exert anti-inflammatory and anticoagulant effects, however, is unclear. One explanation is that acetaminophen preferentially inhibits CNS prostaglandin production but has little effect on peripheral cyclooxygenase activity.[42,58] Thus, analgesia and antipyresis are produced by specifically limiting prostaglandin production in central pain interpretation and thermoregulatory centers, respectively. Tissue inflammation and platelet aggregation are peripheral events that would be unaffected by acetaminophen, according to this theory.

PHARMACOKINETICS OF NSAIDS
AND ACETAMINOPHEN

Aspirin is administered orally and is absorbed readily from the stomach and small intestine. Approximately 80 to 90 percent of aspirin remains bound to plasma proteins such as albumin. The remaining 10 to 20 percent is widely distributed throughout the body. The unbound or free drug exerts the therapeutic effects. Aspirin itself (acetylsalicylic acid) is hydrolyzed to an active metabolite, salicylic acid. This biotransformation occurs primarily in the bloodstream, and the salicylic acid is further metabolized by oxidation or conjugation in the liver. Excretion of salicylic acid and its metabolites occurs through the kidney. Although there is some pharmacokinetic variability within the nonaspirin NSAIDs, these drugs generally follow a pattern of absorption, protein binding, metabolism, and excretion similar to that of aspirin.

Acetaminophen is also absorbed rapidly and completely from the upper gastrointestinal tract. Plasma protein binding with acetaminophen is highly variable (20 to 50 percent) but is considerably less than with aspirin. Metabolism of acetaminophen occurs in the liver via conjugation with endogenous substrates, and the conjugated metabolites are excreted through the kidney. When high doses are ingested, a considerable amount of acetaminophen is converted in the liver to a highly reactive intermediate by-product known as N-acetyl-p-benzoquinoneimine. When present in sufficient amounts, this metabolite induces hepatic necrosis by binding to and inactivating certain liver proteins.

SPECIAL CONCERNS IN REHABILITATION PATIENTS

Aspirin and the other NSAIDs are among the most frequently used drugs in the rehabilitation population. Aside from the possibility of stomach discomfort, these drugs have a remarkable lack of adverse effects that directly interfere with physical therapy and occupational therapy. When used for various types of musculoskeletal pain and inflammation, these drugs can often provide analgesia without the sedation and psychomimetic (hallucinogenic, etc.) effects associated with narcotic analgesics. Thus, the therapy session can be conducted with the benefit of pain relief but without the loss of patient attentiveness and concentration. In inflammatory conditions, NSAIDs can be used for prolonged periods without the serious side effects associated with the steroidal drugs (see Chaps. 16 and 29). Of course, the limitation of NSAIDs is that they may not be as effective in moderate-to-severe pain or in severe, progressive inflammation. Still, these agents are a beneficial adjunct in many painful conditions and can usually help facilitate physical rehabilitation by relieving pain. The other clinical uses of these drugs (antipyresis, anticoagulation) may also be encountered in some patients, and these effects are also usually achieved with a minimum of adverse effects.

Acetaminophen is also frequently employed for pain relief in many physical therapy patients. Remember that this drug is equal to NSAIDs in analgesic properties but lacks anti-inflammatory effects. Because both aspirin and acetaminophen are available without prescription, the patient may inquire about the differences between these two drugs. Therapists should be able to provide an adequate explanation of the differential effects of aspirin and acetaminophen but should also remember that the suggested use of these agents should ultimately come from the physician.

CASE STUDY

NONSTEROIDAL ANTI-INFLAMMATORY DRUGS

Brief History. D.B., a 38-year-old man, began to develop pain in his right shoulder. He was employed as a carpenter and had recently been working rather long hours building a new house. The increasing pain required medical attention. The patient was evaluated by a physician, and a diagnosis of subacromial bursitis was made. The patient was also referred to physical therapy, and a program of heat, ultrasound, and exercise was initiated to help resolve this condition.

Problem/Influence of Medication. During the initial physical therapy evaluation, the therapist asked if the patient was taking any medication for the bursitis.

The patient responded that he had been advised by the physician to take aspirin as needed to help relieve the pain. When asked if he had done this, the patient said that he had taken some aspirin once or twice, especially when his shoulder pain kept him awake at night. When he was asked specifically what type of aspirin he had taken, he named a commercial acetaminophen preparation. Evidently the patient was unaware of the difference between acetaminophen and aspirin (acetyl-salicylate).

Decision/Solution. The therapist explained the difference between aspirin and acetaminophen to the patient, pointing out that acetaminophen lacks any significant anti-inflammatory effects. After consulting with the physician to confirm that aspirin was recommended for this patient, the therapist suggested that the patient should take the recommended dosage at regular intervals to help decrease the inflammation in the bursa, as well as to provide analgesia. The patient had taken aspirin in the past without any problem, but the therapist cautioned the patient to contact his physician if any adverse effects were noted (e.g., gastrointestinal distress or tinnitus).

SUMMARY

Aspirin and similarly acting drugs comprise a group of therapeutic agents that are usually referred to as NSAIDs. In addition to their anti-inflammatory effects, these drugs are also known for their ability to decrease mild-to-moderate pain (analgesia), alleviate fever (antipyresis), and inhibit platelet aggregation (anticoagulation). These drugs seem to exert all of their therapeutic effects by inhibiting the function of the cellular cyclo-oxygenase enzyme, which results in decreased prostaglandin and thromboxane synthesis. Aspirin is the prototypical NSAID, and the newer prescription and nonprescription drugs appear to be similar to aspirin in terms of pharmacologic effect and therapeutic efficacy. Acetaminophen also seems to be similar to aspirin in analgesic and antipyretic effects, but acetaminophen lacks anti-inflammatory and anticoagulant properties. These drugs are seen frequently in patients requiring physical therapy, and they usually provide beneficial effects (analgesia, decreased inflammation, etc.) without interfering with the rehabilitation program.

REFERENCES

1. Ahnen, DJ: Colon cancer prevention by NSAIDs: What is the mechanism of action? Eur J Surg Suppl 582:111, 1998.
2. Allison, MC, et al: Gastrointestinal damage associated with the use of nonsteroidal anti-inflammatory drugs. N Engl J Med 327:749, 1992.
3. Antiplatelet Trialists' Collaboration: Secondary prevention of vascular disease by prolonged antiplatelet treatment. BMJ 296:320, 1988.
4. Asad, SI, et al: Effect of aspirin in "aspirin sensitive" patients. BMJ 288:745, 1984.
5. Austen, KF: The role of arachidonic acid metabolites in local and systemic inflammatory processes. Drugs 33(Suppl 1):10, 1987.
6. Bassleer, C, Henrotin, Y, and Franchimnot, P: Effects of sodium naproxen on differentiated human chondrocytes cultivated in clusters. Clin Rheumatol 11:60, 1992.
7. Baumann TJ: Pain management. In DiPiro, JT, et al (eds): Pharmacotherapy: A Pathophysiologic Approach, ed 4. Appleton & Lange, Stamford, CT, 1999.
8. Bjarnason, I: Forthcoming non-steroidal anti-inflammatory drugs: Are they really devoid of side effects? Ital J Gastroenterol Hepatol 31(Suppl 1):S27, 1999.
9. Bjorkman, D: Nonsterioidal anti-inflammatory drug-associated toxicity of the liver, lower gastrointestinal tract, and esophagus. Am J Med 105(Suppl 5A):17S, 1998.

10. Bjorkman, DJ: The effect of aspirin and nonsteroidal anti-inflammatory drugs on prostaglandins. Am J Med 105(Suppl 1B):8S, 1998.
11. Brooks, P: Use and benefits of nonsteroidal anti-inflammatory drugs. Am J Med 104(Suppl 3A):9S, 1998.
12. Brooks, PM and Day, RO: Drug therapy: Nonsteroidal anti-inflammatory drugs—differences and similarities. N Engl J Med 324:1716, 1991.
13. Brooks, PM and Yeomans, ND: Nonsteroidal anti-inflammatory drug gastropathy: Is it preventable? Aust N Z J Med 22:685, 1992.
14. Calverley, DC and Roth, GJ: Antiplatelet therapy. Aspirin, ticlopidine/clopidogrel, and anti-integrin agents. Hematol Oncol Clin North Am 12:1231, 1998.
15. Campbell, WB and Haluska, PV: Lipid-derived autacoids: Eicosanoids and platelet-activating factor. In Hardman, JG, et al (eds): The Pharmacological Basis of Therapeutics, ed 9. McGraw-Hill, New York, 1996.
16. Cashman, JN: Non-steroidal anti-inflammatory drugs versus postoperative pain. J R Soc Med 86:464, 1993.
17. Cataldo, PA, Senagore, AJ, and Kilbride, MJ: Ketorolac and patient controlled analgesia in the treatment of postoperative pain. Surg Gynecol Obstet 176:435, 1993.
18. Chan, PS and Cervoni, P: Prostaglandins, prostacyclin, and thromboxane in cardiovascular disease. Drug Dev Res 7:341, 1986.
19. Chan, WY: Prostaglandins and nonsteroidal anti-inflammatory drugs in dysmenorrhea. Annu Rev Pharmacol Toxicol 23:131, 1983.
20. Ciabattoni, G, et al: Effects of sulindac on renal and extrarenal eicosanoid synthesis. Clin Pharmacol Ther 41:380, 1987.
21. Ciccone, CD and Zambraski, EJ: Effects of prostaglandin inhibition on renal function in deoxycorticosterone-acetate hypertensive yucatan miniature swine. Prostaglandins Med 7:395, 1981.
22. Clive, DM and Stoff, JS: Renal syndromes associated with nonsteroidal antiinflammatory drugs. N Engl J Med 310:563, 1984.
23. Coceani, F and Akarsu, ES: Prostaglandin E2 in the pathogenesis of fever: An update. Ann N Y Acad Sci 856:76, 1998.
24. Collier, S and Ghosh, P: Comparison of the effects of NSAIDs on proteoglycan synthesis by articular cartilage explant and chondrocyte monolayer cultures. Biochem Pharmacol 41:1375, 1991.
25. Committee on Infectious Diseases: Aspirin and Reye's syndrome. Pediatrics 69:810, 1982.
26. Creamer, P, Flores, R, and Hochberg, MC: Management of osteoarthritis in older adults. Clin Geriatr Med 14:435, 1998.
27. Cryer, B and Feldman, M: Cyclooxygenase-1 and cyclooxygenase-2 selectivity of widely used nonsteroidal anti-inflammatory drugs. Am J Med 104:413, 1998.
28. Cryer, B and Kimmey, MB: Gastrointestinal side effects of nonsteroidal anti-inflammatory drugs. Am J Med 105(Suppl 1B):20S, 1998.
29. David, MJ, et al: Effects of NSAIDs on glycosyltransferase activity from human osteoarthritic cartilage. Br J Rheumatol 31(Suppl 1):13, 1992.
30. Day, RO, et al: Non-steroidal anti-inflammatory drug induced upper gastrointestinal haemorrhage and bleeding. Med J Aust 157:810, 1992.
31. Deandrade, JR, et al: The use of ketorolac in the management of postoperative pain. Orthopedics 17:157, 1994.
32. Diener, HC: Antiplatelet drugs in secondary prevention of stroke. Int J Clin Pract 52:91, 1998.
33. Dubois, RN, et al: Cyclooxygenase in biology and disease. FASEB J 12:1063, 1998.
34. Dunn, M: The role of arachidonic acid metabolites in renal hemostasis. Drugs 33(Suppl 1):56, 1987.
35. Dunn, MJ: Nonsteroidal antiinflammatory drugs and renal function. Annu Rev Med 35:411, 1984.
36. Dutch TIA Trial Study Group: A comparison of two doses of aspirin (30 mg vs. 283 mg a day) in patients after a transient ischemic attack or minor ischemic stroke. N Engl J Med 325:1261, 1991.
37. Easton, JD: What have we learned from recent antiplatelet trials? Neurology 51(Suppl 3):S36, 1998.
38. Eriksson, L-O, Beerman, B, and Kallner, M: Renal function and tubular transport effects of sulindac and naproxen in congestive heart failure. Clin Pharmacol Ther 42:646, 1987.
39. Fiedler, MA: Clinical implications of ketorolac for postoperative analgesia. J Perianesth Nurs 12:426, 1997.
40. Fischer, SM: Prostaglandins and cancer. Front Biosci 2:482, 1997.
41. Fletcher JR: Eicosanoids: Critical agents in the physiological process and cellular injury. Arch Surg 128:1192, 1993.
42. Flower, RJ and Vane, JR: Inhibition of prostaglandin synthetase in brain explains the anti-pyretic action of paracetamol (4-acetamidophenol). Nature 240:410, 1972.
43. Foegh, ML, et al: The eicosanoids: Prostaglandins, thromboxanes, leukotrienes, and related compounds. In Katzung, BG (ed): Basic and Clinical Pharmacology, ed 7. Appleton & Lange, Stamford, CT, 1998.
44. Fort, J: Celecoxib, a COX-2 specific inhibitor: The clinical data. Am J Orthop 28(Suppl):13, 1999.
45. Freeland, GR, et al: Hepatic safety of two analgesics used over the counter: Ibuprofen and aspirin. Clin Pharmacol Ther 43:473, 1988.
46. Fretland, DJ: Review: Potential role of prostaglandins and leukotrienes in multiple sclerosis and experimental allergic encephalomyelitis. Prostaglandins Leukot Essent Fatty Acids 45:249, 1992.
47. Fung, HB and Kirschenbaum, HL: Selective cyclooxygenase-2 inhibitors for the treatment of arthritis. Clin Ther 21:1131, 1999.

48. Geis, GS: Update on clinical developments with celecoxib, a new specific COX-2 inhibitor: What can we expect? J Rheumatol 26(Suppl 56):31, 1999.
49. Goetzl, EJ, An, S, and Smith, WL: Specificity of expression and effects of eicosanoid mediators in normal physiology and human diseases. FASEB J 9:1051, 1995.
50. Golden, BD and Abramson, SB: Selective cyclooxygenase inhibitors. Rheum Dis Clin North Am 25:359, 1999.
51. Greene, JM and Winickoff, RN: Cost-conscious prescribing of nonsteroidal anti-inflammatory drugs for adults with arthritis: A review and suggestions. Arch Intern Med 152:1995, 1992.
52. Henrich, WL: Analgesic nephropathy. Trans Am Clin Climatol Assoc 109:147, 1998.
53. Henrotin, Y, Bassleer, C, and Franchimont, P: In vitro effects of etodolac and acetylsalicylic acid on human chondrocyte metabolism. Agents Actions 36:317, 1992.
54. Higgs, GA and Vane, JR: Inhibition of cyclo-oxygenase and lipoxygenase. Br Med Bull 39:265, 1983.
55. Hochberg, MC: Association of nonsteroidal anti-inflammatory drugs with upper gastrointestinal disease: Epidemiologic and economic considerations. J Rheumatol 19(Suppl 36):63, 1992.
56. Hollingworth, P: Paediatric rheumatology review: The use of nonsteroidal anti-inflammatory drugs in paediatric rheumatic diseases. Br J Rheumatol 32:73, 1993.
57. Hugenberg, ST, Brandt, KD, and Cole, CA: Effects of sodium salicylate, aspirin, and ibuprofen on enzymes required by the chondrocyte for synthesis of chondrotin sulfate. J Rheumatol 29:2128, 1993.
58. Insel, P: Analgesic-antipyretic and anti-inflammatory agents and drugs employed in the treatment of gout. In Hardman, JG, et al (eds): The Pharmacologic Basis of Therapeutics, ed 9. McGraw-Hill, New York, 1996.
59. Kimmey, MB: NSAID, ulcers, and prostaglandins. J Rheumatol 19(Suppl 36):68, 1992.
60. Kincaid-Smith, P: Effects of non-narcotic analgesics on the kidney. Drugs 32(Suppl 4):109, 1986.
61. La Corte, R, et al: Prophylaxis and treatment of NSAID-induced gastroduodenal disorders. Drug Saf 20:527, 1999.
62. Lanas, A: Non-steroidal anti-inflammatory drugs and gastrointestinal bleeding. Ital J Gastroenterol Hepatol 31(Suppl 1):S37, 1999.
63. Lanas, A and Hirschowitz, BI: Toxicity of NSAIDs in the stomach and duodenum. Eur J Gastroenterol Hepatol 11:375, 1999.
64. Langman, MJ: Risks of anti-inflammatory drug-associated damage. Inflamm Res 48:236, 1999.
65. Larsen, GL and Henson, PM: Mediators of inflammation. Annu Rev Immunol 1:335, 1983.
66. Lasagna, L and McMahon, FG: Introduction: Aspirin's infinite variety. Am J Med 74(Suppl 6A):1, 1983.
67. Lefkowith, JB: Cyclooxygenase-2 specificity and its clinical implications. Am J Med 106(Suppl 5B):43S, 1999.
68. Lewis, HD, et al: Protective effects of aspirin against acute myocardial infarction and death in men with unstable angina. N Engl J Med 309:396, 1983.
69. Lewis, RA, Austen, KF, and Soberman, RJ: Mechanisms of disease: Leukotrienes and other products of the 5-lipoxygenase pathway—biochemistry and relation to pathophysiology in human diseases. N Engl J Med 323:645, 1990.
70. Lipsky, LP, et al: The classification of cyclooxygenase inhibitors. J Rheumatol 25:2298, 1998.
71. Logan, RFA, et al: Effect of aspirin and non-steroidal anti-inflammatory drugs on colorectal adenomas: Case-control study of subjects participating in the Nottingham faecal occult blood screening programme. BMJ 307:285, 1993.
72. Lysak, SZ, et al: Postoperative effects of fentanyl, ketorolac, and piroxicam as analgesics for outpatient laparoscopic procedures. Obstet Gynecol 83:270, 1994.
73. Marks, F, Furstenberger, G, and Muller-Decker, K: Metabolic targets of cancer chemoprevention: Interruption of tumor development by inhibitors of arachidonic acid metabolism. Recent Results Cancer Res 151:45, 1999.
74. Mason, JC: NSAIDs and the oesophagus. Eur J Gastroenterol Hepatol 11:369, 1999.
75. McGuire, DA, Sanders, K, and Hendricks, SD: Comparison of ketorolac and opioid analgesics in postoperative ACL reconstruction outpatient pain control. Arthroscopy 9:653, 1993.
76. McKenna, F: COX-2: separating myth from reality. Scand J Rheumatol Suppl 109:19, 1999.
77. Muller, B: Pharmacology of thromboxane A2, prostacyclin and other eicosanoids in the cardiovascular system. Therapie 46:217, 1991.
78. Muller-Peddinghaus, R: Potential anti-inflammatory effects of 5-lipoxygenase inhibition exemplified by the leukotriene synthesis inhibitor BAY X 1005. J Physiol Pharmacol 48:529, 1997.
79. Nissen, I, Jensen, KA, and Ohrstrom, JK: Indomethacin in the management of postoperative pain. Br J Anaesth 69:304, 1992.
80. O'Byrne, PM: Asthma treatment: antileukotriene drugs. Can Respir J 5(Suppl A):64A, 1998.
81. O'Hara, DA, et al: Ketorolac tromethamine as compared with morphine sulfate for treatment of postoperative pain. Clin Pharmacol Ther 41:556, 1987.
82. Owen, PR: Prostaglandin synthetase inhibitors in the treatment of primary dysmenorrhea. Am J Obstet Gynecol 148:96, 1984.
83. Patrono, C: Prevention of myocardial infarction and stroke by aspirin: Different mechanisms? Different dosage? Thromb Res 92(Suppl 1):S7, 1998.
84. Pedersen, P, Nielsen, KD, and Jensen, PE: The efficacy of Na$^+$-naproxen after diagnostic and therapeutic arthroscopy of the knee joint. Arthroscopy 9:170, 1993.

85. Peskar, BM and Maricic, N: Role of prostaglandins in gastroprotection. Dig Dis Sci 43(Suppl):23S, 1998.
86. Peters, BH, Fraim, CJ, and Masel, BE: Comparison of 650 mg aspirin and 1000 mg acetaminophen with each other, and with placebo in moderately severe headache. Am J Med 74(Suppl 6A):36, 1983.
87. Pincus, T, et al: Long-term drug therapy for rheumatoid arthritis in seven rheumatology private practices. 1. Nonsteroidal anti-inflammatory drugs. J Rheumatol 19:1874, 1992.
88. Piper, PJ: Pharmacology of leukotrienes. Br Med Bull 39:255, 1983.
89. Prescott, LF: Effects of non-narcotic analgesics on the liver. Drugs 32(Suppl 4):129, 1986.
90. Prigge, ST, et al: Structure and mechanism of lipoxygenases. Biochimie 79:629, 1997.
91. Raskin, JB: Gastrointestinal effects of nonsteroidal anti-inflammatory therapy. Am J Med 106(Suppl 5B):3S, 1999.
92. Rasmussen, S, et al: The clinical effect of naproxen sodium after arthroscopy of the knee: A randomized, double-blind, prospective study. Arthroscopy 9:375, 1993.
93. Redden, RJ: Ketorolac tromethamine: An oral/injectable nonsteroidal anti-inflammatory for postoperative pain control. J Oral Maxillofac Surg 50:1310, 1992.
94. Reilly, MP, Lawson, JA, and FitzGerald, GA: Eicosanoids and isoeicosanoids: Indices of cellular function and oxidant stress. J Nutr 128:434S, 1998.
95. Robinson, DR: Regulation of prostaglandin synthesis by antiinflammatory drugs. J Rheumatol Suppl 47:32, 1997.
96. Rubin, BR: Specific cyclooxygenase-2 (COX-2) inhibitors. J Am Osteopath Assoc 99:322, 1999.
97. Russell, RI: Defining patients at risk of non-steroidal anti-inflammatory drug gastropathy. Ital J Gastroenterol Hepatol 31(Suppl 1):S14, 1999.
98. Salgia, AD and Kosnik, SD: When acetaminophen use becomes toxic. Treating acute accidental and intentional overdose. Postgrad Med 105:81, 1999.
99. Samuelsson, B: An elucidation of the arachadonic acid cascade. Discovery of prostaglandins, thromboxane and leukotrienes. Drugs 33(Suppl 1):2, 1987.
100. Samuelsson, B: Leukotrienes: Mediators of immediate hypersensitivity reactions and inflammation. Science 220:568, 1983.
101. Savage, RL, et al: Variations in the risk of peptic ulcer complications with nonsteroidal antiinflammatory drug therapy. Arthritis Rheum 36:84, 1993.
102. Schafer, AI: Effects of nonsteroidal anti-inflammatory therapy on platelets. Am J Med 106(Suppl 5B):25S, 1999.
103. Scheiman, J and Isenberg, J: Agents used in the prevention and treatment of nonsteroidal anti-inflammatory drug-associated symptoms and ulcers. Am J Med 105(Suppl 5A):32S, 1998.
104. Schmassmann, A: Mechanisms of ulcer healing and effects of nonsteroidal anti-inflammatory drugs. Am J Med 104(Suppl 3A):43S, 1998.
105. Seibert, K, et al: Distribution of COX-1 and COX-2 in normal and inflamed tissues. Adv Exp Med Biol 400A:167, 1997.
106. Settipane, GA: Aspirin and allergic diseases: A review. Am J Med 74(Suppl 6A):102, 1983.
107. Sharma, S and Sharma, SC: An update on eicosanoids and inhibitors of cyclooxygenase enzyme systems. Indian J Exp Biol 35:1025, 1997.
108. Sperling, RI: Eicosanoids in rheumatoid arthritis. Rheum Dis Clin North Am 21:741, 1995.
109. Stalnikowicz, R and Rachmilewitz, D: NSAID-induced gastroduodenal damage: Is prevention needed. A review and meta-analysis. J Clin Gastroenterol 17:238, 1993.
110. Steering Committee of the Physicians' Health Study Research Group: Final report on the aspirin component of the ongoing physicians' health study. N Engl J Med 321:129, 1989.
111. Subbaramaiah, K, et al: Inhibition of cyclooxygenase: A novel approach to cancer prevention. Proc Soc Exp Biol Med 216:201, 1997.
112. Suh, O, Mettlin, C, and Petrelli, NJ: Aspirin use, cancer, and polyps of the large bowel. Cancer 72:1171, 1993.
113. Tan, RA: The role of antileukotrienes in asthma management. Curr Opin Pulm Med 4:25, 1998.
114. Thun, MJ, et al: Aspirin use and risk of fatal cancer. Cancer Res 53:1322, 1993.
115. Tolman, KG: Hepatotoxicity of non-narcotic analgesics. Am J Med 105(Suppl 1B):13S, 1998.
116. Turner, D and Berkel, HJ: Nonsteroidal anti-inflammatory drugs for the prevention of colon cancer. Can Med Assoc J 149:595, 1993.
117. Vane, JR, Bahkle, YS, and Botting, RM: Cyclooxygenases 1 and 2. Annu Rev Pharmacol Toxicol 38:97, 1998.
118. Vane, JR and Botting, RM: Anti-inflammatory drugs and their mechanism of action. Inflamm Res 47(Suppl 2):S78, 1998.
119. Vane, JR and Botting, RM: Mechanism of action of nonsteroidal anti-inflammatory drugs. Am J Med 104(Suppl 3A):2S, 1998.
120. Venturini, CM, Isakson, P, and Needlemen, P: Non-steroidal anti-inflammatory drug-induced renal failure: A brief review of the role of cyclo-oxygenase isoforms. Curr Opin Nephrol Hypertens 7:79, 1998.
121. Walt, RP: Drug therapy: Misoprostol for the treatment of peptic ulcer and antiinflammatory drug-induced gastroduodenal ulceration. N Engl J Med 327:1575, 1992.
122. Ward, MR: Reye's syndrome: An update. Nurse Pract 22:45, 1997.
123. Weller, JM: Medical modifiers of sports injury: The use of nonsteroidal anti-inflammatory drugs (NSAIDs) in sports soft-tissue injury. Clin Sports Med 11:625, 1992.

124. Wenzel, SE: New approaches to anti-inflammatory therapy for asthma. Am J Med 104:287, 1998.
125. Whelton, A: Nephrotoxicity of nonsteroidal anti-inflammatory drugs: Physiologic foundations and clinical implications. Am J Med 106(Suppl 5B):13S, 1999.
126. Willard, JE, Lange, RA, and Hillis, LD: Current concepts: The use of aspirin in ischemic heart disease. N Engl J Med 327:175, 1992.
127. Willkens, RF: The selection of a nonsteroidal antiinflammatory drug: Is there a difference? J Rheumatol 19(Suppl 36):9, 1992.

CHAPTER 16

Pharmacologic Management of Rheumatoid Arthritis and Osteoarthritis

Rheumatoid arthritis and osteoarthritis represent the two primary pathologic conditions that affect joints and periarticular structures. Although the causes underlying these conditions are quite different from one another, both conditions can cause severe pain and deformity in various joints in the body. Likewise, pharmacologic management plays an important role in the treatment of each disorder. Because physical therapists and other rehabilitation specialists often work with patients who have rheumatoid arthritis or osteoarthritis, an understanding of the types of drugs used to treat these diseases is important.

This chapter will begin by describing the etiology of rheumatoid joint disease and the pharmacologic treatment of rheumatoid arthritis. An analogous discussion of osteoarthritis will follow. These descriptions will hopefully provide rehabilitation specialists with an understanding of the role of drug therapy in arthritis and the impact drug therapy can have on physical therapy and occupational therapy.

RHEUMATOID ARTHRITIS

Rheumatoid arthritis is a chronic, systemic disorder that affects many different tissues in the body but is characterized primarily by synovitis and the destruction of articular tissue.[53,105] This disease is associated with pain, stiffness, and inflammation in the small synovial joints of the hands and feet, as well as in larger joints such as the knee. Although marked by periods of exacerbation and remission, rheumatoid arthritis is often progressive in nature, with advanced stages leading to severe joint destruction and bone erosion.

Specific criteria for the diagnosis of rheumatoid arthritis in adults are listed in Table 16–1. In addition to the adult form of this disease, there is also a form of arthritis that occurs in children (i.e., juvenile rheumatoid arthritis). Juvenile rheumatoid arthritis differs from the adult form of this disease, with the age of onset (younger than 16 years) and

TABLE 16–1 Criteria for the Classification of Rheumatoid Arthritis*

Criterion	Definition
1. Morning stiffness	Morning stiffness in and around the joints, lasting at least 1 hr before maximal improvement.
2. Arthritis of 3 or more joint areas	At least 3 joint areas simultaneously have had soft tissue swelling or fluid (not bony overgrowth alone) observed by a physician. The 14 possible areas are right or left PIP, MCP, wrist, elbow, knee, ankle, and MTP joints.†
3. Arthritis of hand joints	At least 1 area swollen (as defined above) in a wrist, MCP, or PIP joint.
4. Symmetric arthritis	Simultaneous involvement of the same joint areas (as defined in 2) on both sides of the body (bilateral involvement of PIPs, MCPs, or MTPs is acceptable without absolute symmetry).
5. Rheumatoid nodules	Subcutaneous nodules over bony prominences or extensor surfaces, or in juxtaarticular regions, observed by a physician.
6. Serum rheumatoid factor	Demonstration of abnormal amounts of serum rheumatoid factor by any method for which the result has been positive in <5% of normal control subjects.
7. Radiographic changes	Radiographic changes typical of rheumatoid arthritis on posteroanterior hand and wrist radiographs, which must include erosions or unequivocal bony decalcification; localized in or most marked adjacent to the involved joints (osteoarthritis changes alone do not qualify).

*For classification purposes, a patient shall be said to have rheumatoid arthritis if he or she has satisfied at least 4 of these 7 criteria. Criteria 1 through 4 must have been present for at least 6 weeks.

†PIP = proximal interphalangeal; MCP = metacarpophalangeal; MTP = metatarsophalangeal.

Source: Arnett, et al: The American Rheumatism Association 1987 Revised Criteria for the Classification of Rheumatoid Arthritis. Arthritis and Rheumatism 31:315–324, 1988. Reprinted from ARTHRITIS AND RHEUMATISM Journal, copyright 1988. Used by permission of the American College of Rheumatology.

other criteria helping to differentiate these two types of rheumatoid joint disease.[43,53,86] The drug treatment of adult and juvenile rheumatoid arthritis is fairly similar, however, with the exception that some drugs (e.g., glucocorticoids) are used more cautiously in children.[122] Consequently, in this chapter most of the discussion of the management of rheumatoid arthritis is directed toward the adult form of this disease.

Rheumatoid arthritis affects about 1.0 percent of the population worldwide.[31,53,81] This disease occurs three times more often in women than in men, with women between the ages of 20 and 40 especially susceptible to the onset of rheumatoid joint disease.[43,53,105] Rheumatoid arthritis often causes severe pain and suffering, frequently devastating the patient's family and social life as well as his or her job situation.[81,83] The economic impact of this disease is also staggering, with the medical costs and loss of productivity exceeding $1 billion annually in the United States.[83] Consequently, rheumatoid arthritis is a formidable and serious problem in contemporary health care.

Immune Basis for Rheumatoid Arthritis

The initiating factors in rheumatoid arthritis are not known. It is apparent, however, that the underlying basis of this disease consists of some type of autoimmune response in genetically susceptible individuals.[54,87,93,105,109] Some precipitating factor (possibly a virus or other infectious agent) appears to initiate the formation of antibodies that are later recognized by the host as antigens.[53,105,109] Subsequent formation of new antibodies to these antigens then initiates a complex chain of events involving a variety of immune system components such as mononuclear phagocytes, T lymphocytes, and B lymphocytes.[39,53,109] These cells basically interact with each other to produce a number of arthritogenic mediators, including cytokines (interleukins, growth factors), eicosanoids (prostaglandins, leukotrienes), and destructive enzymes (proteases, collagenases).[37,38,54,75,87,109] These substances act either directly or through other cellular components of the immune system to induce synovial cell proliferation and destruction of articular cartilage and bone.[53,105] Thus, the joint destruction in rheumatoid arthritis is the culmination of a series of events that result from an inherent defect in the immune response in patients with this disease.[54,109]

Overview of Drug Therapy in Rheumatoid Arthritis

The drug treatment of rheumatoid arthritis has two goals: (1) to decrease joint inflammation and (2) to arrest the progression of this disease. Three general categories of drugs are available to accomplish these goals: (1) nonsteroidal anti-inflammatory drugs (NSAIDs), (2) glucocorticoids, and (3) a diverse group of agents known as *disease-modifying antirheumatic drugs* (DMARDs) (Table 16–2).[11,21,108] The NSAIDs and glucocorticoids are used primarily to decrease joint inflammation, but these agents do not necessarily halt the progression of rheumatoid arthritis. The DMARDs attempt to slow or halt the advancement of this disease, usually by interfering with the immune response that seems to

TABLE 16–2 Drug Categories Used in Rheumatoid Arthritis

I. Nonsteroidal Anti-Inflammatory Drugs

Aspirin (many trade names)	Meclofenamate (Meclomen)
Celecoxib (Celebrex)*	Nabumetone (Relafen)
Diclofenac (Voltaren)	Naproxen (Anaprox, Naprosyn)
Diflunisal (Dolobid)	Oxaprozin (Daypro)
Etodolac (Lodine)	Phenylbutazone (Butazolidin, Cotylbutazone, others)
Fenoprofen (Nalfon)	Piroxicam (Feldene)
Flurbiprofen (Ansaid)	Rofecoxib (Vioxx)*
Ibuprofen (many trade names)	Sulindac (Clinoril)
Indomethacin (Indocin)	Tolmetin (Tolectin)
Ketoprofen (Orudis, others)	

II. Glucocorticoids

Betamethasone (Celestone)	Methylprednisolone (Medrol, others)
Cortisone (Cortone acetate)	Prednisolone (Prelone, others)
Dexamethasone (Decadron, others)	Prednisone (Deltasone, others)
Hydrocortisone (Cortef, others)	Triamcinolone (Aristocort, others)

III. Disease-Modifying Antirheumatic Drugs

Auranofin (Ridaura)	Gold sodium thiomalate (Myochrysine)
Aurothioglucose (Solganal)	Hydroxychloroquine (Plaquenil)
Azathioprine (Imuran)	Leflunomide (Arava)
Chloroquine (Aralen)	Methotrexate (Rheumatrex, others)
Cyclophosphamide (Cytoxan)	Penicillamine (Cuprimine, Depen)
Cyclosporine (Neoral, Sandimmune)	Sulfasalazine (Azulfidine)
Etanercept (Enbrel)	

*Subclassified as cyclooxygenase type 2 (COX-2) inhibitors; see Chapter 15.

be the primary underlying factor in rheumatoid arthritis.[20] Each of these major drug categories, as well as specific disease-modifying drugs, is discussed in the following sections of this chapter.

Nonsteroidal Anti-Inflammatory Drugs

Aspirin and the other NSAIDs are usually considered the first line of defense in treating rheumatoid arthritis.[2,11,113] Although NSAIDs are not as powerful in reducing inflammation as glucocorticoids, they are associated with fewer serious side effects, and they offer the added advantage of analgesia. Consequently, NSAIDs such as aspirin are often the first drugs employed in treating rheumatoid arthritis; in fact, this disease can often be controlled adequately for extended periods in some patients solely by the use of an NSAID.[98] In patients who continue to experience progressive joint destruction despite NSAID therapy, these drugs are often combined with one of the disease-modifying agents discussed later in this chapter. Usually, it is not advisable to use two different NSAIDs simultaneously because there is an increased risk of side effects without any appreciable increase in therapeutic efficacy. Some amount of trial and error may be involved in selecting the best NSAID, and several agents may have to be given in succession before an optimal drug is found for that patient. As discussed in Chapter 15, aspirin appears to approximately equal the newer, more expensive NSAIDs in terms of anti-inflammatory and analgesic effects, but some of the newer drugs may produce less gastrointestinal discomfort. The choice of a specific NSAID ultimately depends on each individual patient's response to the therapeutic effects and side effects of any given agent.[17,128]

MECHANISM OF ACTION

The pharmacology of the NSAIDs was discussed in Chapter 15. Basically, aspirin and the other NSAIDs exert most or all of their anti-inflammatory and analgesic effects by inhibiting the synthesis of prostaglandins.[10,59,118] Certain prostaglandins (i.e., prostaglandin E_2 [PGE_2]) are believed to participate in the inflammatory response by increasing local blood flow and vascular permeability and by exerting a chemotactic effect on leukocytes.[17] Prostaglandins are also believed to sensitize pain receptors to the nociceptive effects of other pain mediators such as bradykinin.[59] Aspirin and other NSAIDs prevent the production of prostaglandins by inhibiting the cyclooxygenase (COX) enzyme that initiates prostaglandin synthesis. As discussed in Chapter 15, aspirin and most other NSAIDs inhibit all COX forms; that is, these drugs inhibit the COX-1 form of the enzyme that produces beneficial and protective prostaglandins in certain tissues while also inhibiting the COX-2 form that synthesizes prostaglandins in painful and inflamed tissues.[118]

Newer NSAIDs, however, are known as COX-2 inhibitors because these drugs inhibit the specific form of cyclooxygenase (COX-2) that synthesizes prostaglandins during pain and inflammation. COX-2 drugs (celecoxib and rofecoxib; see Table 16–2) spare the production of normal or protective prostaglandins produced by COX-1 in the stomach, kidneys, and platelets (see Chap. 15).[45,50,73,77] Hence, these COX-2 selective drugs may be especially beneficial during long-term use in people with rheumatoid arthritis because they may be less toxic to the stomach and other tissues. The effect of COX-2 selective drugs and other NSAIDs on prostaglandin biosynthesis is discussed in more detail in Chapter 15.

ADVERSE SIDE EFFECTS

The problems and adverse effects of aspirin and other NSAIDs are discussed in Chapter 15. The most common problem with chronic use of most NSAIDs is stomach irritation, which can lead to gastric ulceration and hemorrhage. This can be resolved to some extent by taking aspirin in an enteric-coated form so that release of the aspirin is delayed until the drug reaches the small intestine. Other pharmacologic interventions such as prostaglandin analogs (misoprostol) and proton pump inhibitors (omeprazole) can also be used if gastropathy continues to be a limiting factor during NSAID use (see Chap. 15). Chronic NSAID use can also produce bleeding problems (because of platelet inhibition) and impaired renal function, especially in the elderly or debilitated patient. As indicated earlier, COX-2 selective drugs may reduce the risk of toxicity to the stomach, kidneys, and other tissues because these drugs spare the production of normal or protective prostaglandins in these tissues. These newer drugs, however, may cause other problems such as diarrhea, heartburn, gastrointestinal cramps, and an increased risk of upper respiratory tract infections. Despite the potential for various side effects, aspirin and other NSAIDs continue to be used extensively by people with rheumatoid arthritis and are often used for extended periods without serious adverse effects.

Glucocorticoids

Glucocorticoids such as prednisone are extremely effective anti-inflammatory agents, but they are associated with a number of serious side effects (see "Adverse Side Effects"). Likewise, glucocorticoids (known also as corticosteroids) are similar to NSAIDs in that they may decrease the inflammatory symptoms of rheumatoid arthritis, but they do not necessarily halt the progression of this disease.[103] Their current use in rheumatoid arthritis is typically reserved for patients whose disease is uncontrolled by NSAIDs and who need relief from the symptoms associated with an acute exacerbation of this disease. In particular, the judicious short-term use of systemic (oral) glucocorticoids can serve as a bridge between an acute flare-up of rheumatoid joint disease and successful management by other drugs such as the disease-modifying agents.[22,71] Glucocorticoids can also be injected directly into the arthritic joint, a technique that can be invaluable in the management of acute exacerbations. There is, of course, considerable controversy about whether intra-articular glucocorticoids will produce harmful catabolic effects in joints that are already weakened by arthritic changes. At the very least, the number of injections into an arthritic joint should be limited, and a common rule of thumb is to not exceed more than four injections into one joint within 1 year.[99] Consequently, glucocorticoids play an important but limited role in managing rheumatoid arthritis. The extended or excessive use of these agents is not advisable, and attempts are usually made to substitute NSAIDs and disease-modifying agents as soon as possible.[71,103]

MECHANISM OF ACTION

The details of the cellular effects of steroids are discussed in Chapter 29. Briefly, glucocorticoids increase the production of several anti-inflammatory proteins while also inhibiting the production of many pro-inflammatory substances.[7,106] These agents, for example, increase the production of proteins such as lipocortin-1.[7,13] Lipocortin-1 inhibits the phospholipase A_2 enzyme that normally liberates fatty acid precursors at the start of prostaglandin and leukotriene biosynthesis. Glucocorticoid-induced production of lipocortin-1 therefore blocks the first step in the synthesis of these pro-inflammatory prostaglandins and leukotrienes.[13] It is interesting to note that glucocorticoids inhibit prostaglandin and leukotriene synthesis, whereas NSAIDs only inhibit prostaglandin production (see the preceding section and Chap. 15). This may help explain why glucocorticoids are superior in treating certain types of leukotriene-induced inflammation, such as the airway inflammation that occurs in asthma.[7] Glucocorticoids likewise increase the production of proteins such as interleukin-10, interleukin-1 receptor antagonist, and neutral endopeptidase.[7] These other proteins contribute to the anti-inflammatory effects by inhibiting, destroying, or blocking various other inflammatory chemicals, peptides, and proteins.[7]

In addition to increasing the synthesis of anti-inflammatory proteins, glucocorticoids also directly inhibit the transcription factors that initiate synthesis of pro-inflammatory cytokines (e.g., interleukins, tumor necrosis factor), enzymes (e.g., Cox-2, nitric oxide synthetase), and receptor proteins (e.g., natural killer receptors).[7,106] Glucocorticoids also appear to have a direct inhibitory effect on macrophages, eosinophils, T lymphocytes, and several other types of cells that are involved in the inflammatory response.[7] Consequently, glucocorticoids affect many aspects of inflammation, and their powerful anti-inflammatory effects in rheumatoid arthritis result from their ability to blunt various cellular and chemical components of the inflammatory response.

ADVERSE SIDE EFFECTS

The side effects of glucocorticoids are numerous (see Chap. 29). These drugs exert a general catabolic effect on all types of supportive tissue (i.e., muscle, tendon, bone). Osteoporosis is a particularly important problem in the patient with arthritis, because many of these patients have significant bone loss before even beginning steroid therapy. Glucocorticoids have been known to increase bone loss in patients with arthritis, even when these drugs are used in fairly low doses.[22,88,99] Glucocorticoids may also cause muscle wasting and weakness, as well as hypertension, aggravation of diabetes mellitus, glaucoma, and cataracts.[22] These side effects emphasize the need to limit glucocorticoid therapy as much as possible when dealing with the patient with arthritis.

Disease-Modifying Antirheumatic Drugs

The fact that NSAIDs and glucocorticoids do not typically slow the progression of rheumatoid arthritis has led to the search for drugs that can alter the progressive nature of this disease. An eclectic group of agents has been identified as being able to arrest, or even reverse, the pathologic changes in some patients with rheumatoid arthritis. These drugs, commonly referred to as DMARDs, are also referred to as slow-acting antirheumatic drugs (SAARDs) to emphasize that a delay of several weeks to several months often occurs between the onset of drug therapy and the onset of clinical benefits.[16] The disease-modifying terminology is more common, so the DMARD acronym will be used here.

Disease-modifying agents currently used in treating rheumatoid arthritis are listed in Table 16–3. As the name implies, DMARDs attempt to induce remission by modifying the pathologic process inherent to rheumatoid arthritis. In general, DMARDs inhibit the immune response thought to be underlying rheumatoid disease. Most of these drugs inhibit the function of monocytes and T and B lymphocytes that are responsible for perpetuating joint inflammation and destruction.[55] However, the exact mechanism of action of these drugs in controlling rheumatoid arthritis is often poorly understood (see later in this chapter).[32]

TABLE 16–3 Disease-Modifying Antirheumatic Drugs

Drug	Trade Name	Usual Dosage	Special Considerations
Antimalarials			
Chloroquine	Aralen	Oral: Up to 4 mg/kg of lean body weight per day.	Periodic ophthalmic exams recommended to check for retinal toxicity.
Hydroxychloroquine	Plaquenil	Oral: Up to 6.5 mg/kg of lean body weight per day.	Similar to chloroquine.
Azathioprine	Imuran	Oral: 1 mg/kg body weight per day; can be increased after 6–8 wk up to maximum dose of 2.5 mg/kg body weight.	Relatively high toxicity; should be used cautiously in debilitated patients or patients with renal disease.
Cyclophosphamide	Cytoxan	Oral: 1.5–2 mg/kg body weight per day; can be increased to a maximum daily dose of 3 mg/kg body weight.	Long-term use is limited because of potential for carcinogenicity.
Cyclosporine	Neoral, Sandimmune	Oral: 2.5 mg/kg body weight per day; can be increased after 8 wk by 0.5–0.75 mg/kg body weight per day. Dose can be increased after another 4 wk to a maximum daily dose of 4 mg/kg body weight per day.	May cause nephrotoxicity and gastrointestinal problems.
Etanercept	Enbrel	Subcutaneous injection: 25 mg twice each week.	Relatively low incidence of serious side effects compared with other immunosuppressants.
Gold compounds			
Auranofin	Ridaura	Oral: 6 mg once each day or 3 mg BID.	May have a long latency (6–9 mo) before onset of benefits.
Aurothioglucose	Solganal	Intramuscular: 10 mg the 1st wk, 25 mg the 2nd and 3rd wk, then 25–50 mg each wk until total dose of 1 g. Maintenance doses of 25–50 mg every 2–4 wk can follow.	Effects occur somewhat sooner than oral gold, but still has long delay (4 mo).
Gold sodium thiomalate	Myochrysine	Similar to aurothioglucose.	Similar to aurothioglucose.
Leflunomide	Arava	Oral: 100 mg/day for the first 3 days; continue with a maintenance dose of 20 mg/day thereafter.	May decrease joint erosion and destruction with relatively few side effects during short-term use; effects of long-term use remain to be determined.
Methotrexate	Rheumatrex, others	Oral: 2.5–5 mg every 12 hr for total of 3 doses/wk or 10 mg once each week. Can be increased up to a maximum of 20–25 mg/wk.	Often effective in halting joint destruction, but long-term use limited by toxicity.
Penicillamine	Cuprimine, Depen	Oral: 125 or 250 mg once each day; can be increased to a maximum of 1.5 g/day.	Relatively high incidence of toxicity with long-term use.
Sulfasalazine	Azulfidine	Oral: 0.5–1.0 g/day for the first week; dose can be increased by 500 mg each week up to a maximum daily dose of 2–3 g/day.	Relatively high toxicity; may produce serious hypersensitivity reactions and blood dyscrasias.

232

Hence, disease-modifying drugs are typically used to control synovitis and erosive changes during the active stages of rheumatoid joint disease.[99,113] There is still considerable concern, however, over the safety and efficacy of DMARDs. These drugs are often ineffective in halting disease progression in some patients, and many DMARDs can produce serious side effects such as hepatic and renal toxicity.[62,76,113] Despite these limitations, there has been a definite trend both to use DMARDs more frequently and to use these drugs earlier in the course of rheumatoid arthritis before excessive joint destruction has occurred.[60,84] The pharmacology of specific DMARDs is discussed here.

ANTIMALARIAL DRUGS

Originally used in the treatment of malaria, the drugs chloroquine (Aralen) and hydroxychloroquine (Plaquenil) have also been found to be effective in treating rheumatoid arthritis. In the past, these drugs have been used reluctantly because of the fear of retinal toxicity (see "Adverse Side Effects").[102] There is now evidence, however, that these agents can be used safely and effectively, and some clinicians feel that these drugs should be considered as a reasonable first choice when selecting a disease-modifying drug.[44,62,76]

Mechanism of Action. Antimalarials exert a number of effects, although it is unclear exactly which of these contribute to their ability to halt the progression in rheumatoid disease. These drugs are known to increase pH within certain intracellular vacuoles in macrophages and other immune-system cells.[42] This effect is believed to disrupt the ability of these cells to process antigenic proteins and present these antigens to T cells.[104] Decreased T-cell stimulation results in immunosuppression and attenuation of the arthritic response.[42] Antimalarials have also been shown to stabilize lysosomal membranes and impair DNA and RNA synthesis, although the significance of these effects in their role as antiarthritics remains unclear.[79]

Adverse Side Effects. Chloroquine and hydroxychloroquine are usually considered the safest DMARDs.[44] The major concern with antimalarial use is that high doses of these drugs can produce irreversible retinal damage. Retinal toxicity is rare, however, when daily dosages are maintained below the levels typically used to treat rheumatoid arthritis (i.e., less than 3.5 to 4.0 mg/kg per day for chloroquine and less than 6.0 to 6.5 mg/kg per day for hydroxychloroquine).[80] Ocular exams should be scheduled periodically, however, to ensure the safe and effective use of these drugs during prolonged administration.[59] Other side effects such as headache and gastrointestinal distress can occur, but these are relatively infrequent and usually transient.

AZATHIOPRINE

Azathioprine (Imuran) is an **immunosuppressant** drug that is often used to prevent tissue rejection following organ transplants. Because of its immunosuppressant properties, this drug has been employed in treating cases of severe, active rheumatoid arthritis that have not responded to other agents.

Mechanism of Action. The mechanism of action of azathioprine is not known. This drug has been shown to impair the synthesis of DNA and RNA precursors, but it is unclear exactly how (or if) this is related to its immunosuppressant effects. Azathioprine can inhibit immune responses mediated by T cells and other immunocompetent cells, but the pharmacologic mechanism of these effects is not known.[113]

Adverse Side Effects. Azathioprine is relatively toxic, with more frequent and more severe side effects than other DMARDs.[16,44] The primary side effects include fever, chills, sore throat, fatigue, loss of appetite, and nausea or vomiting; these effects often limit the use of this drug as an antiarthritic.

ETANERCEPT

Etanercept (Enbrel) binds to a specific component of the inflammatory response known as tumor necrosis factor (TNF) and thereby reduces the ability of TNF to contribute to joint inflammation.[51] Preliminary reports suggest that etanercept is remarkably successful in decreasing rheumatoid disease activity even in people who have not responded to other DMARDs.[64,89,90] Etanercept likewise has a relatively low incidence of side effects.[89] One drawback at the present time is that etanercept must be given parenterally, usually by subcutaneous injection twice each week. Nonetheless, etanercept is the first TNF inhibitor approved for clinical use, and this drug and similar agents promise to be an important addition to the antirheumatic armamentarium.[65,78]

Mechanism of Action. As indicated, etanercept binds selectively to TNF.[51] This action prevents TNF from binding to surface receptors located on other inflammatory cells. TNF is therefore unable to activate other inflammatory cells that cause inflammation and joint destruction in rheumatoid arthritis.[51]

Adverse Side Effects. Etanercept itself causes relatively few side effects; that is, this drug does not cause extensive adverse reactions by interacting directly with specific tissues and organs. There is, however, concern that patients taking this drug may be prone to upper respiratory tract infections and other serious infections, including sepsis.[64] This increased risk of infection probably occurs because this drug inhibits a key component of the immune response—namely, TNF. This drug is therefore contraindicated in people with infections, and administration should be discontinued if an infection develops after beginning etanercept. Parenteral administration may also cause irritation around the injection site.[64]

GOLD THERAPY

Compounds containing elemental gold were among the first drugs identified as DMARDs (Fig. 16–1). Specific compounds such as aurothioglucose (Solganal) and gold sodium thiomalate (Myochrysine) have been used in the past and are usually administered by intramuscular injection. An orally active gold compound, auranofin (Ridaura), has also been developed and offers the advantage of oral administration.[24,87] Auranofin is also somewhat better tolerated than parenteral gold compounds in terms of severe adverse side effects.[16,87] Gold therapy can arrest further progression of rheumatoid joint disease in many patients, but these drugs do not reverse damage that has already occurred. Hence, these drugs are now used fairly early in the course of rheumatoid arthritis, before excessive joint destruction takes place.

Mechanism of Action. Although the exact mechanism is not fully understood, gold compounds probably induce remission in patients with rheumatoid arthritis by inhibiting the maturation and function of mononuclear phagocytes.[28,59,117] These drugs accumulate in the lysosomes of macrophages and other synovial cells and thereby suppress the action of key components in the cellular immune reaction inherent in this disease.[1,24,121] A number of additional cellular effects have been noted (decreased lysosomal enzyme release, decreased influence of reactive oxygen species), and these effects may also contribute to the effectiveness of gold compounds in treating rheumatoid arthritis.[1,55,113]

Adverse Side Effects. Adverse effects are relatively common with gold therapy, with approximately one third of patients experiencing some form of toxic effect.[66] The primary side effects caused by gold compounds are gastrointestinal distress (diarrhea, indigestion), irritation of the oral mucosa, and rashes and itching of the skin.[66,127] Other side effects include proteinuria, conjunctivitis, and **blood dyscrasias** (e.g., thrombo-

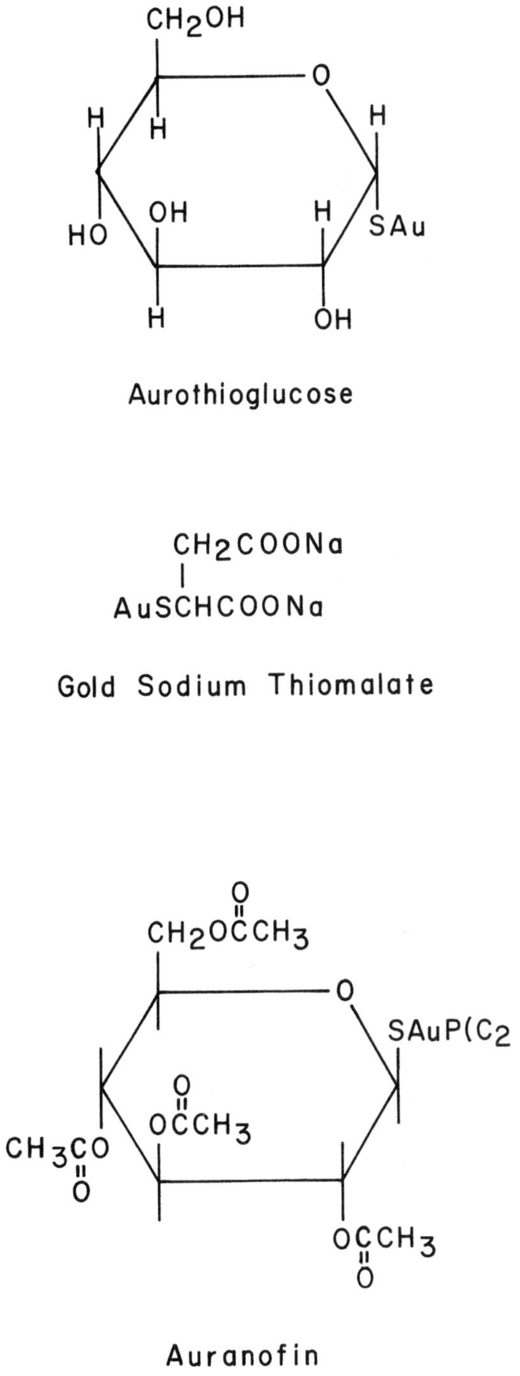

CH_2OH

Aurothioglucose

CH_2COONa
|
$AuSCHCOONa$

Gold Sodium Thiomalate

O
‖
CH_2OCCH_3

$SAuP(C_2$

O
‖
$OCCH_3$

CH_3CO
‖
O

$OCCH_3$
‖
O

Auranofin

FIGURE 16–1. Gold compounds used to treat rheumatoid arthritis.

cytopenia, leukopenia). As mentioned earlier, auranofin may be safer than parenteral gold compounds because it produces fewer cutaneous and potentially serious hematologic side effects, but auranofin tends to produce more gastrointestinal irritation than injected forms of gold.[109] Certain patients with rheumatoid arthritis may be genetically predisposed to the toxic side effects of gold compounds.[52,114] This is interesting in that it may be possible to predict via genetic screening which patients will not tolerate these drugs, thus sparing the patient from an unpleasant and possibly harmful toxic episode. Screening for genetic susceptibility has not been instituted on a routine basis, however, and drug therapy with gold compounds continues to be done by trial and error.

LEFLUNOMIDE

Leflunomide (Arava) is a relative newcomer to the antirheumatic drug arsenal. This drug helps decrease pain and inflammation in rheumatoid joint disease, and leflunomide has been shown to slow the formation of bone erosions in arthritic joints.[100,109] Leflunomide is also fairly well tolerated by most patients and may produce beneficial effects fairly soon (1 month) after beginning treatment.[108] This drug is therefore a potential alternative to other DMARDs that are more toxic or take much longer to produce antirheumatic effects.

Mechanism of Action. Leflunomide acts primarily by inhibiting the synthesis of RNA precursors in lymphocytes.[41] When stimulated, lymphocytes must radically increase their RNA synthesis to proliferate and become activated during the inflammatory response. Leflunomide blocks a key enzyme responsible for RNA synthesis, so that these lymphocytes cannot progress to a more activated state and cannot cause as much joint inflammation.[41]

Adverse Side Effects. Leflunomide's primary side effects include gastrointestinal distress, allergic reactions (rashes), and hair loss.[100] This drug can also affect the liver, and liver function may need to be monitored periodically in some patients.

METHOTREXATE

Methotrexate (Folex, Mexate, Rheumatrex) is an antimetabolite used frequently in the treatment of cancer (see Chap. 36). There is considerable evidence that this drug is also one of the most effective DMARDs.[57,70,92,124] Methotrexate has been shown to slow the effects of rheumatoid arthritis as evidenced by decreased synovitis, decreased bone erosion, and less narrowing of the joint space in patients treated with this drug.[46,123,124] The therapeutic effects of methotrexate have also been reported as equal to, or better than, other DMARDs, such as oral gold or azathioprine, and methotrexate may offer somewhat of an advantage in terms of a more rapid onset than other DMARDs.[3,109,123] Hence, methotrexate's popularity as a DMARD has increased during the past few years, and this drug continues to be used more commonly to treat rheumatoid arthritis in both adults and children.[49,92,94,99,112]

Mechanism of Action. The ability of methotrexate and similar anticancer drugs to impair DNA and RNA synthesis is well known (see Chap. 36). Methotrexate inhibits the synthesis of folic acid and thus inhibits the formation of nucleoproteins that serve as DNA precursors.[47] This action inhibits cellular replication by impairing the cell's ability to produce new genetic material, an effect that helps attenuate tumor cell replication in cancer. It was originally believed that methotrexate was beneficial in rheumatoid arthritis by an analogous antiproliferative effect on rapidly replicating cells (monocytes, lymphocytes) that constitute the immune response underlying rheumatic joint disease.[63] Evidence now suggests that most of methotrexate's anti-inflammatory and antirheumatic effects are mediated through adenosine.[27,111] Methotrexate increases the release of endogenous adenosine, and adenosine in turn inhibits various components of the immune response.[27,111] Regardless of the exact mechanism, methotrexate has become a mainstay in the management of rheumatoid arthritis.

Adverse Side Effects. Methotrexate is a relatively toxic drug, and a number of adverse side effects can occur.[44] The primary problems involve the gastrointestinal tract and include loss of appetite, nausea, and other forms of gastrointestinal distress (including intragastrointestinal hemorrhage).[109,110] Long-term methotrexate use in patients with rheumatoid arthritis has also been associated with pulmonary problems, hematologic disorders, liver dysfunction, and hair loss.[23,110,126] These side effects often limit the use of methotrexate in patients with rheumatoid arthritis, and most patients who stop using this drug do so because of an adverse side effect rather than a loss of the drug's effectiveness.[19,85,119] Methotrexate does, however, offer a favorable benefit-to-risk ratio in many patients and continues to gain popularity as a DMARD.

PENICILLAMINE

Penicillamine (Cuprimine), a derivative of penicillin, is officially classified as a chelating agent that is often used in the treatment of heavy metal intoxication (e.g., lead poisoning). In addition, this drug has been used in patients with severe rheumatoid arthritis who have not responded to other measures such as gold therapy.[91]

Mechanism of Action. The basis for the antiarthritic effects of penicillamine is unknown. Reductions in serum immunoglobulin M rheumatoid factor have been observed with penicillamine, and this drug has been shown to depress T-cell function.[113,125] These and similar findings suggest that penicillamine works by suppressing the immune response in rheumatoid arthritis, but the exact mechanisms remain to be determined.

Adverse Side Effects. Penicillamine is considered to be moderately toxic when compared with other DMARDs.[44] Side effects that have been reported as occurring more frequently include fever, joint pain, skin rashes and itching, and swelling of lymph glands. Other adverse effects that may occur less frequently are bloody or cloudy urine, swelling of feet and legs, unusual weight gain, sore throat, and excessive fatigue.

OTHER DMARDs

Because of the autoimmune basis of rheumatoid arthritis, various other drugs that affect the immune response are currently being used on a limited basis to treat this disease. For instance, cyclosporine (Sandimmune), an immunosuppressant agent that is used to prevent rejection of organ transplants (see Chap. 37), is sometimes used to treat patients with rheumatoid arthritis who have not responded to other measures.[29,115] Sulfasalazine (Azulfidine), a drug that is typically used to treat inflammatory bowel disease, may also be helpful in treating rheumatoid arthritis because of its immunosuppressant effects.[109,113] Cyclophosphamide (Cytoxan) is used primarily to treat cancer, but this agent can be used to suppress the immune system in severe cases of rheumatoid arthritis.

In general, these drugs are more toxic and are usually reserved for patients who have not responded to more traditional DMARDs such as methotrexate. Drugs with immunosuppressant activity may also be used in combination with more traditional DMARDs to provide optimal benefits in certain patients. Combination drug therapy in rheumatoid arthritis is addressed in the next section.

DMARD Combinations Used in Rheumatoid Arthritis

There has been a great deal of interest in using several DMARDs simultaneously to achieve optimal effects in treating rheumatoid arthritis. The strategy of combination therapy is to attack the underlying disease process from several pharmacologic vantage points, in much the same way that combination therapies are commonly used in other disorders such as hypertension (Chap. 21) and cancer (Chap. 36). Although the benefits of combining DMARDs has been questioned in the past, most practitioners currently advocate a combination of two or more drugs so that optimal benefits can be achieved with a relatively lower dose of each drug.[69,92] Likewise, the best way to combine specific DMARDs is still being investigated, with various combinations of new and old DMARDs being studied for efficacy and toxicity.[18,68] At present, methotrexate is typically the cornerstone of treatment, with other DMARDs added, depending on the needs of each patient.[68,101] For example, a triple combination of methotrexate with hydroxychloroquine and sulfasalazine is currently advocated as an effective treatment for many patients.[92,120]

The drawback of combination therapy is, of course, an increased risk of toxicity and drug interactions when several DMARDs are used simultaneously.[69] This fact is understandable, considering that many DMARDs have a relatively high risk of toxicity when used alone, and combining these drugs will certainly increase the risk of adverse drug reactions. Nonetheless, combination therapy continues to gain acceptance, and the use of two or three DMARDs may provide patients with the best hope for halting the progression of rheumatoid arthritis.[116] Continued research will hopefully lend additional insight to the best way that DMARDs can be combined to safely and effectively treat patients with rheumatoid arthritis.

Dietary Implications for Rheumatoid Arthritis

There is an ongoing search for other pharmacologic and nonpharmacologic interventions that can help arrest the progression of rheumatoid joint disease. There is some evidence, for example, that dietary manipulation can alleviate the symptoms of rheumatoid arthritis. Diets that are high in fish oil and certain fatty acids (e.g., gammalinolenic acid) have been advocated for patients with rheumatoid arthritis because these diets may supply precursors that enhance the biosynthesis of certain endogenous antiinflammatory and immunosuppressant compounds.[33,74] Hence, dietary changes used in combination with drug therapy may provide additional benefits for some people with rheumatoid arthritis.

OSTEOARTHRITIS

Osteoarthritis far exceeds rheumatoid arthritis as the most common form of joint disease. The prevalence of osteoarthritis increases with age. Approximately 50 to 80 percent of people age 65 have osteoarthritis to some extent, and virtually everyone over age 75 has some degree of osteoarthritic joint disease.[12,53,72] In contrast to rheumatoid joint disease, osteoarthritis does not seem to be caused by an immune response but rather seems to be associated with an intrinsic defect in the joint cartilage. This defect causes a slow, progressive deterioration of articular cartilage that is accompanied by degenerative bony changes, including thickening of the subchondral bone, creation of subchondral bone cysts, and formation of large bony protrusions (osteophytes) at the joint margins.[31,53,105] Osteoarthritis typically occurs in large weight-bearing joints such as the knees and hips, as well as some of the smaller joints in the hands and feet.[31] Patients are described as having primary osteoarthritis when there is no apparent reason for the onset of joint destruction; in secondary osteoarthritis, a factor such as previous joint trauma, infection, or metabolic disease is responsible for triggering the articular changes associated with this disease. Obesity and genetic susceptibility have also been implicated as predisposing factors in osteoarthritis.[12,31,40,53]

Clearly, osteoarthritis is a different form of joint disease than rheumatoid arthritis. Hence, treatment of these conditions also differs somewhat. As discussed previously, rheumatoid arthritis is characterized by a severe inflammatory response that is perpetuated by a cellular immune reaction. Thus, drug therapy in rheumatoid disease consists of agents that are focused on directly relieving these inflammatory symptoms (i.e., NSAIDs or glucocorticoids) or drugs that attempt to arrest the cellular immune response that causes this inflammation (DMARDs). Treatment of joint inflammation is not a major focus of drug therapy in osteoarthritis, however. A mild inflammatory synovitis does occur in osteoarthritis, but this is secondary to the articular damage inherent to this disease.[53] Also, drug therapy represents one of the primary interventions in rheumatoid arthritis, whereas treatment of osteoarthritis is dominated by nonpharmacologic measures such as physical therapy, weight loss, and joint replacement in the advanced stages of this disease.[105]

Hence, drug therapy is often not initiated during the early stages of osteoarthritis.[36] When joint pain begins to be a problem, simple analgesics such as acetaminophen and the NSAIDs have been the major form of drug therapy. Newer pharmacologic strategies are also emerging that attempt to slow or reverse the pathologic changes in osteoarthritis. These newer strategies use disease-modifying osteoarthritic drugs (DMOADs) rather than drugs that treat only the symptoms of osteoarthritis.[15] Two types of DMOADs will be addressed: drugs that attempt to directly improve the viscosity and function of synovial fluid (**viscosupplementation**) and agents that serve as precursors to the normal constituents of joint tissues (glucosamine and chondroitin sulfate).

Acetaminophen and NSAIDs

Acetaminophen is often the first drug used to treat osteoarthritis.[26,72,107] As indicated in Chapter 15, acetaminophen is as effective as NSAIDs in controlling pain, but acetaminophen does not have anti-inflammatory effects. The lack of anti-inflammatory effects is of less concern when acetaminophen is used in osteoarthritis versus rheumatoid arthritis because the inflammatory symptoms are much milder in osteoarthritis. Acetaminophen is therefore successful in reducing pain, and because this drug does not cause gastric irritation, acetaminophen is often considered the drug of choice in mild-to-moderate osteoarthritis.[4,36] Hence, acetaminophen provides a relatively safe and effective form of analgesia for patients with osteoarthritis, especially when this drug needs to be administered for long periods of time.[14,36]

NSAIDs are also used for the symptomatic treatment of pain in osteoarthritis.[9,36,72] These drugs are used primarily for their analgesic properties, although the anti-inflammatory effects of the NSAIDs can help control the mild synovitis that typically occurs in advanced osteoarthritis secondary to joint destruction.[14,36] If the primary goal is pain reduction, however, NSAIDs do not provide any advantages over acetaminophen. As indicated earlier, acetaminophen is often a better choice than traditional NSAIDs because most NSAIDs cause gastric irritation. The newer COX-2 selective NSAIDs (see Chap. 15) do not appear to cause gastric irritation, and these COX-2 drugs may be a valuable alternative to acetaminophen and traditional NSAIDs in the long-term treatment of osteoarthritis.

Regardless of the exact drug used, there is no doubt that the analgesia produced by NSAIDs or acetaminophen plays a valuable role in the management of osteoarthritis. These drugs can allow the patient to maintain a more active lifestyle and participate in various activities, including exercise programs and other forms of physical and occupational therapy. However, these drugs do not alter the progressive course of joint destruction and osteoarthritic changes. There is preliminary evidence, in fact, that some of the NSAIDs may actually impair cartilage formation by inhibiting the synthesis of proteoglycans and other key cartilaginous components (see Chap. 15).[8,25,34,56,58,95] At the present time, however, acetaminophen and NSAIDs remain the cornerstone of the pharmacologic treatment of joint pain in osteoarthritis.

Viscosupplementation

Viscosupplementation is a clinical procedure that is being used increasingly in the treatment of osteoarthritis. This technique uses a substance known as hyaluronan to restore the lubricating properties of synovial fluid in osteoarthritic joints.[72,96] Hyaluronan is a polysaccharide that can be injected into an arthritic joint to help restore the normal viscosity of the synovial fluid.[61] This treatment helps reduce joint stresses and thus limits the progression of articular destruction seen in osteoarthritis.[48] This technique can provide substantial benefits in 65 to 80 percent of the patients receiving treatment.[97]

When used to treat osteoarthritis, viscosupplementation typically consists of 2 to 10 weekly injections of hyaluronan. Patients often experience a decrease in pain within a few days after injection, and pain continues to diminish within the first few weeks after beginning treatment. Duration of relief is variable, but most patients who respond to viscosupplementation experience beneficial effects for 6 months to 1 year after a series of injections.[5,97]

Hence, viscosupplementation may actually attenuate the progressive changes in joint structure and function typically seen in osteoarthritis. This fact suggests that viscosupplementation may represent one of the first DMOADs available for treating osteoarthritic joints.[36] Future clinical studies will be needed to determine if viscosupplementation provides long-term benefits without excessive adverse effects in patients with osteoarthritis.

Glucosamine and Chondroitin Sulfate

It has been suggested that dietary supplements such as glucosamine and chondroitin sulfate may help protect articular cartilage and halt or reverse joint degeneration in osteoarthritis. These two compounds are key ingredients needed for the production of several components of articular cartilage and synovial fluid, including glycosaminoglycans, proteoglycans, and hyaluronic acid.[67,82] It seems reasonable that increased amounts of these ingredients should facilitate the repair of joint tissues, improve synovial fluid viscosity, and help restore joint function in conditions like osteoarthritis. Hence, several products containing glucosamine or glucosamine combined with chondroitin sulfate are currently available as nonprescription dietary supplements. These supplements typically contain oral daily dosages of 1500 mg glucosamine and 1200 mg chondroitin sulfate.[35]

The exact effects of dietary chondroitin and glucosamine, however, remain to be determined. Some poorly controlled clinical studies have suggested that these supplements may help decrease pain and increase joint mobility in people with osteoarthritis.[6,30] There is little evidence, however, that taking these dietary supplements has a direct beneficial effect on the structure and composition of articular cartilage and synovial fluid. It is also unrealistic to assume that oral supplements available without prescription will produce benefits similar to those seen when these compounds are administered in higher doses or by parenteral routes (intra-articularly, intramuscularly). Likewise, dietary supplements may not contain adequate amounts of these compounds, and some preparations may not even contain the dose that is claimed on the package.[35]

The idea of taking dietary supplements containing glucosamine, chondroitin, or similar substances therefore remains controversial. Although the rationale for taking these compounds is logical, more information is needed about the absorption, distribution, and ultimately the intra-articular changes associated with daily oral dosages available without prescription. There are likewise no long-term studies on the efficacy or potential side effects when these supplements are taken for extended periods. Nonetheless, these compounds are readily available to consumers, and people with osteoarthritis will probably continue to take these supplements even in the absence of definitive evidence of their efficacy.

SPECIAL CONCERNS FOR ANTIARTHRITIC DRUG THERAPY IN REHABILITATION PATIENTS

Drugs used to treat rheumatoid arthritis and osteoarthritis often play a vital role in permitting optimal rehabilitation of patients with joint disease. By decreasing pain and inflammation, these drugs help facilitate a more active and vigorous program of exercise and functional activity. Some drugs, such as the disease-modifying drugs used in rheumatoid arthritis and osteoarthritis, appear to be able to impair or even halt the progression of joint destruction. This may enable the therapist to help restore muscle strength and joint function rather than simply employ a program of maintenance therapy during a steady downward progression in patients with arthritis.

The influence of antiarthritic drugs on the rehabilitative process depends primarily on the type of drugs used. Beginning with the NSAIDs, there is little concern for adverse effects on physical therapy procedures. These drugs are relatively safe and are not usually associated with the type of side effects that will directly influence the physical therapy of patients with rheumatoid arthritis or osteoarthritis. If the glucocorticoids are used, the therapist must be aware of the many adverse side effects of these drugs. In particular, the catabolic effects of these agents on supporting tissues (muscle, tendon, bone, skin) must be considered. Range-of-motion and strengthening programs must be used judiciously to avoid fractures and soft-tissue injuries. Care must also be taken to prevent skin breakdown, especially when splints and other protective orthotic devices are employed.

The disease-modifying agents used in rheumatoid arthritis are each associated with a number of side effects that could influence rehabilitation. Some of these drugs, such as the gold compounds and methotrexate, may cause headache and nausea, which may be bothersome during the therapy session. Joint pain and swelling may also occur with drugs such as methotrexate and penicillamine, and these effects may also become a problem during rehabilitation. A variety of other side effects can occur, depending on the particular DMARD being used and the sensitivity of the individual patient. Therapists should be aware of any change in patient response, not only when a new drug is being started but also during the prolonged use of DMARDs.

Finally, the use of DMOADs (viscosupplementation, glucosamine, chondroitin) to restore joint function in osteoarthritis is fairly new, and it is not yet clear if these techniques will have any side effects that will have a direct impact on physical rehabilitation. Likewise, it remains to be seen if there are any rehabilitation techniques (exercise, physical agents) that could enhance the effectiveness of DMOADs. It is hoped that these techniques will work synergistically with physical therapy to improve function in patients with osteoarthritic joints.

CASE STUDY

RHEUMATOID ARTHRITIS

Brief History. A.T., a 75-year-old woman, was diagnosed several years ago with rheumatoid joint disease. Currently she is being seen three times each week in physical therapy as an outpatient for a program of paraffin and active exercise to her wrists and hands. Resting splints were also fabricated for both hands, and these are worn at night to prevent joint deformity. The patient was also instructed in a home exercise program to maintain joint mobility in both upper extremities. Pharmacologic management in this patient originally consisted of NSAIDs, beginning with aspirin and later switching to ibuprofen. Six months ago, she was also placed on auranofin (Ridaura), which was instituted in an attempt to halt the progressive arthritic changes. This orally administered gold compound was given at a dosage of 3 mg twice each day.

Problem/Influence of Medication. The combination of an NSAID and a disease-modifying drug, along with the physical therapy program, seemed to be helping to decrease the patient's pain and joint stiffness. However, she began to develop skin rashes and itching on her arms and legs. The therapist noticed this while preparing the patient for her paraffin treatment. It seemed that these rashes might be occurring as a side effect of the auranofin. The therapist brought this to the attention of the physician, who concurred that this was probably a side effect of the gold therapy.

Decision/Solution. The patient was temporarily removed from auranofin therapy to see if this skin reaction would subside. In the interim, the therapist discontinued paraffin so that the rashes and itching on the distal forearm would not be exacerbated. To continue to provide gentle heat, a warm whirlpool (100°F) was substituted for the paraffin bath. Also, the night splints were temporarily discontinued to prevent irritation to the affected areas. After 2 weeks, the skin rashes had virtually disappeared, and the original physical therapy program was resumed. After another week, the physician restarted auranofin administration. No other adverse effects were noted, and the patient continued to notice improvements in her arthritic condition.

SUMMARY

Rheumatoid arthritis and osteoarthritis represent two distinct forms of joint disease that can produce devastating effects on the structure and function of synovial joints. Fortunately, management of these conditions has improved substantially through advancements in drug therapy. Rheumatoid arthritis can be treated pharmacologically with NSAIDs, glucocorticoids, and various DMARDs. NSAIDs, including aspirin, represent the primary form of drug therapy in the early stages of this disease, and these drugs are often used in conjunction with other drugs as the arthritic condition increases in severity. Glucocorticoids are often effective in decreasing the joint inflammation typically found in rheumatoid arthritis, but long-term use of these agents is limited because of their many toxic effects. Disease-modifying drugs can slow or halt the progressive nature of rheumatoid arthritis by suppressing the immune response inherent in this disease. Although there is some concern about the efficacy and safety of these drugs, DMARDs have been a welcome addition to the rather limited arsenal of drugs used to treat rheumatoid arthritis.

Drug treatment of osteoarthritis differs somewhat from that of rheumatoid arthritis, with management of pain by using NSAIDs and acetaminophen constituting the major form of drug therapy. A newer technique known as viscosupplementation has also been used to help restore the lubricating properties of the synovial fluid in osteoarthritic joints. It remains to be seen, however, if this technique will become widely accepted as a safe and effective treatment for osteoarthritis. In any event, drug therapy along with nonpharmacologic measures such as physical therapy can provide an effective way of dealing with the potentially devastating effects of rheumatoid arthritis and osteoarthritis.

REFERENCES

1. Aaseth, J, Haugen, M, and Forre, O: Rheumatoid arthritis and metal compounds: Perspectives on the role of oxygen radical detoxification. Analyst 123:3, 1998.
2. Agambar, L and Flower, R: Anti-inflammatory drugs. Physiotherapy 76:198, 1990.
3. Alarcon, GS, et al: Radiographic evidence of disease progression in methotrexate treated and non-methotrexate disease modifying antirheumatic drug treated rheumatoid arthritis patients: A meta-analysis. J Rheumatol 19:1868, 1992.
4. Bagge, E and Brooks, P: Osteoarthritis in older patients. Optimum treatment. Drugs Aging 7:176, 1995.
5. Balazs, EA and Denlinger, JL: Viscosupplementation: A new concept in the treatment for osteoarthritis. J Rheumatol 20(Suppl 39):3, 1993.
6. Barclay, TS, Tsourounis, C, and McCart, GM: Glucosamine. Ann Pharmacother 32:574, 1998.
7. Barnes, PJ: Anti-inflammatory actions of glucocorticoids: Molecular mechanisms. Clin Sci (Colch) 94:557, 1998.
8. Bassleer, C, Henrotin, Y, and Franchimont, P: Effects of sodium naproxen on differentiated human chondrocytes cultivated in clusters. Clin Rheumatol 11:60, 1992.
9. Bird, HA: When are NSAIDs appropriate in osteoarthritis? Drugs Aging 12:87, 1998.
10. Bjorkman, DJ: The effect of aspirin and nonsteroidal anti-inflammatory drugs on prostaglandins. Am J Med 105(Suppl 1B):8S, 1998.
11. Blackburn, WD: Management of osteoarthritis and rheumatoid arthritis: Prospects and possibilities. Am J Med 100(Suppl 2A):24S, 1996.
12. Boh, LE: Osteoarthritis. In DiPiro, JT, et al (eds): Pharmacotherapy: A Pathophysiologic Approach. Appleton & Lange, Stamford, CT, 1999.
13. Bomalaski, JS and Clark, MA: Review: Phospholipase A_2 and arthritis. Arthritis Rheum 36:190, 1993.
14. Bradley, JD, et al: Treatment of knee osteoarthritis: Relationship of clinical features of joint inflammation to the response to a nonsteroidal antiinflammatory drug or pure analgesic. J Rheumatol 19:1950, 1992.
15. Brady, SJ, et al: Pharmacotherapy and osteoarthritis. Baillieres Clin Rheumatol 11:749, 1997.
16. Brooks, PM: The use of suppressive agents for the treatment of rheumatoid arthritis. Aust N Z J Med 23:193, 1993.
17. Brooks, PM and Day, RO: Drug therapy: Nonsteroidal anti-inflammatory drugs—differences and similarities. N Engl J Med 324:1716, 1991.
18. Brooks, PM and Schwarzer, AC: Combination chemotherapy in rheumatoid arthritis. Ann Rheum Dis 50:507, 1991.
19. Buchbinder, R, et al: Methotrexate therapy in rheumatoid arthritis: A life table review of 587 patients treated in community practice. J Rheumatol 20:639, 1993.
20. Byrne, J: Rheumatology. Part 2: The role of medication. Prof Nurse 14:353, 1999.
21. Calabrese, LH: Rheumatoid arthritis and primary care: the case for early diagnosis and treatment. J Am Osteopath Assoc 99:313, 1999.
22. Caldwell, JR and Furst, DE: The efficacy and safety of low-dose corticosteroids for rheumatoid arthritis. Semin Arthritis Rheum 21:1, 1991.

23. Cannon, GW: Methotrexate pulmonary toxicity. Rheum Dis Clin North Am 23:917, 1997.
24. Chaffman, M, et al: Auranofin: A preliminary review of its pharmacologic properties and therapeutic use in rheumatoid arthritis. Drugs 27:378, 1984.
25. Collier, S and Ghosh, P: Comparison of the effects of NSAIDs on proteoglycan synthesis by articular cartilage explant and chondrocyte monolayer cultures. Biochem Pharmacol 41:1375, 1991.
26. Creamer, P, Flores, R, and Hochberg, MC: Management of osteoarthritis in older adults. Clin Geriatr Med 14:435, 1998.
27. Cronstein, BN: The mechanism of action of methotrexate. Rheum Dis Clin North Am 23:739, 1997.
28. Crooke, ST and Mirabelli, CK: Molecular mechanisms of action of auranofin and other gold complexes as related to their biological activities. Am J Med 75(Suppl 6A):109, 1983.
29. Cush, JJ, et al: US consensus guidelines for the use of cyclosporine A in rheumatoid arthritis. J Rheumatol 26:1176, 1999.
30. Da Camara, CC and Dowless, GV: Glucosamine sulfate for osteoarthritis. Ann Pharmacother 32:580, 1998.
31. Damjanov, I: Pathology for the Health-Related Professions. WB Saunders, Philadelphia, 1996.
32. Danning, CL and Boumpas, DT: Commonly used disease-modifying antirheumatic drugs in the treatment of inflammatory arthritis: An update on mechanisms of action. Clin Exp Rheumatol 16:595, 1998.
33. Darlington, LG and Ramsey, NW: Review of dietary therapy for rheumatoid arthritis. Br J Rheumatol 32:507, 1993.
34. David, MJ, et al: Effects of NSAIDs on glycosyltransferase activity from human osteoarthritic cartilage. Br J Rheumatol 31(Suppl 1):13, 1992.
35. Deal, CL and Moskowitz, RW: Neutraceuticals as therapeutic agents in osteoarthritis. The role of glucosamine, chondroitin sulfate, and collagen hydrolysate. Rheum Dis Clin North Am 25:379, 1999.
36. Dieppe, P: Drug treatment of osteoarthritis. J Bone Joint Surg Br 75:673, 1993.
37. Dinarello, CA and Wolff, SM: The role of interleukin-1 in disease. N Engl J Med 328:106, 1993.
38. Dooley, MA, et al: The effects of nonsteroidal drug therapy in early rheumatoid arthritis on serum levels of soluble interleukin-2 receptor, CD4, and CD8. J Rheumatol 20:1857, 1993.
39. Fathman, CG: What a rheumatologist needs to know about T cell receptor structure and function. J Rheumatol 19(Suppl 32):12, 1992.
40. Felson, DT, et al: Obesity and knee osteoarthritis. Ann Intern Med 109:18, 1988.
41. Fox, RI: Mechanism of action of leflunomide in rheumatoid arthritis. J Rheumatol Suppl 53:20, 1998.
42. Fox, RI: Mechanism of action of hydroxychloroquine as an antirheumatic drug. Semin Arthritis Rheum 23(Suppl 1):82, 1993.
43. Frazier, MS, Drzymkowski, JA, and Doty, SJ: Essentials of Human Diseases and Conditions. WB Saunders, Philadelphia, 1996.
44. Fries, JF, et al: The relative toxicity of alternate therapies for rheumatoid arthritis: Implications for the therapeutic progression. Semin Arthritis Rheum 23(Suppl 1):68, 1993.
45. Fung, HB and Kirschenbaum, HL: Selective cyclooxygenase-2 inhibitors for the treatment of arthritis. Clin Ther 21:1131, 1999.
46. Furst, DE: The rationale use of methotrexate in rheumatoid arthritis and other rheumatic diseases. Br J Rheumatol 36:1196, 1997.
47. Furst, DE and Kremer, JM: Methotrexate in rheumatoid arthritis. Arthritis Rheum 31:305, 1988.
48. Ghosh, P, et al: The effects of intraarticular administration of hyaluronan in a model of early osteoarthritis in sheep. II. Cartilage composition and proteoglycan metabolism. Semin Arthritis Rheum 22(Suppl 1):31, 1993.
49. Giannini, EH, et al: Comparative safety and efficacy of advanced drug therapy in children with juvenile rheumatoid arthritis. Semin Arthritis Rheum 23:34, 1993.
50. Golden, BD and Abramson, SB: Selective cyclooxygenase-2 inhibitors. Rheum Dis Clin North Am 25:359, 1999.
51. Goldenberg, MM: Etanercept, a novel drug for the treatment of patients with severe, active rheumatoid arthritis. Clin Ther 21:75, 1999.
52. Hakala, M, et al: Association of different HLA antigens with various toxic effects of gold salts in rheumatoid arthritis. Ann Rheum Dis 45:177, 1986.
53. Hansen, M: Pathophysiology: Foundations of Disease and Clinical Intervention. WB Saunders, Philadelphia, 1998.
54. Harris, ED: Mechanisms of disease: Rheumatoid arthritis: Pathophysiology and implications for therapy. N Engl J Med 322:1277, 1990.
55. Harth, M: Mechanisms of action of disease modifying antirheumatic drugs. J Rheumatol 19(Suppl 32):100, 1993.
56. Henrotin, Y, Bassleer, C, and Franchimont, P: In vitro effects of etodolac and acetylsalicylic acid on human chondrocyte metabolism. Agents Actions 36:317, 1992.
57. Hillson, JL and Furst, DE: Pharmacology and pharmacokinetics of methotrexate in rheumatic disease. Practical issues in treatment and design. Rheum Dis Clin North Am 23:757, 1997.
58. Hugenberg, ST, Brandt, KD, and Cole, CA: Effect of sodium salicylate, aspirin, and ibuprofen on enzymes required by the chondrocyte for synthesis of chondroitin sulfate. J Rheumatol 20:2128, 1993.
59. Insel, PA: Analgesic-antipyretic and antiinflammatory agents and drugs employed in the treatment of gout. In Hardman, JG, et al (eds): The Pharmacologic Basis of Therapeutics, ed 9. McGraw-Hill, New York, 1996.

60. Irvine, S, Munro, R, and Porter, D: Early referral, diagnosis, and treatment of rheumatoid arthritis: Evidence for changing medical practice. Ann Rheum Dis 58:510, 1999.
61. Iwata, H: Pharmacologic and clinical aspects of intraarticular injection of hyaluronate. Clin Orthop 289:285, 1993.
62. Jackson, CG and Williams, HJ: Disease-modifying antirheumatic drugs. Using their clinical pharmacological effects as a guide to their selection. Drugs 56:337, 1998.
63. Jaffe, IA: New approaches to the management of rheumatoid arthritis. J Rheumatol 19(Suppl 36):2, 1992.
64. Jarvis, B and Faulds, D: Etanercept: A review of its use in rheumatoid arthritis. Drugs 57:945, 1999.
65. Jones, RE and Moreland, LW: Tumor necrosis factor inhibitors for rheumatoid arthritis. Bull Rheum Dis 48:1, 1999.
66. Katzung, BG and Furst, DE: Nonsteroidal anti-inflammatory drugs; disease-modifying antirheumatic drugs; nonopioid analgesics; drugs used in gout. In Katzung, BG (ed): Basic and Clinical Pharmacology, ed 7. Appleton & Lange, Stamford, CT, 1998.
67. Kelly, GS: The role of glucosamine sulfate and chondroitin sulfates in the treatment of degenerative joint disease. Altern Med Rev 3:27, 1998.
68. Kremer, JM: Methotrexate and leflunomide: Biochemical basis for combination therapy in the treatment of rheumatoid arthritis. Semin Arthritis Rheum 29:14, 1999.
69. Kremer, JM: Methotrexate and emerging therapies. Rheum Dis Clin North Am 24:651, 1998.
70. Kremer, JM: Long-term methotrexate therapy in rheumatoid arthritis: A review. J Rheumatol 12(Suppl 12):25, 1985.
71. Laan, RF, Jansen, TL, and van Riel, PL: Glucocorticosteroids in the management of rheumatoid arthritis. Rheumatology 38:6, 1999.
72. Lane, NE and Thompson, JM: Management of osteoarthritis in the primary-care setting: An evidence-based approach to treatment. Am J Med 103(Suppl 6A):25S, 1997.
73. Lefkowith, JB: Cyclooxygenase-2 specificity and its clinical implications. Am J Med 106(Suppl 5B):43S, 1999.
74. Leventhal, LJ, Boyce, EG, and Zurier, RB: Treatment of rheumatoid arthritis with gammalinolenic acid. Ann Intern Med 119:867, 1993.
75. Lewis, RA, Austen, KF, and Soberman, RJ: Mechanisms of disease: Leukotrienes and other products of the 5-lipoxygenase pathway—biochemistry and relation to pathophysiology in human diseases. N Engl J Med 323:645, 1990.
76. Li, E, Brooks, P, and Conaghan, PG: Disease-modifying antirheumatic drugs. Curr Opin Rheumatol 10:159, 1998.
77. Lipsky, LP, et al: The classification of cyclooxygenase inhibitors. J Rheumatol 25:2298, 1998.
78. Lorenz, HM and Kalden, JR: Biologic agents in the treatment of inflammatory rheumatic diseases. Curr Opin Rheumatol 11:179, 1999.
79. Mackenzie, AH: Antimalarial drugs for rheumatoid arthritis. Am J Med 75(Suppl 6A):49, 1983.
80. Mackenzie, AH: Dose refinements in long-term therapy of rheumatoid arthritis with antimalarials. Am J Med 75(Suppl 1A):40, 1983.
81. Markenson, JA: Worldwide trends in the socioeconomic impact and long-term prognosis of rheumatoid arthritis. Semin Arthritis Rheum 21(Suppl 1):4, 1991.
82. McCarty, MF: Enhanced synovial production of hyaluronic acid may explain rapid clinical response to high-dose glucosamine in osteoarthritis. Med Hypotheses 50:507, 1998.
83. McDuffie, FC: Morbidity impact of rheumatoid arthritis on society. Am J Med 78(Suppl 1A):1, 1985.
84. McGuire, JL and Ridgway, WM: Aggressive drug therapy for rheumatoid arthritis. Hosp Pract 28:45, 1993.
85. McKendry, RJR and Dale, P: Adverse effects of low-dose methotrexate therapy in rheumatoid arthritis. J Rheumatol 20:1850, 1993.
86. Miller, ML: Clinical aspects of juvenile rheumatoid arthritis. Curr Opin Rheumatol 9:423, 1997.
87. Moncur, C and Williams, HJ: Rheumatoid arthritis: Status of drug therapies. Phys Ther 75:511, 1995.
88. Morand, EF: Corticosteroids in the treatment of rheumatologic diseases. Curr Opin Rheumatol 10:179, 1998.
89. Moreland, LW: Inhibitors of tumor necrosis factor for rheumatoid arthritis. J Rheumatol 26(Suppl 57):7, 1999.
90. Moreland, LW: Soluble tumor necrosis factor receptor (p75) fusion protein (ENBREL) as a therapy for rheumatoid arthritis. Rheum Dis Clin North Am 24:579, 1998.
91. Munro, R and Capell, HA: Penicillamine. Br J Rheumatol 36:104, 1997.
92. O'Dell, JR: Triple therapy with methotrexate, sulfasalazine, and hydroxychloroquine in patients with rheumatoid arthritis. Rheum Dis Clin North Am 24:465, 1998.
93. Panayi, GS: The immunopathogenesis of rheumatoid arthritis. Br J Rheumatol 32(Suppl 1):4, 1993.
94. Passo, MH and Hashkes, PJ: Use of methotrexate in children. Bull Rheum Dis 47:1, 1998.
95. Pelletier, JP: The influence of tissue cross-talking on OA progression: Role of nonsteroidal antiiflammatory drugs. Osteoarthritis Cartilage 7:374, 1999.
96. Pelletier, J-P and Martel-Pelletier, J: The pathophysiology of osteoarthritis and the implications of the use of hyaluronan and hylan as therapeutic agents in viscosupplementation. J Rheumatol 20(Suppl 39):19, 1993.
97. Peyron, JG: Intraarticular hyaluronan injections in the treatment of osteoarthritis: State-of-the-art review. J Rheumatol 20(Suppl 39):10, 1993.

98. Pincus, T, et al: Long-term drug therapy for rheumatoid arthritis in seven rheumatology private practices. 1. Nonsteroidal anti-inflammatory drugs. J Rheumatol 19:1874, 1992.
99. Porter, DR and Sturrock, RD: Fortnightly review: Medical management of rheumatoid arthritis. BMJ 307:425, 1993.
100. Rozman, B: Clinical experience with leflunomide in rheumatoid arthritis. J Rheumatol Suppl 53:27, 1998.
101. Ryan, L and Brooks, P: Disease-modifying antirheumatic drugs. Curr Opin Rheumatol 11:161, 1999.
102. Rynes, RI: Ophthalmologic safety of long-term hydroxychloroquine treatment. Am J Med 75(Suppl 1A):35, 1983.
103. Saag, KG: Low-dose corticosteroid therapy in rheumatoid arthritis: Balancing the evidence. Am J Med 103(Suppl 6A):31S, 1997.
104. Salmeron, G and Lipsky, PE: Immunosuppressive potential of antimalarials. Am J Med 75(Suppl 1A):19, 1983.
105. Schiller, AL: Bones and joints. In Rubin, E and Farber, JL (eds): Pathology, ed 2. JB Lippincott, Philadelphia, 1994.
106. Schimmer, BP and Parker, KL: Adrenocorticotropic hormone: Adrenocortical steroids and their synthetic analogs: Inhibitors of the synthesis and actions of adrenocortical hormones. In Hardman, JG, et al (eds): The Pharmacological Basis of Therapeutics, ed 9. McGraw-Hill, New York, 1996.
107. Schnitzer, TJ: Non-NSAID pharmacologic treatment options for the management of chronic pain. Am J Med 105(Suppl 1B):45S, 1998.
108. Schuna, AA: Update on treatment of rheumatoid arthritis. J Am Pharm Assoc (Wash) 38:728, 1998.
109. Schuna, AA, Schmidt, MJ, and Walbrandt, D: Rheumatoid arthritis. In DiPiro, JT, et al (eds): Pharmacotherapy: A Pathophysiologic Approach. Appleton & Lange, Stamford, CT, 1999.
110. Scully, CJ, Anderson, CJ, and Cannon, GW: Long-term methotrexate therapy for rheumatoid arthritis. Semin Arthritis Rheum 20:317, 1991.
111. Seitz, M: Molecular and cellular effects of methotrexate. Curr Opin Rheumatol 11:226, 1999.
112. Singsen, BH and Goldbach-Mansky, R: Methotrexate in the treatment of juvenile rheumatoid arthritis and other pediatric rheumatoid and nonrheumatoid disorders. Rheum Dis Clin North Am 23:811, 1997.
113. Spencer-Green, G: Drug treatment of arthritis: Update on conventional and less conventional methods. Postgrad Med 93:129, 1993.
114. Stockman, A, et al: Genetic markers in rheumatoid arthritis: Relationship to toxicity from d-penicillamine. J Rheumatol 13:269, 1986.
115. Symposium (various authors): An international consensus report: The use of cyclosporin A in rheumatoid arthritis. Br J Rheumatol 32(Suppl 1):1, 1993.
116. Symposium (various authors): Combination therapy in the treatment of rheumatoid arthritis. Semin Arthritis Rheum 23(Suppl 1):1, 1993.
117. Tsokos, GC: Immunomodulatory treatment in patients with rheumatic diseases: Mechanisms of actions. Semin Arthritis Rheum 17:24, 1987.
118. Vane, JR and Botting, RM: Anti-inflammatory drugs and their mechanism of action. Inflamm Res 47(Suppl 2):S78, 1998.
119. Van Ede, AE, et al: Methotrexate in rheumatoid arthritis: An update with focus on mechanisms involved in toxicity. Semin Arthritis Rheum 27:277, 1998.
120. Verhoeven, AC, Boers, M, and Tugwell, P: Combination therapy in rheumatoid arthritis: Updated systematic review. Br J Rheumatol 37:612, 1998.
121. Walz, DT, et al: Biologic actions and pharmacokinetic studies of auranofin. Br J Med 75(Suppl 6A):90, 1983.
122. Ward, DJ and Tidswell, ME: Rheumatoid arthritis and juvenile chronic arthritis. In Downie, PA (ed): Cash's Textbook of Orthopaedics and Rheumatology for Physiotherapists. JB Lippincott, Philadelphia, 1984.
123. Weinblatt, ME, et al: The effects of drug therapy on radiographic progression of rheumatoid arthritis. Results of a 36-week randomized trial comparing methotrexate and auranofin. Arthritis Rheum 36:613, 1993.
124. Weinstein, A, et al: Low-dose methotrexate treatment of rheumatoid arthritis: Long-term observations. Am J Med 79:331, 1985.
125. Wernick, R, et al: IgG and IgM rheumatoid factors in rheumatoid arthritis. Arthritis Rheum 26:593, 1983.
126. West, SG: Methotrexate hepatotoxicity. Rheum Dis Clin North Am 23:883, 1997.
127. Wilkinson, SM, et al: Suspected cutaneous drug toxicity in rheumatoid arthritis: An evaluation. Br J Rheumatol 32:798, 1993.
128. Willkens, RF: The selection of a nonsteroidal antiinflammatory drug: Is there a difference? J Rheumatol 19(Suppl 36):9, 1992.

CHAPTER 17

Patient-Controlled Analgesia

Patient-controlled analgesia (PCA) was first introduced into clinical practice in the early 1980s as an alternative way to administer analgesic medications. The basic principle behind PCA is that the patient can self-administer small doses of the drug (usually an opioid) at relatively frequent intervals to provide optimal pain relief.[27] These small doses are typically delivered intravenously or into the spinal canal by some type of machine (pump) that is controlled by the patient. Patient-controlled analgesia has several apparent advantages over more traditional dosing regimens. In particular, PCA systems often provide equivalent or increased analgesic effects with the use of less drug and a lower incidence of side effects.[14,22] This fact has generated a great deal of interest and increased use of PCA in a variety of clinical situations. For instance, PCA systems have been used to help manage acute pain following surgery, and PCAs have also been used to treat pain in patients with cancer and other conditions associated with chronic pain.[22,27,31]

Hence, PCA continues to gain acceptance as an optimal method for treating pain. Because PCA is used extensively to treat acute and chronic pain, rehabilitation specialists should be aware of some of the fundamental principles governing PCA. This chapter begins by discussing the basic concepts and strategies of PCA, followed by some of the practical aspects of PCA, including the types of analgesics used, the possible routes of administration, and the types of machines used to administer the drugs. An indication of why PCA is often clinically superior to more traditional methods of analgesia is then presented. Finally, potential problems associated with PCA and the specific ways that PCA can affect patients receiving physical therapy and occupational therapy are discussed. It is hoped that this will provide the reader with a better understanding of why PCA systems are often a preferred method of managing pain in contemporary practice.

PHARMACOKINETIC BASIS FOR PCA

To provide optimal management of pain, analgesic drugs should be delivered into the bloodstream or other target tissues (epidural space, intrathecal space) in a predictable and fairly constant manner. The goal is to maintain drug levels within a fairly well-defined range, or **therapeutic window.**[17,27] Such a therapeutic window for analgesia is represented schematically by the shaded area in Figure 17–1. If drug levels are below this

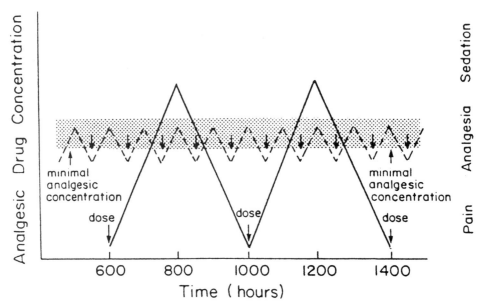

FIGURE 17–1. Pharmacokinetic model for PCA using opioid drugs. Conventional intramuscular injection is indicated by the long solid lines, PCA is indicated by the short dashed lines, and the therapeutic window for analgesia is indicated by the shaded area. (From Ferrante, et al,[17] pp 457–461, with permission.)

window, the analgesic is below the minimum analgesic concentration, and the patient is in pain. Drug levels above the window may produce adequate analgesia but may also produce side effects such as sedation. The traditional method of administering analgesics is to give relatively large doses with relatively large time intervals between each dosage. For instance, opioid analgesics are typically injected intramuscularly every 3 to 4 hours to manage severe pain, thus creating large fluctuations in the amount of drug present in the body. These large fluctuations are illustrated by the dark, solid lines in Figure 17–1. As illustrated in Figure 17–1, this traditional method of administration is associated with long periods of time when the drug concentration falls below the therapeutic window, allowing pain to occur, or above the therapeutic window, causing sedation.

Figure 17–1 also illustrates why PCA systems are better at maintaining drug levels within the therapeutic (analgesic) window. Systems using some form of PCA deliver small doses of the analgesic on a relatively frequent basis, as indicated by the dashed lines in Figure 17–1. Drug levels are maintained within the analgesic range; there are shorter periods of time when the drug concentration falls below the therapeutic window (i.e., below the shaded area), and there is virtually no time when side effects occur because the concentration rises above the therapeutic window. Hence, analgesia can be achieved more effectively with a reduced incidence of side effects.

PCA DOSING STRATEGIES AND PARAMETERS

The fact that PCA enables the patient to self-deliver small doses of the analgesic at frequent intervals illustrates the need for specific dosing parameters that control the amount and frequency of analgesic administration. Several terms are used to describe these parameters and indicate each parameter's role in safeguarding against excessive drug delivery.[16,27] The basic terms that describe PCA dosing strategies are indicated here.

Loading Dose

A single large dose is given initially to establish analgesia. This **loading dose** is used to bring levels of the analgesic to the therapeutic window illustrated by the shaded area in Figure 17–1.

Demand Dose

The amount of drug that is self-administered by the patient each time he or she activates the PCA delivery mechanism is known as the **demand dose.** The magnitude of these doses for some commonly used opioid analgesics are listed in Table 17–1.

Lockout Interval

The minimum amount of time allowed between each demand dose is called the **lockout interval.** After the patient self-administers a dose, the PCA delivery system will not deliver the next dose until the lockout interval has expired. Typical lockout intervals for commonly used opioids are listed in Table 17–1.

1- and 4-Hour Limits

Some PCA systems can be set to limit the total amount of drug given in a 1- or 4-hour period. The use of these parameters is somewhat questionable, however, because other parameters such as the demand dose and lockout interval automatically limit the total amount of drug that can be given in a specific period of time.

Background Infusion Rate

In some patients, a small amount of the analgesic is infused continuously to maintain a low, background level of analgesia. Demand doses are superimposed on the background infusion whenever the patient feels an increase in pain (e.g., the so-called breakthrough pain that may occur when the patient coughs or changes position). The use of background infusion basically combines the technique of continuous infusion with PCA, which may provide optimal analgesia with minimal side effects.[25,30,31]

Successful versus Total Demands

Successful demands occur when the patient activates the PCA delivery system and actually receives a demand dose of the drug. Demands made during the lockout interval would not be successful but would be added to the number of successful demands to indicate the total demands. A large number of unsuccessful demands may indicate

TABLE 17–1 Parameters for PCA Using Opioid Medications

Drug (Concentration)	Demand Dose	Lockout Interval (min)
Fentanyl (10 μg/mL)	10–20 μg	5–10
Hydromorphone (0.2 mg/mL)	0.05–0.25 mg	5–10
Meperidine (10 mg/mL)	5–30 mg	5–12
Methadone (1 mg/mL)	0.5–2.5 mg	8–20
Morphine (1 mg/mL)	0.5–3.0 mg	5–12
Nalbuphine (1 mg/mL)	1–5 mg	5–10
Oxymorphone (0.25 mg/mL)	0.2–0.4 mg	8–10

Source: Ferrante,[16] p 292, with permission.

that the PCA parameters are not effective in providing adequate analgesia. Most PCA systems therefore record the number of total demands so that the demand dose can be adjusted if a large number of unsuccessful demands are being made.

TYPES OF ANALGESICS USED FOR PCA

Opioid analgesics (see Chap. 14) are the primary medications used during PCA.[16] Opioids such as morphine, meperidine, and fentanyl are powerful analgesics that act primarily on the spinal cord and brain to inhibit the transmission and perception of nociceptive impulses. Opioids must be used cautiously because these drugs can cause serious side effects and because the potential for overdose with opioids is fairly high. As explained earlier, PCA often provides a safer and more effective way to administer these powerful drugs by preventing large fluctuations in plasma opioid levels.

Local anesthetics such as bupivacaine have also been used during PCA (see Chap. 12). These drugs, which block transmission along afferent sensory neurons, can be administered epidurally to block sensation at the spinal cord level. Local anesthetics have been used as the single anesthetic agent when PCA is used during labor and childbirth.[18,19] These drugs have also been mixed with opioids to provide optimal PCA during labor or following surgery.[11,21,23,29] Hence, local anesthetics serve as an alternative or adjunct to opioids during PCA.

ADMINISTRATION ROUTES DURING PCA

Intravenous PCA

Perhaps the simplest and most common method of PCA administration is through the peripheral IV route. When PCA will be needed for a fairly short period of time (e.g., for the first few days after surgery), typically a needle is inserted into a peripheral vein and then is connected to a catheter or IV line. Small intermittent doses of the analgesic can then be administered through the catheter and delivered directly into the systemic circulation.

When IV PCA will be needed for longer periods, a catheter can be implanted surgically in a large central vein with the tip of the catheter advanced to the right atrium of the heart. The catheter is then tunneled through subcutaneous tissues and brought out through the patient's skin to allow administration of PCA. Alternatively, the catheter can be connected to a small container known as an *access port* that is implanted subcutaneously within the patient's body (Fig. 17–2). This type of catheter-port system is used to provide a method of IV drug delivery that is located primarily within the patient's body. Injections can be made through the skin and into the port through a self-sealing silicone rubber septum located on the port. When these ports are used during PCA, the external PCA source is connected to the port via a special (Huber) needle that is inserted through the skin and into the port (see Fig. 17–2). The analgesic drug is then given from the PCA pump through a catheter into the port and ultimately into the systemic circulation. This provides an effective way of getting small, frequent doses of the drug into the bloodstream with less risk of infection or displacement of the intravenous catheter. This type of PCA-port delivery also enables the patient to be disconnected from the PCA delivery system for short periods of time by removing the needle from the port. This allows the patient to bathe or get dressed without risking damage to the indwelling port-IV system.[6]

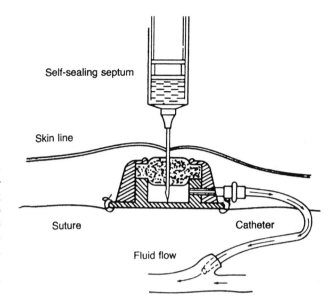

FIGURE 17–2. Schematic representation of an implantable vascular access port that can be used with PCA. The port can be connected to a PCA pump via a percutaneous needle, and a catheter leads from the port to a large central vein. (From Knox, LS: Implantable venous access devices. Crit Care Nurse 7:71, 1987, with permission.)

Epidural and Intrathecal PCA

PCA can also be achieved by administering drugs directly into the spaces surrounding the spinal cord.[29] This is typically done by inserting a small catheter so that the tip of the catheter lies in either the epidural space or the subarachnoid space at a specific level of the spinal cord (Fig. 17–3). Delivery of the drug into the subarachnoid space is usually referred to as **intrathecal administration** because the catheter is placed within the sheath of membranes that surrounds the spinal cord (intrathecal means "within a sheath"; see Chap. 2). If this type of PCA is intended for fairly short-term use, the catheter can be externalized through the skin on the midline of the patient's back and held in place by surgical tape. For longer-term use, the catheter is often tunneled through the subcutaneous tissues in the patient's abdominal wall, after which the catheter can either be brought out through the skin on the patient's side (see Fig. 17–3) or connected to some type of implanted access port or drug reservoir. In either case, PCA is then achieved by delivering the drug through the catheter and into the area directly surrounding the spinal cord.

Administration of drugs into the epidural or intrathecal space is obviously more difficult than simple intravenous delivery using a peripheral vein. Spinal delivery does, however, offer advantages in terms of providing effective analgesia with less drug. For instance, it is estimated that epidural morphine is 5 to 10 times more potent than IV morphine, indicating that much more drug must be administered by the IV route to achieve adequate analgesia.[6] Likewise, a study involving women who had undergone caesarean delivery showed that the amount of opioid (hydromorphone) required to provide analgesia during the first and second postoperative day was three to four times higher when administered via the IV route as compared with the epidural route.[28] In addition, intrathecal administration often requires even less drug than with the epidural route because the analgesic is being delivered within the spinal membranes and into the CSF. Analgesic requirements can be as much as 10 times lower when hydrophilic drugs like morphine are administered intrathecally versus epidurally because these drugs do not pass easily through the dura mater.[6]

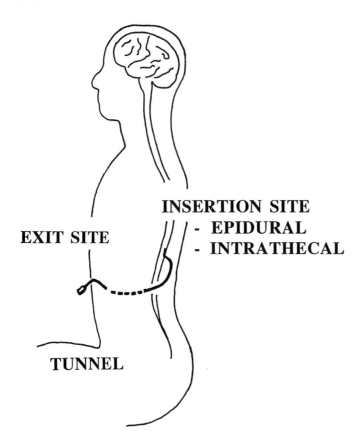

INSERTION SITE
- **EPIDURAL**
- **INTRATHECAL**

EXIT SITE

TUNNEL

FIGURE 17–3. Schematic illustration of PCA spinal delivery. The catheter delivers the analgesic into either the epidural or intrathecal (subarachnoid) space. Catheters for long-term use are tunneled under the skin *(dashed line)* and can exit on the anterior-lateral flank for connection to the PCA pump.

Hence, the route of administration used during PCA can have dramatic effects on the amount of drug needed to provide adequate analgesia. Therefore, selection of the desired route will depend on several factors, including how long PCA will be required and whether the more complex methods (i.e., spinal delivery, surgically implanted catheters and ports) will offer substantial benefits over simpler techniques that use a peripheral IV route.

PCA Pumps

The increase in popularity and use of PCA has been largely because of the development of infusion devices that can administer the analgesic in a safe and accurate manner. These devices, or *pumps,* vary in technologic sophistication and cost, but they all share some common features.[33] These features are summarized in Table 17–2. PCA pumps essentially allow the practitioner to set specific parameters of drug delivery (demand dose, lockout interval, etc.). The pump must then provide features to safeguard the patient against pump malfunction and warn the patient or caregiver if drug delivery is interrupted.

Pumps used for PCA fall into two basic categories: external and internal (implantable) pumps.[33] The most basic type of external pump is a simple syringe driver (Fig. 17–4). A syringe containing the medication is placed in a viselike machine that advances the syringe a small amount when the patient activates the pump. A second type of pump uses some

TABLE 17–2 Basic Features of Some Common PCA Pumps

Feature	Abbott PMP	Bard Ambulatory PCA Infuser	Pharmacia/Deltec Infuser
Size	6.75 9× 4.0 × 23	4.75 × 3.4 × 1.2 (100-mL container) 4.75 × 3.4 × 2.75 (250-mL container)	1.1 × 3.5 × 6.3 (50-mL cassette) 1.1 × 3.5 × 7.8 (100-mL cassette)
Power source	Wall plug in AC 2 × 9 alkaline battery; attachable battery pack	Lithium 3 × 3 V battery	Alkaline 9 V
Drive mechanism	Rotary peristaltic	Linear peristaltic	Linear peristaltic
Bolus dose	0.1–25 mL (or mg/hr)	0.1–20 mL (or mg/hr)	0.1–6 mL (or mg/ml)
Reservoir	0.1–1000 mL (or mg or μg)	Maximum of 240 mL	50–100 mL
Lockout	5–99 min	3 min–10 hr	5–999 min
Hourly limit	Maximum 25 mL	1–30 mL	0–6 mL

Source: Adapted from Shaw,[33] p 3422, with permission.

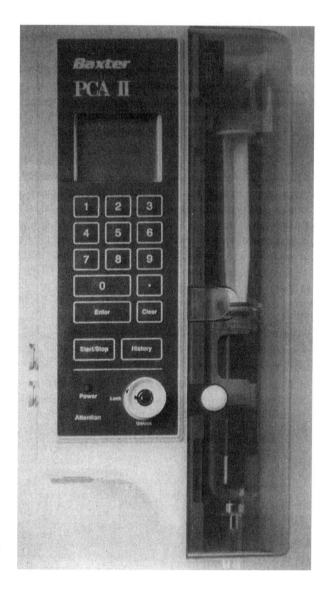

FIGURE 17–4. An example of a syringe driver pump that is commonly used with PCA.

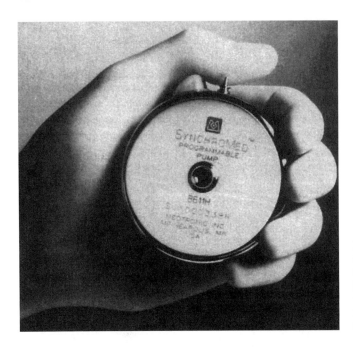

FIGURE 17–5. An example of an implantable, electronically controlled PCA pump. This pump is implanted surgically in the patient's abdomen and can be refilled periodically through a self-sealing septum.

sort of peristaltic action that sequentially compresses a piece of tubing to milk the medication through the tubing toward the patient. A third type of pump known as a cassette system works by drawing the medication into a fluid container within the pump and then expelling the selected amount of medication out of the chamber into tubing that leads to the patient. In most cases, these external pumps are activated when the patient pushes a button located on the end of a pendant that is connected to the pump (see Fig. 17–4).

Internal, or implantable, pumps are placed surgically beneath the patient's skin and connected to a catheter that leads to the patient's bloodstream or perispinal spaces (epidural or intrathecal). This basically creates a closed system within the patient's body. These pumps typically contain a reservoir that is filled with the medication. The reservoir can be refilled by inserting a Huber needle through the skin and into the pump via a resealable septum located on the outside of the pump (Fig. 17–5). Some implantable pumps use a rotatory peristaltic mechanism to milk the medication out of the pump. Other pumps use a bellows system to compress a chamber within the pump, thus expelling a given quantity of the drug from the pump. Implantable pumps are often programmed through the skin with some sort of electronic control device.

The type of pump selected for a given patient depends primarily on which method (external or implantable) will best serve the patient's needs, as well as on other factors, including cost and availability of a given type of pump. Advances in pump technology will continue to improve the devices that are available, and future developments will undoubtedly provide devices that are even more efficient in providing PCA.

COMPARISON OF PCA TO TRADITIONAL METHODS OF ANALGESIC ADMINISTRATION

From the pharmacokinetic perspective discussed previously, it is apparent that giving small, frequent doses of analgesic through PCA should be superior to administering large doses at infrequent intervals. Many clinical studies have attempted to verify this by comparing IV PCA using opioid drugs with traditional IM opioid injection. Although some studies have not shown any clear advantages or disadvantages of PCA,[10,17,26,32] most controlled trials indicate that PCA provided improved analgesia without an increase in side effects.[1,3,4,12,14,20,35,37,38] Several studies also reported that patients were more satisfied with the pain control provided by PCA versus traditional IM dosing, which seems to be related to the increased feeling of control over their pain offered to patients receiving PCA.[3,4,7,34,35] Some studies also suggested that patients receiving opioid PCA are generally able to ambulate sooner and tend to have shorter hospital stays than patients receiving opioids by the traditional IM route.[8,9,38] Other studies, however, failed to find a significant difference in factors such as length of stay[38] or ability to ambulate sooner.[5] The discrepancies in the results from specific studies are understandable, considering that these studies often differed in their research design and patient populations (various types of surgical procedures, and so forth). Nonetheless, the preponderance of evidence suggests that PCA systems afford some obvious advantages in certain patients over more traditional methods such as periodic IM injection.

One must then consider how PCA-like administration would compare with continuous infusion of an analgesic drug. As discussed in Chapter 14, it is sometimes feasible to administer opioid analgesics by slow, continuous infusion into the bloodstream or into some other area such as the epidural or intrathecal space. Continuous infusion would obviously provide the best way of maintaining drug concentration within a given therapeutic range. Studies have indeed shown that continuous infusion of opioids into the epidural space may produce somewhat better pain relief than IV PCA.[2,23,36] This is understandable considering that epidural delivery places the drug much closer to the spinal cord than does IV delivery. It would be more helpful to compare continuous epidural infusion with analogous PCA delivery into the epidural space. Studies that have made the comparison of continuous epidural infusion with epidural PCA have failed to show any clear advantage of continuous infusion.[19,21,24] In fact, continuous epidural infusion was often associated with the need for more drug than epidural PCA to provide an equivalent level of analgesia.[6,19,24] Hence, epidural PCA seems to be superior to continuous delivery of analgesics into the epidural space.

Thus, PCA has been shown to have certain advantages over more traditional methods such as intermittent IM injection or continuous epidural infusion. One must also consider that PCA decreases the need for other health professionals (physicians, nurses, pharmacists) to be directly involved in administering analgesics or adjusting the rate of analgesic delivery. IM injection, for instance, requires that the nurse be available at the proper time to inject the proper amount of the correct drug into the correct patient. This clearly takes the locus of control out of the patient's hands and makes the patient feel more dependent on an outside person to provide pain relief. When PCA systems are used appropriately, pain control is literally in the patient's hands. Likewise, continuous infusion often requires frequent adjustments by a qualified person who must attempt to match the dose of analgesic to the patient's pain level. This is especially difficult if pain levels are changing, such as in the patient recovering from surgery. With PCA, the patient is able to automatically titrate the amount of analgesia according to his or her pain. Again, this underscores a key advantage of PCA: this technique is superior to more traditional methods of analgesia because the person most qualified to judge his or her pain is empowered to self-administer the analgesic according to his or her own needs.

PROBLEMS AND SIDE EFFECTS OF PCA

Pharmacologic Side Effects

Side effects typically seen when opioids are used for PCA include sedation, pruritus, and gastrointestinal problems (nausea, vomiting). The incidence of these side effects, however, is not significantly increased during PCA versus more traditional methods of opioid administration such as intermittent intramuscular dosing.[3,41] Respiratory depression is another common side effect of opioid use, but again, there is no increased incidence of this problem when opioids are given via PCA.[3,15] In fact, the risk of respiratory depression is believed to be negligible when opioids are administered through spinal routes (epidural and intrathecal).[6] Hence, there does not seem to be an increase in the side effects commonly seen when PCA techniques are used to administer opioids, and the side effects commonly associated with these drugs may even be reduced during certain types of PCA application.

The incidence of side effects during PCA with local anesthetics is not well defined. Local anesthetics could conceivably cause sensory loss and motor weakness below the level of spinal administration. The possibility of these effects is directly dependent on the dose and site of administration, with the likelihood greater when higher doses of local anesthetic are administered into the subarachnoid space.[40] Also, administration of local anesthetics with a vasoconstrictor (epinephrine) has been shown to cause excessive inhibition of motor function (dense motor block) because the anesthetic is not dispersed as easily by the local circulation.[21] Hence, transient sensory and motor loss must always be considered as a potential side effect when local anesthetics are used during PCA.

Problems with PCA Delivery

Other problems that can occur with PCA systems include errors on the part of the operator (nurse, physician, etc.) or the patient and mechanical problems with the pump-delivery system.[39] These problems are summarized in Table 17–3. Operator errors typically occur because the pump is not programmed correctly or some other error occurs in loading the analgesic into the pump.[13] Errors on the part of the patient can occur if the patient is not properly educated in PCA use or if the patient lacks adequate cognitive skills to use the PCA correctly. Problems can likewise occur if the patient intentionally tries to administer more drug than is necessary to adequately control pain; that is, the

TABLE 17–3 Summary of Problems That Can Occur during PCA Therapy

Operator Errors	Patient Errors	Mechanical Problems
Misprogramming PCA device	Failure to understand PCA therapy	Failure to deliver on demand
Failure to clamp or unclamp tubing	Misunderstanding PCA pump device	Cracked drug vials or syringes
Improperly loading syringe or cartridge	Intentional analgesic abuse	Defective one-way valve at Y connector
Inability to respond to safety alarms		Faulty alarm system
Misplacing PCA pump key		Malfunctions (e.g., lock)

Source: White,[39] p 81, with permission.

patient attempts to use the PCA as a form of drug abuse. Although the safeguards provided by the device (small demand dose, appropriate lockout interval) should prevent addiction, these PCA systems are not usually as successful in controlling pain in people with a history of opioid addiction because of the potential for abuse and misuse. Finally, mechanical problems, including pump malfunction and clogging or displacement of the delivery tubing, may preclude delivery of the analgesic. Members of the health-care team should be alert for signs that the drug is being overdelivered during PCA, as evidenced by an increase in analgesic side effects, or that the analgesic is being underdelivered, as indicated by inadequate pain control.

SPECIAL CONCERNS FOR PCA IN REHABILITATION PATIENTS

When used appropriately, PCA offers several advantages to patients receiving physical therapy and occupational therapy. As discussed previously, PCA often provides analgesia with a lower chance of certain side effects such as sedation. Patients will be more alert and have a clearer sensorium while still receiving optimal pain control. Likewise, PCA prevents large fluctuations in plasma analgesic concentration and helps maintain analgesic concentration within a more finite range (see Fig. 17–1). This decreases the need to schedule rehabilitation at the time when analgesic concentrations are at optimal levels because concentrations should always be within the appropriate range. Patients may also be more mobile using various PCA systems as compared with more traditional analgesic methods. The use of PCA may allow patients to begin ambulation sooner following surgery, and PCA systems can help decrease the need for the patient to be bed-bound for long periods because of severe pain or the side effects from high, intermittent doses of analgesics.[33,37] Rehabilitation specialists should therefore acknowledge the advantages of PCA and capitalize on these advantages whenever possible in patients receiving PCA.

Rehabilitation specialists should also be aware of potential problems that can occur in patients receiving PCA. In particular, by monitoring the patient's signs and symptoms, therapists can help detect problems in PCA delivery. Therapists should use visual analog scales or some other valid measurement tool to routinely assess pain in patients receiving PCA. Patients exhibiting inadequate pain management or an unexplained increase in pain may be using a PCA system that is underdelivering the analgesic drug. The medical and nursing staff should be notified so that the delivery problem can be identified and rectified. Conversely, signs of respiratory depression or excessive sedation may indicate that the patient is being overdosed by the PCA system. This can obviously be a life-threatening situation that requires immediate attention. Hence, it is the responsibility of all health-care workers including rehabilitation specialists to look for signs of PCA malfunction every time they interact with the patient.

CASE STUDY

PATIENT-CONTROLLED ANALGESIA

Brief History. S.G., a 61-year-old man, was being treated for severe osteoarthritis in the right knee. Following an unsuccessful course of conservative therapy, S.G. was admitted to the hospital for a total knee replacement. The surgery was performed successfully, and PCA was instituted for postoperative pain management. PCA consisted of an external syringe pump connected to an IV catheter. The analgesic used was meperidine at a concentration of 10 mg/mL. Parameters for PCA were set by the physician to allow a demand dose of 1 mL (10 mg) with a lockout interval of 10 minutes. An initial or loading dose of 10 mg was also provided at the conclusion of the surgery. Physical therapy was initiated at the patient's bedside on the afternoon following surgery. The therapist found the patient groggy from the surgery, but the patient was coherent and able to understand simple commands. Pain, as assessed by a visual analog scale (VAS), was rated in the 4- to 5-cm range of a 10-cm scale (10 cm being equivalent to "worst pain imaginable"). The patient was observed using his PCA during the therapy session, and he seemed to understand how to use this device properly.

Problem/Influence of Drug Therapy. When seen at the bedside on the day following surgery, the patient was in obvious discomfort. Pain was rated in the 8- to 9-cm range of the VAS. The patient stated that he had been using the PCA as instructed and that the device had been recording his successful attempts with an audible signal. Upon closer inspection, however, the therapist noticed that the syringe was not properly engaged in the pump mechanism. Hence, the syringe was not being propelled forward, and the demand dose was not being administered.

Decision/Solution. The PCA malfunction was brought to the attention of the nursing staff, and the problem was quickly rectified. The syringe containing the opioid had apparently been refilled earlier in the day and had not been installed properly into the pump's syringe driver. The patient was given an initial 10-mg infusion, and PCA was then resumed according to the original dosing parameters. The remainder of the patient's recovery was uneventful, and he was able to participate actively and enthusiastically in the rehabilitation sessions.

SUMMARY

PCA allows the patient to self-administer a small amount of analgesic medication on a relatively frequent basis. This technique has been used to administer drugs such as opioids and local anesthetics. PCA can often provide better pain control with smaller quantities of the drug and a lower incidence of side effects. The patient is allowed to self-administer a small dose of the drug by pressing a button that is connected to some type of pump. These PCA pumps vary in their cost, level of sophistication, and location (external versus surgically implanted), but all pumps are capable of being programmed to prevent the patient from exceeding certain dosing parameters. PCA systems continue to increase in popularity and are now used in a variety of clinical situations to manage acute and chronic pain. Rehabilitation specialists should be aware that PCA can provide improved pain control and enhance the patient's recovery. Human error or mechanical malfunction during PCA, however, may cause excessive or inadequate drug delivery, so therapists should also be alert for any signs that patients are receiving too much or too little analgesic during PCA.

REFERENCES

1. Albert, JM and Talbott, TM: Patient-controlled analgesia versus conventional intramuscular analgesia following colon surgery. Dis Colon Rectum 31:83, 1988.

2. Allaire, PH, et al: A prospective randomized comparison of epidural infusion of fentanyl and intravenous administration of morphine by patient-controlled analgesia after radical retropubic prostatectomy. Mayo Clin Proc 67:1031, 1992.

3. Ballantyne, JC, et al: Postoperative patient-controlled analgesia: Meta-analysis of initial randomized controlled trials. J Clin Anesth 5:182, 1993.

4. Boldt, J, et al: Pain management in cardiac surgery patients: Comparison between standard therapy and patient-controlled analgesia regimen. J Cardiothorac Vasc Anesth 12:654, 1998.

5. Choiniere, M, et al: Efficacy and costs of patient-controlled analgesia versus regularly administered intramuscular opioid therapy. Anesthesiology 89:1377, 1998.

6. Chrubasik, J, Chrubasik, S, and Martin, E: Patient-controlled spinal opiate analgesia in terminal cancer. Drugs 43:799, 1992.

7. Chumbley, GM, Hall, GM, and Salmon, P: Patient-controlled analgesia: An assessment by 200 patients. Anaesthesia 53:216, 1998.

8. Conner, M and Deane, D: Patterns of patient-controlled analgesia and intramuscular analgesia. Appl Nurs Res 8:67, 1995.

9. Cowan, T: Patient-controlled analgesia devices. Prof Nurse 13:119, 1997.

10. Dahl, JB, et al: Patient-controlled analgesia: A controlled trial. Acta Anaesthesiol Scand 31:744, 1987.

11. De Leon-Casasola, OA and Lema, MJ: Postoperative epidural opioid analgesia: What are the choices? Anesth Analg 83:867, 1996.

12. D'Haese, J, et al: Pharmaco-economic evaluation of a disposable patient-controlled analgesia device and intramuscular analgesia in surgical patients. Eur J Anaesthesiol 15:297, 1998.

13. Eade, DM: Patient-controlled analgesia: Eliminating errors. Nurs Manage 28:38, 1997.

14. Etches, RC: Patient-controlled analgesia. Surg Clin North Am 79:297, 1999.

15. Etches, RC: Respiratory depression associated with patient-controlled analgesia: A review of eight cases. Can J Anaesth 41:125, 1994.

16. Ferrante, FM: Patient-controlled analgesia. Anesthesiol Clin North Am 10:287, 1992.

17. Ferrante, FM, et al: A statistical model for pain in patient-controlled analgesia and conventional intramuscular opioid regimens. Anesth Analg 67:457, 1988.

18. Gambling, DR, et al: Comparison of patient-controlled epidural analgesia and conventional intermittent "top-up" injections during labor. Anesth Analg 70:256, 1990.

19. Gambling, DR, et al: A comparative study of patient-controlled epidural analgesia (PCEA) and continuous infusion epidural analgesia (CIEA) during labour. Can J Anaesth 35:249, 1988.

20. Hecker, BR and Albert, L: Patient-controlled analgesia: A randomized, prospective comparison between two commercially available PCA pumps and conventional analgesic therapy for postoperative pain. Pain 35:115, 1988.

21. Lysak, SZ, Eisenach, JC, and Dobson, CE: Patient-controlled epidural analgesia during labor: A comparison of three solutions with a continuous infusion control. Anesthesiology 72:44, 1990.

22. Ma, CS and Lin, D: Patient controlled analgesia: Drug options, infusion schedules, and other considerations. Hosp Formul 26:198, 1991.

23. Madej, TH, et al: Hypoxaemia and pain relief after lower abdominal surgery: Comparison of extradural and patient-controlled analgesia. Br J Anaesth 69:554, 1992.

24. Marlowe, S, Englstrom, R, and White, PF: Epidural patient-controlled analgesia (PCA): An alternative to continous epidural infusions. Pain 37:97, 1989.

25. McCoy, EP, Furness, G, and Wright, PMC: Patient-controlled analgesia with and without background infusion: Analgesia assessed using the demand-delivery ratio. Anaesthesia 48:256, 1993.

26. McGrath, D, et al: Comparison of one technique of patient-controlled postoperative analgesia with intramuscular meperidine. Pain 37:265, 1989.

27. Nolan, MF and Wilson, MC: Patient-controlled analgesia: A method for the controlled self-administration of opioid pain medications. Phys Ther 75:374, 1995.

28. Parker, RK and White, PF: Epidural patient-controlled analgesia: An alternative to intravenous patient-controlled analgesia for pain relief after cesarean delivery. Anesth Analg 75:245, 1992.

29. Rawal, N: Epidural and spinal agents for postoperative analgesia. Surg Clin North Am 79:313, 1999.

30. Rayburn, WF, et al: Combined continuous and demand narcotic dosing for patient-controlled analgesia after cesarean section. Anesthesiol Rev 17:58, 1990.

31. Ripamonti, C and Bruera, E: Current status of patient-controlled analgesia in cancer patients. Oncology 11:373, 1997.

32. Rosen, DM, et al: Analgesia following major gynecological laparoscopic surgery: PCA versus intermittent intramuscular injection. J Soc Laparoendosc Surg 2:25, 1998.

33. Shaw, HL: Treatment of intractable cancer pain by electronically controlled parenteral infusion of analgesic drugs. Cancer 72(Suppl):3416, 1993.

34. Snell, CC, Fothergill-Bourbonnais, F, and Durocher-Hendriks, S: Patient controlled analgesia and intramuscular injections: A comparison of patient pain experiences and postoperative outcomes. J Adv Nurs 25:681, 1997.

35. Spetzler, B and Anderson, L: Patient-controlled analgesia in the total joint arthroplasty patient. Clin Orthop 215:122, 1987.

36. Tsui, SL, et al: Epidural infusion of bupivacaine 0.0625% plus fentanyl 3.3 micrograms/ml provides bet-

ter postoperative analgesia than patient-controlled analgesia with intravenous morphine after gynaeco-
logical laparotomy. Anaesth Intensive Care 25:476, 1997.
37. Wasylak, TJ, et al: Reduction of postoperative morbidity following patient-controlled morphine. Can J
    Anaesth 37:726, 1990.
38. White, CL, Pokrupa, RP, and Chan, MH: An evaluation of the effectiveness of patient-controlled analge-
    sia after spinal surgery. J Neurosci Nurs 30:225, 1998.
39. White, PF: Mishaps with patient-controlled analgesia. Anesthesiology 66:81, 1987.
40. Wild, L and Coyne, C: Epidural analgesia. Am J Nurs 4:26, 1992.
41. Woodhouse, A and Mather, LE: Nausea and vomiting in the postoperative patient-controlled analgesia
    environment. Anaesthesia 52:770, 1997.

SECTION V

Autonomic and Cardiovascular Pharmacology

CHAPTER 18

Introduction to Autonomic Pharmacology

The human nervous system can be divided into two major functional areas: the somatic nervous system and the autonomic nervous system (ANS). The somatic division is concerned primarily with voluntary function—that is, control of the skeletal musculature. The ANS is responsible for controlling bodily functions that are largely involuntary, or automatic, in nature. For instance, the control of blood pressure (BP) and other aspects of cardiovascular function is under the influence of the ANS. Other involuntary, or vegetative, functions such as digestion, elimination, and thermoregulation are also controlled by this system.

Considering the potential problems that can occur in various systems, such as the cardiovascular and digestive systems, the use of therapeutic drugs to alter autonomic function is one of the major areas of pharmacology. Drugs affecting autonomic function are prescribed routinely to many patients, including those individuals seen for physical and occupational therapy. The purpose of this chapter is to review some of the primary anatomic and physiologic aspects of the ANS. This review is intended to provide rehabilitation specialists with a basis for understanding the pharmacologic effects and clinical applications of the autonomic drugs, which are discussed in subsequent chapters.

ANATOMY OF THE AUTONOMIC NERVOUS SYSTEM: SYMPATHETIC AND PARASYMPATHETIC DIVISIONS

The ANS can be roughly divided into two areas: the sympathetic and parasympathetic nervous systems.[17] The *sympathetic*, or thoracolumbar, division arises primarily from neurons located in the thoracic and upper lumbar regions of the spinal cord. The *parasympathetic*, or craniosacral, division is composed of neurons originating in the midbrain, brainstem, and sacral region of the spinal cord. There are many other anatomic and functional characteristics differentiating these two divisions, which are briefly discussed later in this chapter. For a more detailed discussion of the anatomic and functional organization of the ANS, the reader is referred to several excellent sources listed at the end of this chapter.[11,13,14,22]

263

Preganglionic and Postganglionic Neurons

The somatic nervous system uses one neuron to reach from the CNS to the periphery. In the somatic motor system, for instance, the alpha motor neuron begins in the spinal cord and extends all the way to the skeletal muscle; that is, it does not synapse until it reaches the muscle cell. In both the sympathetic and parasympathetic divisions, however, two neurons are used in sequence to reach from the CNS (i.e., brain or spinal cord) to the peripheral organ or tissue that is being supplied. The first neuron begins somewhere in the CNS and extends a certain distance toward the periphery before synapsing with a second neuron, which completes the journey to the final destination. The synapse of these two neurons is usually in one of the autonomic ganglia (see "Sympathetic Organization" and "Parasympathetic Organization"). Hence, the first neuron in sequence is termed the *preganglionic neuron,* and the second is referred to as the *postganglionic neuron.*

In both the sympathetic and parasympathetic divisions, preganglionic fibers are myelinated type B fibers, and postganglionic fibers are the small, unmyelinated type C fibers. In the sympathetic division, preganglionic neurons tend to be relatively short, whereas the sympathetic postganglionic neurons are relatively long. The opposite is true for the parasympathetic division, with the preganglionic neurons being relatively long and the postganglionic neurons short. The location of preganglionic and postganglionic fibers in each autonomic division is presented here.

Sympathetic Organization

The cell bodies for the sympathetic preganglionic fibers arise from the intermediolateral gray columns of the thoracic and upper lumbar spinal cord. The preganglionic fibers leave the spinal cord via the ventral root of the spinal nerve and end in a sympathetic ganglion. The sympathetic ganglia are located in three areas: (1) the paired paravertebral, or chain, ganglia, which lie bilaterally on either side of the vertebral column; (2) a group of unpaired prevertebral ganglia, which lie anterior to the aorta (e.g., the celiac plexus, the superior and inferior mesenteric ganglia); and (3) a small number of terminal ganglia, which lie directly in the tissue that is innervated (e.g., the bladder and rectum).

When the preganglionic fiber reaches one of the sympathetic ganglia, it synapses with a postganglionic fiber. Actually, one sympathetic preganglionic neuron may synapse with many postganglionic fibers. (The ratio of preganglionic to postganglionic fibers in the sympathetic chain ganglia is usually 1:15 to 20.)[22] The postganglionic fiber then leaves the ganglion to travel to the effector tissue that it supplies (e.g., the heart, peripheral arteriole, sweat gland).

Parasympathetic Organization

Parasympathetic preganglionic neurons originate in the midbrain and brainstem (cranial portion) or the sacral region of the spinal cord. Neurons comprising the cranial portion of the parasympathetics exit the CNS via cranial nerves III, VII, IX, and X. Cranial nerve X (vagus nerve) is particularly significant because it contains approximately 75 percent of the efferent component of the entire parasympathetic division. Neurons that are the preganglionic fibers of the sacral portion exit the spinal cord via the pelvic splanchnic nerves.

As in the sympathetic division, parasympathetic preganglionic neurons synapse in the periphery with a postganglionic fiber. This synapse usually takes place in a terminal ganglion that is located directly in the organ or tissue supplied by the postganglionic neuron. Consequently, the parasympathetic ganglia are usually embedded directly in the organ or tissue that is innervated.

FUNCTIONAL ASPECTS OF THE SYMPATHETIC AND PARASYMPATHETIC DIVISIONS

Except for skeletal muscle, virtually all tissues in the body are innervated in some way by the ANS.[17] Table 18–1 summarizes the innervation and effects of the sympathetic and parasympathetic divisions on some of the major organs and tissues in the body. As indicated in Table 18–1, some organs, such as the heart, are innervated by both sympathetic and parasympathetic neurons. Other tissues, however, may be supplied by only the sympathetic division. The peripheral arterioles, for instance, are innervated by the sympathetic division but receive no parasympathetic innervation.

If an organ *is* innervated by both the sympathetic and parasympathetic divisions, a physiologic antagonism typically exists between these divisions; that is, if both divisions innervate the tissue, one division usually increases function, whereas the other decreases activity. For instance, the sympathetics increase heart rate and stimulate cardiac output, whereas the parasympathetics cause bradycardia. However, it is incorrect to state that the sympathetics are always excitatory in nature and that the parasympathetics are always inhibitory. In tissues such as the gastrointestinal tract, the parasympathetics tend

TABLE 18–1 Response of Effector Organs to Autonomic Stimulation

Organ	Sympathetic*	Parasympathetic†
Heart	Increased contractility (beta-1) Increased heart rate (beta-1)	Decreased heart rate (musc) Slight decrease in contractility (musc)
Arterioles	Vasoconstriction of skin and viscera (alpha-1) Vasodilation of skeletal muscle and liver (beta-2)	No parasympathetic innervation
Lung	Bronchodilation (beta-2)	Bronchoconstriction (musc)
Eye		
Radial muscle	Contraction (alpha-1)	Relaxation (musc)
Ciliary muscle	Relaxation (beta-2)	Contraction (musc)
Gastrointestinal function	Decreased motility (alpha-1,-2; beta-1,-2)	Increased motility and secretion (musc)
Kidney	Increased renin secretion (alpha-1, beta-1)	No parasympathetic innervation
Urinary bladder		
Detrusor	Relaxation (beta-2)	Contraction (musc)
Trigone and sphincter	Contraction (alpha-1)	Relaxation (musc)
Sweat glands	Increased secretion (musc‡)	No parasympathetic innervation
Liver	Glycogenolysis and gluconeogenesis (alpha-1, beta-2)	Glycogen synthesis (musc)
Fat cells	Lipolysis (alpha-2, beta-1)	No parasympathetic innervation

*The primary receptor subtypes that mediate each response are listed in parentheses (e.g, alpha-1, beta-2).
†Note that all organ responses to parasympathetic stimulation are mediated via muscarinic (musc) receptors.
‡Represents response due to sympathetic postganglionic cholinergic fibers.

to increase intestinal motility and secretion, whereas the sympathetics slow down intestinal motility. The effect of each division on any tissue must be considered according to the particular organ or gland in question.

One generalization that can be made regarding sympathetic and parasympathetic function is that the sympathetic division tends to mobilize body energy, whereas the parasympathetic division tends to conserve and store body energy. Typically, sympathetic discharge is increased when the individual is faced with some stressful situation. This situation initiates the classic fight-or-flight scenario in which the person must either flee or defend himself or herself. Sympathetic discharge causes increased cardiac output, decreased visceral blood flow (thus leaving more blood available for skeletal muscle), increased cellular metabolism, and several other physiologic changes that facilitate vigorous activity. In contrast, the parasympathetic division tends to have the opposite effect. Parasympathetic discharge slows down the heart and generally brings about changes that encourage inactivity. Parasympathetic discharge tends to increase intestinal digestion and absorption, an activity that stores energy for future needs.

Finally, activation of the sympathetic division tends to result in a more massive and diffuse reaction than does parasympathetic activation. Parasympathetic reactions tend to be fairly discrete and to affect only one organ or tissue. For instance, the parasympathetic fibers to the myocardium can be activated to slow down the heart without a concomitant emptying of the bowel through an excitatory effect on the lower gastrointestinal tract. When the sympathetic division is activated, effects are commonly observed on many tissues throughout the body. The more diffuse sympathetic reactions routinely produce a simultaneous effect on the heart, total peripheral vasculature, general cellular metabolism, and so on.

FUNCTION OF THE ADRENAL MEDULLA

The adrenal medulla synthesizes and secretes norepinephrine and epinephrine directly into the bloodstream. Typically, the secretion from the adrenal medulla contains about 20 percent norepinephrine and 80 percent epinephrine.[11] These two hormones are fairly similar in action, except that **epinephrine** increases cardiac function and cellular metabolism to a greater extent than **norepinephrine** because epinephrine has a higher affinity for certain receptors than norepinephrine (i.e., epinephrine binds more readily to the beta subtype of adrenergic receptors; see "Autonomic Receptors").[11]

The adrenal medulla is innervated by sympathetic neurons. During normal, resting conditions, the adrenal medulla secretes small amounts of epinephrine and norepinephrine. During periods of stress, however, a general increase in sympathetic discharge causes an increased release of epinephrine and norepinephrine from the adrenal medulla. Because these hormones are released directly into the bloodstream, they tend to circulate extensively throughout the body. Circulating epinephrine and norepinephrine can reach tissues that are not directly innervated by the sympathetic neurons, thus augmenting the general sympathetic effect. Also, the circulating epinephrine and norepinephrine are removed from the body more slowly than norepinephrine that is produced locally at the sympathetic postganglionic nerve terminals. As a result, adrenal release of epinephrine and norepinephrine tends to prolong the effect of the sympathetic reaction.

Consequently, the adrenal medulla serves to augment the sympathetic division of the ANS. In situations that require a sudden increase in sympathetic function (i.e., the fight-or-flight scenario), the adrenal medulla works with the sympathetics to produce a more extensive and lasting response.

AUTONOMIC INTEGRATION AND CONTROL

Most of the autonomic control over various physiologic functions is manifested through autonomic reflexes; that is, homeostatic control of BP, thermoregulation, and gastrointestinal function depend on the automatic reflex adjustment in these systems through the sympathetic and parasympathetic divisions.[17] Autonomic reflexes are based on the following strategy: some peripheral sensor monitors a change in the particular system. This information is relayed to a certain level of the CNS, where it is integrated. An adjustment is made in the autonomic discharge to the specific organ or tissue, which will alter its activity to return physiologic function back to the appropriate level.

A practical example of this type of autonomic reflex control is the so-called baroreceptor reflex, which is important in the control of BP. In this particular example, pressure sensors (i.e., baroreceptors) located in the large arteries of the thorax and neck monitor changes in BP and heart rate. A sudden drop in BP is sensed by these baroreceptors, and this information is relayed to the brainstem. In the brainstem, this information is integrated, a compensatory increase occurs in sympathetic discharge to the heart and peripheral vasculature, and parasympathetic outflow to the heart is decreased. The result is an increase in cardiac output and an increase in peripheral vascular resistance, which effectively bring BP back to the appropriate level. The baroreceptor reflex works in the opposite fashion when BP suddenly increases, with the ultimate result a return to normal pressure levels because of a decrease in sympathetic outflow and an increase in cardiac parasympathetic discharge.

The baroreceptor response is just one example of the type of reflex activity employed by the ANS. The control of other involuntary functions usually follows a similar pattern of peripheral monitoring, central integration, and altered autonomic discharge. Body temperature, for instance, is monitored by thermoreceptors located in the skin, viscera, and hypothalamus. When a change in body temperature is monitored by these sensors, this information is relayed to the hypothalamus, and appropriate adjustments are made in autonomic discharge in order to maintain thermal homeostasis (e.g., sweating is increased or decreased, and blood flow is redistributed). Many other autonomic reflexes that control other visceral and involuntary functions operate in a similar manner.

Integration of autonomic responses is often fairly complex and may occur at several levels of the CNS. Some reflexes, such as emptying of the bowel and bladder, are integrated primarily at the level of the sacral spinal cord. Other reflexes, such as the baroreceptor reflex previously discussed, are integrated at higher levels in the so-called vasomotor center located in the brainstem. Also, the hypothalamus is important in regulating the ANS, and many functions, including body temperature, water balance, and energy metabolism, are controlled and integrated at the hypothalamus. To add to the complexity, higher levels of the brain such as the cortex and limbic system may also influence autonomic function through their interaction with the hypothalamus, brainstem, and spinal cord. This information is important pharmacologically because drugs that act on the CNS have the potential to alter autonomic function by influencing the central integration of autonomic responses. Drugs that affect the cortex, limbic system, and brainstem may indirectly alter the response of some of the autonomic reflexes by altering the relationship between afferent input and efferent sympathetic and parasympathetic outflow.

AUTONOMIC NEUROTRANSMITTERS

Acetylcholine and Norepinephrine

There are four sites of synaptic transmission in the efferent limb of the ANS: (1) the synapse between preganglionic and postganglionic neurons in the sympathetic division, (2) the analogous preganglionic-postganglionic synapse in the parasympathetic division, (3) the synapse between the sympathetic postganglionic neuron and the effector cell, and (4) the parasympathetic postganglionic–effector cell synapse. Figure 18–1 summarizes the chemical neurotransmitter that is present at each synapse.

As indicated in Figure 18–1, the transmitter at the preganglionic-postganglionic synapse in both divisions is acetylcholine. The transmitter at the parasympathetic postganglionic–effector cell synapse is also acetylcholine. The transmitter at the sympathetic postganglionic–effector cell synapse is usually norepinephrine. A small number of sympathetic postganglionic fibers, however, also use acetylcholine as their neurotransmitter.

Consequently, all preganglionic neurons and parasympathetic postganglionic neurons are said to be cholinergic in nature because of the presence of acetylcholine at their respective synapses. Most sympathetic postganglionic neurons use norepinephrine and are referred to as **adrenergic**. (Norepinephrine is sometimes referred to as noradrenaline, hence the term "adrenergic.") An exception to this scheme is the presence of certain sympathetic postganglionic fibers that use acetylcholine as their neurotransmitter. These sympathetic cholinergic neurons innervate sweat glands and certain blood vessels in the face, neck, and lower extremities.

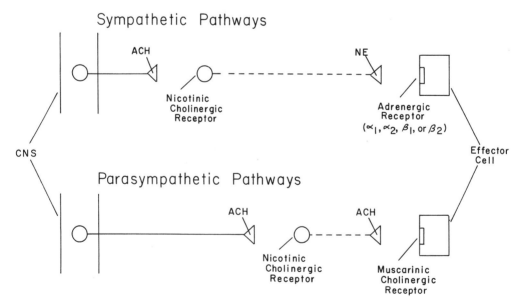

FIGURE 18–1. Autonomic neurotransmitters and receptors. Preganglionic neurons *(solid lines)* release acetylcholine (ACh). Postganglionic neurons *(dashed lines)* release ACh in the parasympathetic pathways and norepinephrine (NE) in the sympathetic pathways.

Other Autonomic Neurotransmitters

In recent years, it has become apparent that several nonadrenergic, noncholinergic neurotransmitters may also be present in the ANS. Purinergic substances such as adenosine and adenosine triphosphate have been implicated as possible transmitters in the gastrointestinal tract.[12,18,19] Several peptides, such as substance P, vasoactive intestinal polypeptide, and angiotensin II, have been identified as possibly participating in the autonomic control of intestinal and respiratory function.[1–3,8,18] Nitric oxide may also help regulate various peripheral autonomic responses, and this substance may also control CNS autonomic activity.[4,16]

Whether all of these nonadrenergic, noncholinergic substances are true neurotransmitters is still uncertain. They may act as cotransmitters that are released from the synaptic terminal along with the classic autonomic transmitters (i.e., acetylcholine and norepinephrine). These other substances, however, may simply be produced locally and serve to modulate synaptic activity without actually being released from the presynaptic terminal. Additional information will be necessary to fully identify the role of these and other nonadrenergic, noncholinergic substances as autonomic neurotransmitters.

AUTONOMIC RECEPTORS

Because there are two primary neurotransmitters involved in autonomic discharge, there are two primary classifications of postsynaptic receptors. **Cholinergic** receptors are located at acetylcholine synapses, and adrenergic receptors are located at norepinephrine synapses. As indicated in Figure 18–2, each type of receptor has several subclassifications. The location and functional significance of these classifications and subclassifications are presented here.

Cholinergic Receptors

Cholinergic receptors are subdivided into two categories: **nicotinic** and **muscarinic.** Although acetylcholine will bind to all cholinergic receptors, certain receptors bind pref-

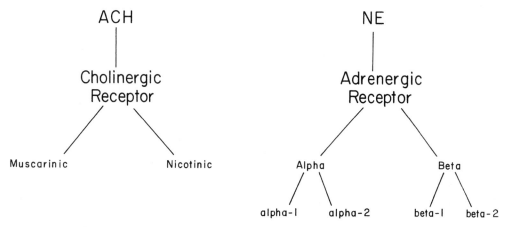

FIGURE 18–2. Receptor classifications and subclassifications for acetylcholine (ACh) and norepinephrine (NE), the two primary neurotransmitters used in the autonomic nervous system.

erentially with the drug nicotine. Other receptors have a specific affinity for muscarine, a naturally occurring compound found in certain poisonous mushrooms. Thus, the terms "nicotinic" and "muscarinic" were derived.

Nicotinic cholinergic receptors are located at the junction between preganglionic and postganglionic neurons in both the sympathetic and parasympathetic pathways (see Fig. 18–1). This fact is significant pharmacologically because any drug that affects these nicotinic receptors will affect activity in both divisions of the ANS. The cholinergic nicotinic receptor located in the ANS is sometimes referred to as a type I (or N_N) nicotinic receptor to differentiate it from the type II (or N_M) nicotinic receptors, which are located at the skeletal neuromuscular junction.

Muscarinic cholinergic receptors are located at all the synapses between cholinergic postganglionic neurons and the terminal effector cell, including all the parasympathetic terminal synapses, as well as the sympathetic postganglionic cholinergic fibers, which supply sweat glands and some specialized blood vessels. Current research suggests that there may be five subtypes of muscarinic receptors; that is, muscarinic subtypes can be classified as M_1, M_2, M_3, and so forth, based on their structural and chemical characteristics.[5,7,9,13,14,20] The exact role of these muscarinic receptor subtypes continues to be elucidated through ongoing research, and future studies will lend more insight into how each receptor subtype participates in normal function and specific diseases.

Thus, cholinergic muscarinic receptors ultimately mediate the effect on the tissue itself. Table 18–2 summarizes the primary physiologic responses when muscarinic receptors are stimulated on various tissues in the body. Note that the specific response to stimulation of a muscarinic cholinergic receptor depends on the tissue in question. Stimulation of muscarinic receptors on the myocardium, for instance, causes a decrease in heart rate, whereas stimulation of muscarinic receptors in the intestinal wall leads to increases in smooth muscle contraction and glandular secretion.

Adrenergic Receptors

As shown in Figure 18–2, the adrenergic receptors are subdivided into two primary categories: alpha- and beta-adrenergic receptors. **Alpha receptors** are further subdivided into alpha-1 and alpha-2 receptors, and **beta receptors** are subdivided into beta-1 and beta-2 receptors.[11] These divisions are based on a different sensitivity of each receptor subcategory to different endogenous and exogenous agents. Alpha-1 receptors, for instance, bind more readily with certain agonists and antagonists, whereas alpha-2 receptors bind preferentially with other agents. Specific agents that bind to each adrenergic receptor subcategory are identified in Chapter 20.

In the ANS, the various types of adrenergic receptors are found on the effector cell in the innervated tissue. In other words, these receptors are located at the terminal synapse between sympathetic postganglionic adrenergic neurons and the tissue they supply. The basic characteristics of each adrenergic receptor subtype are briefly outlined here.

Alpha-1 Receptors. A primary location of these receptors is the smooth muscle located in various tissues throughout the body. Alpha-1 receptors are located on the smooth muscle located in the peripheral vasculature, intestinal wall, radial muscle of the iris, ureters, urinary sphincter, and spleen capsule. The response of each tissue when the alpha-1 receptor is stimulated depends on each tissue (see Table 18–2).

Alpha-2 Receptors. The alpha-2 receptors were originally identified by their presence on the presynaptic terminal of certain adrenergic synapses.[6] These presynaptic alpha-2 receptors appear to modulate the release of neurotransmitters from the pre-

TABLE 18–2 Autonomic Receptor Locations and Responses

Receptor	Primary Location(s)	Response
Cholinergic		
Nicotinic	Autonomic ganglia	Mediate transmission to postganglionic neuron
Muscarinic	All parasympathetic effector cells	
	Visceral and bronchiole smooth muscle	Contraction (generally)
	Cardiac muscle	Decreased heart rate
	Exocrine glands (salivary, intestinal, lacrimal)	Increased secretion
	Sweat glands	Increased secretion
Adrenergic		
Alpha-1	Vascular smooth muscle	Contraction
	Intestinal smooth muscle	Relaxation
	Radial muscle iris	Contraction (mydriasis)
	Ureters	Increased motility
	Urinary sphincter	Contraction
	Spleen capsule	Contraction
Alpha-2	CNS inhibitory synapses	Decreased sympathetic discharge from CNS
	Presynaptic terminal at peripheral adrenergic synapses	Decreased norepinephrine release
	Gastrointestinal tract	Decreased motility and secretion
	Pancreatic islet cells	Decreased insulin secretion
Beta-1	Cardiac muscle	Increased heart rate and contractility
	Kidney	Increased renin secretion
	Fat cells	Increased lipolysis
Beta-2	Bronchiole smooth muscle	Relaxation (bronchodilation)
	Some arterioles (skeletal muscle, liver)	Vasodilation
	Gastrointestinal smooth muscle	Decreased motility
	Skeletal muscle and liver cells	Increased cellular metabolism
	Uterus	Relaxation
	Gallbladder	Relaxation

synaptic terminal; that is, they seem to decrease the release of norepinephrine and other chemicals, thus serving as a form of negative feedback that limits the amount of neurotransmitter released from the pre-synaptic terminal.[13,21] As discussed in Chapter 13, alpha-2 receptors have also been found on spinal interneurons, and stimulation of these alpha-2 receptors may cause decreased neurotransmitter release and diminished stimulation of interneurons that influence the alpha motor neuron. Thus, alpha-2 stimulants (agonists) such as tizanidine have been used to decrease neuronal excitability in the spinal cord and thereby decrease muscle hyperexcitability in conditions such as spasticity (see Chap. 13). Also, alpha-2 receptors have been found postsynaptically on certain CNS adrenergic synapses involved in the control of sympathetic discharge.[15] Stimulation of these centrally located alpha-2 receptors is believed to inhibit sympathetic discharge from the brainstem. The importance of central alpha-2 receptors in controlling cardiovascular function and the possible use of alpha-2 agonists to control BP are discussed in Chapter 21. Alpha-2 receptors are also located in the gastrointestinal tract and pancreas, and stimulation of these receptors at these sites causes decreased intestinal motility and decreased insulin secretion, respectively.

Beta-1 Receptors. These receptors predominate in the heart and kidneys (see Table 18–2).[10] The cardiac beta-1 receptors have received a tremendous amount of attention with regard to pharmacologic antagonism of their function through the use of the so-called beta blockers. Beta-1 receptors are also located on fat cells, and stimulation of these receptors increases fat breakdown (lipolysis).

Beta-2 Receptors. Beta-2 receptors are found primarily on the smooth muscle of certain vasculature, the bronchioles, the gallbladder, and the uterus.[10] Their presence in bronchiole smooth muscle is especially important in the pharmacologic management of respiratory conditions such as asthma (see Chap. 26). These receptors are also responsible for mediating changes in the metabolism of skeletal muscle and liver cells.

Table 18–2 summarizes receptor subtypes that are located on the primary organs and tissues in the body and the associated response when the receptor is stimulated. Exactly which receptor subtype is located on any given tissue depends on the tissue in question. Note that some tissues may have two or more different subtypes of adrenergic receptor (e.g., skeletal muscle arterioles appear to have alpha-1 and beta-2 receptors). Also, the response of a tissue when the receptor is stimulated is dependent on the specific receptor-cell interaction. Stimulation of the vascular alpha-1 receptor, for instance, results in smooth-muscle contraction and vasoconstriction, whereas stimulation of the intestinal alpha-1 receptor results in relaxation and decreased intestinal motility. This difference is caused by the way the receptor is coupled to the cell's internal biochemistry at each location. As discussed in Chapter 4, the surface receptor at one cell may be coupled to the internal enzymatic machinery of the cell so that it stimulates cell function. The same receptor subtype at a different tissue will be linked to inhibitory enzymes that slow down cell function. Refer to Chapter 4 for a more detailed description of how surface receptors are coupled to cell function.

PHARMACOLOGIC SIGNIFICANCE OF AUTONOMIC RECEPTORS

Perhaps no area of research has contributed more to pharmacology than the identification, classification, and subclassification of autonomic receptors. The realization that various tissues have distinct subtypes of receptors has enabled the use of drugs that affect certain tissues and organs while causing minimal effects on other tissues. For instance, a beta-1 antagonist (i.e., a drug that specifically blocks the beta-1 adrenergic receptor) will slow down heart rate and decrease myocardial contractility without causing any major changes in the physiologic functions that are mediated by the other autonomic receptors.

However, several limitations of autonomic drugs must be realized. First, a drug that binds preferentially to one receptor subtype will bind to that receptor at all of its locations. For example, a muscarinic antagonist that decreases activity in the gastrointestinal tract may also decrease bronchial secretions in the lungs and cause urinary retention because of relaxation of the detrusor muscle of the bladder. Also, no drug is entirely specific for only one receptor subtype. For instance, the so-called beta-1–specific antagonists atenolol and metoprolol have a 10- to 20-fold greater affinity for beta-1 receptors than for beta-2 receptors.[10] At high enough concentrations, however, these drugs will affect beta-2 receptors as well. Finally, organs and tissues in the body do not contain only one subtype of receptor. For example, the predominant receptor in the bronchioles is the beta-2 subtype, but some beta-1 receptors are also present. Thus, a patient using a beta-1–specific drug such as metoprolol may experience some respiratory effects as well.[10]

Consequently, many side effects as well as beneficial effects of autonomic drugs can be attributed to the interaction of various agents with different receptors. The significance of autonomic receptor subtypes, as well as the use of specific cholinergic and adrenergic drugs in treating various problems, is covered in more detail in Chapters 19 and 20.

SUMMARY

The ANS is primarily responsible for controlling involuntary, or vegetative, functions in the body. The sympathetic and parasympathetic divisions of the ANS often function as physiologic antagonists to maintain homeostasis of various activities, including BP control, thermoregulation, digestion, and elimination. The primary neurotransmitters used in synaptic transmission within the ANS are acetylcholine and norepinephrine. These chemicals are found at specific locations in each autonomic division, as are their respective cholinergic and adrenergic receptors. The two primary types of autonomic receptors (cholinergic and adrenergic) are subdivided according to differences in drug affinity. Receptor subtypes are located in specific tissues throughout the body and are responsible for mediating the appropriate tissue response. Most autonomic drugs exert their effects by interacting in some way with autonomic synaptic transmission so that a fairly selective and isolated effect is achieved.

REFERENCES

1. Barnes, PJ: Non-adrenergic non-cholinergic neural control of human airways. Arch Int Pharmacodyn Ther 280:208, 1986.
2. Bauer, V and Matusak, O: The non-adrenergic non-cholinergic innervation and transmission in the small intestine. Arch Int Pharmacodyn Ther 280(Suppl):137, 1986.
3. Beaulieu, P and Lambert, C: Peptidic regulation of heart rate and interactions with the autonomic nervous system. Cardiovasc Res 37:578, 1998.
4. Boeckxstaens, GE and Pelckmans, PA: Nitric oxide and the non-adrenergic non-cholinergic neurotransmission. Comp Biochem Physiol A 118:925, 1997.
5. Cortes, R, et al: Muscarinic cholinergic receptor subtypes in the human brain. II. Quantitative autoradiographic studies. Brain Res 362:239, 1986.
6. Davey, MJ: Alpha adrenoceptors: An overview. J Mol Cell Cardiol 18(Suppl 5):1, 1986.
7. Ehlert, FJ, Ostrom, RS, and Sawyer, GW: Subtypes of the muscarinic receptor in smooth muscle. Life Sci 61:1729, 1997.
8. Ferguson, AV and Washburn, DL: Angiotensin II: A peptidergic neurotransmitter in central autonomic pathways. Prog Neurobiol 54:169, 1998.
9. Fryer, AD and Jacoby, DB: Muscarinic receptors and control of airway smooth muscle. Am J Respir Crit Care Med 158(Suppl 3):S154, 1998.
10. Gerber, JG and Nies, AS: Beta-adrenergic blocking drugs. Annu Rev Med 36:145, 1985.
11. Guyton, AC and Hall, JE: Textbook of Medical Physiology, ed 9. WB Saunders, Philadelphia, 1996.
12. Hasko, G and Szabo, C: Regulation of cytokine and chemokine production by transmitters and co-transmitters of the autonomic nervous system. Biochem Pharmacol 56:1079, 1998.
13. Hoffman, BB, Lefkowitz, RJ, and Taylor, P: Neurotransmission: The autonomic and somatic motor nervous systems. In Hardman, JG, et al (eds): The Pharmacological Basis of Therapeutics, ed 9. McGraw-Hill, New York, 1996.
14. Katzung, BG: Introduction to autonomic pharmacology. In Katzung, BG (ed): Basic and Clinical Pharmacology, ed 7. Appleton & Lange, Stamford, CT, 1998.
15. Koss, MC: Review article: Pupillary dilation as an index of central nervous system alpha-2 adrenoceptor activation. J Pharmacol Methods 15:1, 1986.
16. Krukoff, TL: Central actions of nitric oxide in regulation of autonomic functions. Brain Res Brain Res Rev 30:52, 1999.
17. Shields, RW: Functional anatomy of the autonomic nervous system. J Clin Neurophysiol 10:2, 1993.
18. Silverthorn, DV: Human Physiology: An Integrated Approach. Prentice-Hall, Upper Saddle River, NJ, 1998.
19. Su, C: Purinergic neurotransmission and neuromodulation. Annu Rev Pharmacol Toxicol 23:397, 1983.
20. Vickroy, TW, et al: Agonist binding to multiple muscarinic receptors. Fed Proc 43:2785, 1984.
21. Westfall, TC: Evidence that noradrenergic neurotransmitter release is regulated by presynaptic receptors. Fed Proc 43:1352, 1984.
22. Williams, PL, et al (eds): Gray's Anatomy, ed 38. WB Saunders, New York, 1995.

CHAPTER 19

Cholinergic Drugs

This chapter discusses drugs that affect the activity at **cholinergic** synapses—that is, synapses using acetylcholine as a neurotransmitter. These cholinergic synapses are very important in a number of different physiologic systems. As discussed in Chapter 18, acetylcholine is one of the primary neurotransmitters in the autonomic nervous system (ANS), especially the parasympathetic autonomic division. Consequently, many of the drugs discussed in this chapter are administered to alter the response of various tissues to autonomic parasympathetic control. Acetylcholine is also the neurotransmitter at the skeletal neuromuscular junction. Certain cholinergic stimulants are used to treat a specific problem at the skeletal neuromuscular junction (i.e., myasthenia gravis). Cholinergic synapses are also found in specific areas of the brain, and some anticholinergic drugs are used to decrease the symptoms of such diverse problems as parkinsonism and motion sickness. These drugs are therefore used in a variety of clinical situations.

The purpose of this chapter is to present an overview of these drugs in the context that they share a common mode of action; that is, they influence cholinergic activity. Considering the diverse clinical applications of cholinergic and anticholinergic agents, physical therapists and occupational therapists will likely encounter patients taking these agents. Some knowledge of the pharmacodynamics of these medications will enable the rehabilitation specialist to understand the therapeutic rationale behind drug administration, as well as the patient's response to the drug.

Autonomic cholinergic drugs can be divided into two general categories: cholinergic stimulants and anticholinergic drugs. Cholinergic stimulants effectively increase activity at acetylcholine synapses, whereas anticholinergic drugs decrease synaptic activity. Cholinergic stimulants and anticholinergic agents can be further characterized according to functional or pharmacodynamic criteria, and these criteria will be discussed in more detail in this chapter.

CHOLINERGIC RECEPTORS

Many autonomic cholinergic drugs affect synaptic activity by interacting with the acetylcholine receptor located on the postsynaptic membrane. At each cholinergic synapse, postsynaptic receptors are responsible for recognizing the acetylcholine molecule and transducing the chemical signal into a postsynaptic response. As discussed in

Chapter 18, cholinergic receptors can be subdivided into muscarinic and nicotinic receptors according to their affinity for certain drugs.[9]

Muscarinic cholinergic receptors are generally found on the peripheral tissues supplied by parasympathetic postganglionic neurons—that is, on effector organs such as the gastrointestinal tract, urinary bladder, heart, and eye. Acetylcholine synapses found in specific areas of the CNS also use the muscarinic subtype of cholinergic receptor. Nicotinic cholinergic receptors are located in the autonomic ganglia (nicotinic type I or N_N) and at the skeletal neuromuscular junction (nicotinic type II or N_M). Refer to Chapter 18 for a more detailed discussion of cholinergic receptor subclassification.

The existence of different varieties of cholinergic receptors is important pharmacologically. Some drugs are relatively specific for a certain cholinergic receptor subtype, whereas others tend to bind rather indiscriminately to all cholinergic receptors. Obviously, the more specific drugs are preferable because they tend to produce a more precise response with fewer side effects. As this chapter will point out, however, specificity is only a relative term, and drugs that bind preferentially to one receptor subtype may produce a variety of responses.

CHOLINERGIC STIMULANTS

Cholinergic stimulants increase activity at acetylcholine synapses. Chemically, many agents are capable of potently and effectively stimulating cholinergic activity. However, only a few drugs exhibit sufficient safety and relative specificity to be used in clinical situations. These clinically relevant drugs can be subdivided into two categories, depending on their mechanism of action. Direct-acting cholinergic stimulants exert their effects by binding directly with the cholinergic receptor (Fig. 19–1). Indirect-acting cholinergic stimulants increase synaptic activity by inhibiting the acetylcholinesterase enzyme located at the cholinergic synapse (see Fig. 19–1). Table 19–1 lists specific direct-acting and indirect-acting cholinergic stimulants, and the rationale for their use is presented here.

Direct-Acting Cholinergic Stimulants

Direct-acting stimulants bind directly to the cholinergic receptor and activate the receptor, which in turn initiates a cellular response. These stimulants may be considered true cholinergic agonists, and they function in a manner similar to the acetylcholine molecule. By definition, acetylcholine itself is a direct-acting cholinergic stimulant. Exogenously administered acetylcholine is not used therapeutically, however, because it is degraded rapidly and extensively by the acetylcholinesterase enzyme, which is found ubiquitously throughout the body.

As mentioned previously, there are many pharmacologic agents that can directly stimulate cholinergic receptors. A certain degree of drug specificity is desirable, however, when these agents are considered for therapeutic purposes. For instance, drugs that have a greater specificity for the muscarinic cholinergic receptor are more beneficial. These muscarinic cholinergic stimulants will primarily affect the peripheral tissues while exerting a minimal effect on the cholinergic receptors located in the autonomic ganglia and the neuromuscular junction. (Recall that the cholinergic receptors found in the autonomic ganglia and at the skeletal neuromuscular junction are the nicotinic type I and nicotinic type II, respectively.)

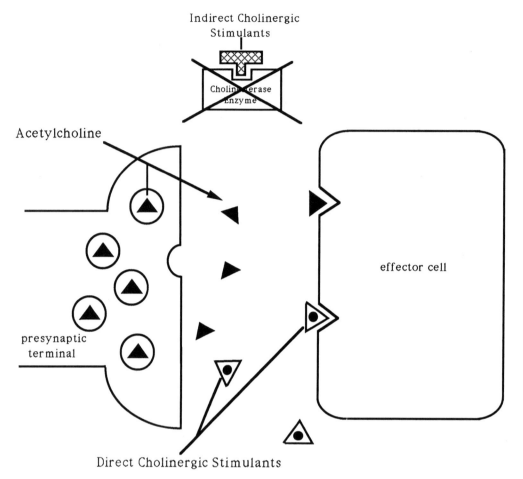

FIGURE 19–1. Mechanism of action of cholinergic stimulants. Direct-acting stimulants bind directly to the postsynaptic cholinergic receptor. Indirect-acting stimulants inhibit the cholinesterase enzyme, thus allowing acetylcholine to remain in the synaptic cleft.

Consequently, only a few agents are suitable for clinical use as direct-acting cholinergic stimulants. For systemic administration, bethanechol (Duvoid, Urecholine) is the primary direct-acting cholinergic stimulant used clinically (see Table 19–1). Bethanechol appears to preferentially stimulate muscarinic cholinergic receptors, although some stimulation of the ganglionic nicotinic receptor may also occur.[1] Other direct-acting cholinergic stimulants such as carbachol and pilocarpine are limited to topical use in ophthalmologic conditions (glaucoma). These antiglaucoma drugs would produce too many side effects if administered systemically but are relatively specific when administered directly to the eye. Clinical applications of direct-acting cholinergic stimulants are summarized in Table 19–1.

Indirect-Acting Cholinergic Stimulants

Indirect-acting stimulants increase activity at cholinergic synapses by inhibiting the acetylcholinesterase enzyme. This enzyme is normally responsible for destroying

TABLE 19–1 Cholinergic Stimulants

Generic Name	Trade Name(s)	Primary Clinical Use(s)*
Direct-Acting (Cholinergic Agonists)		
Bethanechol	Duvoid, Urabeth, Urecholine	Postoperative gastrointestinal and urinary atony
Carbachol	Isopto Carbachol, Miostat	Glaucoma
Pilocarpine	Pilocar, Adsorbocarpine, many others	Glaucoma
Indirect-Acting (Cholinesterase Inhibitors)		
Ambenonium	Mytelase	Myasthenia gravis
Demecarium	Humorsol	Glaucoma
Donepezil	Aricept	Dementia of the Alzheimer type
Echothiophate	Phospholine Iodide	Glaucoma
Edrophonium	Enlon, Reversol, Tensilon	Myasthenia gravis, reversal of neuromuscular blocking drugs
Neostigmine	Prostigmin	Postoperative gastrointestinal and urinary atony, myasthenia gravis, reversal of neuromuscular blocking drugs
Physostigmine	Antilirium, Eserine, Isopto Eserine	Glaucoma, reversal of CNS toxicity caused by anticholinergic drugs
Pyridostigmine	Mestinon	Myasthenia gravis, reversal of neuromuscular blocking drugs
Tacrine	Cognex	Dementia of the Alzheimer type

*Agents used to treat glaucoma are administered topically, that is, directly to the eye. Agents used for other problems are given systemically by oral administration or injection.

acetylcholine after this neurotransmitter is released from the presynaptic terminal. Indirect-acting stimulants inhibit the acetylcholinesterase, thus allowing more acetylcholine to remain at the synapse. The result is an increase in cholinergic synaptic transmission.

Because of their effect on the acetylcholinesterase enzyme, indirect-acting stimulants are also referred to as *cholinesterase inhibitors* or *anticholinesterase agents*. The exact way in which each drug inhibits the acetylcholinesterase enzyme varies. The net effect is similar, however, in that the enzyme's ability to degrade acetylcholine is diminished by these drugs.

Unlike the systemic direct-acting cholinergic stimulants (bethanechol), cholinesterase inhibitors display a relative lack of specificity regarding which cholinergic synapses they stimulate. These drugs tend to inhibit the acetylcholinesterase found at all cholinergic synapses. Thus, they may exert a stimulatory effect on the peripheral muscarinic cholinergic synapses, as well as the cholinergic synapses found at the autonomic ganglia, at the skeletal neuromuscular junction, and within certain areas of the CNS. In appropriate doses, however, certain agents exert some degree of specificity at peripheral versus CNS synapses. Indirect-acting stimulants such as neostigmine, for example, tend to predominantly affect the skeletal neuromuscular junction and peripheral tissues containing muscarinic receptors. In contrast, newer agents such as tacrine and donepezil show more specificity for cholinergic synapses in certain regions of the brain; hence, these newer drugs have been used to boost cholinergic function in conditions such as Alzheimer disease. Still, none of the indirect-acting cholinergic stimulants affect only one type of tissue, and some adverse side effects of these agents will be caused by their relatively nonspecific activity.

The primary indirect-acting cholinergic stimulants currently in use are neostigmine and pyridostigmine. Several other agents are also used therapeutically to treat systemic conditions such as myasthenia gravis, ophthalmologic disorders such as glaucoma, and diminished acetylcholine activity associated with degenerative brain syndromes such as Alzheimer disease. These indirect-acting agents are summarized in Table 19–1.

Clinical Applications of Cholinergic Stimulants

Direct-acting and indirect-acting cholinergic stimulants are used to treat the decrease in smooth-muscle tone that sometimes occurs in the gastrointestinal tract and urinary bladder following abdominal surgery or trauma. Indirect-acting stimulants are also used in the treatment of glaucoma and myasthenia gravis, in Alzheimer disease, and to reverse the effects from an overdose of other drugs such as neuromuscular blocking agents and anticholinergic drugs. Each of these applications is briefly discussed here.

Alzheimer Disease. Alzheimer disease is a progressive neurodegenerative disorder that affects older adults. This disorder is characterized by neuronal atrophy and other pathologic changes in neuron structure and function throughout the brain (neurofibrillary tangles, formation of plaques, and so forth). Included in this neuronal degeneration are cholinergic neurons that are critical in memory, cognition, and other higher cortical functions.[5,15] Although there is no cure for this disease, indirect cholinergic stimulants such as tacrine and donepezil (see Table 19–1) may help decrease some of the symptoms during the early stages of Alzheimer disease.[5,16] By inhibiting acetylcholine breakdown, these drugs prolong the effects of any acetylcholine that is released from neurons that are still functioning in the cerebral cortex.

Regrettably, these drugs do not alter the progression of Alzheimer disease, and they tend to lose effectiveness as this disease develops into the advanced stages.[6,16] This loss of effectiveness makes sense in that these drugs can only prolong the effects of endogenously released acetylcholine; they will have no effect when cortical neurons degenerate to the point where acetylcholine is no longer being synthesized and released within the brain. Nonetheless, drugs such as tacrine and donepezil can help patients retain better cognitive function during the early stages of Alzheimer disease, which can sustain a better quality of life for these patients for as long as possible.[16] Several new cholinesterase inhibitors such as rivastigmine are likewise being developed, and these newer agents may provide longer-lasting effects in people with Alzheimer disease.[8,11]

Gastrointestinal and Urinary Bladder Atony. After surgical manipulation or other trauma to the viscera, there is often a period of atony (i.e., lack of tone) in the smooth muscle of these organs. As a result, intestinal peristalsis is diminished or absent, and the urinary bladder becomes distended, leading to urinary retention. Under normal circumstances, acetylcholine released from parasympathetic postganglionic neurons would stimulate smooth-muscle contraction in these tissues. Consequently, cholinergic agonists (i.e., drugs that mimic or enhance the effects of acetylcholine) are administered to treat this problem. Bethanechol and neostigmine, a direct-acting and an indirect-acting cholinergic stimulant, respectively, are the drugs most frequently used to treat this condition until normal gastrointestinal and urinary function is resumed.

Glaucoma. Glaucoma is an increase in intraocular pressure brought on by an accumulation of aqueous humor within the eye.[12] If untreated, this increased pressure leads to impaired vision and blindness. Cholinergic stimulation via the parasympathetic supply to the eye increases the outflow of aqueous humor, thus preventing excessive accumulation. If evidence of increased intraocular pressure exists, cholinergic stimulants are among the drugs that may be used to treat this problem.[12] Direct-acting and indirect-acting cholinergic drugs (see Table 19–1) are usually applied topically to the eye by placing the drug directly within the conjunctival sac to treat glaucoma. This application concentrates the action of the drug on the eye, thus limiting the side effects that might occur if these agents were given systemically.

Myasthenia Gravis. Myasthenia gravis is a disease affecting the skeletal neuromuscular junction and is characterized by skeletal muscle weakness and profound fatigability.[3] As the disease progresses, the fatigue increases in severity and in the number of muscles involved. In advanced stages, the patient requires respiratory support because of a virtual paralysis of the respiratory musculature. In myasthenia gravis, the number of functional cholinergic receptors located postsynaptically at the neuromuscular junction is diminished.[13] As a result, acetylcholine released from the presynaptic terminal cannot sufficiently excite the muscle cell to reach threshold. Thus, the decreased receptivity of the muscle cell accounts for the clinical symptoms of weakness and fatigue.

Myasthenia gravis appears to be caused by an autoimmune response whereby an antibody to the neuromuscular cholinergic receptor is produced.[13] Although no cure is available, cholinesterase inhibitors such as neostigmine and pyridostigmine may alleviate the muscular fatigue associated with this disease. These indirect-acting cholinergic agonists inhibit the acetylcholinesterase enzyme at the neuromuscular junction, allowing the endogenous acetylcholine released from the presynaptic terminal to remain at the myoneural junction for a longer period of time. The endogenously released acetylcholine is able to provide adequate excitation of the skeletal muscle cell and thus allow a more sustained muscular contraction.

Reversal of Anticholinergic-Induced CNS Toxicity. Indirect-acting cholinergic stimulants (e.g., physostigmine) are sometimes used to reverse the toxic effects of anticholinergic drugs on the CNS. An overdose of anticholinergic drugs may produce toxic CNS effects such as delirium, hallucinations, and coma. By inhibiting acetylcholine breakdown, indirect-acting stimulants enable endogenously released acetylcholine to overcome the anticholinergic drug effects.

Reversal of Neuromuscular Blockage. Drugs that block transmission at the skeletal neuromuscular junction are often used during general anesthesia to maintain skeletal muscle paralysis during surgical procedures (see Chap. 11). These skeletal muscle paralytic agents include curare-like drugs (e.g., tubocurarine, gallamine, pancuronium). Occasionally, the neuromuscular blockage caused by these drugs must be reversed. For instance, an accelerated recovery from the paralytic effects of these neuromuscular blockers may be desired at the end of a surgical procedure. Consequently, indirect-acting cholinergic stimulants are sometimes used to inhibit the acetylcholinesterase enzyme at the neuromuscular junction, thus allowing endogenously released acetylcholine to remain active at the synaptic site and effectively overcome the neuromuscular blockade until the curare-like agents have been metabolized.

Adverse Effects of Cholinergic Stimulants

Cholinergic stimulants are frequently associated with a number of adverse side effects caused by the relative nonspecificity of these drugs. Even a drug like bethanechol, which is relatively specific for muscarinic receptors, may stimulate muscarinic receptors on many different tissues. For example, administering bethanechol to increase gastrointestinal motility may also result in bronchoconstriction if this drug reaches muscarinic receptors in the upper respiratory tract. Many indirect-acting stimulants (i.e., the cholinesterase inhibitors) show even less specificity and may increase synaptic activity in all synapses that they reach, including nicotinic cholinergic synapses.

The adverse effects associated with both the direct-acting and indirect-acting cholinergic stimulants mimic the effects that would occur during exaggerated parasympathetic activity. This notion is logical considering that the parasympathetic autonomic division exerts its effects on peripheral tissues by releasing acetylcholine from postganglionic neurons. Consequently, the primary adverse effects of cholinergic stimulants include gastrointestinal distress (nausea, vomiting, diarrhea, abdominal cramping), increased salivation, bronchoconstriction, bradycardia, and difficulty in visual accommodation. Increased sweating and vasodilation of facial cutaneous blood vessels (flushing) may also occur because of an effect on the tissues supplied by special sympathetic postganglionic neurons that release acetylcholine. The incidence of these side effects varies from patient to patient, but the onset and severity of these adverse effects increase as higher drug doses are administered.

ANTICHOLINERGIC DRUGS

In contrast to drugs that stimulate cholinergic activity, anticholinergic drugs attempt to diminish the response of tissues to cholinergic stimulation. In general, these drugs are competitive antagonists of the postsynaptic cholinergic receptors; that is, they bind reversibly to the cholinergic receptor but do not activate it. This binding blocks the receptor from the effects of endogenously released acetylcholine, thus diminishing the cellular response to cholinergic stimulation. (See Chapter 4 for a more detailed description of the mechanism by which drugs function as competitive antagonists.)

Anticholinergic drugs can be classified as antimuscarinic or antinicotinic agents, depending on their specificity for the two primary subtypes of cholinergic receptors. This chapter focuses on the antimuscarinic agents; the antinicotinic drugs are discussed at length in Chapters 11 and 21. Antinicotinic drugs such as mecamylamine and trimethaphan, for example, are relatively specific for the nicotinic type I receptor located in the autonomic ganglia. These nicotinic type I antagonists are sometimes used to treat extremely high blood pressure. The use of antinicotinic drugs in treating hypertensive emergencies is discussed in Chapter 21. Antinicotinic drugs that block the skeletal neuromuscular junction (i.e., the nicotinic type II drugs) are sometimes used as an adjunct in general anesthesia and are used to produce skeletal muscle paralysis during surgery. These so-called neuromuscular blockers are discussed in Chapter 11.

Source and Mechanism of Action of Antimuscarinic Anticholinergic Drugs

The prototypical antimuscarinic anticholinergic drug is atropine (Fig. 19–2). *Atropine* is a naturally occurring substance that can be obtained from the extract of plants such as belladonna and jimsonweed. Other natural, semisynthetic, and synthetic antimuscarinic anticholinergic agents have been developed that are similar in structure or function to atropine.

As mentioned previously, antimuscarinic anticholinergic drugs all share the same basic mechanism of action: they block the postsynaptic cholinergic muscarinic receptor.

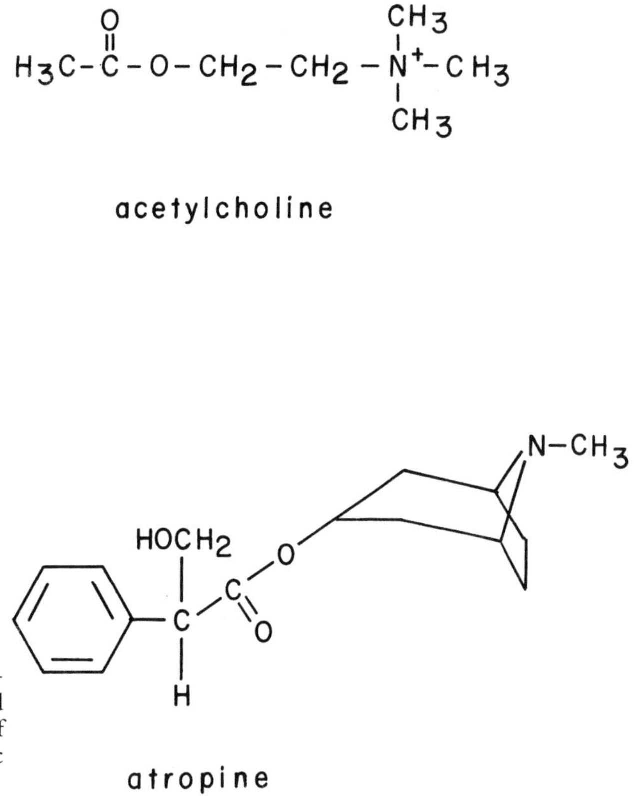

$$H_3C-\overset{\overset{O}{\|}}{C}-O-CH_2-CH_2-\overset{\overset{CH_3}{|}}{\underset{\underset{CH_3}{|}}{N^+}}-CH_3$$

acetylcholine

FIGURE 19–2. Structures of acetylcholine and atropine. Atropine and similar agents antagonize the effects of acetylcholine by blocking muscarinic cholinergic receptors.

atropine

However, certain antimuscarinic agents seem to preferentially affect some tissues more than others. For instance, certain antimuscarinics seem to preferentially antagonize gastrointestinal muscarinic receptors, whereas others have a predominant effect on CNS cholinergic synapses. This fact suggests some degree of specificity of these drugs, which may be because of differences in the muscarinic receptor at gastrointestinal versus central synapses. Indeed, there is evidence that as many as five muscarinic receptor subtypes may exist at different locations in the body; these subtypes are designated M_1, M_2, M_3, M_4, and M_5 receptors.[1,4,10,17] Some drugs may be more selective for a certain receptor subtype than for others. This drug-receptor specificity is far from complete, however, and virtually every antimuscarinic drug will antagonize cholinergic receptors on a number of different tissues, leading to a number of side effects with these drugs (see "Side Effects of Anticholinergic Drugs"). Perhaps as more is learned about muscarinic receptor subtypes, more selective anticholinergic drugs may be developed.

Clinical Applications of Antimuscarinic Drugs

The primary clinical applications of antimuscarinic anticholinergic drugs include the treatment of certain gastrointestinal disorders. These drugs may also be helpful in managing Parkinson disease. In addition, they have been used to treat a variety of other clinical disorders involving many other physiologic systems.[7] The clinical applications of antimuscarinic agents are discussed here, and specific drugs used in various clinical situations are outlined in Table 19–2.

TABLE 19–2 Common Anticholinergic Drugs*

Generic Name	Trade Name(s)	Primary Clinical Use(s)*
Anisotropine	Valpin	Peptic ulcer
Atropine	Generic	Peptic ulcer, irritable bowel syndrome, preoperative antisecretory agent, cardiac arrhythmias (e.g., sinus bradycardia, post-myocardial infarction, asystole), reversal of neuromuscular blockade, antidote to cholinesterase inhibitor poisoning
Belladonna	Generic	Peptic ulcer, irritable bowel syndrome, dysmenorrhea, nocturnal enuresis
Clidinium	Quarzan	Peptic ulcer, irritable bowel syndrome
Cyclopentolate	AK-Pentolate, Cyclogyl, Ocu-Pentolate	Induces mydriasis for ophthalmologic procedures
Dicyclomine	Bentyl, others	Irritable bowel syndrome
Glycopyrrolate	Robinul	Peptic ulcer, preoperative antisecretory agent, antidiarrheal, reversal of neuromuscular blockade
Homatropine	Homapin	Peptic ulcer
Hyoscyamine	Cystospaz, Levsin, others	Peptic ulcer, irritable bowel syndrome, urinary bladder hypermotility
Ipratropium	Atrovent	Bronchodilator
Mepenzolate	Cantil	Peptic ulcer
Methantheline	Banthine	Peptic ulcer, neurogenic bladder
Oxybutynin	Ditropan	Neurogenic bladder
Propantheline	Pro-Banthine	Peptic ulcer, irritable bowel syndrome
Scopolamine	Transderm-Scop	Motion sickness, peptic ulcer, preoperative antisecretory agent

*Clinical uses listed for a specific agent reflect that agent's approved indication(s). Actual clinical use, however, may be limited because anticholinergics have generally been replaced by agents that are more effective and better tolerated. Anticholinergic drugs used specifically to treat Parkinson disease are listed in Table 10–2, Chapter 10.

Cardiovascular System. Atropine is sometimes used to block the effects of the vagus nerve (cranial nerve X) on the myocardium. Release of acetylcholine from vagal efferent fibers slows heart rate and the conduction of the cardiac action potential throughout the myocardium. Atropine reverses the effects of excessive vagal discharge and is used to treat the symptomatic bradycardia that may accompany myocardial infarction.[1] Atropine may also be useful in treating other cardiac arrhythmias, such as atrioventricular nodal block and ventricular asystole.

Cholinergic Poisoning. Cholinergic poisoning can occur in several situations, such as eating wild mushrooms, being exposed to certain insecticides, or being exposed to certain types of chemical warfare.[10] These potentially life-threatening occurrences typically require emergency treatment with atropine or an analogous anticholinergic agent. In cases of severe poisoning, fairly high doses of these drugs must often be administered for several days.

Eye. Atropine and similar antimuscarinics block the acetylcholine-mediated contraction of the pupillary sphincter muscle, thus causing dilation of the pupil (mydriasis).[7] During an ophthalmologic exam, these drugs may be applied topically in order to dilate the pupil, thus allowing a more detailed inspection of internal eye structures such as the retina.

Gastrointestinal System. Stimulation of the gastrointestinal tract via parasympathetic cholinergic neurons generally produces an increase in gastric secretions and an increase in gastrointestinal motility. Consequently, certain antimuscarinic anticholinergics tend to reverse this stimulation by blocking the effects of endogenously released acetylcholine. Clinically, these drugs are used as an adjunct in peptic ulcer. The rationale is that they will limit secretion of gastric acid, thus reducing irritation of the stomach mucosa. Also, antimuscarinic anticholinergic drugs have been approved for treatment of irritable bowel syndrome. This condition is characterized by hyperactivity of gastrointestinal smooth muscle and includes problems such as irritable colon and spastic colon. These antimuscarinic agents are sometimes referred to as *antispasmodics* because of their reported ability to decrease gastrointestinal smooth-muscle tone or spasms.

Drugs used to treat peptic ulcer and irritable bowel syndrome are listed in Table 19–2. Although these agents are approved for use in these conditions, considerable doubt exists as to how effective they are in actually resolving these gastrointestinal disorders. Their use in treating peptic ulcer has essentially been replaced by other agents such as the H_2 histamine receptor blockers (see Chap. 27), but antimuscarinic anticholinergics may still be used if other drugs are ineffective or poorly tolerated.[1] These drugs will not cure peptic ulcer or prevent its recurrence when the medication is discontinued. In essence, they treat only a symptom of the problem (increased gastric secretion), without really addressing the cause of the increased secretion (e.g., emotional stress).

Finally, antimuscarinic anticholinergic drugs used to treat gastrointestinal problems are often combined with other agents such as antianxiety drugs. Librax, for instance, is the trade name for a combination of chlordiazepoxide and clidinium (an antianxiety agent and an anticholinergic agent, respectively). These combination products are supposedly better at relieving gastrointestinal problems in which emotional factors are also present.

Motion Sickness. Antimuscarinics (scopolamine in particular) are used frequently in the treatment of motion sickness. Scopolamine appears to block cholinergic transmission from areas of the brain and brainstem that mediate motion-related nausea and vomiting (i.e., the vestibular system and reticular formation).[14] These drugs are often administered transdermally via small patches that adhere to the skin.[7]

Parkinson Disease. The pharmacologic management of Parkinson disease is discussed in detail in Chapter 10. Consequently, the use of anticholinergic drugs in this disorder will be mentioned only briefly at this time. Parkinsonism is a movement disorder caused by a deficiency of the neurotransmitter dopamine in the basal ganglia. This deficiency leads to overactivity of central cholinergic synapses. Hence, anticholinergic drugs should be beneficial in helping resolve this increase in central cholinergic influence.[7]

Certain anticholinergic drugs such as benztropine, biperiden, and trihexyphenidyl are approved for use in treating Parkinson disease (see Chap. 10, Table 10–2 for a more complete list). As mentioned, these drugs seem to preferentially block the central muscarinic cholinergic synapses involved in parkinsonism. This does not mean that these drugs do not affect other peripheral muscarinic receptors. Indeed, these antiparkinsonian drugs are associated with a number of side effects, such as dry mouth, constipation, and urinary retention, which are caused by their antagonistic effect on muscarinic receptors located outside the brain. Their primary effect, however, is to decrease the influence of central cholinergic synapses in parkinsonism.

Preoperative Medication. Atropine and related antimuscarinics are occasionally used preoperatively to decrease respiratory secretions during general anesthesia. Their use in this capacity has declined considerably, however, because the newer inhalation forms of general anesthesia do not stimulate bronchial secretions to the same extent as earlier general anesthetics (see Chap. 11).[7] Antimuscarinics may also be administered to prevent bradycardia during surgery, especially in children.

Respiratory Tract. Stimulation of the upper respiratory tract via the vagus causes bronchoconstriction. Anticholinergic drugs that block the effects of vagal-released acetylcholine will relax bronchial smooth muscle. Consequently, atropine and some synthetic derivatives have been used to treat the bronchospasm that occurs in patients with asthma and chronic obstructive pulmonary disease (COPD).[1] Although anticholinergics are not usually the initial drugs used to treat bronchoconstriction, they may be used in combination with other drugs or as a second choice for patients who are unable to tolerate more conventional forms of bronchodilators such as the adrenergic agonists.[2] The use of anticholinergics in treating respiratory disorders is discussed in more detail in Chapter 26.

Urinary Tract. Atropine and several synthetic antimuscarinics have been used to alleviate urinary frequency and incontinence caused by hypertonicity of the urinary bladder.[7] Increased bladder tone results if the normal reflex control of bladder function is disrupted (i.e., the so-called neurogenic bladder syndrome) or a urinary tract infection irritates the bladder. Antimuscarinics inhibit contraction of the bladder detrusor muscle, thus allowing the bladder to fill more normally with a decreased frequency of urination and less chance of incontinence.

Side Effects of Anticholinergic Drugs

Considering the diverse uses of the anticholinergic drugs named previously, these drugs can obviously affect a number of different tissues. A systemically administered anticholinergic agent cannot be targeted for one specific organ without also achieving a response in other tissues as well. For instance, an antimuscarinic drug administered to decrease motility in the gastrointestinal tract may also affect other tissues containing muscarinic receptors (e.g., the bladder, bronchial smooth muscle, eye, heart). As higher doses are administered for any given problem, the chance of additional effects in tissues other than the target organ is also increased.

Consequently, antimuscarinic anticholinergic drugs are associated with a number of side effects. Exactly which symptoms (if any) will be encountered depends on a number of factors, such as the specific anticholinergic agent, the dosage of the drug, and the individual response of each patient. The most common side effects include dryness of the mouth, blurred vision, urinary retention, constipation, and tachycardia. Each of these side effects is caused by blockade of muscarinic receptors on the tissue or organ related to the side effect. Some patients also report symptoms such as confusion, dizziness, nervousness, and drowsiness, presumably because of an interaction of antimuscarinic drugs with CNS cholinergic receptors. These CNS-related symptoms occur more frequently with anticholinergic drugs that readily cross the blood-brain barrier.

SUMMARY

Drugs affecting acetylcholine-mediated responses are classified as cholinergic stimulants and anticholinergic drugs. Cholinergic stimulants increase cholinergic activity by binding to the acetylcholine receptor and activating the receptor (direct-acting stimulants) or by inhibiting the acetylcholinesterase enzyme, thus allowing more acetylcholine to remain active at the cholinergic synapse (indirect-acting stimulants). Anticholinergic drugs inhibit cholinergic activity by acting as competitive antagonists; that is, they bind to the cholinergic receptor but do not activate it.

Cholinergic stimulants and anticholinergic drugs affect many tissues in the body and are used to treat a variety of clinical problems. Cholinergic stimulants are often administered to increase gastrointestinal and urinary bladder tone; to treat conditions such as glaucoma, myasthenia gravis, and Alzheimer disease; and to reverse the neuromuscular blockade produced by curare-like drugs. Anticholinergic drugs are used principally to decrease gastrointestinal motility and secretions and to decrease the symptoms of Parkinson disease, but they may also be used to treat problems in several other physiologic systems. Because of the ability of cholinergic stimulants and anticholinergic drugs to affect many different tissues, these drugs may be associated with a number of side effects. Considering the diverse clinical applications of cholinergic stimulants and anticholinergic drugs, physical and occupational therapists may frequently encounter patients taking these drugs. Rehabilitation specialists should be aware of the rationale for drug administration, as well as possible adverse side effects of cholinergic stimulants and anticholinergic agents.

REFERENCES

1. Brown, JH and Taylor, P: Muscarinic receptor agonists and antagonists. In Hardman, JG, et al (eds): The Pharmacological Basis of Therapeutics, ed 9. McGraw-Hill, New York, 1996.
2. Demirkan, K, et al: Can we justify ipratropium therapy as initial management of acute exacerbations of COPD? Pharmacotherapy 19:838, 1999.
3. Drachman, DB: Myasthenia gravis. N Engl J Med 330:1797, 1994.
4. Ehlert, FJ, Ostrom, RS, and Sawyer, GW: Subtypes of the muscarinic receptor in smooth muscle. Life Sci 61:1729, 1997.
5. Emilien, G, et al: Prospects for pharmacological intervention in Alzheimer disease. Arch Neurol 57:454, 2000.
6. Francis, PT, et al: The cholinergic hypothesis of Alzheimer's disease: A review of progress. J Neurol Neurosurg Psychiatry 66:137, 1999.
7. Hoover, DB: Muscarinic blocking drugs. In Craig, CR and Stitzel, RE (eds): Modern Pharmacology and Clinical Applications, ed 5. Little Brown, New York, 1997.
8. Jann, MW: Rivastigmine, a new-generation cholinesterase inhibitor for the treatment of Alzheimer's disease. Pharmacotherapy 20:1, 2000.
9. Katzung, BG: Introduction to autonomic pharmacology. In Katzung, BG (ed): Basic and Clinical Pharmacology, ed 7. Appleton & Lange, Stamford, CT, 1998.
10. Katzung, BG: Cholinoceptor-blocking drugs. In Katzung, BG (ed): Basic and Clinical Pharmacology, ed 7. Appleton & Lange, Stamford, CT, 1998.
11. Krall, WJ, Sramek, JJ, and Cutler, NR: Cholinesterase inhibitors: A therapeutic strategy for Alzheimer disease. Ann Pharmacother 33:441, 1999.
12. Lesar, TS: Glaucoma. In DiPiro, JT, et al (eds): Pharmacology: A Pathophysiologic Approach, ed 4. Appleton & Lange, Stamford, CT, 1999.
13. Lindstorm, JM: Acetylcholine receptors and myasthenia. Muscle Nerve 23:453, 2000.
14. Price, NM, et al: Transdermal scopolamine in the prevention of motion sickness at sea. Clin Pharmacol Ther 29:414, 1981.
15. Sugimoto, H, et al: Donepezil hydrochloride (E2020) and other acetylcholinesterase inhibitors. Curr Med Chem 7:303, 2000.
16. Tune, LE and Sunderland, T: New cholinergic therapies: Treatment tools for the psychiatrist. J Clin Psychiatry 59(Suppl 13):31, 1998.
17. Wess, J, et al: Muscarinic acetylcholine receptors: Structural basis of ligand binding and G protein coupling. Life Sci 56:915, 1995.

CHAPTER **20**

Adrenergic Drugs

The purpose of this chapter is to describe drugs that either stimulate activity at norepinephrine synapses (adrenergic agonists) or inhibit norepinephrine influence (adrenergic antagonists). To be more specific, this chapter will focus on drugs that primarily influence activity in the sympathetic nervous system through their effect on adrenergic synapses. Norepinephrine is usually the neurotransmitter at the junction between sympathetic postganglionic neurons and peripheral tissues. Consequently, most of the adrenergic agonists discussed in this chapter are used to augment sympathetic responses, and the adrenergic antagonists are used to attenuate sympathetic-induced activity. In fact, adrenergic agonists are sometimes referred to as **sympathomimetic,** and antagonists are referred to as **sympatholytic,** because of their ability to increase and decrease sympathetic activity, respectively.

As in Chapter 19, the drugs discussed here are categorized according to a common mode of action rather than according to common clinical applications. Most of the drugs introduced in this chapter will again appear throughout this text when they are classified according to their use in treating specific problems. For instance, the beta-selective adrenergic antagonists (i.e., beta blockers; see "Beta Antagonists") are collectively introduced in this chapter. Individual beta blockers, however, are also discussed in subsequent chapters with regard to their use in specific problems, such as hypertension (see Chap. 21), angina pectoris (see Chap. 22), cardiac arrhythmias (see Chap. 23), and congestive heart failure (see Chap. 24).

The drugs described in this chapter are used to treat a variety of disorders, ranging from severe cardiovascular and respiratory problems to the symptoms of the common cold. Because of the widespread use of these drugs in cardiovascular disease and other disorders, many patients seen in physical and occupational therapy will be taking adrenergic agonists or antagonists. In this chapter, the basic pharmacodynamic mechanisms, clinical applications, and adverse effects of these drugs are introduced. The relevance of specific adrenergic drugs to physical rehabilitation is addressed in more detail in subsequent chapters that categorize their use according to specific disorders (hypertension, angina, asthma, etc.).

Many adrenergic agonists and antagonists exert their effects by binding directly to the appropriate postsynaptic receptor. Because a great deal of the specificity (or lack of specificity) of these drugs depends on the drug-receptor interaction, adrenergic receptor classes and subclasses are briefly reviewed here.

ADRENERGIC RECEPTOR SUBCLASSIFICATIONS

As discussed in Chapter 18, adrenergic receptors can be divided into two primary categories: alpha and beta receptors. Each category can then be subdivided, so that there are four common receptor subtypes: alpha-1, alpha-2, beta-1, and beta-2.[19] Adrenergic receptor subtypes are located on specific tissues throughout the body, and the response mediated by each receptor depends on the interaction between that receptor and the respective tissue. Refer to Chapter 18 for a more detailed description of adrenergic receptor locations and responses.

The primary uses of adrenergic agonists and antagonists according to their selectivity for individual receptor subtypes are summarized in Table 20–1. In general, a specific agonist is used to mimic or increase the response mediated by that receptor, whereas the antagonist is used to decrease the receptor-mediated response.

Clinically useful adrenergic agonists and antagonists display variable amounts of specificity for each receptor subtype. Some drugs are fairly specific and bind to only one receptor subtype (e.g., a specific alpha-1 agonist such as phenylephrine preferentially stimulates the alpha-1 subtype). Other drugs show a moderate amount of specificity and perhaps affect one major receptor category. An example is the nonselective beta antagonist propranolol, which blocks beta-1 and beta-2 receptors but has little or no effect on alpha receptors. Finally, other drugs such as epinephrine are rather nonspecific and affect alpha and beta receptors fairly equally. In some clinical situations, administering a

TABLE 20–1 Summary of Adrenergic Agonist and Antagonist Use According to Receptor Specificity

Primary Receptor Location: Response When Stimulated	Agonist Use(s)*	Antagonist Use(s)*
Alpha-1 receptor		
Vascular smooth muscle: vasoconstriction	Hypotension Nasal congestion Paroxysmal supraventricular tachycardia	Hypertension
Alpha-2 receptor		
CNS synapses (inhibitory): decreased sympathetic discharge (brainstem effect); inhibited neuronal excitation (spinal cord effect)	Hypertension Spasticity	No significant clinical use
Beta-1 receptor		
Heart: increased heart rate and force of contraction	Cardiac decompensation	Hypertension Arrhythmias Angina pectoris Heart failure Prevention of reinfarction
Beta-2 receptor		
Bronchioles: bronchodilation Uterus: relaxation	Prevent bronchospasm Prevent premature labor	No significant clinical use

*Primary clinical condition(s) that the agonists or antagonists are used to treat. See text for specific drugs in each category and a discussion of treatment rationale.

fairly selective drug may be desirable, whereas other problems may benefit from a drug that interacts with more than one receptor subtype. Use of selective versus nonselective adrenergic drugs is considered in the sections that describe "Adrenergic Agonists" and "Adrenergic Antagonists" in this chapter.

"Receptor selectivity," however, is a relative term. Even though an adrenergic drug is reported to be selective for only one receptor subtype, a certain affinity for other receptor subtypes may also occur to a lesser degree. A beta-1–specific drug, for instance, binds preferentially to beta-1 receptors but may also show some slight affinity for beta-2 receptors. Selectivity is also dose-related, with the relative degree of receptor selectivity decreasing as higher doses are administered. Consequently, some side effects of the so-called selective drugs may be caused by stimulation of other receptor subtypes, especially at higher drug doses.

ADRENERGIC AGONISTS

Drugs that stimulate the adrenergic receptors are presented here according to their relative specificity for each receptor subtype. The drugs that primarily activate alpha receptors are discussed first, followed by beta-selective drugs, and finally drugs that have mixed alpha and beta agonist activity.

Alpha Agonists

ALPHA-1–SELECTIVE AGONISTS

General Indications

Alpha-1 agonists bind directly to and activate the alpha-1 receptor that is located primarily on vascular smooth muscle, thus leading to smooth-muscle contraction and vasoconstriction. Because of their vasoconstrictive properties, these drugs are able to increase blood pressure by increasing peripheral vascular resistance. Consequently, certain alpha-1 agonists are administered systemically to treat acute hypotension that may occur in emergencies such as shock or during general anesthesia. A second common clinical application of these drugs is the treatment of nasal congestion (i.e., the runny nose, stuffy head feelings often associated with the common cold). In appropriate doses, alpha-1 agonists preferentially constrict the vasculature in the nasal and upper respiratory mucosa, thus decreasing the congestion and mucosal discharge. A third application of alpha-1 agonists is to decrease heart rate during attacks of paroxysmal supraventricular tachycardia. By increasing peripheral vascular resistance, these drugs bring about a reflex decrease in heart rate through the cardiac baroreceptor reflex.

Specific Agents

Mephentermine (Wyamine):   This alpha-1 stimulant is used primarily to maintain or restore blood pressure during hypotensive episodes that may occur during spinal anesthesia. It is typically administered by intravenous or intramuscular injection to allow a rapid onset.

Methoxamine (Vasoxyl):   This drug is used primarily to increase and maintain blood pressure in severe, acute hypotension, especially during general anesthesia and spinal anesthesia. It is usually administered by injection (intramuscularly or intravenously).

Oxymetazoline (Afrin, Visine, many others):   This drug is used in nose drops and nasal sprays to decrease nasal congestion through alpha-1–mediated vasoconstriction. Higher or systemic doses may also cause hypotension, presumably because of stimulation of CNS alpha-2 receptors in a manner similar to clonidine (see "Alpha-2–Selective Agonists"). Oxymetazoline can also be administered as eye drops to decrease redness and minor irritation of the eye.

Phenylephrine (Neo-Synephrine, others):   Like methoxamine, phenylephrine can be administered systemically to treat hypotension, and phenylephrine can also be used to terminate certain episodes of supraventricular tachycardia. In addition, phenylephrine is administered topically to treat nasal congestion and is found in many over-the-counter spray decongestants.

Pseudoephedrine (Novafed, Sudafed, many others):   Pseudoephedrine is administered orally for its decongestant effects, is found in many over-the-counter preparations, and is commonly used to help relieve cold symptoms.

Xylometazoline (Otrivin, Inspire Nasal Spray, others):   This drug is used primarily as a nasal spray to decrease congestion during colds and allergies.

Adverse Effects

The primary side effects associated with alpha-1–specific agonists are caused by excessive stimulation of alpha-adrenergic responses. Some of the more frequent side effects include increased blood pressure, headache, and an abnormally slow heart rate (because of reflex bradycardia). Some patients also report feelings of chest pain, difficulty breathing, and feelings of nervousness. These side effects are quite variable from patient to patient and are usually dose-related (i.e., they occur more frequently at higher doses).

ALPHA-2–SELECTIVE AGONISTS

General Indications

Alpha-2–selective drugs are used in the treatment of hypertension and for the treatment of spasticity. When treating hypertension, these drugs stimulate alpha-2 receptors located in the brain and brainstem. When stimulated, these central alpha-2 receptors exert an *inhibitory* effect on sympathetic discharge from the vasomotor center in the brainstem.[32] Diminished sympathetic discharge results in a decrease in blood pressure. The use of alpha-2 agonists in lowering blood pressure is discussed in more detail in Chapter 21.

Alpha-2 receptors have also been identified on interneurons in the spinal cord. Stimulation of these receptors causes inhibition of these interneurons, and a subsequent decrease in excitability of motor neurons supplied by these interneurons.[8,10] Alpha-2 agonists have therefore been used to normalize neuronal activity in conditions such as spasticity, and the use of these drugs as antispasticity agents is discussed in more detail in Chapter 13.

Consequently, alpha-2 agonists appear to exert their antihypertensive effects and antispasticity effects by preferentially stimulating alpha-2 receptors in the brain and spinal cord, respectively. In both situations, it is unclear whether alpha-2 agonists exert their primary effects on presynaptic or postsynaptic receptors. Stimulation of presynaptic alpha-2 receptors located at adrenergic synapses results in a decrease in norepinephrine release from the presynaptic terminal.[10] Similarly, alpha-2 receptors have also been identified postsynaptically at specific central synapses, and these postsynaptic receptors are believed to directly inhibit neuronal excitation.[10,16] Thus, alpha-2 agonists may exert their effects by stimulating either central presynaptic or postsynaptic receptors or by acting on inhibitory presynaptic and postsynaptic receptors simultaneously.

Specific Agents

Clonidine (Catapres, Duraclon):   Clonidine is used primarily as an antihypertensive and as an analgesic. Clonidine's antihypertensive effects occur because this drug stimulates alpha-2 receptors in the vasomotor center of the brainstem and decreases sympathetic discharge to the heart and vasculature. Clonidine, however, is not usually successful when used alone in the long-term treatment of essential hypertension. This drug is usually reserved for short-term management or in combination with other antihypertensive drugs, especially in patients who are unable to tolerate alpha-1 antagonists such as prazosin (see "Alpha Antagonists"). As indicated, clonidine can also be used as an analgesic, and this drug is sometimes combined with other analgesics (opioids) for treating severe pain in people with cancer. Clonidine's analgesic effects are probably mediated by stimulation of alpha-2 receptors located in the spinal cord. Because of its effects on alpha-2 receptors in the spinal cord, clonidine also has antispasticity effects. Use of this drug in spasticity, however, is often limited because it also causes hypotension. Finally, clonidine has sedative properties and has been used on occasion as an antianxiety drug or an adjunct in general anesthesia.

Guanabenz (Wytensin):   Guanabenz is used primarily to decrease blood pressure via its effect on alpha-2 receptors in the brainstem. As an antihypertensive, this drug is similar to clonidine in efficacy and clinical use.

Methyldopa (Aldomet):   Methyldopa has been used as an antihypertensive drug for some time, but its mechanism of action is poorly understood. Currently, methyldopa is believed to exert its effects by being converted to alpha-methylnorepinephrine in the body.[26] Alpha-methylnorepinephrine is a potent alpha-2 agonist that lowers blood pressure by stimulating inhibitory central adrenergic receptors in a manner similar to clonidine and guanabenz.

Tizanidine (Zanaflex):   Tizanidine is used primarily for treating spasticity.[22,23] This drug is similar to clonidine but has less vasomotor effect and is therefore less likely to cause hypotension and other cardiovascular problems. As indicated earlier, tizanidine stimulates alpha-2 receptors in the spinal cord, which results in decreased excitatory input onto the alpha motor neuron. Decreased excitation of the alpha motor neuron results in decreased spasticity of the skeletal muscle supplied by that neuron. Use of tizanidine as an antispasticity drug is addressed in more detail in Chapter 13.

Adverse Effects

Use of alpha-2–specific drugs may be associated with some relatively minor side effects such as dizziness, drowsiness, and dry mouth. More pronounced adverse effects such as difficulty in breathing, an unusually slow heart rate, and persistent fainting may indicate a toxic accumulation or overdose of these drugs.

Beta Agonists

BETA-1–SELECTIVE AGONISTS

General Indications

The beta-1 receptor is located primarily on the myocardium, and stimulation of the receptor results in increased heart rate and increased force of myocardial contraction (i.e., increased cardiac output). Consequently, beta-1 agonists are used primarily to increase cardiac output in emergency situations such as cardiovascular shock or if complications develop during cardiac surgery. Beta-1 agonists may also be used to increase cardiac function in the short-term treatment of certain types of heart disease, including heart failure.

Specific Agents

Dobutamine (Dobutrex): Dobutamine is used for short-term management of cardiac decompensation that sometimes occurs during exacerbations of heart disease or following cardiac surgery. This drug is often administered via intravenous pump infusion to allow relatively stable plasma levels.

Dopamine (Intropin): In addition to its ability to stimulate dopamine receptors, this drug directly stimulates beta-1–adrenergic receptors. At higher doses, dopamine may also indirectly stimulate adrenergic activity by increasing the release of norepinephrine from presynaptic storage sites. Clinically, this drug is used to treat cardiac decompensation in a manner similar to dobutamine. Dopamine is also used to increase cardiac output in acute or severe hypotension. Dopamine is especially useful in the management of hypotension with decreased renal blood flow. Dopamine is able to increase cardiac output by stimulating beta-1 adrenoceptors on the myocardium while vasodilating the renal vasculature through an effect on renal dopamine receptors. This effectively increases blood pressure and renal perfusion, thus facilitating normal kidney function.

Adverse Effects

Because of their cardiostimulatory effects, beta-1–selective drugs may induce side effects such as chest pain and cardiac arrhythmias in some patients. Shortness of breath and difficulty in breathing (i.e., feelings of chest constriction) have also been reported.

BETA-2–SELECTIVE AGONISTS

General Indications

One important location of beta-2 receptors is on bronchiole smooth muscle. When stimulated, the receptor mediates relaxation of the bronchioles. Consequently, most beta-2 agonists are administered to treat the bronchospasm associated with respiratory ailments such as asthma, bronchitis, and emphysema.[6,11,33] Because a nonselective beta agonist will also stimulate the myocardium (beta-1 effect), beta-2–selective agonists are often used preferentially in treating asthma, especially if the patient also has some cardiac abnormality such as ischemia or arrhythmias.[11] Another clinically important location of beta-2 receptors is on uterine muscle. When stimulated, these receptors cause inhibition or relaxation of the uterus. As a result, drugs such as ritodrine and terbutaline are used to inhibit premature uterine contractions during pregnancy, thus preventing premature labor and delivery.[4,5]

Specific Agents

Beta-2–selective bronchodilators: This group of drugs includes albuterol (Proventil, Ventolin), bitolterol (Tornalate), fenoterol (Berotec), isoetharine (Bronkometer, Bronkosol, others), metaproterenol (Alupent, others), pirbuterol (Maxair), procaterol (Pro-Air), and salmeterol (Serevent). These agents are similar pharmacologically and are used for their ability to stimulate beta-2 receptors located on pulmonary smooth muscle, thus causing bronchodilation in patients with asthma and similar conditions. Isoproterenol (Isuprel) can also be included with this group, but this drug is somewhat less beta-2–selective and affects beta-1 receptors as well. Beta-2 bronchodilators are often administered by oral inhalation so that the drug is applied directly to bronchial membranes. Albuterol and similar agents, for example, are packaged in small aerosol inhalers so that the patient can self-administer the drug at the onset of a bronchospastic attack. The use of these drugs in treating respiratory conditions is addressed in more detail in Chapter 26.

Ritodrine (Yutopar):   The primary clinical application of this drug is to inhibit premature labor.[4] Ritodrine activates uterine beta-2 receptors, which mediate relaxation of uterine muscle. This drug is usually administered initially via intravenous pump infusion, and maintenance therapy is accomplished through oral administration.

Terbutaline (Brethine, Bricanyl):   Terbutaline is usually administered by oral inhalation for the treatment of bronchospasm (i.e., similar to albuterol). Terbutaline has also been administered systemically to inhibit premature labor and thus prolong pregnancy (i.e., similar to ritodrine).

Adverse Effects

The primary side effects associated with beta-2–specific drugs include nervousness, restlessness, and trembling. These adverse symptoms may be caused by stimulation of central beta-adrenergic receptors. There is also some suggestion that excessive use of beta-2 agonists may cause increased airway hyperresponsiveness that could lead to severe and possibly fatal asthmatic attacks.[6,35] This fact has generated debate about the safe and effective use of these drugs in treating asthma, and the contemporary use of beta-2 agonists, along with other antiasthmatic drugs, is described in Chapter 26. When used to prevent premature labor, drugs such as ritodrine have also been associated with increases in maternal heart rate and systolic blood pressure, as well as maternal pulmonary edema. These changes in maternal cardiopulmonary function can be quite severe and may be fatal to the mother.

Drugs with Mixed Alpha and Beta Agonist Activity

GENERAL INDICATIONS

Several drugs are available that display a rather mixed agonistic activity with regard to adrenergic receptor subtypes. Some drugs such as epinephrine appear to be able to stimulate all four adrenergic receptor subtypes. Other drugs such as norepinephrine bind to both types of alpha receptors, bind to beta-1 receptors to a lesser extent, and show little or no affinity for beta-2 receptors. Another group of indirect adrenergic agonists (ephedrine, metaraminol) appear to act as nonselective agonists because of their ability to increase the release of norepinephrine from presynaptic storage sites. Because of the ability of many of these multiple-receptor drugs to affect a number of adrenoceptor subtypes, their clinical uses are quite varied. Specific agents with mixed agonistic activity and their respective applications are presented here.

SPECIFIC AGENTS

Amphetamines: Drugs such as amphetamine (generic), dextroamphetamine (Dexedrine, others), and methamphetamine (Desoxyn) are known for their powerful sympathomimetic effects. These drugs appear to increase norepinephrine release and decrease norepinephrine reuptake and breakdown at adrenergic synapses, thus increasing activity at synapses with norepinephrine-sensitive receptors (i.e., alpha-1, alpha-2, and beta-1 receptors). These drugs may also exert similar effects on certain dopaminergic synapses. Amphetamines are used on a limited basis to treat attention-deficit disorder in children and to increase mental alertness in adults with narcolepsy. Use of these drugs to suppress appetite or to combat normal sleepiness is discouraged because of their high potential for abuse, and these drugs are classified in the United States as schedule II controlled substances (see Chap. 1 for a description of controlled substance classification).

Ephedrine (generic): Ephedrine appears to preferentially stimulate alpha-1, alpha-2, and beta-1 adrenoceptors by increasing the release of norepinephrine at synapses that use these receptor subtypes. This drug is used primarily for its alpha-1 effects and can be used to treat severe, acute hypotension. When treating hypotension in emergency situations (e.g., shock), ephedrine is administered systemically by injection (intravenously, intramuscularly, or subcutaneously). Because of its ability to stimulate alpha-1 receptors in the nasal mucosa, ephedrine is also used as a nasal decongestant. As a decongestant, ephedrine is typically combined with other agents (antitussives, antihistamines) to form cough and cold products. Ephedrine is also sometimes administered as a bronchodilator (beta-2 agonist effect), but the use of this drug in asthma and related conditions has generally been replaced by safer agents (see Chap. 26). Finally, ephedrine has been administered to produce a general excitatory effect on central adrenergic receptors and has been used to treat conditions associated with a decrease in CNS arousal (e.g., narcolepsy).

Epinephrine (Adrenalin, Bronkaid Mist, Primatene Mist, others): Epinephrine appears to directly stimulate all adrenergic receptor subtypes and is administered for a variety of reasons. Epinephrine is found in many antiasthmatic inhalation products because of its ability to stimulate beta-2 receptors on the bronchi. Because it stimulates vascular alpha-1 receptors, epinephrine may be applied topically to produce local vasoconstriction and control bleeding during minor surgical procedures (e.g., suturing superficial wounds). Likewise, epinephrine may be mixed with a local anesthetic when the anesthetic is injected during minor surgical and dental procedures. The vasoconstriction produced by the epinephrine prevents the anesthetic from being washed away by the local blood flow, thus prolonging the effects of the anesthetic. Because of a potent ability to stimulate the heart (beta-1 effect), epinephrine is frequently administered during cardiac arrest to re-establish normal cardiac rhythm. Finally, epinephrine is often the drug of choice in treating anaphylactic shock. Anaphylactic shock is a hypersensitive allergic reaction marked by cardiovascular collapse (decreased cardiac output, hypotension) and severe bronchoconstriction. Epinephrine is ideally suited to treat this problem because of its ability to stimulate the heart (beta-1 effect), vasoconstrict the periphery (alpha-1 effect), and dilate the bronchi (beta-2 effect).

Metaraminol (Aramine): Metaraminol appears to act like ephedrine; that is, metaraminol increases the release of presynaptic norepinephrine and thereby stimulates alpha-1, alpha-2, and beta-1 receptors. This drug is usually administered by injection (intramuscularly, intravenously, or subcutaneously) to treat hypotension occurring in shock or general anesthesia.

Norepinephrine (Levophed): Norepinephrine stimulates both types of alpha receptors as well as beta-1 receptors but displays very little agonistic activity toward beta-2 receptors. It is usually administered intravenously to treat hypotension during shock or general anesthesia.

Phenylpropanolamine (Acutrim, Dexatrim, Propagest, others):   The exact mechanism of this drug is unclear. Although it may directly stimulate alpha and beta receptors, this drug probably exerts its effects by increasing the release of presynaptic norepinephrine; thus, phenylpropanolamine is an indirect-acting, nonselective agonist. Because of its alpha-1 agonist properties, phenylpropanolamine can be used as a nasal decongestant. Phenylpropanolamine also appears to act as an appetite suppressant or "diet" drug by increasing the release of norepinephrine within the hypothalamus. In this regard, it is similar to amphetamine-like compounds, which may also suppress feeding behavior by increasing adrenergic influence in the brain. Finally, this drug can help treat urinary incontinence, presumably because of an effect on alpha receptors that inhibit contraction of the bladder. Phenylpropanolamine is taken orally for nasal decongestion, appetite suppression, or urinary incontinence.

ADVERSE EFFECTS

Because of the general ability of many of the drugs described previously to produce CNS excitation, some of the primary side effects are nervousness, restlessness, and anxiety. Because these agents also tend to stimulate the cardiovascular system, prolonged or excessive use may also lead to complications such as hypertension, arrhythmias, and even cardiac arrest. When used to treat bronchospasm, prolonged administration via inhalation may also cause some degree of bronchial irritation with some agents.

ADRENERGIC ANTAGONISTS

Adrenergic antagonists or blockers bind to adrenergic receptors but do not activate the receptor. These agents are often referred to as sympatholytic drugs because of their ability to block the receptors that typically mediate sympathetic responses (i.e., alpha and beta receptors). Clinically useful adrenergic antagonists usually show a fairly high degree of specificity for one of the major receptor classifications. They tend to bind preferentially to either alpha- or beta-adrenergic receptors. Specific drugs may show an additional degree of specificity within the receptor class. For instance, a beta blocker may bind rather selectively to only beta-1 receptors, or it may bind fairly equally to both beta-1 and beta-2 receptors.

The general clinical applications of alpha antagonists and beta antagonists are presented here. Specific agents within each major group are also discussed.

Alpha Antagonists

GENERAL INDICATIONS

Alpha antagonists are administered primarily to reduce peripheral vascular tone by blocking the alpha-1 receptors located on vascular smooth muscle. When stimulated by endogenous catecholamines (norepinephrine, epinephrine), the alpha-1 receptor initiates vasoconstriction.

Consequently, alpha antagonists are used in conditions where peripheral vasodilation would be beneficial. A principal application of these agents, for instance, is in treating hypertension.[12,36] These drugs seem to attenuate the peripheral vasoconstriction mediated by excessive adrenergic influence, thus decreasing blood pressure through a decrease in peripheral vascular resistance. These agents may also be used in patients with a pheochromocytoma, which is a tumor that produces large quantities of epinephrine and norepinephrine. Alpha antagonists are often administered prior to and during the removal of such a tumor, thus preventing the hypertensive crisis that may occur from excessive alpha-1 stimulation from catecholamines released from the tumor. Similarly, alpha antagonists have been used to successfully prevent and treat the sudden increase in blood pressure that often occurs during an autonomic crisis. These drugs have been used to promote vasodilation in conditions of vascular insufficiency, including peripheral vascular disease and Raynaud phenomenon. However, the success of these drugs in treating vascular insufficiency has been somewhat limited.

A group of drugs known collectively as *ergot alkaloids* display some alpha-blocking ability as well as other unique properties. Ergot alkaloids, which include the ergoloid mesylates and ergotamine, are used clinically for diverse problems, including treatment of vascular headache and improvement of mental function in presenile dementia.

Because the primary uses of alpha antagonists involve their ability to decrease vascular tone, the clinically useful alpha antagonists tend to be somewhat alpha-1 selective. Alpha-2 receptors should not be selectively antagonized because this event may ultimately lead to an *increase* in peripheral vascular tone through an increase in sympathetic discharge. Certain alpha-2 receptors are located in the brainstem, and stimulation of these receptors appears to decrease sympathetic outflow from the vasomotor center. Thus, blocking these centrally located alpha-2 receptors is counterproductive when a decrease in vascular tone is desired.

SPECIFIC AGENTS

Ergoloid mesylates (Gerimal, Hydergine):   These compounds, also known as dihydrogenated ergot alkaloids, exhibit some ability to produce peripheral vasodilation by blocking peripheral alpha-1 receptors. The primary clinical application of ergoloid mesylates is to increase mental acuity and alertness in geriatric patients with dementia related to Alzheimer disease. These drugs supposedly increase mental function by increasing cerebral blood flow or by increasing oxygen utilization in the brain. The mechanism of action of these drugs is probably a moot point, however, because there is no evidence that they produce any significant clinical benefits in treating dementia of the Alzheimer type.[39] These drugs are usually administered orally or sublingually.

Ergotamine (Ergomar, Ergostat):   Ergotamine and similar drugs such as dihydroergotamine exert a number of complex effects. At higher doses, these drugs act as competitive alpha antagonists, hence their inclusion here. However, these drugs appear to produce vasoconstriction in blood vessels that have low vascular tone and vasodilation in vessels that have high vascular tone. Exactly how they accomplish these rather contradictory effects is unclear, but these drugs essentially function as partial agonists because they display agonistic (stimulatory) activity in vessels with low tone and antagonistic (inhibitory) activity in vessels with high tone. Clinically, these drugs are used for their ability to prevent or abort vascular headaches (migraine, cluster headaches) by vasoconstricting cerebral vessels[28]; that is, their alpha-agonistic ability in dilated cerebral vessels may explain their primary clinical usefulness. These drugs can also stimulate 5-hydroxytryptamine (serotonin) receptors, and some, if not all, of their antimigraine effects have been attributed to an agonistic effect on vascular serotonin receptors.[30,31] When used in headache suppression, these drugs are administered by a number of routes, including oral, oral inhalation, sublingual, rectal, and even injection. These drugs are sometimes combined with other agents (caffeine, belladonna, barbiturates, antihistamines) for treatment of vascular headaches.

Phenoxybenzamine (Dibenzyline): Phenoxybenzamine is a noncompetitive alpha-1 blocker, which essentially means that it binds irreversibly to the alpha-1 receptor. This drug tends to have a slow onset, but its effects last much longer than those of the competitive blockers (e.g., phentolamine and prazosin). Phenoxybenzamine is used primarily to control blood pressure prior to and during the removal of a pheochromocytoma. This drug is not typically used for the long-term management of hypertension, however, because it produces several side effects including reflex tachycardia. Other indications for phenoxybenzamine include treatment of urinary retention in benign prostatic hypertrophy and treatment of vasospastic disease (Raynaud phenomenon). Phenoxybenzamine is usually administered orally.

Phentolamine (Regitine): Phentolamine is a competitive alpha antagonist used primarily to control blood pressure during management of pheochromocytoma. The drug is usually administered via intravenous or intramuscular injection. Phentolamine is not usually used to treat essential hypertension because with prolonged use, effectiveness tends to decrease and patients begin to develop adverse side effects such as hypotension, cardiac arrhythmias, and myocardial ischemia.

Prazosin (Minipress): Prazosin is a competitive alpha-1 antagonist that has emerged as one of the primary alpha-1 selective agents. It tends to produce vasodilation in both arteries and veins, and is used primarily in the long-term management of essential hypertension.[38] Prazosin has also been used to reduce alpha-1 receptor-mediated activity in congestive heart failure, Raynaud phenomenon, pheochromocytoma, and benign prostatic hypertrophy. Prazosin is administered orally.

Other alpha-1 receptor antagonists: Several new alpha-1–selective antagonists have been developed, and some of the more promising agents include doxazosin (Cardura)[14,37,38] and terazosin (Hytrin).[20,36] These drugs are gaining favor in treating hypertension because they lower blood pressure while producing beneficial effects on serum lipid profiles (decreased total cholesterol, decreased triglycerides) and on glucose metabolism.[12,20,36–38] These drugs are typically administered orally, and their role in treating hypertension will be discussed in more detail in Chapter 21.

ADVERSE EFFECTS OF ALPHA-1 ANTAGONISTS

One of the primary adverse effects associated with alpha antagonists is reflex tachycardia. By blocking alpha-1 receptors, these drugs tend to decrease blood pressure by decreasing peripheral vascular resistance. As blood pressure falls, a compensatory increase in cardiac output is initiated via the baroreceptor reflex. The increased cardiac output is mediated in part by an increase in heart rate, hence the reflex tachycardia. A second major problem with these drugs is orthostatic hypotension. Dizziness and syncope following changes in posture are quite common because of the decrease in peripheral vascular tone. With alpha antagonists, orthostatic hypotension may be a particular problem just after drug therapy is initiated, in geriatric patients, or following exercise.

Beta Antagonists

GENERAL INDICATIONS

Beta antagonists are generally administered for their effect on the beta-1 receptors that are located on the heart.[15,17] When stimulated, these receptors mediate an increase in cardiac contractility and rate of contraction. By blocking these receptors, beta antagonists reduce the rate and force of myocardial contractions. Consequently, beta antagonists are frequently used to decrease cardiac workload in conditions such as hypertension and certain types of angina pectoris. Beta blockers may also be used to normalize heart rate in certain forms of cardiac arrhythmias. Specific clinical applications of individual beta blockers are summarized in Table 20–2.

Another important function of beta blockers is their ability to limit the extent of myocardial damage following a heart attack and to reduce the risk of fatality following myocardial infarction.[7,9,18,25] Apparently, these drugs help reduce the workload of the damaged heart, thus allowing the heart to recover more completely following infarction. Likewise, there is increasing evidence that some beta blockers can help improve cardiac function in certain types of heart failure,[3,24,27] and this idea is addressed in more detail in Chapter 24.

Clinically useful beta antagonists are classified as beta-1 selective if they predominantly affect the beta-1 subtype, or beta nonselective if they have a fairly equal affinity for beta-1 and beta-2 receptors (see Table 20–2). Beta-1–selective drugs are also referred to as *cardioselective* because of their preferential effect on the myocardium. Even if a beta antagonist is nonselective (i.e., blocks both beta-1 and beta-2 receptors), the beta-1 blockade is clinically beneficial. When stimulated, beta-2 receptors, which are found primarily on bronchial smooth muscle, cause bronchodilation. Blockade of these beta-2 receptors may lead to smooth-muscle contraction and bronchoconstriction. Thus, drugs that selectively block beta-2 receptors have no real clinical significance because they promote bronchoconstriction.[34]

Currently, a number of beta blockers are used clinically; selection of a specific agent depends on factors such as cardioselectivity, duration of action (half-life), and several other ancillary properties of each drug. Certain beta blockers, for instance, produce added effects such as mild peripheral vasodilation or stabilization of cardiac membranes that

TABLE 20–2 Summary of Common Beta Blockers

Generic Name	Trade Name(s)	Selectivity	Primary Indications*
Acebutolol	Sectral	Beta-1	Hypertension, arrhythmias
Atenolol	Tenormin	Beta-1	Angina pectoris, hypertension, prevent reinfarction
Betaxolol	Kerlone	Beta-1	Hypertension
Bisoprolol	Zebeta	Beta-1	Hypertension
Carteolol	Cartrol	Nonselective	Hypertension
Labetalol	Normodyne, Trandate	Nonselective	Hypertension
Metoprolol	Lopressor, Toprol-XL	Beta-1	Angina pectoris, hypertension, prevent reinfarction
Nadolol	Corgard	Nonselective	Hypertension, angina pectoris
Penbutolol	Levatol	Nonselective	Hypertension
Pindolol	Visken	Nonselective	Hypertension
Propranolol	Inderal	Nonselective	Angina pectoris, arrhythmias, hypertension, prevent reinfarction, prevent vascular headache
Sotalol	Betapace	Nonselective	Arrhythmias
Timolol	Blocadren	Nonselective	Hypertension, prevent reinfarction, prevent vascular headache

*Only indications listed in the United States product labeling are included in this table. All drugs are fairly similar pharmacologically, and some may be used for appropriate cardiovascular conditions not specifically listed in product labeling.

can be beneficial in treating certain cardiovascular conditions.[13,34,40] Primary indications and the relative selectivity of these drugs are summarized in Table 20–2. Clinical applications of specific beta blockers are discussed in more detail in Chapters 21 through 24.

SPECIFIC AGENTS

Acebutolol (Sectral):   Acebutolol is described as a relatively cardioselective beta blocker that tends to bind preferentially to beta-1 receptors at lower doses but binds to both types of beta receptors as dosages increase. This drug also exerts mild to moderate intrinsic sympathomimetic activity, which means that acebutolol not only blocks the beta receptor from the effects of endogenous catecholamines but also stimulates the receptor to some extent (i.e., it acts as a partial beta agonist). This advantage protects the beta receptor from excessive endogenous stimulation while still preserving a low level of background sympathetic activity. Primary clinical applications are for treatment of hypertension and for prevention and treatment of cardiac arrhythmias. The drug is usually administered orally.

Atenolol (Tenormin):   Like acebutolol, atenolol is regarded as beta-1 selective but tends to be less beta specific at higher doses. The drug is administered orally for the long-term treatment of hypertension and chronic, stable angina. Atenolol is also administered immediately following a myocardial infarction to prevent reinfarction and promote recovery of the myocardium.

Betaxolol (Kerlone):   This drug is a relatively beta-1–selective agent that is administered orally for treating hypertension.

Bisoprolol (Zebeta):   This drug is similar to betaxolol.

Carteolol (Cartrol):   Carteolol is a nonselective beta blocker that also has moderate intrinsic sympathomimetic activity. It is typically administered orally to treat hypertension.

Labetalol (Normodyne, Trandate):   Labetalol is a nonselective beta blocker. This drug also appears to have some alpha-1–selective blocking effects. Labetalol is used primarily in the management of hypertension and, although usually given orally, may be injected intravenously in emergency hypertensive situations.

Metoprolol (Lopressor, Toprol-XL):   Metoprolol is considered a cardioselective beta blocker and has been approved for treating hypertension, for preventing angina pectoris, and for preventing myocardial reinfarction. As an antihypertensive and antianginal, metoprolol is usually administered orally. In the prevention of reinfarction, metoprolol is initiated by intravenous injection and then followed up by oral administration.

Nadolol (Corgard):   Nadolol is a nonselective beta blocker that is administered orally as an antihypertensive and antianginal agent. This drug has somewhat of an advantage over other nonselective beta blockers (propranolol) in that nadolol often needs to be taken only once each day.

Penbutolol (Levatol):   This drug is similar to carteolol.

Pindolol (Visken):   Pindolol is a nonselective beta blocker that also exhibits the highest level of intrinsic sympathomimetic activity of the beta blockers. Pindolol is used primarily in the long-term management of hypertension, but this drug may also be used to prevent certain types of angina pectoris.

Propranolol (Inderal):   Propranolol, the classic nonselective beta blocker, is approved for use in hypertension, angina pectoris, cardiac arrhythmias, and prevention of myocardial reinfarction. In addition, propranolol has been used in the prevention of vascular headache and as an adjunct to alpha blockers in treating pheochromocytoma. Propranolol is usually administered orally for the long-term management of the conditions listed previously, but it may be administered via intravenous injection for the immediate control of arrhythmias.

Sotalol (Betapace): This drug is a nonselective beta blocker that is administered primarily to treat arrhythmias, although it is also sometimes used as an antihypertensive or antianginal agent. It is administered orally.

Timolol (Blocadren): This nonselective beta blocker is administered orally for treatment of hypertension and prevention of myocardial reinfarction. It may also be used to treat angina or prevent vascular headaches.

ADVERSE EFFECTS

When nonselective beta blockers are used, some antagonism of beta-2 receptors also occurs.[2] The antagonism of beta-2 receptors on bronchiole smooth muscle often leads to some degree of bronchoconstriction and an increase in airway resistance. Although this event is usually not a problem in individuals with normal pulmonary function, patients with respiratory problems such as asthma, bronchitis, and emphysema may be adversely affected by nonselective beta antagonists. In these patients, one of the beta-1–selective drugs should be administered.

Selective and nonselective beta blockers are also associated with several other adverse effects. The most serious of these effects results from excessive depression of cardiac function.[29] By slowing down the heart too much, these agents can lead to cardiac failure, especially if there is some pre-existing cardiac disease. Because of their antihypertensive properties, beta blockers may produce orthostatic hypotension, and dizziness and syncope may occur following abrupt changes in posture. Patients taking beta blockers for prolonged periods have also been reported to have an increase in centrally related side effects such as depression, lethargy, and sleep disorders.[1,21] These behavioral side effects may be because of interaction of the beta blockers with CNS receptors.

Various other relatively minor side effects have also been reported, including gastrointestinal disturbances (nausea, vomiting) and allergic responses (fever, rash). However, these are fairly uncommon and tend to be resolved by adjusting the dosage or the specific type of medication.

Other Drugs That Inhibit Adrenergic Neurons

GENERAL INDICATIONS

Several agents are available that inhibit activity at adrenergic synapses by interfering with the release of norepinephrine. Rather than directly blocking the postsynaptic receptor, these drugs typically inhibit or deplete the presynaptic terminal of stored norepinephrine. These drugs are used primarily to decrease peripheral adrenergic influence and to treat problems such as hypertension and cardiac arrhythmias.

SPECIFIC AGENTS

Bretylium (Bretylol): Bretylium appears to directly inhibit the release of norepinephrine from adrenergic nerve terminals. With prolonged use, this drug may also replace presynaptic norepinephrine in a manner similar to guanadrel and guanethidine (see the next two agent listings in this section). Bretylium is used primarily in the treatment of cardiac arrhythmias (see Chap. 23). In addition to its effect on norepinephrine release, bretylium also appears to have a direct stabilizing effect on cardiac muscle cells that contributes to this drug's antiarrhythmic properties. Although usually given orally for the long-term management of ventricular arrhythmias, bretylium is injected intravenously for the emergency treatment of ventricular tachycardia and ventricular fibrillation.

Guanadrel (Hylorel):   Guanadrel is taken up by the presynaptic terminal and appears to directly inhibit the release of norepinephrine. With prolonged use, guanadrel slowly replaces norepinephrine in the presynaptic vesicles. This substitution of guanadrel for norepinephrine further inhibits activity at postsynaptic adrenergic synapses by creating a false neurotransmitter. Guanadrel also replaces stored norepinephrine in the adrenal medulla, thus decreasing adrenal influence on cardiovascular function. Guanadrel is administered orally for management of hypertension.

Guanethidine (Ismelin):   Similar in action and effects to guanadrel, this drug is actively transported into the presynaptic terminal by the norepinephrine pump, where it inhibits norepinephrine release and later replaces stored norepinephrine. Unlike guanadrel, guanethidine selectively affects postganglionic sympathetic adrenergic nerve terminals and does not affect release of norepinephrine from the adrenal medulla. Guanethidine is usually administered orally for the management of moderate-to-severe hypertension.

Metyrosine (Demser):   Metyrosine inhibits the enzyme that initiates catecholamine synthesis (epinephrine, norepinephrine), and this drug is used to diminish catecholamine stores prior to removal of a catecholamine-producing tumor (pheochromocytoma).

Rauwolfia alkaloids: This chemical group includes reserpine (Serpalan), deserpidine (Harmonyl), and rauwolfia serpentina (Raudixin, Rauval, others). These drugs all inhibit the synthesis of catecholamines (norepinephrine, epinephrine) as well as 5-hydroxytryptamine (serotonin) in peripheral and CNS sympathetic nerve endings. This inhibition eventually causes a depletion of presynaptic neurotransmitter stores in several tissues including postganglionic nerve terminals, adrenal medulla, and brain. Unlike guanethidine and guanadrel, these agents do not appear to actually replace the presynaptic neurotransmitter but simply prevent more transmitter from being resynthesized. Reserpine and the other rauwolfia alkaloids are administered orally to treat mild-to-moderate hypertension. The antihypertensive effects of these drugs are caused, in part, by the inhibition of peripheral adrenergic nerve terminals, although some of their antihypertensive effects may also be because of the inhibition of CNS catecholamine activity.

ADVERSE EFFECTS

Orthostatic hypotension is occasionally a problem with the aforementioned drugs, and dizziness and syncope sometimes occur after a sudden change in posture. Some patients also experience gastrointestinal disturbances including nausea, vomiting, and diarrhea. Peripheral edema, as evidenced by swelling in the feet and legs, has also been reported.

SUMMARY

This chapter classifies and describes a variety of drugs according to their stimulatory (agonistic) or inhibitory (antagonistic) effect on adrenergic function. In general, adrenergic agonists are administered according to their ability to evoke specific tissue responses via specific adrenergic receptors. Alpha-1–adrenergic agonists are used as antihypotensive agents because of their ability to increase peripheral vascular resistance; they may also be used as nasal decongestants because of their ability to vasoconstrict the nasal mucosa. Agonists selective for alpha-2 receptors are administered to treat hypertension and spasticity because of their ability to inhibit neuronal activity in the brainstem and spinal cord, respectively. Cardioselective beta-1 agonists are used primarily for their ability to stimulate the heart, and beta-2 agonists are used in the treatment of asthma and premature labor because of their ability to relax bronchiole and uterine smooth muscle, respectively.

Alpha-adrenergic antagonists are used primarily as antihypertensive drugs because of their ability to block vascular alpha-1 receptors. Beta-adrenergic antagonists (beta blockers) are administered primarily for their inhibitory effects on myocardial function and are used in the prevention and treatment of hypertension, angina pectoris, arrhythmias, heart failure, and myocardial reinfarction. Many of the drugs introduced in this chapter are discussed further in later chapters that deal with specific clinical conditions (e.g., hypertension, asthma).

REFERENCES

1. Avorn, J, Everitt, DE, and Weiss, S: Increased antidepressant use in patients prescribed beta-blockers. JAMA 255:357, 1986.
2. Bauer, K, Rakusen, S, and Kaik, G: Pulmonary effects of long-term beta-2 blockade in healthy subjects: Comparative study of oral metoprolol OROS. Am Heart J 120(Suppl):473, 1990.
3. Bristow, MR: Pathophysiologic and pharmacologic rationales for clinical management of chronic heart failure with beta-blocking agents. Am J Cardiol 71:C12, 1993.
4. Canadian Preterm Labor Investigators Group: Treatment of preterm labor with the beta-adrenergic agonist ritodrine. N Engl J Med 327:308, 1992.
5. Caritis, SN: Treatment of preterm labour. A review of therapeutic options. Drugs 26:243, 1983.
6. Chung, KF: The current debate concerning beta-agonists in asthma. A review. J R Soc Med 86:96, 1993.
7. Ciccone, CD: Current trends in cardiovascular pharmacology. Phys Ther 76:481, 1996.
8. Coward, DM: Tizanidine: Neuropharmacology and mechanism of action. Neurology 44(Suppl 9):S6, 1994.
9. Cruickshank, JM: Beta-blockers: Primary and secondary prevention. J Cardiovasc Pharmacol 20(Suppl 11):S55, 1992.
10. Delwaide, PJ and Pennisi, G: Tizanidine and electrophysiologic analysis of spinal control mechanisms in humans with spasticity. Neurology 44(Suppl 9):S21, 1994.
11. Executive Committee, American Academy of Allergy and Immunology: Inhaled beta-2 adrenergic agonists in asthma. J Allergy Clin Immunol 91:1234, 1993.
12. Frishman, WH and Kotob, F: Alpha-adrenergic blocking drugs in clinical medicine. J Clin Pharmacol 39:7, 1999.
13. Frolich, ED: Vasodilating beta-blockers: Systemic and regional hemodynamic effects. Am Heart J 121:1012, 1991.
14. Fulton, B, Wagstaff, AJ, and Sorkin, EM: Doxazosin. An update of its clinical pharmacology and therapeutic applications in hypertension and benign prostatic hyperplasia. Drugs 49:295, 1995.
15. Gerber, JG and Nies, AS: Beta-adrenergic blocking drugs. Annu Rev Med 36:145, 1985.
16. Gillis, RA, Gatti, PJ, and Quest, JA: Mechanism of the anti-hypertensive effect of alpha-2 agonists. J Cardiovasc Pharmacol 7(Suppl 8):S38, 1985.
17. Hansson, L: Review of state-of-the-art beta-blocker therapy. Am J Cardiol 67:43B, 1991.
18. Held, P: Effects of beta-blockers on ventricular dysfunction after myocardial infarction: Tolerability and survival effects. Am J Cardiol 71:39C, 1993.
19. Hoffman, BB: Adrenoceptor-activating and other sympathomimetic drugs. In Katzung, BG (ed): Basic and Clinical Pharmacology, ed 7. Appleton & Lange, Stamford, CT, 1998.
20. Horky, K: Alpha-1 blockade in the management of hypertension. J Clin Pharmacol 33:874, 1993.
21. Koella, WP: CNS-related effects of beta-blockers with special reference to mechanisms of action. Eur J Clin Pharmacol 28(Suppl 1):55, 1985.
22. Lataste, X, et al: Comparative profile of tizanidine in the management of spasticity. Neurology 44(Suppl 9):S53, 1994
23. Lawson, K: Tizanidine: A therapeutic weapon for spasticity? Physiotherapy 84:418, 1998.

24. Leung, W-H, et al: Improvement in exercise performance and hemodynamics by labetalol in patients with idiopathic dilated cardiomyopathy. Am Heart J 119:884, 1990.
25. Levy, S: Secondary prevention after myocardial infarction: In favor of beta-blockers. J Cardiovasc Pharmacol 16(Suppl 6):S50, 1990.
26. Oates, JA: Antihypertensive agents and the drug therapy of hypertension. In Hardman, JG, et al (eds): The Pharmacological Basis of Therapeutics, ed 9. McGraw-Hill, New York, 1996.
27. Packer, M: Beta-adrenergic blockade in chronic heart failure: Principles, progress, and practice. Prog Cardiovasc Dis 41(Suppl 1):39, 1998.
28. Peatfield, R: Migraine. Current concepts of pathogenesis and treatment. Drugs 26:364, 1983.
29. Peel, C and Mossberg, KA: Effects of cardiovascular medications on exercise responses. Phys Ther 75:387, 1995.
30. Peroutka, SJ: 5-Hydroxytryptamine receptor subtypes and the pharmacology of migraine. Neurology 43(Suppl 3):34, 1993.
31. Raskin, NJ: Acute and prophylactic treatment of migraine: Practical approaches and pharmacologic rationale. Neurology 43(Suppl 3):39, 1993.
32. Reid, JL, et al: Clinical pharmacology of drugs acting on imidazoline and adrenergic receptors. Studies with clonidine, moxonidine, rilmenidine, and atenolol. Ann N Y Acad Sci 763:673, 1995.
33. Sears, MR: Asthma treatment: Inhaled beta-agonists. Can Respir J 5(Suppl A):54A, 1998.
34. Shanks, RG: Clinical pharmacology of vasodilating beta-blocking drugs. Am Heart J 121:1006, 1991.
35. Spitzer, WO, et al: The use of beta-agonists and the risk of death and near death from asthma. N Engl J Med 326:501, 1992.
36. Symposium (various authors): Clinical application of alpha$_1$-receptor blockade: Terazosin in the management of hypertension. J Clin Pharmacol 33:866, 1993.
37. Symposium (various authors): Management of coronary heart disease risk factors in hypertensive patients: Clinical experience with doxazosin. Am Heart J 121:245, 1991.
38. Taylor, SH and Grimm, RH: New developments in the role of alpha$_1$-adrenergic receptors in cardiovascular disease. Am Heart J 119:655, 1990.
39. Thompson, TL, et al: Lack of efficacy of hydergine in patients with Alzheimer's disease. N Engl J Med 323:445, 1990.
40. Turner, P: Which ancillary properties of beta-adrenoceptor blocking drugs influence their therapeutic or adverse effects: A review. J R Soc Med 84:672, 1991.

CHAPTER 21

Antihypertensive Drugs

Hypertension is defined as a sustained, reproducible increase in blood pressure. Hypertension is one of the most common diseases affecting adults living in industrialized nations. In the United States, for example, hypertension occurs in approximately 26 percent of white men and 17 percent of white women who are between 35 and 45 years of age.[7] The prevalence of this disease in 35- to 45-year-old black men and black women is estimated at 44 and 37 percent, respectively.[7] If left untreated, the sustained increase in blood pressure associated with hypertension can lead to cardiovascular problems (stroke, heart failure), renal disease, and blindness.[25,44,49,51,102] These and other medical problems ultimately lead to an increased mortality rate in hypertensive individuals.

Although there is a general consensus regarding the adverse effects of hypertension, some debate exists as to exactly how much of an increase in blood pressure constitutes hypertension. Generally, diastolic values greater than 90 mm Hg and/or systolic values greater than 140 mm Hg warrant a diagnosis of hypertension. A more detailed classification scheme is shown in Table 21–1. Patients are often classified as having stage 1, stage 2, or stage 3, depending on the extent of their elevated blood pressure. As might be expected, the incidence of morbidity and mortality increases as the hypertension becomes more severe. Hence, pharmacologic and nonpharmacologic methods are often implemented to decrease blood pressure to diastolic values between 80 and 85 mm Hg and systolic values between 130 and 140 mm Hg.[44]

Hypertension is often described as a silent killer because of the lack of symptoms throughout most of the course of this disease. Patients may feel perfectly well into the advanced stages of hypertension. Rehabilitation specialists dealing with hypertensive patients are usually treating some problem other than the increased blood pressure (i.e., hypertension is not the reason the patient is referred to physical therapy and occupational therapy). Considering the prevalence of hypertension, however, many patients receiving therapy for various other problems will also be taking antihypertensive drugs, so some knowledge of the pharmacology of these agents is essential.

The pharmacologic management of hypertension has evolved to where blood pressure can be controlled for extended periods in most patients. There are currently several major categories of antihypertensive agents, and new drugs are continually being added to the antihypertensive arsenal. Each group of antihypertensive drugs is discussed under the appropriate section in this chapter, as well as how several different drugs can be used together when treating hypertension. To better understand how these drugs work

TABLE 21–1 Classification of BP*

Category	Systolic BP (mm Hg)	Diastolic BP (mm Hg)
Optimal	<120	<80
Normal	<130	<85
High normal	130–139	85–89
Hypertension		
Stage 1	140–159	90–99
Stage 2	160–179	100–109
Stage 3	≥180	≥110

*The diastolic pressure is the primary value used to make a diagnosis of stage 1, 2, or 3 hypertension. "Isolated" hypertension indicates an increase in only the systolic value, with the diastolic pressure remaining relatively normal.

Source: From The Sixth Report of the National Committee on Detection, Evaluation, and Treatment of High Blood Pressure (JNC-VI). Arch Intern Med 157:2413, 1997, with permission.

in decreasing blood pressure, the normal control of blood pressure and the possible mechanisms that generate a hypertensive state are briefly discussed here.

NORMAL CONTROL OF BLOOD PRESSURE

Blood pressure is normally maintained by the complex interaction of several physiologic systems.[43] Short-term control of blood pressure is accomplished primarily by the baroreceptor reflex[48] (see Chap. 18). The baroreceptor reflex monitors and corrects changes in blood pressure within a matter of seconds by altering cardiac output and peripheral vascular resistance. The more long-term management of blood pressure is accomplished primarily by the kidneys through their control of fluid balance. Changes in blood pressure through the renal handling of fluid and electrolytes usually take place over a period of several hours to several days. Humoral factors such as circulating catecholamines (from the adrenal gland), arginine vasopressin (from the pituitary gland), and angiotensin II (from a reaction involving the kidney) can also play a role in regulating blood pressure, especially if blood pressure decreases suddenly. Together, these various systems interact to maintain blood pressure within a fairly narrow range.

Although the control of blood pressure is a fairly complex subject, the actual factors that determine blood pressure can be simplified somewhat. At any given time, blood pressure is the product of cardiac output and the total resistance in the peripheral vasculature. This relationship is illustrated by the following equation:

$$BP = (CO) \times (TPR)$$

where BP = blood pressure, CO = cardiac output, and TPR = total peripheral resistance in the systemic vasculature. As indicated by this equation, BP can be maintained at a relatively constant level by changes in either CO or TPR. A decrease in CO, for instance, can potentially be offset by an increase in TPR so that BP does not appreciably change. Conversely, a sudden fall in TPR will necessitate an increase in CO if BP is to be maintained.

The relevance of this simple equation to antihypertensive therapy will become apparent as different drugs are discussed. Some antihypertensive drugs exert their effects primarily by acting on CO, others primarily affect TPR, and some agents decrease both factors in an attempt to lower blood pressure.

PATHOGENESIS OF HYPERTENSION

Essential versus Secondary Hypertension

Hypertension can be divided into two major categories: secondary hypertension and primary, or essential, hypertension. In secondary hypertension, the elevated blood pressure can be attributed to some specific abnormality such as renal artery stenosis, catecholamine-producing tumors, endocrine disorders, or cerebral damage. The treatment of secondary hypertension is rather straightforward, with efforts focused on correcting the underlying pathology (e.g., the cause of the problem can be dealt with directly by surgery). Secondary hypertension, however, accounts for only about 5 percent of the patients diagnosed with hypertension.[47] The remaining 95 percent of hypertensive individuals are classified as having primary, or essential, hypertension. In essential hypertension, there is no clear, readily discernible cause of the elevated blood pressure.

Consequently, the exact cause of hypertension in the majority of patients is unknown. Many theories have been proposed to explain how blood pressure increases and eventually becomes sustained in essential hypertension. Some of the major factors that may account for the increased blood pressure in essential hypertension are presented here.

Possible Mechanisms in Essential Hypertension

The voluminous literature dealing with potential causes and mechanisms of essential hypertension cannot be fully reviewed here. As stated previously, the exact cause of hypertension in most patients is not known. There appears to be a rather complex interaction of genetic and environmental factors that ultimately leads to adaptive changes in the cardiovascular system of the patient with essential hypertension.[32,38,84,92] Diet, stress, and other external factors, for example, are associated with increased blood pressure. These factors seem to be more influential in certain patients, suggesting a possible genetic predisposition to hypertension. Other risk factors such as cigarette smoking and alcohol abuse clearly play a role in potentiating the onset and maintenance of hypertension. The point is that essential hypertension is probably not caused by only one factor but rather by a subtle, complex interaction of many factors. The exact way in which these factors interact probably varies from person to person, so that the cause of this disease really must be regarded individually rather than according to one common etiology.

Despite the fact that the actual cause of hypertension is unknown, studies in humans and in animal models that mimic essential hypertension have suggested that the sympathetic nervous system may be a final common pathway in mediating and perpetuating the hypertensive state; that is, the factors described earlier may interact in such a way as to cause a general increase in sympathetic activity, which then becomes the common denominator underlying the elevated blood pressure in essential hypertension.[22,26,59,71,128] Increased sympathetic activity should produce a hypertensive effect because of the excitatory effect of sympathetic neurons on the heart and peripheral vasculature. Increased sympathetic drive may initially increase blood pressure by increasing cardiac output. In later stages, cardiac output often returns to normal levels, with the increased blood pressure then due to an increase in vascular resistance. The reasons for this shift from elevated cardiac output to elevated peripheral vascular resistance are somewhat unclear. A sustained increase in sympathetic activity, however, may be the initiating factor that begins a sequence of events ultimately resulting in essential hypertension.

Once blood pressure does become elevated, hypertension seems to become self-perpetuating to some extent. Mechanisms that control blood pressure (the baroreceptor reflex), for example, may decrease in sensitivity, thus blunting the normal response to elevated pressure.[48] Increased sympathetic discharge to the kidneys and altered renal hemodynamics may also cause changes in renal function that contribute to the sustained increase in blood pressure.[16,62] Metabolic changes, including decreased sensitivity to insulin and problems with lipid metabolism, may also occur, and these changes seem to play a role in perpetuating hypertension.[56,95]

The increased blood pressure may also invoke adaptive changes in the peripheral vasculature so that peripheral vessels become less compliant and vascular resistance increases[88,107,109]; that is, increased pressure on the vascular wall causes thickening of the wall, which further increases the resistance to blood flow through the thickened vessels. The peripheral vasculature may also become more reactive to pressor substances such as norepinephrine and angiotensin II.[6,17] Hypertension is likewise associated with a defect in the production of vasoactive substances by the cells lining the peripheral vasculature (i.e., the vascular endothelium). The vascular endothelium normally produces several vasoactive substances, including vasodilators (nitric oxide, bradykinin, prostaglandin I_2) and vasoconstrictors (angiotensin II, endothelin I).[74,105] These endothelial-derived substances help maintain local control over vascular resistance.[5,76] In hypertension, however, there may be a defect in the production of these substances, especially decreased production of nitric oxide.[4,9,74,78,82,85] A relative deficiency of this vasodilator would result in increased vascular resistance, which helps increase the hypertension.

The possible factors involved in initiating and maintaining essential hypertension are summarized in Figure 21–1. Ultimately, certain environmental factors may turn on the sympathetic division of the autonomic nervous system in susceptible individuals. Increased sympathetic discharge then creates a vicious cycle whereby increased sympathetic effects in conjunction with the increased blood pressure itself help perpetuate the hypertension. Exactly how various factors initiate the increased sympathetic discharge is not fully understood and may in fact vary from patient to patient. It is hoped that future studies will elaborate on the exact role of such factors in causing essential hypertension and that treatment can then be focused on preventing the changes that initially increase blood pressure.

DRUG THERAPY

Several major categories of drugs exist for the treatment of essential hypertension. These categories include diuretics, sympatholytic drugs, vasodilators, drugs that inhibit the renin-angiotensin system, and calcium channel blockers. The primary sites of action and effects of each category are summarized in Table 21–2. The mechanism of action, rationale for use, specific agents, and adverse effects of drugs in each category are discussed in the next few sections of this chapter.

DIURETICS

Mechanism of Action and Rationale for Use

Diuretics increase the formation and excretion of urine. These drugs are used as antihypertensive agents because of their ability to increase the renal excretion of water and

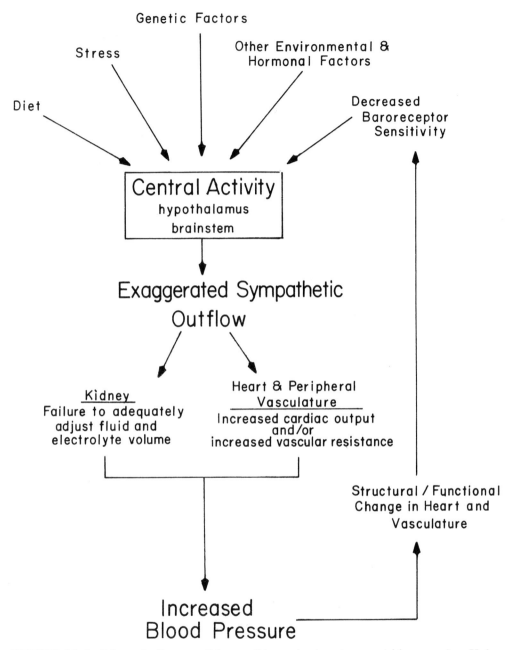

FIGURE 21–1. Schematic diagram of the possible mechanisms in essential hypertension. Various factors interact to turn on sympathetic outflow to the kidneys, heart, and peripheral vasculature, resulting in elevated blood pressure. Hypertension also causes structural and functional changes in the vasculature that help maintain the elevated pressure.

sodium, thus decreasing the volume of fluid within the vascular system. This situation is somewhat analogous to the decrease in pressure that would occur inside a balloon if some of the air inside the balloon were allowed to leak out. Consequently, diuretics appear to have a rather direct effect on blood pressure through their ability to simply decrease the amount of fluid in the vascular system.

TABLE 21–2 Antihypertensive Drug Categories

Category	Primary Site(s) of Action	Primary Antihypertensive Effect(s)
Diuretics	Kidneys	Decrease plasma fluid volume
Sympatholytics	Various sites within the sympathetic division of the autonomic nervous system	Decrease sympathetic influence on the heart and/or peripheral vasculature
Vasodilators	Peripheral vasculature	Lower vascular resistance by directly vasodilating peripheral vessels
Inhibition of the renin-angiotensin system (ACE inhibitors and angiotensin II receptor blockers)	Peripheral vasculature and certain organs with a functional renin-angiotensin system (heart, kidneys)	ACE inhibitors: prevent the conversion of angiotensin I to angiotensin II. Angiotensin II receptor blockers: block the effects of angiotensin II on the vasculature and various other tissues
Calcium channel blockers	Limit calcium entry into vascular smooth muscle and cardiac muscle	Decrease vascular smooth-muscle contraction; decrease myocardial force and rate of contraction

Diuretics are often the first type of drugs used to treat hypertension.[15,51,93] They are relatively inexpensive and seem to work well for a large percentage of patients with mild-to-moderate hypertension.[40] The use of diuretics alone and in conjunction with other antihypertensives is discussed in more detail in "Stepped-Care Approach to Hypertension" later in this chapter.

Although they differ chemically, all diuretics exert their beneficial effects by acting directly on the kidneys to increase water and sodium excretion.[1,69] Diuretic drugs can be subclassified according to their chemical structure or the manner in which they affect kidney function. The primary subclassifications of diuretics are listed here.

Classification of Diuretics

Thiazide Diuretics. Thiazide drugs share a common chemical nucleus as well as a common mode of action. These drugs act primarily on the early portion of the distal tubule of the nephron, where they inhibit sodium reabsorption. By inhibiting sodium reabsorption, more sodium is retained within the nephron, creating an osmotic force that also retains more water in the nephron. Because more sodium and water are passed through the nephron, from which they will ultimately be excreted from the body, a diuretic effect is produced. Thiazides are the most frequently used type of diuretic for hypertension. Specific types of thiazide drugs are listed in Table 21–3.

Loop Diuretics. These drugs act primarily on the ascending limb of the loop of Henle within the nephron (hence the term "loop diuretic"). They exert their diuretic effect by inhibiting the reabsorption of sodium and chloride from the nephron, thereby also preventing the reabsorption of water that follows these electrolytes. Specific types of loop diuretics are listed in Table 21–3.

Potassium-Sparing Diuretics. Several different drugs with diuretic properties are classified as potassium-sparing because of their ability to prevent potassium secretion into the distal tubule of the nephron. Normally, a sodium-potassium exchange occurs in the distal tubule, whereby sodium is reabsorbed and potassium is secreted. Potassium-sparing agents interfere with this exchange in various ways (depending on the specific

TABLE 21–3 Diuretic Drugs Used to Treat Hypertension

Thiazide diuretics	Loop diuretics
Bendroflumethiazide (Naturetin)	Bumetanide (Bumex)
Chlorothiazide (Diuril)	Ethacrynic acid (Edecrin)
Chlorthalidone (Hygroton, others)	Furosemide (Lasix, others)
Hydrochlorothiazide (Esidrix, others)	*Potassium-sparing diuretics*
Hydroflumethiazide (Diucardin, Saluron)	
Methyclothiazide (Enduron, others)	Amiloride (Midamor)
Metolazone (Diulo, Zaroxolyn)	Spironolactone (Aldactone)
Polythiazide (Renese)	Triamterene (Dyrenium)
Quinethazone (Hydromox)	
Trichlormethiazide (Metahydrin, Naqua)	

drug) so that potassium is spared from secretion and sodium remains in the tubule, from which it is excreted. Although these agents do not produce a diuretic effect to the same extent as the loop and thiazide drugs, potassium-sparing drugs have the advantage of reducing potassium loss and thus preventing potassium depletion (hypokalemia). Specific potassium-sparing drugs are listed in Table 21–3.

Adverse Effects of Diuretics

The most serious side effects of diuretics are fluid depletion and electrolyte imbalance.[1,113] By the very nature of their action, diuretics decrease extracellular fluid volume as well as produce sodium depletion (**hyponatremia**) and potassium depletion (**hypokalemia**). Hypokalemia is a particular problem with the thiazide and loop diuretics but occurs less frequently when the potassium-sparing agents are used. Hypokalemia and other disturbances in fluid and electrolyte balance can produce serious metabolic and cardiac problems and may even prove fatal to some individuals. Consequently, patients must be monitored closely, and the drug dosage should be maintained at the lowest effective dose. Also, potassium supplements are used in some patients to prevent hypokalemia.

Fluid depletion may also be a serious problem during diuretic therapy. A decrease in blood volume may cause a reflex increase in cardiac output and peripheral vascular resistance because of activation of the baroreceptor reflex (see Chap. 18). This occurrence may produce an excessive demand on the myocardium, especially in patients with cardiac disease. Decreased blood volume may also activate the renin-angiotensin system, thereby causing further peripheral vasoconstriction and increased cardiac workload. Again, these effects of fluid depletion may be especially serious in patients with certain types of heart failure.

Less serious, but bothersome, side effects of diuretic therapy include gastrointestinal disturbances and weakness and fatigue. **Orthostatic hypotension** may occur because of the relative fluid depletion produced by these drugs. Changes in mood and confusion may also develop in some patients.

SYMPATHOLYTIC DRUGS

As discussed previously, the preponderance of evidence indicates that an increase in sympathetic activity may be an underlying factor in essential hypertension. Conse-

TABLE 21–4 Sympatholytic Drugs Used to Treat Hypertension

Beta blockers

    Acebutolol (Sectral)
    Atenolol (Tenormin)
    Betaxolol (Kerlone)
    Bisoprolol (Zebeta)
    Carteolol (Cartrol)
    Labetalol (Normodyne; Trandate)
    Metoprolol (Lopressor, others)
    Nadolol (Corgard)
    Oxprenolol (Trasicor)
    Penbutolol (Levatol)
    Pindolol (Visken)
    Propranolol (Inderal)
    Sotalol (Betapace)
    Timolol (Blocadren)

Alpha blockers

    Doxazosin (Cardura)
    Phenoxybenzamine (Dibenzyline)
    Prazosin (Minipress)
    Terazosin (Hytrin)

Presynaptic adrenergic inhibitors

    Guanadrel (Hylorel)
    Guanethidine (Ismelin)
    Reserpine (Serpalan, others)

Centrally acting agents

    Clonidine (Catapres)
    Guanfacine (Tenex)
    Guanabenz (Wytensin)
    Methyldopa (Aldomet)

Ganglionic blockers

    Mecamylamine (Inversine)
    Trimethaphan (Arfonad)

quently, drugs that interfere with sympathetic discharge (i.e., sympatholytic agents) should be valuable as antihypertensive agents. These sympatholytic drugs can be classified according to where and how they interrupt sympathetic activity. Sympatholytic drugs used to treat hypertension include beta-adrenergic blockers, alpha-adrenergic blockers, presynaptic adrenergic neurotransmitter depletors, centrally acting drugs, and ganglionic blockers (Table 21–4). Each of these categories is discussed here.

Beta Blockers

MECHANISM OF ACTION AND RATIONALE FOR USE

Beta-adrenergic blockers have been used extensively to decrease blood pressure and are a mainstay of antihypertensive therapy in many patients.[46,61,63] Beta blockers exert their primary effect on the heart, where they decrease the heart rate and force of myocardial contraction. In hypertensive patients, these drugs lower blood pressure by slowing down the heart and reducing cardiac output. This statement, however, is probably an oversimplification of how beta blockers produce an antihypertensive effect. In addition to their direct effect on the myocardium, beta blockers also produce a general decrease in sympathetic tone.[47] Exactly how this decrease in sympathetic activity occurs remains to be determined. Some theories suggest (1) that beta blockers may have a central inhibitory effect on sympathetic activity, (2) that they influence renin release from the kidneys and within the CNS, (3) that they impair sympathetic activity in the ganglia or at the presynaptic adrenergic terminals, or (4) that they act by a combination of these and other factors.[47] Regardless of the exact mechanism of their action, beta blockers continue to be used extensively in treating hypertension, and these agents seem to be especially helpful in reducing the risk of certain hypertension-related complications such as myocardial infarction and stroke.[61,63]

SPECIFIC AGENTS

Beta-adrenergic blockers that are approved for use in hypertension are listed in Table 21–4. These drugs are all effective in decreasing blood pressure, but certain beta blockers have additional properties that make them more suitable in specific patients.[120] As discussed in Chapter 20, some beta blockers are relatively selective for beta-1 receptors (cardioselective) and tend to affect the heart more than the lungs and other tissues (see Table 20–2). Certain beta blockers such as pindolol and acebutolol function as partial agonists and are said to have *intrinsic sympathomimetic activity* because they block the effects of excessive endogenous catecholamines while still producing a normal background level of sympathetic stimulation to the heart.[21,33] Some agents such as labetalol and propranolol are able to normalize the excitability of the cardiac cell membrane; these drugs are said to have *membrane-stabilizing activity*.[21,120] Finally, carvedilol and some of the newer "third-generation" beta blockers produce peripheral vasodilation as well as cardiac beta blockade, making these drugs especially useful in decreasing blood pressure.[30,35,87,111,116] Some newer agents may likewise have other beneficial side effects such as antioxidant properties and the ability to decrease lipid abnormalities and insulin resistance.[30,56,87,104] Hence, selection of a specific beta blocker is based on these additional properties, along with consideration for the individual needs of each patient.

ADVERSE EFFECTS

Nonselective beta blockers (i.e., those with a fairly equal affinity for beta-1 and beta-2 receptors) may produce bronchoconstriction in patients with asthma and similar respiratory disorders. Cardiovascular side effects include excessive depression of heart rate and myocardial contractility as well as orthostatic hypotension. Other side effects include depression, fatigue, gastrointestinal disturbances, and allergic reactions. Beta blockers are generally well tolerated by most patients, however, and the incidence of severe side effects is relatively low.

Alpha Blockers

MECHANISM OF ACTION AND RATIONALE FOR USE

Drugs that block the alpha-1–adrenergic receptor on vascular smooth muscle will promote a decrease in vascular resistance.[11,34] Because total peripheral vascular resistance often increases in essential hypertension, blocking vascular adrenergic receptors should be an effective course of action. In a sense, alpha blockers act directly on the tissues that ultimately mediate the increased blood pressure—that is, the peripheral vasculature. In the past, the use of alpha blockers in mild-to-moderate essential hypertension was somewhat limited because these drugs are sometimes *too* effective and tended to cause problems with hypotension.[31]

It is now recognized that alpha-1 antagonists may offer specific advantages in treating hypertension, including an ability to improve blood lipid profiles (decreased triglycerides and total cholesterol, increased high-density lipoprotein–cholesterol ratio) and produce a favorable effect on glucose metabolism and insulin resistance.[11,34,54,55,115,122] Newer agents such as doxazosin also appear to have fewer adverse cardiovascular side effects, such as reflex tachycardia, presumably because these agents are longer-acting and do not cause a sudden fall in blood pressure.[36] Hence, alpha-1 blockers are gaining acceptance in the treatment of mild-to-moderate hypertension; they are also included in the antihypertensive regimen of patients with more severe cases of high blood pressure.

Alpha-1 blockers can also be used to treat the symptoms of benign prostatic hypertrophy because they decrease sympathetic-mediated contraction of smooth muscle located in the prostate gland.[36,97] Reduction of muscle tone in the prostate decreases constriction of the ureter, thereby improving urinary flow and the ability to empty the bladder.

SPECIFIC AGENTS

The characteristics of individual alpha blockers are discussed in Chapter 20. Basically, these drugs can be differentiated according to their relative alpha-1 selectivity, duration of action, and other pharmacokinetic properties. Prazosin has been the primary alpha blocker used in the past, but newer agents such as doxazosin and terazosin are gaining acceptance in treating hypertension. Prazosin and other alpha blockers approved as antihypertensives are listed in Table 21–4.

ADVERSE EFFECTS

One of the primary problems with alpha blockers is reflex tachycardia. When peripheral vascular resistance falls because of the effect of these drugs, the baroreceptor reflex often responds by generating a compensatory increase in heart rate. This tachycardia may be a significant problem, especially if there is any history of cardiac disease. To prevent reflex tachycardia, a beta blocker may be administered with the alpha blocker. The beta blocker will negate the increase in heart rate that is normally mediated through the sympathetic innervation to the heart. Alternatively, use of a longer-acting drug (doxazosin) may reduce the risk of reflex tachycardia because these agents produce a milder and more prolonged decrease in blood pressure following administration. Hence, reflex mechanisms that control blood pressure (i.e., the baroreflex) are not suddenly activated, as would be the case if blood pressure was reduced more rapidly with a shorter-acting drug.

The other major adverse effect with alpha blockers is orthostatic hypotension. Blockade of alpha-1 receptors in peripheral arteries and veins often promotes pooling of blood in the lower extremities when a patient stands up. Therapists should be alert for the symptoms of orthostatic hypotension (i.e., dizziness and syncope), especially for the first few days that an alpha blocker is administered.

Presynaptic Adrenergic Inhibitors

MECHANISM OF ACTION AND RATIONALE FOR USE

Drugs that inhibit the release of norepinephrine from the presynaptic terminals of peripheral adrenergic neurons may be used effectively in some individuals with hypertension. Some agents, such as reserpine, inhibit the presynaptic synthesis and storage of norepinephrine in peripheral and CNS adrenergic neurons.[47,124] Other agents (guanadrel, guanethidine) replace norepinephrine in peripheral sympathetic neurons, thus creating a false neurotransmitter.[91] In either case, depletion of norepinephrine from the presynaptic terminal decreases sympathetic-mediated excitation of the heart and peripheral vasculature, resulting in decreased blood pressure.

SPECIFIC AGENTS

Drugs that inhibit the presynaptic synthesis and storage of norepinephrine are discussed in Chapter 20. The drugs in this category used to treat hypertension are listed in Table 21–4. These drugs are often used in conjunction with other agents in the stepped-care approach to hypertension (see "Stepped-Care Approach to Hypertension").

ADVERSE EFFECTS

Orthostatic hypotension is sometimes a problem with these agents. Other bothersome side effects include gastrointestinal disturbances such as nausea, vomiting, and diarrhea.

Centrally Acting Agents

MECHANISM OF ACTION AND RATIONALE FOR USE

Several drugs currently available seem to inhibit sympathetic discharge from the brainstem. Sympathetic discharge from the vasomotor center appears to be influenced by two types of neuronal receptors located in the brainstem: alpha-2 adrenergic receptors and imidazoline type I1 receptors. Stimulation of these receptors results in a *decrease* in sympathetic discharge to the heart and vasculature. Centrally acting sympatholytics are therefore characterized as agonists for either one type or possibly both types of these receptors. Clonidine, for example, is considered to be primarily an alpha-2 agonist, although this drug also has some ability to stimulate imidazoline receptors.[42,124] Newer agents in this category such as moxonidine and rilmenidine seem to be more selective for imidazoline receptors.[24,108,127] In either case, stimulation of these centrally located receptors results in a decrease in sympathetic outflow and a subsequent decrease in cardiovascular stimulation and blood pressure.[99,103,108,127] Consequently, centrally acting drugs offer a unique approach to hypertension because these drugs limit sympathetic activity at the source (brainstem vasomotor center) rather than at the periphery (cardiovascular neuroeffector junction).

SPECIFIC AGENTS

The primary drugs in this category are clonidine, guanabenz, guanfacine, and methyldopa (see Table 21–4). The first three drugs act directly primarily on the alpha-2 receptor, whereas methyldopa acts as an alpha-2 agonist after being converted in vivo to alpha-methylnorepinephrine. As indicated, moxonidine and rilmenidine act primarily on imidazoline receptors. These imidazoline-specific drugs are still fairly experimental at the present time, and these agents may gain more widespread acceptance in the future.

ADVERSE EFFECTS

At therapeutic doses, these drugs are associated with some troublesome but relatively minor side effects, including dry mouth, dizziness, and sedation. The incidence of sedation seems to be related to the alpha-2 stimulatory effects of these drugs. Hence, agents that are more selective for imidazoline receptors seem to be tolerated better because patients are more alert and have less psychomotor slowing.[24,99,103,124,127]

Ganglionic Blockers

MECHANISM OF ACTION AND RATIONALE FOR USE

Drugs that block synaptic transmission at autonomic ganglia will dramatically and effectively reduce blood pressure by decreasing systemic sympathetic activity.[119] These agents are essentially nicotinic cholinergic antagonists (see Chap. 18), which block transmission at the junction between presynaptic and postsynaptic neurons in sympathetic and parasympathetic pathways. Because of the effect of these agents on both divisions of the autonomic nervous system, ganglionic blockers are used very sparingly in treating hypertension. Currently, these drugs are used primarily to reduce blood pressure in emergency situations, such as a hypertensive crisis.[8]

SPECIFIC AGENTS

Ganglionic blockers currently used to decrease blood pressure in a hypertensive crisis are listed in Table 21–4.

ADVERSE EFFECTS

As might be expected, ganglionic blockers produce a multitude of side effects because of the inhibition of both sympathetic and parasympathetic responses. Some adverse effects include gastrointestinal discomfort (nausea, constipation), urinary retention, visual disturbances, and orthostatic hypotension. At higher doses, they may even exhibit some neuromuscular blocking activity. These and other side effects may be quite severe in some patients. Fortunately, ganglionic blockers are usually not used for extended periods of time because the patient is placed on other antihypertensive drugs when the hypertensive crisis is resolved.

VASODILATORS

Mechanism of Action and Rationale for Use

Drugs that directly vasodilate the peripheral vasculature will produce an antihypertensive effect by decreasing peripheral vascular resistance.[47,129] Although other drugs such as the alpha blockers may ultimately produce vasodilation by interrupting adrenergic supply to the vasculature, the vasodilators exert an inhibitory effect directly on vascular smooth-muscle cells. Vasodilators are believed to inhibit smooth-muscle contraction by increasing the intracellular production of second messengers such as cyclic guanosine monophosphate (cyclic GMP) (see Chap. 4). Increased amounts of cyclic GMP inhibit the function of the contractile process in the vascular smooth-muscle cell, thus leading to vasodilation.

Specific Agents

The primary vasodilators used in hypertension are hydralazine (Apresoline) and minoxidil (Loniten) (Table 21–5). These drugs are not usually the first medications used in patients with hypertension but tend to be added to the drug regimen if other agents

TABLE 21–5 Antihypertensive Vasodilators, ACE Inhibitors,
Angiotensin II Receptor Blockers, and Calcium Channel Blockers

Vasodilators	
Diazoxide (Hyperstat)	Minoxidil (Loniten)
Hydralazine (Apresoline)	Nitroprusside (Nipride, Nitropress)

ACE Inhibitors	
Benazepril (Lotensin)	Moexipril (Univasc)
Captopril (Capoten)	Quinapril (Accupril)
Enalapril (Vasotec)	Ramipril (Altace)
Fosinopril (Monopril)	Trandolapril (Mavik)
Lisinopril (Prinivil, Zestril)	

Angiotensi2.n II Receptor Blockers	
Candesartan (Atacand)	Losartan (Cozaar)
Irbesartan (Avapro)	Valsartan (Diovan)

Calcium Channel Blockers	
Diltiazem (Cardizem)	Nicardipine (Cardene)
Felodipine (Plendil)	Nifedipine (Adalat, Procardia)
Isradipine (DynaCirc)	Verapamil (Calan, Isoptin)

(diuretics, beta blockers) prove inadequate.[67] Hydralazine is likewise used to lower blood pressure in emergency situations such as severe pre-eclampsia or malignant hypertension.[67,98] Other vasodilators include diazoxide (Hyperstat) and nitroprusside (Nipride, Nitropress), but these drugs are usually given only in emergency situations to treat a patient in hypertensive crisis.[67]

Nitric oxide also produces vasodilation in vascular smooth muscle. As indicated earlier, hypertension may be perpetuated by a defect in the production of nitric oxide by the vascular endothelium. It follows that providing nitric oxide directly or administering precursors for nitric oxide production may help reduce vascular resistance and decrease arterial pressure in specific hypertensive syndromes.[78] To date, inhaled nitric oxide has been used to treat acute pulmonary hypertension associated with respiratory distress syndrome in newborns and adults.[29,66] Future studies are needed to determine if nitric oxide administration may also be an effective way to treat systemic (essential) hypertension.

Adverse Effects

Although vasodilators are effective in lowering blood pressure, these drugs are associated with a number of adverse effects. Reflex tachycardia often occurs because of baroreflex responses that attempt to compensate for the fall in vascular resistance produced by these drugs. This side effect is analogous to the increased heart rate that often occurs when alpha blockers are used to decrease peripheral vascular resistance. Other common reactions include dizziness, postural hypotension, weakness, nausea, fluid retention, and headaches. Minoxidil also increases hair growth on the face, ears, forehead, and other hairy body surfaces. This increased hair growth is often a cause for discontinued use of this drug by women. Some men, however, have applied minoxidil cutaneously to treat baldness, and a topical preparation of this drug (Rogaine) is marketed as a potential hair-growth stimulant.

INHIBITION OF THE RENIN-ANGIOTENSIN SYSTEM

Mechanism of Action and Rationale for Use

The renin-angiotensin system involves several endogenous components that help regulate vascular tone in various organs and tissues.[43] In the systemic circulation, the renin-angiotensin system acts by a sequence of events that are summarized in Figure 21–2. Renin is an enzyme produced primarily in the kidneys. When blood pressure falls, renin is released from the kidneys into the systemic circulation. Angiotensinogen is a peptide that is produced by the liver and circulates continually in the bloodstream. When renin contacts angiotensinogen, angiotensinogen is transformed into angiotensin I. The circulating angiotensin I is then transformed by angiotensin-converting enzyme into angiotensin II. The converting enzyme is located in the vasculature of many tissues, especially the lung. Angiotensin II is an extremely potent vasoconstrictor. Consequently, the fall in blood pressure that activated the renin-angiotensin system is rectified by the increase in vascular resistance caused by angiotensin II.

The sequence of events just described illustrates the role of the systemic renin-angiotensin system in normal blood pressure regulation. Exactly what goes wrong with this system in patients with essential hypertension is not fully understood. Some patients display increased levels of circulating renin, hence their classification as having

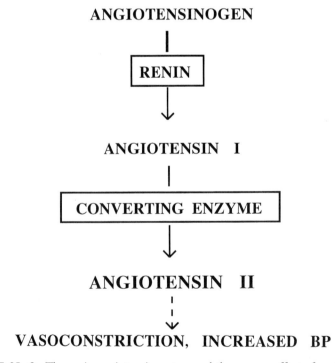

FIGURE 21–2. The renin-angiotensin system and the pressor effect of angiotensin II.

high-renin hypertension. Why plasma renin production is elevated in these patients, however, is often unclear. In addition to problems in circulating levels of renin and angiotensin II, there may also be problems with the renin-angiotensin system in specific tissues or organs. For instance, a complete, functioning renin-angiotensin system has been identified within the brain[28,37] and in the heart and vascular walls.[121,126] This fact suggests that some of the hypertensive effects of this system may be mediated through CNS mechanisms or by changes directly in the vascular tissues.

Nonetheless, activation of the renin-angiotensin system is extremely detrimental in people with high blood pressure. Excess production of angiotensin II causes vasoconstriction that perpetuates the hypertensive condition. More important, angiotensin II is a powerful stimulant of vascular tissue growth, and sustained production of angiotensin II results in thickening and hypertrophy of the vascular wall.[39,88] The thickened vascular wall causes a decrease in the lumen of the vessel, thereby causing additional resistance to blood flow and increased hypertension. In other words, angiotensin II causes abnormal remodeling of the vascular wall that results in a rather permanent increase in vascular resistance.[39]

Fortunately, two pharmacologic strategies have been developed to inhibit the effects of abnormal renin-angiotensin system activation. The first strategy involves drugs that inhibit the enzyme that converts angiotensin I to angiotensin II. Hence, these drugs are commonly referred to as angiotensin-converting enzyme (ACE) inhibitors. ACE inhibitors therefore decrease the hypertensive effects of angiotensin II by limiting the production of this compound. More recently, a second strategy has emerged in the form of drugs that block angiotensin II receptors on various tissues.[60,90] Angiotensin II stimulates vascular and other tissues by binding to a protein receptor (specifically, the AT1 angiotensin II receptor) on these tissues.[123] Newer drugs, known as angiotensin II blockers or antagonists, have therefore been developed to block these receptors, thereby negating the harmful effects of angiotensin II on vascular and other tissues.

ACE inhibitors and angiotensin II blockers have been important additions to the antihypertension arsenal. These drugs can be used alone or in conjunction with other drugs for the long-term control of high blood pressure.[52] In fact, these drugs appear to have several advantages over other antihypertensives, such as a lower incidence of cardiovascular side effects (i.e., less reflex tachycardia and orthostatic hypotension).[57,106] The ability of these drugs to inhibit angiotensin II–induced vascular hypertrophy and remodeling is also recognized as an important benefit during treatment of high blood pressure.[13,72,121] These drugs are likewise extremely beneficial in decreasing morbidity and mortality associated with congestive heart failure, and use of these drugs in heart failure will be addressed in Chapter 24.

Specific Agents

ACE inhibitors and angiotensin II blockers used to treat hypertension are listed in Table 21–5. These drugs have been shown to be effective in many cases of mild-to-moderate essential hypertension, and they may be used alone or in combination with beta blockers or diuretics.

Adverse Effects

ACE inhibitors are generally well tolerated in most patients. Some individuals may experience an allergic reaction as evidenced by skin rash. This reaction usually disappears when the dosage is reduced or when administration is discontinued. Patients may also experience a persistent dry cough that is annoying but relatively harmless. Other problems (gastrointestinal discomfort, dizziness, chest pain) may occur in some patients, but major adverse effects are relatively rare.

Angiotensin II blockers are also well tolerated, and these drugs do not cause the cough associated with ACE inhibitors.[60,90,101,123] Hence, the angiotensin II blockers appear to be as effective as ACE inhibitors but may be better tolerated in patients who experience side effects such as coughing.[50,64]

CALCIUM CHANNEL BLOCKERS

Drugs that selectively block calcium entry into vascular smooth muscle cells were originally developed to treat certain forms of angina pectoris and cardiac arrhythmias (Chaps. 22 and 23, respectively). Calcium channel blockers are now recognized as beneficial in the treatment of essential hypertension.[14,19,53] Calcium appears to play a role in activating the contractile element in smooth muscle much in the same way that calcium initiates actin-myosin interaction in skeletal muscle cells. Drugs that block calcium entry into vascular smooth muscle will inhibit the contractile process, leading to vasodilation and decreased vascular resistance.[45,68,100] Calcium channel blockers also tend to decrease heart rate and myocardial contraction force, and some of their antihypertensive properties may derive from their inhibitory effect on the heart.[45,65] Consequently, calcium channel blockers have gained popularity over the last several decades as one of the primary treatments for high blood pressure.[117]

Some issues, however, have developed fairly recently regarding the safety of these drugs in treating hypertension. Several studies noted that use of certain calcium channel blockers was associated with an increased risk of myocardial infarction when these drugs were administered to certain hypertensive people (older adults, people with diabetes, patients with unstable angina).[12,73,83] Even though these findings occurred with only certain types of calcium channel blockers (e.g., the short-acting form of nifedipine), the possibility that these drugs could increase the risk of cardiovascular problems caused a great deal of debate about the general safety of this group of drugs.[81] Likewise, other studies suggested that calcium channel blockers may increase the risk of cancer, presumably because these drugs interfere with the normal role that calcium plays in regulating cell growth and turnover.[80] Subsequent studies, however, have failed to establish a clear link between calcium channel blockers and cancer.[23,73,80,83]

Consequently, the popularity of calcium channel blockers as antihypertensives has diminished somewhat over the past few years. These drugs still play a prominent role in the antihypertensive arsenal, but practitioners are more cautious about using these drugs to lower blood pressure in certain types of patients.[12,114] It has also been recommended that longer-acting or sustained-release forms of these drugs be used whenever possible, because they do not cause as sudden a change in blood pressure as their short-acting counterparts and may therefore be somewhat safer.[12,112]

Specific Agents

The primary calcium channel blockers used to treat hypertension are listed in Table 21–5. These agents differ somewhat, and they can be subclassified into several categories according to their chemistry and how they block calcium channels.[75,96] Despite their chemical diversity, however, calcium channel blockers all act by limiting calcium entry into cardiovascular tissues.[100] These agents have all been shown to be effective in treating hypertension, and selection of a specific agent is typically based on the side effect profile of each drug and the individual needs of each patient. As mentioned earlier, several agents are also available in longer-acting (sustained-release) forms, and use of these longer-acting agents may help reduce the risk of certain cardiovascular side effects (reflex tachycardia, orthostatic hypotension). Because calcium channel blockers are also important in treating angina, the pharmacology of these drugs is discussed in more detail in Chapter 22.

Adverse Effects

These drugs may cause excessive vasodilation, as evidenced by swelling in the feet and ankles, and some patients may also experience orthostatic hypotension. Abnormalities in heart rate (too fast, too slow, irregular) may also occur, and reflex tachycardia, caused by excessive peripheral vasodilation, has been noted with certain drugs such as the short-acting form of nifedipine. Other bothersome side effects include dizziness, headache, and nausea.

STEPPED-CARE APPROACH TO HYPERTENSION

In many hypertensive patients, more than one type of drug must be given to successfully control blood pressure.[86,94,125] In general, the more severe the hypertension, the greater the need for a combination of several agents. To provide some type of rationale for effective drug use, a stepped-care approach is often implemented. The object of a stepped-care approach is to begin drug therapy with certain types of drugs and then, if additional drugs are needed, to follow a logical progression in each patient. One type of stepped-care system is outlined in Table 21–6. Typically, drug therapy is initiated with either a thiazide diuretic, a beta blocker, an ACE inhibitor, or a calcium channel blocker (step 1). If blood pressure is not adequately controlled, other types of antihypertensive drugs are instituted as outlined in steps 2 through 4 (see Table 21–6).

TABLE 21–6 Stepped-Care Approach to Hypertension

STEP 1: In patients with mild hypertension, drug therapy is usually initiated with a single agent (monotherapy) from one of the following classes: a diuretic, a beta blocker, an ACE inhibitor, or a calcium channel blocker.

STEP 2: If a single drug is unsuccessful in reducing blood pressure, a second agent is added. The second drug can be from one of the initial classes not used in step 1, or it can be from a second group that includes the centrally acting agents (clonidine, guanabenz), presynaptic adrenergic inhibitors (reserpine, guanethidine), alpha-1 blockers (prazosin, doxazosin), and vasodilators (hydralazine, minoxidil).

STEP 3: A third agent is added, usually from one of the classes listed in step 2 that has not already been used. Three different agents from three different classes are often administered concurrently in this step.

STEP 4: A fourth drug is added from still another class.

A stepped-care approach is generally regarded as the most effective way to use different types of antihypertensive drugs.[77] The stepped-care approach is not a set protocol, however, but only a guideline for drug administration. Specific programs can (and should) be tailored to individual patients by substituting various drugs at each step.[10,52]

NONPHARMACOLOGIC TREATMENT OF HYPERTENSION

Although several effective and relatively safe drugs exist for treating hypertension, the use of nondrug methods in decreasing blood pressure should not be overlooked, especially in cases of mild or borderline hypertension.[18,58,79,118] Certain dietary modifications such as sodium restriction, low-fat diets, and diets high in certain fish oils have been helpful to some patients.[3,51,89] Decreasing the use of alcohol and tobacco may also help lower blood pressure. Generally, a decrease in body weight will produce an antihypertensive effect.[20,51,70,84,110] Regular exercise may help decrease blood pressure by decreasing body weight or by mechanisms unrelated to weight loss.[2,18] Many forms of behavior modification and stress management techniques have also been suggested as nonpharmacologic methods of blood pressure control.

Considerable debate exists as to whether mild hypertension should be treated initially with drugs or if a trial with one or more nonpharmacologic techniques should be employed first.[41] This decision must be made on an individual basis, with consideration given to the patient's lifestyle and chance of compliance with a nondrug approach. There is ample evidence, however, that optimal results are obtained when lifestyle changes are combined with antihypertensive drug therapy.[18,27,70,84,89] Hence, changes in lifestyle and behavior should be encouraged in all hypertensive patients, regardless of whether drug therapy is initiated. Patients should be encouraged to quit smoking, lose weight, manage stress, and modify their diet, even if blood pressure is reduced pharmacologically.

SPECIAL CONCERNS IN REHABILITATION PATIENTS

Considering the prevalence of hypertension, therapists will undoubtedly work with many patients taking blood pressure medications. These drugs produce a diverse array of side effects that can influence the rehabilitation session. Primary among these are hypotension and orthostatic hypotension. Because the major action of these drugs is to lower blood pressure, physical therapists and occupational therapists should be cautious when their patients change posture suddenly or engage in other activities that may lower blood pressure.

Activities that produce widespread vasodilation must be avoided or used very cautiously, especially if vasodilating drugs are used. Systemically applied heat (whirlpool, Hubbard tank), for instance, may cause blood pressure to fall precipitously if alpha blockers, calcium channel blockers, or direct-acting vasodilators are being administered. Similarly, exercise may cause vasodilation in skeletal musculature, which may potentiate the peripheral vasodilation induced by these antihypertensive drugs. Also, if beta blockers are given, cardiac responses to exercise (i.e., increased heart rate and cardiac output) may be somewhat blunted because the myocardial response to sympathetic stimulation will be diminished.

Aside from being aware of the side effects of antihypertensive drugs, therapists may also play an important role in encouraging patient compliance in dealing with high blood pressure. Although drug therapy can control blood pressure in many individuals, patients are often forgetful or hesitant about taking their medications, largely because hypertension is usually asymptomatic until the late stages of this disease. The patient will probably feel fine even when the drug is not taken, or the patient may actually avoid taking the drug because of some bothersome side effect (i.e., the patient may actually feel better without the drug). The idea that hypertension is a silent killer must be reinforced continually in many patients. Through their close contact with the patient, rehabilitation specialists are often in a good position to remind the patient of the consequences of non-compliance. Also, therapists can help suggest and supervise nonpharmacologic methods of lowering blood pressure (e.g., exercise programs, stress management, relaxation techniques). Physical therapists and occupational therapists can play a valuable role in helping patients realize the importance of long-term pharmacologic and nonpharmacologic management of hypertension.

CASE STUDY

HYPERTENSION

Brief History. H.C. is a 55-year-old man who works as an attorney for a large corporation. He is consistently faced with a rather demanding work schedule, often working 12- to 14-hour days, 6 days each week. In addition, he is 25 to 30 pounds overweight and is a habitual cigarette smoker. He has a long history of high blood pressure, which has been managed fairly successfully over the past 15 years through the use of different drugs. Currently, H.C. is in step 3 of the stepped-care approach to hypertensive therapy, and three drugs are being administered to control his blood pressure. He is receiving a diuretic (furosemide, 100 mg/day), a cardioselective beta blocker (metoprolol, 200 mg/day), and a vasodilator (minoxidil, 20 mg/day).

While rushing to a business luncheon, H.C. was hit by an automobile as he was crossing the street. He was admitted to the hospital, where radiologic examination revealed a fracture of the right pelvis. Further examination did not reveal any other significant internal injuries. The pelvic fracture appeared stable at the time of admission, and internal fixation was not required. H.C. remained in the hospital and was placed on bed rest. Two days after admission, a physical therapist was called in to consult on this case. The physical therapist suggested a progressive ambulation program using the facility's therapeutic pool. The buoyancy provided by the pool would allow a gradual increase in weight bearing while protecting the fracture site.

Problem/Influence of Medication. To guard against patient hypothermia, the water temperature in the therapeutic pool was routinely maintained at 95°F. The therapist was concerned that immersing the patient in the pool would cause excessive peripheral vasodilation. Because the patient was taking a vasodilating drug (minoxidil), the additive effect of the warm pool and vasodilating agent might cause profound hypotension because of a dramatic decrease in total peripheral resistance. Also, because this patient was taking a cardioselective beta blocker (metoprolol), his heart would not be able to sufficiently increase cardiac output to offset the decreased peripheral resistance.

Decision/Solution. When the patient was in the pool, the therapist monitored heart rate and blood pressure at frequent, regular intervals. Blood pressure did decrease when the patient was ambulating in the pool, but not to a point of concern because the patient's active leg muscle contractions facilitated venous return, and the buoyancy of the water decreased the effects of gravity on venous pooling in the lower extremities. In fact, only at the end of the rehabilitation session, when the patient came out of the pool, did hypotension become a potential problem. The patient was still experiencing peripheral vasodilation because of the residual effects of the warm water, but he no longer had the advantage of active muscle contractions and water buoyancy to help maintain his blood pressure. To prevent a hypotensive episode at the end of the session, the therapist placed the patient supine on a stretcher as soon as he came out of the water. Also, the patient's legs were quickly toweled dry, and vascular support stockings were placed on the patient's legs as soon as possible. These precautions allowed the patient to progress rapidly through his rehabilitation without any adverse incidents. When he was eventually discharged from the hospital, he was ambulating with crutches, with partial weight bearing on the side of the pelvic fracture.

SUMMARY

Hypertension is a common disease marked by a sustained increase in blood pressure. If untreated, hypertension leads to serious problems such as stroke, renal failure, and problems in several other physiologic systems. Although the cause of hypertension is discernible in a small percentage of patients, the majority of hypertensive individuals are classified as having essential hypertension, which means that the cause of their elevated blood pressure is unknown. Fortunately, several types of drugs are currently available to adequately control blood pressure in essential hypertension. Diuretics, sympatholytics (alpha blockers, beta blockers, etc.), vasodilators, renin-angiotensin system inhibitors, and calcium channel blockers have all been used in treating hypertension. These agents are usually prescribed according to a stepped-care protocol, in which therapy is initiated with one drug and subsequent agents are added as required. Rehabilitation specialists should be aware of the potential side effects of these drugs. Physical and occupational therapists assume an important role in making patients aware of the sequelae of hypertension, and therapists should actively encourage patients to comply with pharmacologic and nonpharmacologic methods of lowering blood pressure.

REFERENCES

1. Antes, LM and Fernandez, PC: Principles of diuretic therapy. Dis Mon 44:254, 1998.
2. Arroll, B and Beaglehole, R: Does physical activity lower blood pressure: A critical review of the clinical trials. J Clin Epidemiol 45:439, 1992.
3. Bonaa, KH, et al: Effect of eicosapentaenoic and docosahexaenoic acids on blood pressure in hypertension. N Engl J Med 322:795, 1990.
4. Boulanger, CM: Secondary endothelial dysfunction: hypertension and heart failure. J Mol Cell Cardiol 31:39, 1999.
5. Britten, MB, Zeiher, AM, and Schachinger, V: Clinical importance of coronary endothelial vasodilator dysfunction and therapeutic options. J Intern Med 245:315, 1999.
6. Buhler, FR, et al: Elevated adrenaline and increased alpha-adrenoceptor mediated vasoconstriction in essential hypertension. J Cardiovasc Pharmacol 4(Suppl I):S134, 1982.
7. Burt, VL, et al: Prevalence of hypertension in the United States adult population: Results from the third National Health and Nutrition Examination Survey, 1988–1991. Hypertension 25:305, 1995.
8. Calhoun, DA and Oparil, S: Current concepts: Treatment of hypertensive crisis. N Engl J Med 323:1177, 1990.

9. Cardillo, C and Panza, JA: Impaired endothelial regulation of vascular tone in patients with systemic arterial hypertension. Vasc Med 3:138, 1998.
10. Caro, JJ: Stepped care for hypertension: Are the assumptions valid? J Hypertens Suppl 15:S35, 1997.
11. Cauffield, JS, Gums, JG, and Curry, RW: Alpha blockers: A reassessment of their role in therapy. Am Fam Physician 54:263, 1996.
12. Cheng, JW and Behar, L: Calcium channel blockers: Association with myocardial infarction, mortality, and cancer. Clin Ther 19:1255, 1997.
13. Chevalier, B, et al: Molecular basis for regression of cardiac hypertrophy. Am J Cardiol 73:10c, 1994.
14. Chobanian, AV (ed): Symposium: Role of calcium channel blockers in the management of hypertension. Am J Med 81(Suppl 6a):1, 1986.
15. Chou, CM: Evaluation and treatment of hypertension. Rheum Dis Clin North Am 25:521, 1999.
16. Ciccone, CD and Zambraski, EJ: Effects of acute renal denervation on kidney function in deoxycorticosterone acetate-hypertensive swine. Hypertension 8:925, 1986.
17. Ciccone, CD and Zambraski, EJ: Effects of phenoxybenzamine, metoprolol, captopril, and meclofenamate on cardiovascular function in deoxycorticosterone acetate hypertensive Yucatan miniature swine. Can J Physiol Pharmacol 61:149, 1983.
18. Cleroux, J, Feldman, RD, and Petrella, RJ: Lifestyle modifications to prevent and control hypertension. 4. Recommendations on physical exercise training. CMAJ 160(Suppl):S21, 1999.
19. Conlin, PR and Williams, GH: Use of calcium channel blockers in hypertension. Adv Intern Med 43:533, 1998.
20. Cutler, J: The effects of nonpharmacologic interventions on blood pressure of persons with high normal levels: Results of the trials of hypertension prevention, phase I. JAMA 267:1213, 1992.
21. DeBono, G, et al: Acebutolol: 10 years of experience. Am Heart J 109:1211, 1985.
22. De Champlain, J, et al: Effects of antihypertensive therapies on the sympathetic nervous system. Can J Cardiol 15(Suppl A):8A, 1999.
23. Dong, EW, et al: A systematic review and meta-analysis of the incidence of cancer in randomized, controlled trials of verapamil. Pharmacotherapy 17:1210, 1997.
24. Dontenwill, M, et al: Role of imidazoline receptors in cardiovascular regulation. Am J Cardiol 74:3A, 1994.
25. Doyle, AE and Donnan, GA: Stroke as a clinical problem in hypertension. J Cardiovasc Pharmacol 15(Suppl 1):S34, 1990.
26. Esler, M and Kaye, D: Increased sympathetic nervous system activity and its therapeutic reduction in arterial hypertension, portal hypertension, and heart failure. J Auton Nerv Syst 72:210, 1998.
27. Fagerberg, B, et al: Cardiovascular effects of weight reduction versus antihypertensive drug treatment: A comparative, randomized, 1-year study of obese men with mild hypertension. J Hypertens 9:431, 1991.
28. Ferrario, CM: The renin-angiotensin system: Importance in physiology and pathology. J Cardiovasc Pharmacol 15(Suppl 3):S1, 1990.
29. Ferreira, E and Shalansky, SJ: Nitric oxide for ARDS—What's the evidence? Pharmacotherapy 19:60, 1999.
30. Feuerstein, GZ, Bril, A, and Ruffolo, RR: Protective effects of carvedilol in the myocardium. Am J Cardiol 80(Suppl 11A):41L, 1997.
31. Freis, ED: Current status of diuretics, beta-blockers, alpha-blockers, and alpha-beta-blockers in the treatment of hypertension. Med Clin North Am 81:1305, 1997.
32. Friedman, GD, et al: Precursors of essential hypertension: Body weight, alcohol and salt use, and parental history of hypertension. Prev Med 17:387, 1988.
33. Frishman, WH: Pindolol: A new beta-adrenoceptor antagonist with partial agonist activity. N Engl J Med 308:940, 1983.
34. Frishman, WH and Kotob, F: Alpha-adrenergic blocking drugs in clinical medicine. J Clin Pharmacol 39:7, 1999.
35. Frohlich, ED: Vasodilating beta-blockers: Systemic and regional hemodynamic effects. Am Heart J 121:1012, 1991.
36. Fulton, B, Wagstaff, AJ, and Sorkin, EM: Doxazosin. An update of its clinical pharmacology and therapeutic applications in hypertension and benign prostatic hyperplasia. Drugs 49:295, 1995.
37. Ganong, WF: The brain renin-angiotensin system. Annu Rev Physiol 46:17, 1984.
38. Gavras, I and Gavras, H: Salt in hypertension: Physiological and molecular aspects. Recent Prog Horm Res 53:1, 1998.
39. Gibbons, GH: The pathophysiology of hypertension: The importance of angiotensin II in cardiovascular remodeling. Am J Hypertens 11(Part 2):177S, 1998.
40. Gifford, RW: The role of diuretics in the treatment of hypertension. Am J Med 77(Suppl 4a):102, 1984.
41. Gifford, RW, et al: The dilemma of "mild" hypertension: Another viewpoint of treatment. JAMA 250:3171, 1983.
42. Guyenet, PG: Is the hypotensive effect of clonidine and related drugs due to imidazoline binding sites? Am J Physiol 273:R1580, 1997.
43. Guyton, AC and Hall, JF: Textbook of Medical Physiology, ed 9. WB Saunders, Philadelphia, 1996.
44. Hansson, L: The Hypertension Optimal Treatment study and the importance of lowering blood pressure. J Hypertens Suppl 17:S9, 1999.
45. Hansson, L: Calcium antagonists: An overview. Am Heart J 122:308, 1991.
46. Hansson, L: Review of state-of-the-art beta-blocker therapy. Am J Cardiol 67:43B, 1991.

47. Hawkins, DW, Bussey, HI, and Prisant, LM: Hypertension. In Dipiro, JT, et al (eds): Pharmacotherapy: A Pathophysiologic Approach. Appleton & Lange, Stamford, CT, 1999.

48. Head, GA: Baroreflexes and cardiovascular regulation in hypertension. J Cardiovasc Pharmacol 26(Suppl 2):S7, 1995.

49. Hebert, PR, et al: Recent evidence on drug therapy of mild to moderate hypertension and decreased risk of coronary heart disease. Arch Intern Med 153:578, 1993.

50. Hedner, T: Management of hypertension: The advent of a new angiotensin II receptor antagonist. J Hypertens Suppl 17:S21, 1999

51. Hennekens, CH: Lessons from hypertension trials. Am J Med 104(Suppl 6A):50S, 1998.

52. Hollenberg, NK: Treatment of hypertension: The place of angiotensin converting enzyme inhibitors in the nineties. J Cardiovasc Pharmacol 20(Suppl 10):S29, 1992.

53. Hollenberg, NK (ed): Symposium: Calcium channel blockers: New insights into their role in the management of hypertension. Am J Med 82(Suppl 3b):1, 1987.

54. Horky, K: Alpha$_1$-blockade in the management of hypertension. J Clin Pharmacol 33:874, 1993.

55. Houston, MC: Alpha 1-blocker combination therapy for hypertension. Postgrad Med 104:167, 1998.

56. Jacob, S, Rett, K, and Henriksen, EJ: Antihypertensive therapy and insulin sensitivity: Do we have to redefine the role of beta-blocking agents? Am J Hypertens 11:1258, 1998.

57. Johnston, CI, Arnolda, L, and Hiwatari, M: Angiotensin-converting enzyme inhibitors in the treatment of hypertension. Drugs 27:271, 1984.

58. Joint National Committee on Detection, Evaluation, and Treatment of High Blood Pressure: The 1984 report. Arch Intern Med 144:1045, 1984.

59. Julius, S: Autonomic nervous system dysregulation in human hypertension. Am J Cardiol 67:3B, 1991.

60. Kaplan, NM: Angiotensin II receptor antagonists in the treatment of hypertension. Am Fam Physician 60:1185, 1999.

61. Kaplan, NM: Beta blockade in the primary prevention of hypertensive cardiovascular events with focus on sudden cardiac death. Am J Cardiol 80(Suppl 9B):20J, 1997.

62. Katholi, RE: Renal nerves in the pathogenesis of hypertension in experimental animals and humans. Am J Physiol 245:F1, 1983.

63. Kendall, MJ: Beta-blockers: a time for reappraisal. J Hum Hypertens 12:803, 1998.

64. Kendall, MJ: Therapeutic advantages of AT1 blockers in hypertension. Basic Res Cardiol 93(Suppl 2):47, 1998.

65. Kenny, J: Calcium channel blocking agents and the heart. BMJ 291:1150, 1985.

66. Kinsella, JP and Abman, SH: Recent developments in inhaled nitric oxide therapy of the newborn. Curr Opin Pediatr 11:121, 1999.

67. Kirsten, R, et al: Clinical pharmacokinetics of vasodilators. Part I. Clin Pharmacokinet 34:457, 1998.

68. Klaus, D: The role of calcium antagonists in the treatment of hypertension. J Cardiovasc Pharmacol 20(Suppl 6):S5, 1992.

69. Kokko, JP: Site and mechanism of action of diuretics. Am J Med 77(Suppl 4a):11, 1984.

70. Langford, HG, et al: Effect of drug and diet treatment of mild hypertension on diastolic blood pressure. Hypertension 17:210, 1991.

71. Leenen, FH: Cardiovascular consequences of sympathetic hyperactivity. Can J Cardiol 15(Suppl A):2A, 1999.

72. Levy, BI, et al: Long-term effects of angiotensin-converting enzyme inhibitors on the arterial wall of adult spontaneous hypertensive rats. Am J Cardiol 71:8E, 1993.

73. Lubsen, J: The calcium channel antagonist debate: Recent developments. Eur Heart J 19(Suppl I):I3, 1998.

74. Luscher, TF and Barton, M: Biology of the endothelium. Clin Cardiol 20(Suppl 2):II-3, 1997.

75. Luscher, TF and Cosentino, F: The classification of calcium antagonists and their selection in the treatment of hypertension. A reappraisal. Drugs 55:509, 1998.

76. Lyons, D: Impairment and restoration of nitric oxide–dependent vasodilation in cardiovascular diseases. Int J Cardiol 62(Suppl 2):S101, 1997.

77. Mancia, G and Grassi, G: Antihypertensive treatment: Past, present, and future. J Hypertens Suppl 16:S1, 1998.

78. Marin, J and Rodriguez-Martinez, MA: Role of vascular nitric oxide in physiological and pathological conditions. Pharmacol Ther 75:111, 1997.

79. Marley, J, Davis, N, and Joy, M: Is the non-pharmacological treatment of hypertension neglected? J R Soc Med 84:540, 1991.

80. Mason, RP: Effects of calcium channel blockers on cellular apoptosis: Implications for carcinogenic potential. Cancer 85:2093, 1999.

81. Massie, BM: The safety of calcium channel blockers. Clin Cardiol 21(Suppl 2):II12, 1998.

82. McHugh, J and Cheek, DJ: Nitric oxide and regulation of vascular tone: Pharmacological and physiological considerations. Am J Crit Care 7:131, 1998.

83. Messerli, FH and Grossman, E: The calcium antagonist controversy: A posthumous commentary. Am J Cardiol 82(Suppl 9B):35R, 1998.

84. Mikhail, N, Golub, MS, and Tuck, ML: Obesity and hypertension. Prog Cardiovasc Dis 42:39, 1999.

85. Mombouli, JV and Vanhoutte, PM: Endothelial dysfunction: From physiology to therapy. J Mol Cell Cardiol 31:61, 1999.

86. Moser, M and Black, HR: The role of combination therapy in the treatment of hypertension. Am J Hypertens 11(Part 2):73S, 1998.
87. Moser, M and Frishman, W: Results of therapy with carvedilol, a beta-blocker vasodilator with antioxidant properties, in hypertensive patients. Am J Hypertens 11(Part 2):15S, 1998.
88. Mulvaney, MJ: Effects of angiotensin-converting enzyme inhibition on vascular remodeling of resistance vessels in hypertensive patients. Metabolism 47(Suppl 1):20, 1998.
89. Neaton, JD, et al: Treatment of mild hypertension study: Final results. JAMA 270:713, 1993.
90. Neutel, JM: Safety and efficacy of angiotensin II receptor antagonists. Am J Cardiol 84(Suppl 2A):13K, 1999.
91. Oates, JA: Antihypertensive agents and the drug therapy of hypertension. In Hardman, JG, et al (eds): The Pharmacological Basis of Therapeutics, ed 9. McGraw-Hill, New York, 1996.
92. O'Byrne, S and Caulfield, M: Genetics of hypertension. Therapeutic implications. Drugs 56:203, 1998.
93. Oglivie, RI, et al: Report of the Canadian Hypertension Society consensus conference: Pharmacologic treatment of essential hypertension. Can Med Assoc J 149:575, 1993.
94. Opie, LH: Principles of combination therapy for hypertension: What we learn from the HOT and other studies—A personal point of view. Cardiovasc Drugs Ther 12:425, 1998.
95. Osei, K: Insulin resistance and systemic hypertension. Am J Cardiol 84(Suppl 1A):33J, 1999.
96. Pitt, B: Diversity of calcium antagonists. Clin Ther 19(Suppl A):3, 1997.
97. Pool, JL: Doxazosin: A new approach to hypertension and benign prostatic hyperplasia. Br J Clin Pract 50:154, 1996.
98. Powers, DR, Papadakos, PJ, and Wallin, JD: Parenteral hydralazine revisited. J Emerg Med 16:191, 1998.
99. Prichard, BN, Owens, CW, and Graham, BR: Pharmacology and clinical use of moxonidine, a new centrally acting sympatholytic antihypertensive agent. J Hum Hypertens 11(Suppl 1):S29, 1997.
100. Prisant, LM: Calcium antagonists: Pharmacologic considerations. Ethn Dis 8:98, 1998.
101. Pylypchuk, GB: ACE inhibitor- versus angiotensin II blocker-induced cough and angioedema. Ann Pharmacother 32:1060, 1998.
102. Reaven, GM: Treatment of hypertension: Focus on prevention of coronary artery disease. J Clin Endocrinol Metab 76:537, 1993.
103. Reid, JL, et al: Clinical pharmacology of drugs acting on imidazoline and adrenergic receptors. Studies with clonidine, moxonidine, rilmenidine, and atenolol. Ann N Y Acad Sci 763:673, 1995.
104. Ruffolo, RR, Feuerstein, GZ, and Ohlstein, EH: Recent observations with beta-adrenoceptor blockade. Beneficial effects in hypertension and heart failure. Am J Hypertens 11(Part 2):9S, 1998.
105. Ruschitzka, F, et al: A rationale for treatment of endothelial dysfunction in hypertension. J Hypertens Suppl 17:S25, 1999.
106. Sassano, P, et al: Antihypertensive effect of enalapril as first-step treatment of mild and moderate uncomplicated essential hypertension. Am J Med 77(Suppl 2a):18, 1984.
107. Schachter, M: Drug-induced modification of vascular structure: Effects of antihypertensive drugs. Am Heart J 122:316, 1991.
108. Schafer, SG, et al: Why imidazoline receptor modulation in the treatment of hypertension? Ann N Y Acad Sci 763:659, 1995.
109. Schiffrin, EL: Vascular remodeling and endothelial function in hypertensive patients: Effects of antihypertensive therapy. Scand Cardiovasc J Suppl 47:15, 1998.
110. Schotte, DE and Stunkard, AJ: The effects of weight reduction on blood pressure in 301 obese patients. Arch Intern Med 150:1701, 1990.
111. Shanks, RG: Clinical pharmacology of vasodilating beta-blocking drugs. Am Heart J 121:1006, 1991.
112. Silvestry, FE and St John Sutton, MG: Sustained-release calcium channel antagonists in cardiovascular disease: Pharmacology and current therapeutic use. Eur Heart J 19(Suppl I):I8, 1998.
113. Spital, A: Diuretic-induced hyponatremia. Am J Nephrol 19:447, 1999.
114. Straka, RJ and Swanson, AL: Calcium channel antagonists: Morbidity and mortality—What's the evidence? Am Fam Physician 57:1551, 1998.
115. Symposium (various authors): Clinical applications of alpha$_1$-receptor blockade: Terazosin in the management of hypertension. J Clin Pharmacol 33:866, 1993.
116. Symposium (various authors): Clinical challenges in hypertension: Therapeutic applications of new vasodilating beta-blockers. J Cardiovasc Pharmacol 18(Suppl 4):S1, 1991.
117. Symposium (various authors): Expanding the role of calcium antagonists in hypertension. J Cardiovasc Pharmacol 17(Suppl 4):S1, 1991.
118. Symposium (various authors): New vistas on nonpharmacological approaches to hypertension. J Cardiovasc Pharmacol 16(Suppl 8):S1, 1990.
119. Taylor, P: Agents acting at the neuromuscular junction and autonomic ganglia. In Hardman, JG, et al (eds): The Pharmacological Basis of Therapeutics, ed 9. McGraw-Hill, New York, 1996.
120. Turner, P: Which ancillary properties of beta-adrenoceptor blocking drugs influence their therapeutic and adverse effects: A review. J R Soc Med 84:672, 1991.
121. Unger, TU and Gohlke, P: Tissue renin-angiotensin systems in the heart and vasculature: Possible involvement in the cardiovascular actions of converting enzyme inhibitors. Am J Cardiol 65:31, 1990.
122. Veelken, R and Schmieder, RE: Overview of alpha 1-adrenoceptor antagonism and recent advances in hypertensive therapy. Am J Hypertens 9:139S, 1996.

123. Weber, MA: Comparison of type 1 angiotensin II blockers and angiotensin converting enzyme inhibitors in the treatment of hypertension. J Hypertens Suppl 15:S31, 1997.
124. Webster, J and Koch, HF: Aspects of tolerability of centrally acting antihypertensive drugs. J Cardiovasc Pharmacol 27(Suppl 3):S49, 1996.
125. Weir, MR: The rationale for combination versus single-entity therapy in hypertension. Am J Hypertens 11:163S, 1998.
126. Yamazaki, T and Yazaki, Y: Role of tissue angiotensin II in myocardial remodelling induced by mechanical stress. J Hum Hypertens 13(Suppl 1):S43, 1999.
127. Yu, A and Frishman, WH: Imidazoline receptor agonist drugs: A new approach to the treatment of hypertension. J Clin Pharmacol 36:98, 1996.
128. Zambraski, EJ, Ciccone, CD, and Izzo, JL: The role of the sympathetic nervous system in 2-kidney DOCA-hypertensive Yucatan miniature swine. Clin Exp Hypertens [A] 8:411, 1986.
129. Zsoter, TT: Vasodilators. Can Med Assoc J 129:424, 1983.

CHAPTER 22

Treatment of Angina Pectoris

Angina pectoris is pain in the chest region that occurs during ischemic heart disease. Attacks of angina pectoris begin suddenly and are often described as a sensation of intense compression and tightness in the retrosternal region, with pain sometimes radiating to the jaw or left arm. In many patients, episodes of angina pectoris are precipitated by physical exertion. Some forms of angina, however, may occur spontaneously even when the patient is at rest or asleep.

The basic problem in angina pectoris is that the supply of oxygen to the heart is insufficient to meet myocardial demands at a given point in time, which results in an imbalance between myocardial oxygen supply and demand (Fig. 22–1).[16,57,77] This imbalance leads to myocardial ischemia, which results in several metabolic, electrophysiologic, and contractile changes in the heart. The painful symptoms inherent in angina pectoris seem to result from the accumulation of metabolic by-products such as lactic acid. Presumably, these metabolic by-products act as nociceptive substances and trigger the painful compressive sensations characteristic of angina pectoris.

Although angina pectoris is thought to be caused by the build-up of lactic acid and other metabolites, the exact mechanisms responsible for mediating anginal pain remain unknown. Also, the emotional state of the patient and other factors that influence central pain perception play an obvious role in angina pectoris. In fact, the majority of anginal attacks may be silent in many patients, and myocardial ischemia may frequently occur without producing any symptoms.[15,17,52,61,77] Clearly, there is much information regarding the nature of angina pectoris still remaining to be clarified.

Considering the prevalence of ischemic heart disease in the United States, many patients receiving physical therapy and occupational therapy may suffer from angina pectoris. These patients may be undergoing rehabilitation for a variety of clinical disorders, including, but not limited to, coronary artery disease. This chapter describes the three primary drug groups used to treat angina pectoris, as well as the pharmacologic management of specific forms of angina. Physical therapists and occupational therapists should be aware of the manner in which these drugs work and the ways in which antianginal drugs can influence patient performance in rehabilitation sessions.

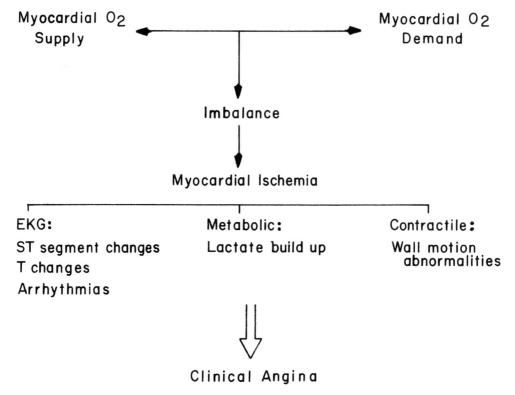

FIGURE 22–1. Myocardial ischemia equation. (Adapted from Miller, AB: Mixed ischemic subsets. Comparison of the mechanism of silent ischemia and mixed angina. Am J Med 79(Suppl 3a):25, 1985, with permission.)

DRUGS USED TO TREAT ANGINA PECTORIS

Three drug groups are typically used to treat angina pectoris: organic nitrates, beta blockers, and calcium channel blockers. These drugs exert various effects that help restore or maintain the balance between myocardial oxygen supply and myocardial oxygen demand. The effects of these drug categories and specific agents within each category are presented here.

ORGANIC NITRATES

Mechanism of Action and Rationale for Use

Organic nitrates consist of drugs such as nitroglycerin and isosorbide dinitrate (Table 22–1). The ability of these agents to dilate vascular smooth muscle is well established. Nitrates are actually drug precursors (prodrugs) that become activated when they are converted to nitrous oxide within vascular smooth muscle.[14,26,56] Nitrous oxide causes vasodilation by increasing the production of cyclic guanosine monophosphate (cyclic GMP) within the muscle cell. Cyclic GMP acts as a second messenger that inhibits smooth-muscle contraction, probably by initiating the phosphorylation of specific contractile proteins.[38,68]

TABLE 22–1 Organic Nitrates

Dosage Form	Onset of Action	Duration of Action
Nitroglycerin		
Oral	20–45 min	4–6 hr
Buccal (extended release)	2–3 min	3–5 hr
Sublingual	1–3 min	30–60 min
Ointment	30 min	4–8 hr
Transdermal patches	Within 30 min	8–24 hr
Isosorbide dinitrate		
Oral	15–40 min	4–6 hr
Oral (extended release)	30 min	12 hr
Chewable	2–5 min	1–2 hr
Sublingual	2–5 min	1–2 hr
Isosorbide mononitrate		
Oral	30–60 min	6–8 hr
Erythrityl tetranitrate		
Oral	30 min	Up to 6 hr
Chewable	Within 5 min	2hr
Buccal	Within 5 min	2hr
Sublingual	Within 5 min	2–3 hr
Pentaerythritol tetranitrate		
Oral	20–60 min	4–5 hr
Amyl nitrite		
Inhaled	30 sec	3–5 min

For years, nitrates were believed to relieve angina attacks by dilating the coronary arteries; that is, they supposedly increased blood flow to the myocardium, thereby increasing myocardial oxygen supply. We now know, however, that these drugs exert their primary antianginal effects by producing a general vasodilation in the vasculature throughout the body, not just the coronary vessels.[20,68] By producing dilation in the systemic venous system, nitrates decrease the amount of blood returning to the heart (*cardiac preload*). By dilating systemic peripheral arterioles, these drugs decrease the pressure against which the heart must pump (*cardiac afterload*). A decrease in cardiac preload and afterload decreases the amount of work the heart must perform; hence, myocardial oxygen demand decreases.

Consequently, nitroglycerin and other organic nitrates seem to primarily decrease myocardial oxygen demand rather than directly increase oxygen supply. Nitrates can also dilate the coronary arteries to some extent because an increase in coronary artery flow has been documented with these drugs.[6,57] The *primary* way that these drugs relieve angina pectoris, however, is through their ability to decrease cardiac work, thus decreasing myocardial oxygen demand.

Specific Agents

Nitroglycerin (Nitro-Bid, Nitrostat, Nitro-Dur, many others). In addition to its use as a powerful explosive, nitroglycerin is perhaps the best known of the antianginal drugs. The explosive nature of this agent is rendered inactive by diluting it with lactose, alcohol, or propylene glycol. Nitroglycerin is administered for both the prevention and the treatment of anginal attacks and is available in oral, buccal, sublingual, and transdermal forms (see Table 22–1).

Sublingual administration of nitroglycerin is the best method to treat an acute attack of angina. Placed under the tongue, the drug is rapidly absorbed through the oral mucosa into the systemic circulation. Therapeutic effects usually begin within 2 minutes when nitroglycerin is administered sublingually. Sublingual administration also spares the nitroglycerin from the first-pass effect. The drug is able to reach the systemic circulation before first passing through the liver, where it is inactivated (see Chap. 2).

For the prevention of angina, extended-release versions of this drug, which can be taken buccally—that is, between the cheek and gum—have been developed. Oral preparations have also been developed, but this method of administration is limited because nitroglycerin undergoes extensive first-pass degradation in the liver when absorbed directly from the intestines.

For prophylaxis of angina, nitroglycerin can also be administered transdermally via ointment or medicated patches placed on the skin (see Table 22–1). Nitroglycerin-impregnated patches or disks are applied cutaneously like a small bandage, with the drug slowly and continuously absorbed through the skin and into the systemic circulation.[31,67,77] Transdermal administration of nitroglycerin using these patches has been regarded favorably because of the ease and convenience of administration. By providing fairly continuous and sustained administration, nitroglycerin can also help prevent the onset of an anginal episode in many people.

One problem associated with nitroglycerin patches is that continuous nitroglycerin administration will cause drug tolerance, thus reducing the antianginal effectiveness of this medication.[51,67] Tolerance to nitrate drugs is rather short-lived, however, and normal responses to nitrate drugs can be restored within only a few hours after withdrawing these agents.[40] Consequently, patients may benefit from having intervals during each day when they do not wear their patches. Daily administration, for example, might be optimized by wearing the patch for 12 to 14 hours, followed by a 10- to 12-hour nitrate-free interval.[70,77] This method of intermittent nitroglycerin administration may provide beneficial effects with less chance of developing drug tolerance.[1,2,55,67] The drawback, of course, is that the patient will be more susceptible to angina attacks during the nitrate-free interval. Hence, intermittent nitrate use must be monitored carefully in each patient to make sure that the patch provides adequate protection during the part of the day or night when angina is likely to occur, without leaving the patient especially vulnerable during the nondrug interval.

Nitroglycerin ointment is another way to provide continuous transdermal administration of this drug.[66,77] The ointment is applied directly to the skin on the patient's chest or back, in much the same way as any topical ointment or skin cream. Although somewhat messy and inconvenient, administration of nitroglycerin via an ointment probably results in higher plasma levels of the drug, as well as more prolonged effects, than with medicated patches.[18] This method is not as popular as transdermal patches, however, because patches are much more convenient and easier to apply. Likewise, tolerance may occur if nitroglycerin is applied continually through topical ointments.

Isosorbide Dinitrate. Like nitroglycerin, isosorbide dinitrate is used for the treatment of acute episodes of angina as well as for the prevention of the onset of anginal attacks. The antianginal and hemodynamic effects last longer with isosorbide, however, so this drug is often classified as a long-acting nitrate.[82] For acute attacks, isosorbide is administered sublingually or by chewable tablets (see Table 22–1). For prevention of angina, this drug is usually given by oral tablets.

Isosorbide Mononitrate. This drug is another long-acting nitrate that is similar in structure and function to isosorbide dinitrate. It is typically given orally for prevention of anginal attacks.

Erythrityl Tetranitrate. Erythrityl tetranitrate is also classified as a long-acting nitrate. When administered sublingually, this drug requires somewhat longer to take action, but the effects tend to last longer than with sublingually administered nitroglycerin. Consequently, erythrityl tetranitrate is used primarily for the prevention rather than the acute treatment of anginal attacks. This drug can be administered orally, sublingually, buccally, or by chewable tablets (see Table 22–1).

Pentaerythritol Tetranitrate (Peritrate). Pentaerythritol tetranitrate, a long-acting nitrate similar in function to erythrityl tetranitrate, is used primarily in the prevention of anginal attacks and is administered orally.

Amyl Nitrite. This drug is supplied in small ampules that can be broken open so that the drug is inhaled during acute anginal attacks. Absorption of the drug through the nasal membranes causes peripheral vasodilation and decreased cardiac preload and afterload. Clinical use of inhaled amyl nitrite is very limited, however, and this type of antianginal treatment has generally been replaced by safer and more convenient methods of nitrate administration (e.g., nitroglycerin patches).

Adverse Side Effects of Nitrates

The primary adverse effects associated with the organic nitrates are headache, dizziness, and orthostatic hypotension.[77] These effects are related to the ability of these drugs to dilate peripheral blood vessels and decrease peripheral resistance. Nausea may also be a problem in some patients. As indicated earlier, tolerance to the beneficial effects of nitrates can occur during the continuous administration of these drugs, but providing daily nitrate-free intervals should prevent this problem.

BETA-ADRENERGIC BLOCKERS

Mechanism of Action and Rationale for Use

By antagonizing beta-1 receptors on the myocardium, beta blockers tend to decrease heart rate and the force of myocardial contraction,[21,77] thus producing an obvious decrease in the work the heart must perform and decreasing myocardial oxygen demand. Beta blockers help maintain an appropriate balance between myocardial oxygen supply and demand by preventing an increase in myocardial oxygen demand.

Consequently, beta blockers are given to certain patients with angina to limit the oxygen demands of the heart.[21,34,57,59] This prophylactic administration prevents the onset of an anginal attack. The use of beta blockers in specific forms of angina is reviewed later in this chapter when the various types of angina are discussed.

Specific Agents

Individual beta blockers were discussed in Chapter 20. Beta blockers effective in treating angina pectoris are listed in Table 22–2. Various beta blockers seem to display a fairly equal ability to decrease episodes of angina pectoris.[77] Certain beta blockers may be more favorable in certain patients because the side effects are more tolerable in that patient or because the dosing schedule is more convenient (e.g., the drug needs to be taken only once each day rather than in several doses). Likewise, some of the newer beta

TABLE 22–2 Beta Blockers Used to Treat Angina Pectoris

Generic Name	Trade Name	Usual Oral Dose
Acebutolol	Sectral	200–600 mg 2 times a day
Atenolol	Tenormin	50–100 mg once a day
Carteolol	Cartrol	2.5–10.0 mg once a day
Labetalol	Normodyne, Trandate	200–400 mg 2 times a day
Metoprolol	Lopressor, others	50–200 mg 2 times a day
Nadolol	Corgard	40–240 mg once a day
Penbutolol	Levatol	20 mg once a day
Pindolol	Visken	5–20 mg 2 times a day
Propranolol	Inderal	40–80 mg 2–4 times a day
Sotalol	Betapace	80–160 mg 2 times a day
Timolol	Blocadren	10–30 mg 2 times a day

blockers may have additional properties that might provide added benefits to certain patients. Newer agents such as carvedilol, for example, produce peripheral vasodilation that can be advantageous for people with angina who also have hypertension.[29] The choice of a specific beta blocker therefore depends on the pharmacologic profile of each drug in conjunction with the particular needs of each patient.[78]

Adverse Side Effects

Beta blockers that bind to both beta-1 and beta-2 receptors (nonselective agents; see Table 20–2) may induce bronchoconstriction in patients with asthma or similar respiratory problems. These patients should be given one of the more cardioselective beta antagonists such as atenolol or metoprolol. Beta blockers may also produce excessive cardiac depression in individuals with certain types of cardiac disease. The beta blockers are generally well tolerated in most patients, however, with major problems being fairly infrequent.

CALCIUM CHANNEL BLOCKERS

Mechanism of Action and Rationale for Use

These drugs block the entry of calcium into vascular smooth muscle.[33,63,81] In vascular smooth muscle, calcium ions facilitate contraction by initiating actin-myosin interaction. Calcium channel blockers decrease the entry of calcium into vascular smooth-muscle cells, thus causing relaxation and vasodilation. By blocking calcium entry into coronary artery smooth muscle, these drugs mediate coronary vasodilation, with a subsequent increase in the supply of oxygen to the myocardium. Consequently, a primary role of calcium channel blockers in angina pectoris is to directly increase coronary blood flow, thus increasing myocardial oxygen supply.[48,75,84]

Calcium channel blockers also cause some degree of systemic vasodilation, and some of their antianginal effects may be related to a decrease in myocardial oxygen demand caused by a decrease in cardiac preload and afterload; that is, they may exert some of their beneficial effects in a manner similar to that of organic nitrates.[33] Also, calcium channel blockers limit the entry of calcium into cardiac striated cells, thus decreasing myocardial contractility and oxygen demand. The *primary* beneficial effects of these drugs in angina pectoris, however, are related to their ability to dilate the coronary arteries and peripheral vasculature. Certain calcium channel blockers can also affect myocardial excitability by altering the conduction of electrical activity throughout the myocardium.[62,77] This effect seems to be more important when these drugs are used to treat cardiac arrhythmias (see Chap. 23).

The calcium channel blockers currently used to treat angina pectoris are listed in Table 22–3. Although the chemistry and exact mechanism of action of each drug is somewhat distinct, all of these agents exert their effects by limiting calcium entry into specific cardiovascular tissues. Certain calcium channel blockers are said to be "selective" if they affect vascular smooth muscle but have little or no effect on the heart. Nonselective calcium channel blockers affect the vasculature and also inhibit calcium entry into cardiac muscle cells. Individual agents are discussed here.

Specific Agents

Bepridil (Bepadin, Vascor). Bepridil is a nonselective calcium channel blocker that inhibits calcium influx into vascular smooth muscle and cardiac striated muscle. It can vasodilate coronary and peripheral vessels, hence its use in angina pectoris. Bepridil also decreases heart rate (negative chronotropic effect) and cardiac contractility (negative inotropic effect) through an inhibitory effect on the myocardium. These negative chronotropic and negative inotropic effects can be problematic, especially if this drug is combined with beta blockers or other drugs that inhibit heart rate and contractility.[72]

Diltiazem (Cardizem). Like the other calcium channel blockers, diltiazem is able to vasodilate the coronary arteries and the peripheral vasculature. Diltiazem also produces some depression of electrical conduction in the sinoatrial and atrioventricular nodes, an effect that may cause slight bradycardia. This bradycardia can be worsened by beta blockers or in patients with myocardial conduction problems, and diltiazem should probably be avoided in these individuals.[72]

Mibefradil. Mibefradil represents the first member of a new class of calcium channel blockers known as tetralol derivatives.[5,23,45,62] These drugs are unique because they block the T type of calcium channel located on vascular smooth muscle (all other calcium channel blockers act on the L type of calcium channels).[54] Hence, mibefradil is pharmacologically distinct from other calcium channel blockers, and this drug controls angina by selectively vasodilating the coronary arteries and the peripheral vasculature and by producing a slight decrease in heart rate.[23] More important, mibefradil lacks some of the problems commonly associated with other calcium channel blockers. For example,

TABLE 22–3 Calcium Channel Blockers

Generic Name	Trade Name	Usual Oral Dose
Bepridil	Vascor	200–300 mg once a day
Diltiazem	Cardizem	30–90 mg 3 or 4 times a day
Felodipine	Plendil	10 mg once a day
Isradipine	DynaCirc	2.5–10 mg 2 times a day
Nicardipine	Cardene	20 mg 3 times a day
Nifedipine	Adalat, Procardia	10–30 mg 3 or 4 times a day
Verapamil	Calan, Isoptin	80–160 mg 3 times a day

mibefradil does not depress myocardial contraction force, and it does not cause a reflex increase in heart rate (reflex tachycardia).[5,23,36] Mibefradil is therefore gaining acceptance in treating angina, and use of this drug and similar agents from this category may be more widespread in the future.

Nifedipine (Procardia) and Other Dihydropyridines. Nifedipine and similar drugs are members of the dihydropyridine class of calcium channel blockers. This class is distinguished by drugs with an *-ipine* suffix, including felodipine (Plendil), isradipine (DynaCirc), and nicardipine (Cardene). These drugs are relatively selective for vascular smooth muscle as compared with cardiac striated muscle, and they vasodilate the coronary arteries and peripheral vasculature without exerting any direct effects on cardiac excitability or contractility.[75] These drugs are therefore advantageous for treating patients with angina who also have certain types of cardiac arrhythmias or other problems with cardiac excitation and conduction.[30] Nifedipine and similar drugs may, however, produce reflex tachycardia, which is a compensatory increase in heart rate that occurs when peripheral vascular resistance decreases because of the drug-induced vasodilation. Other nondihydropyridine drugs (diltiazem, verapamil) also lower vascular resistance, but reflex tachycardia is prevented because these drugs also have an inhibitory effect on heart rate (negative chronotropic effect). If reflex tachycardia does occur with nifedipine, this problem can be controlled somewhat by using sustained-release or long-acting forms of these drugs (see "Adverse Side Effects").

Verapamil (Calan, Isoptin). Verapamil has been used to treat angina because of its ability to vasodilate the coronary vessels. Verapamil, however, seems to be only moderately effective compared with the other antianginal drugs, and verapamil also depresses myocardial excitability and decreases heart rate.[77] Because of its negative effects on cardiac excitation, verapamil is probably more useful in controlling certain cardiac arrhythmias (see Chap. 23).

Adverse Side Effects

The primary problems associated with the calcium channel blockers are related to the peripheral vasodilation produced by these agents. Headache, flushing or feelings of warmth, and dizziness may occur in some patients. Peripheral edema, as evidenced by swelling in the feet and legs, may also occur, and nausea may be fairly common. Nonselective calcium channel blockers that affect the myocardium (e.g., bepridil, diltiazem, verapamil) can cause disturbances in cardiac rhythm. As indicated, reflex tachycardia can also be a problem, especially with nifedipine and other dihydropyridine calcium channel blockers ("-ipine" drugs) that selectively decrease vascular resistance without simultaneously inhibiting heart rate.

There has also been some concern about the safety of the calcium channel blockers. In particular, reports indicated that certain calcium channel blockers such as the short-acting form of nifedipine may be associated with an increased risk of myocardial infarction in certain patients (older patients with hypertension, patients with unstable angina).[46,50] The short-acting or immediate-release form of nifedipine and other "-ipine" calcium channel blockers can be problematic because these drugs may cause a fairly rapid decrease in peripheral vascular resistance and blood pressure.[73] A rapid fall in vascular resistance and blood pressure can precipitate reflex hemodynamic changes (increased heart rate, decreased myocardial perfusion) that lead to ischemia and infarction in susceptible patients. Sustained-release or longer-acting forms of nifedipine and similar agents may be somewhat safer because they do not cause as rapid a change in vascular resistance as the short-acting forms of these drugs.[9,42,71]

Preliminary studies also suggested that calcium channel blockers may increase the risk of cancer.[22,44] Intracellular calcium levels are important in regulating cell division. By modifying calcium influx, calcium channel blockers could conceivably accelerate cell proliferation and lead to cancerous growths. Fortunately, the carcinogenic potential of these drugs has not been proven conclusively by subsequent studies. Hence, calcium channel blockers continue to be used cautiously but effectively in large numbers of patients.

USE OF ANTICOAGULANTS IN ANGINA PECTORIS

Angina pectoris is typically associated with some degree of coronary artery occlusion. To help prevent further blockage of the coronary arteries, certain anticoagulant drugs can be administered so that a partially occluded artery does not become completely blocked and cause myocardial infarction.[10] The two most common agents used in this situation are heparin and aspirin.[12,79] The pharmacology and anticoagulant effects of these drugs are discussed in detail in Chapter 25, and their use in angina is addressed briefly here.

Heparin is often used during the initial or acute phase of unstable angina to prevent clot formation at atherosclerotic plaques that may have ruptured in the coronary arteries.[13,85] Heparin is a fast-acting anticoagulant that leads to the inhibition of thrombin, a key component of the clotting mechanism. With regard to their use in angina, low-molecular-weight heparins (LMWH) such as enoxaparin seem to be especially advantageous because they produce a more predictable anticoagulant response and are tolerated better than more traditonal (unfractionated) heparin.[27,32,47,53,65] Heparin must, however, be administered parenterally, and LMWHs are usually given via subcutaneous injection.

Aspirin inhibits platelet-induced clotting in the coronary arteries and other vascular tissues.[58] As discussed in Chapter 15, aspirin inhibits the biosynthesis of prostaglandins, and certain prostaglandins are responsible for activating platelets during the clotting process. In angina pectoris, aspirin administration can prevent platelets from becoming activated in partially occluded coronary vessels and therefore helps maintain blood flow through these vessels.[58] Aspirin is administered orally and is often used for the long-term management of platelet-induced clotting in people with angina.

Aspirin and heparin are therefore used alone or in combination in various forms of angina to help prevent infarction. When administered with the traditional antianginal medications, these anticoagulants can help decrease morbidity and mortality in people with ischemic heart disease.

TREATMENT OF SPECIFIC TYPES OF ANGINA PECTORIS

All forms of angina pectoris are not the same. Traditionally, angina has been subclassified according to the factors that precipitate the angina and the pathophysiologic mechanisms responsible for producing myocardial ischemia.[16] Table 22–4 summarizes the different types of angina and the drugs used in each type. The major forms of angina and the primary drugs used to treat each type are also discussed here.

TABLE 22–4 Types of Angina Pectoris

Classification	Cause	Drug Therapy
Stable angina	Myocardial oxygen demand exceeds oxygen supply; usually brought on by physical exertion.	Usually treated with either a beta blocker or long-acting nitrate.
Variant angina	Myocardial oxygen supply decreases because of coronary vasospasm; may occur with patient at rest.	Treated primarily with a calcium channel blocker.
Unstable angina	Myocardial oxygen supply decreases at the same time that oxygen demand increases; can occur at any time secondary to atherosclerotic plaque rupture within the coronary artery.	May require a combination of drugs (i.e., a calcium channel blocker plus a beta blocker); anticoagulant drugs are also helpful in preventing thrombogenesis and coronary occlusion.

Stable Angina

Stable angina is the most common form of ischemic heart disease.[77] The primary problem in stable angina is that myocardial oxygen demand greatly exceeds oxygen supply. Stable angina is also frequently referred to as effort or exertional angina because attacks are usually precipitated by a certain level of physical exertion. If the patient exercises beyond a certain level of his or her capacity, the coronary arteries are unable to deliver the oxygen needed to sustain that level of myocardial function, and an anginal episode occurs. The inability of the coronary arteries to adequately deliver oxygen in stable angina is usually caused by some degree of permanent coronary artery occlusion (e.g., coronary artery atherosclerosis or stenosis).

Because stable angina is caused primarily by an increase in myocardial oxygen demand, treatment of this form of angina has consisted mainly of beta blockers and organic nitrates.[35] Beta blockers are administered prophylactically to decrease the workload of the heart, thus limiting myocardial oxygen requirements.[57,72] Nitrates can also be given as a preventive measure to blunt myocardial oxygen needs; nitroglycerin can be administered transdermally through patches or ointments, or long-acting nitrates (isosorbide dinitrate, erythrityl tetranitrate) can be administered orally. Nitroglycerin can also be taken sublingually at the onset of an attack or just before activities that routinely precipitate an attack.

Calcium channel blockers can also be given to treat stable angina, especially if beta blockers are not tolerated or are contraindicated in specific patients.[2,49,69] These drugs decrease cardiac workload directly by limiting calcium entry into myocardial cells and indirectly by producing peripheral vasodilation and thus decreasing cardiac preload and afterload.[57] Hence, calcium channel blockers are administered in stable angina primarily for their effect on the myocardium and peripheral vasculature rather than for their ability to dilate the coronary arteries.

Finally, a combination of various antianginal drugs is often used in patients with stable angina.[35] For example, a beta blocker and a long-acting nitrate may be administered together, especially when either drug alone is not completely successful in managing anginal episodes. Likewise, a beta blocker and a calcium channel blocker may be used in combination,[11,25] but care must be taken to avoid excessive negative chronotropic and negative ionotropic effects on the heart (that is, nondihydropyridine calcium channel blockers can decrease heart rate and contraction force, which can add to the inhibitory effects of beta blockers on the heart).[72] Hence, beta blockers are typically combined with nifedipine or another dihydropyridine agent ("-ipine" drugs) when these two types of antianginal agents are used together.[57,72]

Variant Angina (Prinzmetal's Ischemia)

In variant angina, the primary problem is that oxygen supply to the myocardium *decreases* because of coronary artery vasospasm.[16,80] Vasospasm causes oxygen supply to decrease even though oxygen demand has not changed, and this phenomenon can occur even when the patient is at rest. In some patients with variant angina, the coronary arteries appear to be supersensitive to endogenous vasoconstrictive agents, and a variety of emotional or environmental stimuli may trigger coronary vasospasm.[41,76,80] In many patients, however, the reason for this spontaneous coronary vasoconstriction is unknown.

Calcium channel blockers are usually the drugs of choice in treating the variant form of angina.[48,84] These drugs limit the entry of calcium into the coronary vessels, thus attenuating or preventing the vasospasm underlying variant angina.[84] If calcium channel blockers are not tolerated, long-acting nitrates may be used instead. Calcium channel blockers are especially effective in treating variant angina, however, and most patients with this form of angina respond well to these agents. If patients do not respond to calcium channel blockers alone, long-acting nitrates may be added to calcium channel blockers for management of severe variant angina.[48,80,83]

Unstable Angina

"Unstable" angina is a rather ambiguous term used to identify several serious and potentially life-threatening forms of myocardial ischemia.[8] Unstable angina is often initiated by rupture of atherosclerotic plaques within the coronary arteries, which precipitates coronary vasoconstriction and thrombus formation.[13,47,79] These events cause a decrease in myocardial oxygen supply at the same time that oxygen demand increases in the heart; that is, coronary vasoconstriction-thrombosis is superimposed on an increase in myocardial oxygen requirements.[16] Hence, unstable angina is somewhat of a combination of stable and variant angina. As a result, anginal attacks may begin with minimal levels of exertion or even spontaneously when the patient is at rest. Because unstable angina is also associated with thrombosis and increased platelet aggregation in the affected coronary arteries, this type of angina is often a precursor to acute myocardial infarction.[13] Unstable angina is therefore regarded as the most serious and potentially dangerous form of this disease.

Various traditional antianginal drugs have been used alone or in combination to treat unstable angina.[69] Beta blockers, for example, are among the primary drugs in unstable angina because they decrease cardiac workload and thereby prevent subsequent damage to the ischemic myocardium.[39,64] Beta blockers can also be combined with the two other types of traditional antianginal medications (nitrates and calcium channel blockers), depending on the specific needs and responses of each patient.[24,28,69,77] Most important, however, is the recognition that unstable angina is often associated with coronary artery thrombosis and that anticoagulant and antiplatelet therapy is critical in preventing this type of angina from progressing to myocardial infarction.[7,24,47,79] Hence, heparin and aspirin therapy are often administered in the early stages of unstable angina, with aspirin often continued indefinitely to help prevent coronary occlusion.[64]

NONPHARMACOLOGIC MANAGEMENT
OF ANGINA PECTORIS

The drugs used to treat angina are effective and relatively safe for long-term use. These agents, however, really only treat a symptom of heart disease—namely, the pain associated with myocardial ischemia. Antianginal drugs do not cure any cardiac conditions, nor do they exert any beneficial long-term effects on cardiac function. Consequently, efforts are made in many patients with angina to resolve the underlying disorder responsible for causing an imbalance in myocardial oxygen supply and demand.

Nonpharmacologic treatment usually begins by identifying any potentiating factors that might initiate or exacerbate anginal attacks. For instance, hypertension, congestive heart failure, anemia, and thyrotoxicosis may all contribute to the onset of angina. In some cases, treatment of one of these potentiating factors may effectively resolve the angina, thus making subsequent drug therapy unnecessary. Lifestyle changes including exercise, weight control, giving up smoking, and stress management may also be helpful in decreasing or even eliminating the need for antianginal drugs. Finally, a number of surgical techniques that try to increase coronary blood flow may be attempted. Revascularization procedures such as coronary artery bypass and coronary artery angioplasty may be successful in increasing myocardial oxygen supply, thus attenuating anginal attacks in some patients. Regardless of what strategy is pursued, a permanent solution to the factors that precipitate myocardial ischemia should be explored in all patients with angina pectoris.

SPECIAL CONCERNS IN REHABILITATION PATIENTS

Physical therapists and occupational therapists must be aware of patients who are taking medications for angina pectoris and of whether the medications are taken prophylactically or during an attack. For the patient with stable angina who takes nitroglycerin at the onset of an anginal episode, therapists must make sure the drug is always near at hand during therapy sessions. Because many activities in rehabilitation (exercise, functional training, etc.) increase myocardial oxygen demand, anginal attacks may occur during the therapy session. If the nitroglycerin tablets are in the patient's hospital room (inpatients) or were left at home (outpatients), the anginal attack will be prolonged and possibly severe. A little precaution in making sure patients bring their nitroglycerin to therapy can prevent some tense movements while waiting to see if an anginal attack will subside.

For patients taking antianginal drugs prophylactically (i.e., at regular intervals), having the drug actually present during the rehabilitation session is not as crucial, providing that the patient has been taking the medication as prescribed. Therapists must still be aware, however, that many rehabilitation activities may disturb the balance between myocardial oxygen supply and demand, particularly by increasing oxygen demand beyond the ability of the coronary arteries to increase the oxygen supply to the heart. Consequently, therapists must be aware of the cardiac limitations in their patients with angina and use caution in not overtaxing the heart to the extent that the antianginal drugs are ineffective.

Another important consideration in rehabilitation is the effect of antianginal drugs on the response to an exercise bout. Some patients taking these drugs may experience an *increase* in exercise tolerance because the patient is not as limited by symptoms of angina.[4,43,60] Certain drugs, however, may blunt the ability of the heart to respond to an acute exercise bout. Beta blockers and certain calcium channel blockers, for instance, slow down heart rate and decrease myocardial contractility during exercise.[3,19,37,60,74] At any absolute exercise workload, the myocardial response (e.g., heart rate) of the patient taking these drugs will be lower than if the drug was not taken. Consequently, the heart may not be able to handle some workloads. This blunted exercise response must be taken into account when patients engage in cardiac conditioning activities, and exercise workloads should be adjusted accordingly.

Finally, therapists should be aware of how the side effects of the antianginal drugs may affect the therapy session. The nitrates and calcium channel blockers both produce peripheral vasodilation and can lead to hypotension. This decrease in blood pressure may be exaggerated when the patient suddenly sits up or stands up (orthostatic hypotension). Also, conditions that produce peripheral vasodilation, such as heat or exercise, may produce an additive effect on the drug-induced hypotension, thus leading to dizziness and episodes of fainting (syncope). Therapists should be aware that patients taking nitrates and calcium channel blockers may experience hypotension when systemic heat is applied or when their patients perform exercises that use large muscle groups.

CASE STUDY

ANTIANGINAL DRUGS

Brief History. T.M. is a 73-year-old man who is retired from his job as an accountant. He has a long history of diabetes mellitus, which has progressively worsened over the past decade despite insulin treatments. He also has a history of stable (classic) angina, which has been managed by nitroglycerin. The patient self-administers a nitroglycerin tablet sublingually (0.4 mg per tablet) at the onset of an anginal attack. Recently, this patient was admitted to the hospital for treatment of a gangrenous lesion on his left foot. When this lesion failed to respond to conservative treatment, a left below-knee amputation was performed. Following the amputation, the patient was referred to physical therapy for strengthening and a preprosthetic evaluation.

Problem/Influence of Medication. A program of general conditioning and strengthening was initiated at the patient's bedside the day following surgery. The third day following the amputation, the therapist decided to bring the patient to the physical therapy department for a more intensive program, including standing activities with the parallel bars. The patient arrived in the department via wheelchair and began complaining immediately of chest pains. The patient had not brought his nitroglycerin tablets with him to the therapy session. The therapist immediately phoned the nursing floor, and the patient's medication was rushed to the physical therapy department. While waiting for the nitroglycerin to arrive, the patient's vital signs were monitored, and he was placed in a supine position on a mat table. The drug was administered sublingually while the patient remained supine, and his chest pain subsided.

Decision/Solution. Evidently the exertion and apprehension of merely being transported to the physical therapy department were sufficient to trigger an attack of angina in this patient. The fact that his medication was not readily available created a rather anxious situation, which, fortunately, was resolved without any serious incident. To prevent a repeat of this predicament, the therapist contacted the nursing staff and requested that the patient always bring his medication with him to physical therapy. On subsequent occasions when the patient did experience the onset of angina, he was immediately placed in a supine position and the drug was administered sublingually. The patient was placed supine to prevent any orthostatic hypotension that may occur with nitroglycerin. The patient was eventually fitted with a temporary prosthesis and transferred to an extended-care facility to continue his rehabilitation.

SUMMARY

Pain in the chest region, or angina pectoris, is a common symptom of ischemic heart disease. Anginal pain usually occurs because of an imbalance between myocardial oxygen supply and myocardial oxygen demand. Organic nitrates, beta blockers, and calcium channel blockers are the primary drugs used to treat angina pectoris. Organic nitrates and beta blockers exert their effects primarily by decreasing myocardial oxygen demand, whereas calcium channel blockers primarily increase myocardial oxygen supply. Several forms of angina pectoris can be identified, and specific types of antianginal drugs are used alone or in combination to treat or prevent various forms of angina.

Rehabilitation specialists must be aware of any patients who suffer from angina pectoris and the possibility that patients will have an anginal attack during a therapy session. Therapists should also be cognizant of what drugs are being taken to control the patient's angina, as well as the possibility that side effects of antianginal drugs may influence certain rehabilitation procedures.

REFERENCES

1. Abrams, J: Management of myocardial ischemia: Role of intermittent nitrate therapy. Am Heart J 120(Suppl):762, 1990.
2. Asirvatham, S, Sebastian, C, and Thadani, U: Choosing the most appropriate treatment for stable angina. Safety considerations. Drug Saf 19:23, 1998.
3. Bailey, DG and Carruthers, SG: Interaction between oral verapamil and beta blockers during submaximal exercise: Relevance of ancillary properties. Clin Pharmacol Ther 49:370, 1991.
4. Bassan, M: The day-long antianginal effectiveness of nitroglycerin patches. A double-blind study using dose-titration. Chest 99:1120, 1991.
5. Billups, SJ and Carter, BL: Mibefradil: A new class of calcium-channel antagonists. Ann Pharmacother 32:659, 1998.
6. Brown, BG, et al: The mechanism of nitroglycerin action: Stenosis vasodilation as a major component of the drug response. Circulation 64:1089, 1981.
7. Brunnelli, C, et al: Recognition and treatment of unstable angina. Drugs 52:196, 1996.
8. Chai, AU and Crawford, MH: "Traditional" medical therapy for unstable angina. How important? How to use? Cardiol Clin 17:359, 1999.
9. Cheng, JW and Behar, L: Calcium channel blockers: Association with myocardial infarction, mortality, and cancer. Clin Ther 19:1255, 1997.
10. Choy, JB and Armstrong, PW: Anticoagulant therapy in unstable angina. Cardiol Clin 17:327, 1999.
11. Cleophas, TJ, et al: Combination of calcium channel blockers and beta-blockers for patients with exercise-induced angina pectoris: Beneficial effect of calcium channel blockers largely determined by their effect on heart rate. J Clin Pharmacol 39:738, 1999.
12. Cohen, M: Approaches to the treatment of unstable angina and non-Q wave myocardial infarction. Can J Cardiol 14(Suppl E):11E, 1998.
13. Cohen, M: New therapies for unstable angina and non-Q-wave myocardial infarction: Recent clinical trials. Am Heart J 135(part 3 Suppl):S343, 1998.
14. Cohn, JN: Pharmacologic mechanisms of nitrates in myocardial ischemia. Am J Cardiol 70:G38, 1992.
15. Cohn, PF: Rationale for the use of calcium antagonists in the treatment of silent myocardial ischemia. Clin Ther 19(Suppl A):74, 1997.
16. Cohn, PF: Mechanisms of myocardial ischemia. Am J Cardiol 70:14G, 1992.

17. Creel, CA: Silent myocardial ischemia and nursing implications. Heart Lung 23:218, 1994.
18. Curry, SH, et al: Plasma nitroglycerin concentrations and hemodynamics: Effects of sublingual, ointment and controlled-release forms of nitroglycerin. Clin Pharmacol Ther 36:765, 1984.
19. Dargie, HJ, Grant, S, and McLenachan, J: Angina, ischemia, and effort tolerance with vasodilating beta-blockers. Am Heart J 121:1017, 1991.
20. Darius, H: Role of nitrates for the therapy of coronary artery disease patients in the years beyond 2000. J Cardiovasc Pharmacol 34(Suppl 2):S15, 1999.
21. DeMuinck, ED and Lie, KI: Safety and efficacy of beta-blockers in the treatment of stable angina pectoris. J Cardiovasc Pharmacol 16(Suppl 5):S123, 1990.
22. Dong, EW, et al: A systematic review and meta-analysis of the incidence of cancer in randomized, controlled trials of verapamil. Pharmacotherapy 17:1210, 1997.
23. Ernst, ME and Kelly, MW: Mibefradil, a pharmacologically distinct calcium antagonist. Pharmacotherapy 18:463, 1998.
24. Fox, KM, Mulcahy, D, and Purcell, H: Unstable and stable angina. Eur Heart J 14(Suppl F):15, 1993.
25. Frishman, WH, et al: Comparison of controlled-onset, extended-release verapamil with amlodipine and amlodipine plus atenolol on exercise performance and ambulatory ischemia in patients with chronic stable angina pectoris. Am J Cardiol 83:507, 1999.
26. Fung, HL: Clinical pharmacology of organic nitrates. Am J Cardiol 72:C9, 1993.
27. Futterman, LG and Lemberg, L: Low-molecular-weight heparin: An antithrombotic agent whose time has come. Am J Crit Care 8:520, 1999.
28. Gerstenblith, G: Treatment of unstable angina pectoris. Am J Cardiol 70:32G, 1992.
29. Gonzalez Maqueda, I: Treatment of chronic stable angina with carvedilol: A multiple-action neurohormonal antagonist. A review of controlled clinical trials. J Int Med Res 26:107, 1998.
30. Gradman, AH: The evolving role of calcium channel blockers in the treatment of angina pectoris: Focus on felodipine. Can J Cardiol 11(Suppl B):14B, 1995.
31. Greco, R, et al: Long-term efficacy of nitroglycerin patch in stable angina pectoris. Am J Cardiol 65:9J, 1990.
32. Gurfinkel, E, et al: Rationale for the management of coronary syndromes with low-molecular-weight heparins. Am J Cardiol 82(Suppl 5B):15L, 1998.
33. Hansson, L: Calcium antagonists: An overview. Am Heart J 122:308, 1991.
34. Hansson, L: Review of state-of-the-art beta-blocker therapy. Am J Cardiol 67:43B, 1991.
35. Herlitz, J, Brorsson, B, and Werko, L: Factors associated with the use of various medications amongst patients with severe coronary artery disease. SECOR/SBU Project Group. J Intern Med 245:143, 1999.
36. Hermsmeyer, K, et al: Physiologic and pathophysiologic relevance of T-type calcium-ion channels: Potential indications for T-type calcium antagonists. Clin Ther 19(Suppl A):18, 1997.
37. Hughson, RL and Kowalchuk, JM: Beta-blockade and oxygen delivery to muscle during exercise. Can J Physiol Pharmacol 69:285, 1991.
38. Ignarro, LJ and Kadowitz, PJ: The pharmacological and physiological role of cyclic GMP in vascular smooth muscle relaxation. Annu Rev Pharmacol Toxicol 25:171, 1985.
39. Iliadis, EA, et al: Clinical practice guidelines in unstable angina improve clinical outcomes by assuring early intensive medical treatment. J Am Coll Cardiol 34:1689, 1999.
40. Jordan, RA, et al: Rapidly developing tolerance to transdermal nitroglycerin in congestive heart failure. Ann Intern Med 104:295, 1985.
41. Kaski, JC, et al: Local coronary supersensitivity to diverse vasoconstrictive stimuli in patients with variant angina. Circulation 74:1255, 1986.
42. Krum, H: Critical assessment of calcium antagonists. Aust Fam Physician 26:841, 1997.
43. Lai, C, et al: Effect of calcium antagonists on exercise tests. J Cardiovasc Pharmacol 20(Suppl 5):S55, 1992.
44. Mason, RP: Effects of calcium channel blockers on cellular apoptosis: Implications for carcinogenic potential. Cancer 85:2093, 1999.
45. Massie, BM: Mibefradil, a T-type channel-selective calcium antagonist: Clinical trials in chronic stable angina pectoris. Am J Hypertens 11(Suppl 3):95S, 1998.
46. Massie, BM: The safety of calcium channel blockers. Clin Cardiol 21(Suppl 2):II12, 1998.
47. Mattioli, AV, et al: Efficacy and tolerability of a very low molecular weight heparin compared with standard heparin in patients with unstable angina: A pilot study. Clin Cardiol 22:213, 1999.
48. Mayer, S and Hillis, LD: Prinzmetal's variant angina. Clin Cardiol 21:243, 1998.
49. Meluzin, J, et al: Effects of nifedipine and diltiazem on myocardial ischemia in patients with severe stable angina pectoris treated with nitrates and beta-blockers. J Cardiovasc Pharmacol 20:864, 1992.
50. Messerli, FH and Grossman, E: The calcium antagonist controversy: A posthumous commentary. Am J Cardiol 82(Suppl 9B):35R, 1998.
51. Nabel, EG, et al: Effects of dosing intervals on the development of tolerance to high dose transdermal nitroglycerin. Am J Cardiol 63:663, 1989.
52. Nesto, RW and Phillips, RT: Silent myocardial ischemia: Clinical characteristics underlying mechanisms and indications for treatment. Am J Med 81(Suppl 4a):12, 1986.
53. Nobel, S and Spencer, CM: Enoxaparin. A review of its clinical potential in the management of coronary artery disease. Drugs 56:259, 1998.
54. Noli, G and Luscher, TF: Comparative pharmacological properties among calcium channel blockers: T-channel versus L-channel blockade. Cardiology 89(Suppl 1):10, 1998.

55. Paciaroni, E and Luca, C: Discontinuous transdermal nitroglycerin as treatment for stable angina in the elderly: A double-blind multicentre study. Eur Heart J 12:1076, 1991.
56. Parker, JO: Nitrates and angina pectoris. Am J Cardiol 72:3C, 1993.
57. Parmley, WW: Optimum treatment of stable angina pectoris. Cardiovasc Drugs Ther 12(Suppl 1):105, 1998.
58. Parmley, WW: Optimum treatment of stable angina. Cardiology 88(Suppl 3):27, 1997.
59. Pearle, DL: Pharmacologic management of ischemic heart disease with beta-blockers and calcium channel blockers. Am Heart J 120(Suppl):739, 1990.
60. Peel, C and Mossberg, KA: Effects of cardiovascular medications on exercise responses. Phys Ther 75:387, 1995.
61. Pepine, CJ: Clinical aspects of silent myocardial ischemia in patients with angina and other forms of coronary heart disease. Am J Med 80(Suppl 4c):25, 1986.
62. Pitt, B: Diversity of calcium antagonists. Clin Ther 19(Suppl A):3, 1997.
63. Prisant, LM: Calcium antagonists: Pharmacologic considerations. Ethn Dis 8:98, 1998.
64. Prisant, LM, et al: Pharmacotherapy of unstable angina. J Clin Pharmacol 32:390, 1992.
65. Purcell, H and Fox, KM: Current roles and future possibilities for low-molecular-weight heparins in unstable angina. Eur Heart J 19(Suppl K):K18, 1998.
66. Reichek, N, Goldstein, RE, and Redwood, DR: Sustained effects of nitroglycerin ointment in patients with angina pectoris. Circulation 50:348, 1974.
67. Reiniger, G and Lehmann, G: Increasing nitroglycerin release from patches enables circumvention of early nitrate tolerance. Cardiovasc Drugs Ther 12:217, 1998.
68. Robertson, RM and Robertson, D: Drugs used for the treatment of myocardial ischemia. In Hardman, JG, et al (eds): The Pharmacologic Basis of Therapeutics, ed 9. McGraw-Hill, New York, 1996.
69. Rutherford, JD, et al: Pharmacologic management of angina and acute myocardial infarction. Am J Cardiol 72:C16, 1993.
70. Scheidt, S: Angina: Evolution of the role of nitrates. Am Heart J 120(Suppl):757, 1990.
71. Silvestry, FE and St John Sutton, MG: Sustained-release calcium channel antagonists in cardiovascular disease: Pharmacology and current therapeutic use. Eur Heart J 19(Suppl I):I8, 1998.
72. Spaulding, C, Cabanes, L, and Weber, S: Pharmacological and therapeutic basis for combined administration of beta blockers and calcium channel blockers in the treatment of stable chronic angina. Br J Clin Pract Suppl 88:17, 1997.
73. Stason, WB, et al: Safety of nifedipine in angina pectoris: A meta-analysis. Hypertension 33:24, 1999.
74. Stewart, JK, et al: Effects of diltiazem or propranolol during exercise training of hypertensive men. Med Sci Sports Exerc 22:171, 1990.
75. Struyker-Boudier, HAJ, Smits, JFM, and DeMey, JGR: The pharmacology of calcium antagonists: A review. J Cardiovasc Pharmacol 15(Suppl 4):S1, 1990.
76. Symposium (various authors): Triggering and circadian variation of onset of acute cardiovascular disease. Am J Cardiol 66:1G, 1990.
77. Talbert, RL: Ischemic heart disease. In DiPiro, JT, et al (eds): Pharmacotherapy: A Pathophysiologic Approach, ed 4. Appleton & Lange, Stamford, CT, 1999.
78. Turner, P: Which ancillary properties of beta-adrenoceptor blocking drugs influence their therapeutic and adverse effects: A review. J R Soc Med 84:672, 1991.
79. Turpie, AG: Anticoagulants in acute coronary syndromes. Am J Cardiol 84(Suppl 5A):2M, 1999.
80. Vandergoten, P, Benit, E, and Dendale, P: Prinzmetal's variant angina: Three case reports and a review of the literature. Acta Cardiol 54:71, 1999.
81. Van Zwieten, PA: Clinical pharmacology of calcium antagonists as antihypertensive and anti-anginal drugs. J Hypertens Suppl 14:S3, 1996.
82. Waller, DG: Optimal nitrate therapy with once-daily sustained-release formulation of isosorbide mononitrate. J Cardiovasc Pharmacol 34(Suppl 2):S21, 1999.
83. Winniford, MD, et al: Concomitant calcium antagonist plus isosorbide dinitrate therapy for markedly active variant angina. Am Heart J 108:1269, 1984.
84. Zavecz, JH and Bueno, O: Pharmacologic therapy of angina pectoris. J La State Med Soc 147:208, 1995.
85. Zed, PJ, Tisdale, JE, and Borzak, S: Low-molecular-weight heparins in the management of acute coronary syndromes. Arch Intern Med 159:1849, 1999.

CHAPTER 23

Treatment of Cardiac Arrhythmias

An *arrhythmia* can be broadly defined as any significant deviation from normal cardiac rhythm.[3,5] Various problems in the origination and conduction of electrical activity in the heart can lead to distinct types of arrhythmias. If untreated, disturbances in normal cardiac rhythm result in impaired cardiac pumping ability, and certain arrhythmias are associated with cerebrovascular accidents, cardiac failure, and other sequelae that can be fatal.[23,38,46] Fortunately, a variety of drugs are available to help establish and maintain normal cardiac rhythm.

This chapter presents the primary antiarrhythmic drugs and the therapeutic rationale for their use. Many patients seen in rehabilitation are given these drugs to help control and prevent the onset of arrhythmias. Physical therapists and occupational therapists often work directly with cardiac patients in cardiac rehabilitation and fitness programs. Likewise, cardiac patients taking antiarrhythmic drugs may be seen in rehabilitation for any number of other neuromuscular or musculoskeletal disorders. Consequently, therapists should have some knowledge of the clinical use of these drugs.

To understand how antiarrhythmic drugs exert their effects, we first review the origin and spread of electrical activity throughout the heart. This chapter begins with a brief discussion of cardiac electrophysiology, followed by a presentation of the basic mechanisms responsible for producing disturbances in cardiac rhythm and the common types of arrhythmias seen clinically. Finally, antiarrhythmic drugs are presented according to their mechanism of action and clinical use.

CARDIAC ELECTROPHYSIOLOGY

Cardiac Action Potentials

The action potential recorded from a cardiac Purkinje fiber is shown in Figure 23–1. At rest, the interior of the cell is negative relative to the cell's exterior. As in other excitable tissues (neurons, skeletal muscle), an action potential occurs when the cell interior suddenly becomes positive (*depolarizes*), primarily because of the influx of sodium

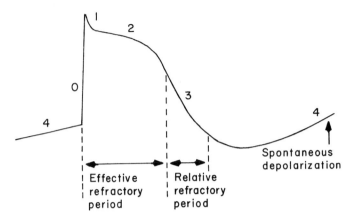

FIGURE 23–1. The cardiac action potential recorded from a Purkinje cell. The effective refractory period is the time during which the cell cannot be depolarized, and the relative refractory period is the time in which a supranormal stimulus is required to depolarize the cell. Action potential phases (0–4) and the ionic basis for each phase are discussed in the text. (From Keefe, DLD, Kates, RE, and Harrison, DC: New antiarrhythmic drugs: Their place in therapy. Drugs 22:363, 1981, with permission.)

ions. The cell interior then returns to a negative potential (*repolarizes*), primarily because of the efflux of potassium ions. The cardiac action potential, however, has several features that distinguish it from action potentials recorded in other nerves and muscles.[2,3] The cardiac action potential is typically divided into several phases (see Fig. 23–1). The ionic movement that occurs in each phase is outlined here.

Phase 0:   Rapid depolarization occurs because of the sudden influx of sodium ions into the cell. At some threshold level, the cell membrane suddenly becomes permeable to sodium ions because of the opening of sodium channels or gates, similar to the spike seen in skeletal muscle depolarization.

Phase 1:   An early, brief period of repolarization occurs because of potassium leaving the cell. Specific potassium channels in the cell membrane open to allow potassium to leave the cell.

Phase 2:   The action potential undergoes a plateau phase, primarily because of the opening of calcium channels and a slow, prolonged influx of calcium ions into the cell. Because the efflux of positively charged potassium ions that occurred in phase 1 is balanced by the influx of positively charged calcium ions, there is no net change in the charge within the cell. Thus, the cell's potential remains relatively constant for a brief period of time, creating the distinctive plateau seen in Figure 23–1. This phase 2 plateau is important in cardiac cells because it prolongs the cell's effective refractory period (i.e., the time interval between successive action potentials). The plateau basically enables the heart to enter a period of rest (*diastole*) so that the cardiac chambers can fill with blood before the next contraction (*systole*).

Phase 3:   At the end of the plateau, repolarization is completed. This is primarily because of the closing (*inactivation*) of the calcium channels, thus terminating the entry of calcium into the cell. Repolarization is completed by the unopposed exit of potassium ions.

Phase 4:   In certain cardiac cells (such as the one shown in Fig. 23–1), phase 4 consists of a slow, spontaneous depolarization. This spontaneous depolarization probably occurs because of the continuous leak of sodium ions into the cell, combined with a gradual decrease in potassium exit from the cell. This combination of sodium entry and decreased potassium exit causes a progressive accumulation of positive charge within the cell, which causes the cell to become more and more positive until it reaches threshold and phase 0 is initiated.[2]

Action potentials recorded from various cardiac cells may vary somewhat from the action potential described previously. Some cells, for instance, may totally lack phase 1 and have a much slower phase 0. Such cells are said to have a slow response as opposed to the fast response just described. Also, action potentials from the nodal cells (see the next section, "Normal Cardiac Rhythm") differ somewhat from the fast-response cells. Nonetheless, the fundamental ionic fluxes that occur during cardiac action potentials are similar in all cardiac cells. This ionic activity is pharmacologically significant because various antiarrhythmic drugs will affect the movement of sodium and other ions in an attempt to establish and maintain normal cardiac rhythm.

Normal Cardiac Rhythm

Certain cardiac cells are able to initiate and maintain a spontaneous automatic rhythm. Even in the absence of any neural or hormonal input, these cells will automatically generate an action potential. They are usually referred to as *pacemaker cells* in the myocardium. Pacemaker cells have the ability to depolarize spontaneously because of a rising phase 4 in the cardiac action potential (see Fig. 23–1). As described previously, the resting cell automatically begins to depolarize during phase 4 until the cell reaches threshold and an action potential is initiated.

Pacemaker cells are found primarily in the sinoatrial (SA) node and in the atrioventricular (AV) node (Fig. 23–2). Although many other cardiac cells also have the ability to generate an automatic rhythm, the pacemaker cells in the SA node usually dominate and control cardiac rhythm in the normal heart.

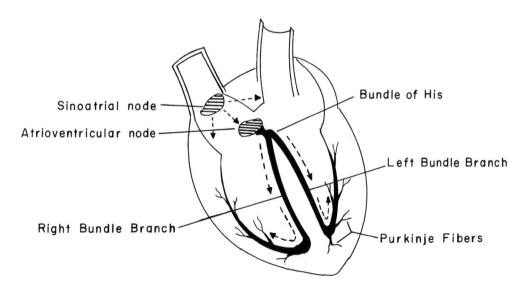

FIGURE 23–2. Schematic representation of the conduction system of the heart. Conduction normally follows the pathways indicated by the dashed lines. Impulses originate in the sinoatrial node and are transmitted to the atrioventricular node. Impulses are then conducted from the atrioventricular node to the ventricles by the bundle of His and the bundle branches.

Normal Conduction of the Cardiac Action Potential

The cardiac action potential is normally conducted throughout the heart in a coordinated and predictable pattern[5] (see Fig. 23–2). The action potential originates in the SA node and is conducted throughout both atria via the atrial muscle cells. While spreading through the atria, the action potential reaches the AV node. From the AV node, the action potential is passed on to the ventricles via a specialized conducting system known as the *bundle of His*. The bundle of His is primarily made up of specialized conducting cells known as *Purkinje fibers*. As the bundle leaves the AV node, it divides into left and right branches, which supply the respective ventricles. The action potential is distributed to all parts of the ventricles via the bundle branches and Purkinje fibers (see Fig. 23–2).

MECHANISMS OF CARDIAC ARRHYTHMIAS

The origin of the cardiac action potential and the system of action potential propagation represent normal cardiac excitation and conduction. Any number of factors can disrupt the normal cardiac excitation process, however, thus resulting in arrhythmic contractions. Such factors include disease, genetic factors, metabolic and electrolyte imbalances, abnormal autonomic influence on the heart, toxicity from other drugs (e.g., digitalis), and myocardial ischemia and infarction.[5,22,27,34,43] Regardless of what the initiating factor is in producing arrhythmias, the mechanism underlying a disturbance in cardiac rhythm can be attributed to one of the three basic abnormalities listed here.[5]

1. *Abnormal impulse generation:* The normal automatic rhythm of the cardiac pacemaker cells has been disrupted. Injury and disease may directly render the SA and AV cells incapable of maintaining normal rhythm. Also, cells that do not normally control cardiac rhythm may begin to compete with pacemaker cells, thus creating multiple areas of automaticity.
2. *Abnormal impulse conduction:* The conduction of impulses throughout the myocardium has been interrupted. Various diseases and local damage may result in the delay or failure of an action potential to reach certain areas. These conduction impairments or heart blocks can prevent a smooth and synchronous contraction, thus creating an abnormal rhythm.
3. *Simultaneous abnormalities of impulse generation and conduction:* A combination of both factors listed previously may cause cardiac arrhythmias.

TYPES OF ARRHYTHMIAS

Cardiac arrhythmias are described by many different terms according to their site of origin, nature of the disturbed heartbeat, or impairment in cardiac conduction.[2,5,7] This text cannot fully describe all of the various forms of arrhythmias occurring clinically. To understand when various antiarrhythmic drugs are used, however, some basic terms describing cardiac arrhythmias must be defined. Some of the more common arrhythmias are listed in Table 23–1. For a more detailed description of the electrophysiologic nature and diagnosis of these arrhythmias, the reader is referred to other sources on this topic.[3,18]

TABLE 23–1 Common Forms of Arrhythmias

Classification	Characteristic Rhythm
Sinus arrhythmias	
Sinus tachycardia	>100 beats/min
Sinus bradycardia	<60 beats/min
Sick sinus syndrome	Severe bradycardia (<50 beats/min); periods of sinus arrest
Supraventricular arrhythmias	
Atrial fibrillation and flutter	Atrial rate > 300 beats/min
Atrial tachycardia	Atrial rate >140–200 beats/min
Premature atrial contractions	Variable
Atrioventricular junctional arrhythmias	
Junctional rhythm	40–55 beats/min
Junctional tachycardia	100–200 beats/min
Conduction disturbances	
Atrioventricular block	Variable
Bundle branch block	Variable
Fascicular block	Variable
Ventricular arrhythmias	
Premature ventricular contractions	Variable
Ventricular tachycardia	140–200 beats/min
Ventricular fibrillation	Irregular, totally uncoordinated rhythm

CLASSIFICATION OF ANTIARRHYTHMIC DRUGS

Drugs used to treat cardiac arrhythmias are traditionally placed in one of four distinct classes according to their mechanism of action.[30,31,36,45] These classifications are summarized in Table 23–2. The accuracy of this classification system has been criticized because some drugs have characteristics that make it difficult to place them in one specific category. Nonetheless, this method of categorizing antiarrhythmic drugs is still commonly used to describe these drugs.[25,30,44] The mechanism of action and specific agents within each class are described here.

CLASS I: SODIUM CHANNEL BLOCKERS

Mechanism of Action and Rationale for Use

Class I antiarrhythmic drugs are essentially sodium channel blockers.[10,29] These drugs bind to membrane sodium channels in various excitable tissues including myocardial cells. In cardiac tissues, class I drugs control sodium channel function by binding to sodium channels that are open (activated) or closed (inactivated).[36] This action normalizes the rate of sodium entry into cardiac tissues and thereby helps control cardiac excitation and conduction.[10] Many class I agents (e.g., lidocaine) are also used as local anesthetics, and the way that these drugs bind to sodium channels is discussed in more detail in Chapter 12.

TABLE 23–2 Classification of Antiarrhythmic Drugs

Generic Names	Trade Names
Class I: Sodium channel blockers	
Subclass A	
Disopyramide	Norpace
Procainamide	Promine, Pronestyl, Procan
Quinidine	Cardioquin, Quinidex, others
Subclass B	
Lidocaine	Xylocaine
Mexiletine	Mexitil
Moricizine*	Ethmozine
Tocainide	Tonocard
Subclass C	
Flecainide	Tambocor
Propafenone	Rythmol
Class II: Beta blocker	
Acebutolol	Sectral
Atenolol	Tenormin
Metoprolol	Lopressor
Nadolol	Corgard
Propranolol	Inderal
Sotalol	Betapace
Timolol	Blocadren
Class III: Drugs that prolong repolarization	
Amiodarone†	Cordarone
Bretylium	Bretylol
Ibutilide	Corvert
Class IV: Calcium channel blocker	
Diltiazem	Cardizem
Verapamil	Calan, Isoptin

*Also has some class IC properties.
†Also has some class I properties.

Because sodium influx plays an important role during action potential generation in phase 0 of the cardiac action potential, inhibition of sodium channels tends to decrease membrane excitability.[16] Thus, class I drugs help stabilize the cardiac cell membrane and normalize the rate of firing of cardiac cells. Although all class I drugs exert their antiarrhythmic effects by inhibiting sodium channel function, various agents affect myocardial excitation and conduction in slightly different ways. Class I drugs are typically subclassified according to how they influence cardiac electrophysiology[31,36] (see Table 23–2). These subclassifications and specific agents in each group are presented here.

Specific Agents

Class IA. Drugs in this group are similar in that they produce a moderate slowing of phase 0 depolarization and a moderate slowing of action potential propagation throughout the myocardium. These drugs also prolong repolarization of the cardiac cell, thus lengthening the time interval before a second action potential can occur (i.e., they increase the effective refractory period). Class IA agents include quinidine, procainamide, and disopyramide (see Table 23–2). Class IA drugs are used to treat a variety of arrhythmias that originate in the ventricles or the atria.

Class IB. These drugs display only a minimal ability to slow phase 0 depolarization, and they produce only a minimal slowing of cardiac conduction. In contrast to IA drugs, class IB agents usually shorten cardiac repolarization; that is, the effective refractory period is decreased. Class IB drugs include lidocaine, mexiletine, moricizine, and tocainide (see Table 23–2). These drugs are primarily used to treat ventricular arrhythmias such as ventricular tachycardia and premature ventricular contractions (PVCs). Lidocaine can be especially effective in treating some patients with severe ventricular arrhythmias that occur following myocardial infarction and cardiac surgery.[35] Routine use of this drug in all patients who have had an acute myocardial infarction has been questioned, however, and administration of lidocaine and other class I drugs should be considered on a patient-by-patient basis following infarction.[1,41]

Class IC. These drugs produce both a marked decrease in the rate of phase 0 depolarization and a marked slowing of cardiac conduction. They have little effect on repolarization, however. Class IC drugs, which include flecainide and propafenone (see Table 23–2), appear to be best suited to treat ventricular arrhythmias, such as ventricular tachycardia and PVCs.

Adverse Side Effects

Despite their use in treating arrhythmias, the most common side effect of all antiarrhythmic drugs is their tendency to *increase* rhythm disturbances (proarrhythmic effects). While attempting to control one type of arrhythmia, these agents can aggravate or initiate other cardiac rhythm abnormalities.[9,13,14,33] This fact seems especially true for the class I agents.[10,42] Because these drugs affect sodium channel function and cardiac excitability, they may produce some serious proarrhythmic effects in certain patients. For example, patients with heart failure, myocardial ischemia, and structural heart disease (including previous infarction) seem to be especially prone to class I–induced arrhythmias, and these drugs should probably be avoided in these patients.[11,32,40,42] Class I drugs are also associated with a variety of annoying side effects such as dizziness, visual disturbances, and nausea.[33] These symptoms are often important, however, because they may indicate the presence of arrhythmias even when the pulse or ECG is not being directly monitored. Hence, class I drugs are still important in treating certain arrhythmias, but they are used less often and more cautiously than in the past.[10,31]

CLASS II: BETA BLOCKERS

Mechanism of Action and Rationale for Use

Drugs that block beta-1 receptors on the myocardium are one of the mainstays in the treatment of arrhythmias. Beta blockers are effective because they decrease the excitatory effects of the sympathetic nervous system and related catecholamines (norepinephrine and epinephrine) on the heart.[31,36] This effect typically decreases cardiac automaticity and prolongs the effective refractory period, thus slowing the heart rate.[2] Beta blockers also slow down conduction through the myocardium. These drugs are most effective in treating heart rate problems that originate in the atria (supraventricular arrhythmias), especially problems originating in the AV node. Some ventricular arrhythmias may also respond to treatment with beta blockers.

Specific Agents

Individual beta blockers are presented in Chapter 20. Beta blockers shown to be effective in treating arrhythmias include acebutolol, atenolol, metoprolol, nadolol, propranolol, sotalol, and timolol (see Table 23–2). Choice of a specific beta blocker depends to a large extent on the exact type of arrhythmia present and the individual patient's response to the drug.

Adverse Side Effects

Because of the ability of beta blockers to slow down the heart, certain patients with poor cardiac pumping ability may experience heart failure when given these drugs. Also, beta blockers may produce excessive slowing of cardiac conduction in some individuals, resulting in an increase in arrhythmias. Both of these problems are relatively rare, however, and beta blockers when used appropriately to treat arrhythmias are well tolerated by most patients.

CLASS III: DRUGS THAT PROLONG REPOLARIZATION

Mechanism of Action and Rationale for Use

These agents delay repolarization of cardiac cells, thus prolonging the effective refractory period of the cardiac action potential.[16,21,24,31] This delay lengthens the time interval before a subsequent action potential can be initiated, thus slowing and stabilizing the heart rate. The effects of class III drugs are complex, but their ability to lengthen the cardiac action potential is most likely mediated by inhibition of potassium efflux during repolarization[2,24]; that is, these drugs limit the ability of potassium to leave the cell during phases 2 and 3 of the action potential, which prolongs repolarization and prevents the cell from firing another action potential too rapidly. Class III drugs are used to treat ventricular arrhythmias such as ventricular tachycardia and ventricular fibrillation and supraventricular arrhythmias such as postoperative atrial fibrillation.[28] Interest in using these drugs and developing new class III agents has increased recently because they affect both atrial and ventricular problems and because they are relatively safe compared with other agents such as the class I drugs.[8,12,31,40]

Specific Agents

Class III drugs currently in use include amiodarone, bretylium, and ibutilide (see Table 23–2). These drugs all exert their primary effects by prolonging repolarization in cardiac cells. Amiodarone, however, also appears to have some properties similar to drugs in other classes, and it may also help control arrhythmias by inhibiting sodium channel function (class I effect), by beta blockade (class II effect), or even by blocking calcium channels (class IV effect).[30]

Adverse Side Effects

An initial increase in cardiac arrhythmias (proarrhythmic effect) may occur when class III drugs are instituted. The most important proarrhythmia is known as torsades de pointes, which is a form of ventricular tachycardia that can be fatal.[8,42] Specific class III agents are associated with various other side effects. Amiodarone, for example, is also associated with pulmonary toxicity and liver damage. Other drugs such as sotalol may have a more favorable side effect profile but may not be as effective in controlling arrhythmias. Side effects of class III drugs therefore vary from agent to agent, and any untoward effects should be monitored carefully.

CLASS IV: CALCIUM CHANNEL BLOCKERS

Mechanism of Action and Rationale for Use

Class IV drugs have a selective ability to block calcium entry into myocardial and vascular smooth-muscle cells. These drugs inhibit calcium influx by binding to specific channels in the cell membrane.[16,36,37] As discussed previously in this chapter, calcium entry plays an important role in the generation of the cardiac action potential, especially during phase 2. By inhibiting calcium influx into myocardial cells, calcium channel blockers can alter the excitability and conduction of cardiac tissues.

Calcium channel blockers decrease the rate of discharge of the SA node, and they inhibit conduction velocity through the AV node.[2,19] These drugs are most successful in treating arrhythmias caused by atrial dysfunction, such as supraventricular tachycardia and atrial fibrillation.[42]

Specific Agents

The pharmacology of specific calcium channel blockers is presented in Chapter 22. Of the calcium channel blockers currently in use, verapamil and diltiazem are currently approved for treating arrhythmias (Table 23–2). Of these two drugs, verapamil appears to be more effective as an antiarrhythmic,[6,26] and this drug has been used to treat both acute and chronic forms of supraventricular arrhythmias, as well as arrhythmias induced by digitalis.[15] Diltiazem is only moderately effective in treating arrhythmias, and other calcium channel blockers such as nifedipine and similar dihydropyridines (see Chap. 22) do not have any substantial effects on cardiac rhythm. These other calcium channel blockers are more effective in dilating vascular smooth muscle and are used more frequently to treat hypertension and angina pectoris (see Chaps. 21 and 22).

Adverse Side Effects

Because drugs like verapamil slow down heart rate by inhibiting calcium entry into cardiac muscle cells, excessive bradycardia (less than 50 beats per minute) may occur in some patients receiving these drugs. Calcium channel blockers also limit calcium entry into vascular smooth muscle, which may cause peripheral vasodilation and lead to dizziness and headaches in some patients.

NONPHARMACOLOGIC TREATMENT OF ARRHYTHMIAS

Antiarrhythmic drugs often help normalize cardiac rhythm and decrease the symptoms associated with cardiac arrhythmias. These drugs, however, do not usually cure these conditions because they do not typically resolve the source of the arrhythmia. As indicated earlier, many antiarrhythmic drugs are also associated with potentially serious side effects, including the risk of increased arrhythmias.[17] Hence, other interventions have been used to try to treat the cause of the rhythm disturbance. In particular, implantable electronic devices (cardioverter defibrillators) and other surgeries (electrode catheter ablation) have been used increasingly to supplement or replace drug therapy in helping control certain arrhythmias.[4,17,20,39,47] Consequently, drug therapy remains a common treatment for people with arrhythmias, but many patients may also receive nonpharmacologic treatment to help provide a longer-term solution for certain rhythm disturbances.

SPECIAL CONCERNS IN REHABILITATION PATIENTS

The primary problems associated with antiarrhythmic drugs in rehabilitation patients are related to the side effects of these agents. Therapists should be aware of the potential for increased arrhythmias or changes in the nature of arrhythmias with these drugs, especially in patients involved in exercise and cardiac rehabilitation programs. Therapists who supervise such patients often can detect the presence of arrhythmias by monitoring ECG recordings. If an ECG recording is not available, palpation of pulses for rate and regularity may detect rhythm disturbances. Also, the presence of other side effects such as faintness or dizziness may signal the presence of cardiotoxic drug effects and increased arrhythmias. Consequently, therapists treating patients for both cardiac and noncardiac disorders may help detect the cardiotoxic effects of antiarrhythmic drugs by being alert for any side effects. By playing a role in the early detection of increased arrhythmias, therapists can alert the physician to a problem and avert any potentially serious or even fatal consequences.

Other concerns related to the side effects are fairly minor. Hypotension may occur with some agents, especially with bretylium (class III) and the calcium channel blockers (class IV). Therapists should be aware that patients may become dizzy, especially after sudden changes in posture.

CASE STUDY

ANTIARRHYTHMIC DRUGS

Brief History. M.R. is a 48-year-old man with a history of coronary artery disease and cardiac rhythm disturbances. Specifically, he has experienced episodes of paroxysmal supraventricular tachycardia, with his heart rate often exceeding 180 beats per minute. He has been treated for several years with the nonspecific beta blocker propranolol (Inderal). Oral propranolol (60 mg/day) has successfully diminished his episodes of tachycardia. In an effort to improve his myocardial function and overall cardiovascular fitness, the patient recently enrolled as an outpatient in a cardiac rehabilitation program. Under the supervision of a physical therapist, he attended cardiac training sessions three times each week. A typical session consisted of warm-up calisthenics, bicycle ergometry, and cool-down stretching activities. Each session lasted approximately 45 minutes.

Problem/Influence of Medication. Propranolol and the other beta blockers are successful in reducing various supraventricular arrhythmias. These drugs, however, also attenuate the cardiac response to exercise. Heart rate and cardiac output are lower at any absolute workload, and maximal heart rate and cardiac output are attenuated by beta blockade. Consequently, the exercise response of a patient taking a beta blocker will be less than if the patient is not taking the drug. This consideration is important because the exercise prescription for any given patient must take into account the patient's maximal exercise capacity. Typically, patients exercise at some submaximal percentage of their maximal ability. If maximal exercise capacity is influenced by the beta blocker, the exercise prescription must be adjusted accordingly.

Decision/Solution. Prior to beginning the rehabilitation program, the patient underwent a graded exercise test (GXT). All patients with cardiac disorders should undergo a GXT before beginning a cardiac rehabilitation program. Patients taking beta blockers and other drugs that affect cardiac function must also be tested under the conditions in which they will eventually be exercising. The GXT accurately determined the patient's exercise workload while he was taking his normal dosage of propranolol. Consequently, the prescribed exercise workload was adjusted by the therapist for the effect of the beta blocker.

During the cardiac rehabilitation sessions, the therapist periodically monitored heart rate, blood pressure, and ECG. No significant episodes of arrhythmias were noted, and the patient progressed rapidly through the program. He was eventually discharged from the formal program with instructions for how to continue his rehabilitation exercises at home and at a local health club.

SUMMARY

Cardiac arrhythmias may arise because of disturbances in the origination and conduction of electrical activity in the heart. These changes in cardiac rhythm can be controlled to a large extent by several groups of drugs, including sodium channel blockers, beta blockers, calcium channel blockers, and drugs that prolong the cardiac action potential. These agents work by different cellular mechanisms to stabilize heart rate and improve the conduction of electrical impulses throughout the myocardium. Although these drugs are often successful in preventing or resolving arrhythmias, rehabilitation specialists should be cognizant of patients who are taking these agents. Therapists should also be alert for any changes in cardiac function or other side effects that may signal toxicity of these drugs.

REFERENCES

1. Antman, EM and Berlin, JA: Declining incidence of ventricular fibrillation in myocardial infarction: Implications for the prophylactic use of lidocaine. Circulation 86:764, 1992.
2. Bauman, JL and Schoen, MD: Arrhythmias. In DiPiro, JT, et al (eds): Pharmacotherapy: A Pathophysiologic Approach, ed 4. Appleton & Lange, Stamford, CT, 1996.
3. Berne, RM and Levy, MN: Cardiovascular Physiology, ed 6. Mosby Year Book, St Louis, 1992.

4. Bocker, D, et al: Antiarrhythmic therapy: Future trends and forecast for the 21st century. Am J Cardiol 80(Suppl 8A):99G, 1997.
5. Boyden, PA: Cellular electrophysiologic basis of cardiac arrhythmias. Am J Cardiol 78(Suppl 4A):4, 1996.
6. Bush, LR, et al: Comparative effects of verapamil, diltiazem and felodipine during experimental digitalis-induced arrhythmias. Pharmacology 34:111, 1987.
7. Cabo, C and Wit, AL: Cellular electrophysiologic mechanisms of cardiac arrhythmias. Cardiol Clin 15:517, 1997.
8. Camm, AJ and Yap, YG: What should we expect from the next generation of antiarrhythmic drugs? J Cardiovasc Electrophysiol 10:307, 1999.
9. Campbell, TJ: Proarrhythmic actions of antiarrhythmic drugs: A review. Aust N Z J Med 20:275, 1990.
10. Campbell, TJ and Williams, KM: Therapeutic drug monitoring: Antiarrhythmic drugs. Br J Clin Pharmacol 46:307, 1998.
11. Capucci, A, Aschieri, D, and Villani, GQ: Clinical pharmacology of antiarrhythmic drugs. Drugs Aging 13:51, 1998.
12. Capucci, A, et al: Clinical potential of emerging antiarrhythmic agents. Drugs R D 1:279, 1999.
13. Chay, TR: Why are some antiarrhythmic drugs proarrhythmic? Cardiac arrhythmia study by bifurcation analysis. J Electrocardiol 28(Suppl):191, 1995.
14. Dhein, S, et al: Comparative study on the proarrhythmic effects of some antiarrhythmic agents. Circulation 87:617, 1993.
15. Ferraris, VA, et al: Verapamil prophylaxis for postoperative atrial dysrhythmias: A prospective, randomized, double-blind study using drug level monitoring. Ann Thorac Surg 43:530, 1987.
16. Grant, AO: On the mechanism of action of antiarrhythmic agents. Am Heart J 123(part 2):1130, 1992.
17. Guerra, PG, et al: Is there a future for antiarrhythmic drug therapy? Drugs 56:767, 1998.
18. Guyton, AC and Hall, JE: Cardiac arrhythmias and their electrocardiographic interpretation. In Textbook of Medical Physiology, ed 9, WB Saunders, Philadelphia, 1996.
19. Henry, PD: Comparative pharmacology of calcium antagonists: Nifedipine, verapamil and diltiazem. Am J Cardiol 46:1047, 1980.
20. Hindricks, G, et al: Antiarrhythmic surgery for treatment of atrial fibrillation: New concepts. Thorac Cardiovasc Surg 47(Suppl 3):365, 1999.
21. Hondeghem, LM: Development of class III antiarrhythmic agents. J Cardiovasc Pharmacol 20(Suppl 2):S17, 1992.
22. Janse, MJ and Wilde, AA: Molecular mechanisms of arrhythmias. Rev Port Cardiol 17(Suppl 2):II41, 1998.
23. Kochs, M, Eggeling, T, and Hombach, V: Pharmacological therapy in coronary heart disease: Prevention of life-threatening ventricular tachycardias and sudden cardiac death. Eur Heart J 14(Suppl E):107, 1993.
24. Kodama, I, Kamiya, K, and Toyama, J: Amiodarone: Ionic and cellular mechanisms of action of the most promising class III agent. Am J Cardiol 84(Suppl 9A):20R, 1999.
25. Kowey, PR: Pharmacological effects of antiarrhythmic drugs. Review and update. Arch Intern Med 158:325, 1998.
26. Krikler, DM: Verapamil in arrhythmia. Br J Clin Pharmacol 21(Suppl 2):183S, 1986.
27. Miller, MB: Arrhythmias associated with drug toxicity. Emerg Med Clin North Am 16:405, 1998.
28. Morady, F: Prevention of atrial fibrillation in the postoperative cardiac patient: Significance of oral class III antiarrhythmic agents. Am J Cardiol 84(Suppl 9A):156R, 1999.
29. Nattel, S: The molecular and ionic specificity of antiarrhythmic drug actions. J Cardiovasc Electrophysiol 10:272, 1999.
30. Nattel, S: Comparative mechanisms of action of antiarrhythmic drugs. Am J Cardiol 72:F13, 1993.
31. Nattel, S and Singh, BN: Evolution, mechanisms, and classification of antiarrhythmic drugs: Focus on class III actions. Am J Cardiol 84(Suppl 9A):11R, 1999.
32. Pinski, SL and Helguera, ME: Antiarrhythmic drug initiation in patients with atrial fibrillation. Prog Cardiovasc Dis 42:75, 1999.
33. Podrid, PJ: Safety and toxicity of antiarrhythmic drug therapy: Benefit versus risk. J Cardiovasc Pharmacol 17(Suppl 6):S65, 1991.
34. Priori, SG, et al: Genetic and molecular basis of cardiac arrhythmias: Impact on clinical management parts I and II. Circulation 99:518, 1999.
35. Scheinman, MM: Treatment of cardiac arrhythmias in patients with acute myocardial infarction. Am J Surg 145:707, 1983.
36. Scholz, H: Classification and mechanism of action of antiarrhythmic drugs. Fundam Clin Pharmacol 8:385, 1994.
37. Schwartz, A: Molecular and cellular aspects of calcium channel antagonism. Am J Cardiol 70:6F, 1992.
38. Singh, BN: Antiarrhythmic drugs: A reorientation in light of recent developments in the control of disorders of rhythm. Am J Cardiol 81(Suppl 6A):3D, 1998.
39. Singh, BN: Controlling cardiac antiarrhythmias: An overview with a historical perspective. Am J Cardiol 80(Suppl 8A):4G, 1997.
40. Singh, BN, et al: Antiarrhythmic agents for atrial fibrillation: Focus on prolonging atrial repolarization. Am J Cardiol 84(Suppl 9A):161R, 1999.
41. Teo, KK, Yusuf, S, and Furberg, CD: Effects of prophylactic antiarrhythmic drug therapy in acute myocardial infarction: An overview of results from randomized controlled trials. JAMA 270:1589, 1993.

42. Van Gelder, IC, Brugemann, J, and Crijns, HJ: Current treatment recommendations in antiarrhythmic therapy. Drugs 55:331, 1998.
43. Vukmir, RB: Cardiac arrhythmia diagnosis. Am J Emerg Med 13:204, 1995.
44. Williams, EMV: Classifying antiarrhythmic actions: By facts or speculation. J Clin Pharmacol 32:964, 1992.
45. Woosley, RL: Antiarrhythmic drugs. Annu Rev Pharmacol Toxicol 31:427, 1991.
46. Zipes, DP: An overview of arrhythmias and antiarrhythmic approaches. J Cardiovasc Electrophysiol 10:267, 1999.
47. Zivin, A and Bardy, GH: Implantable defibrillators and antiarrhythmic drugs in patients at risk for lethal arrhythmias. Am J Cardiol 84(Suppl 9A):63R, 1999.

CHAPTER 24

Treatment of Congestive Heart Failure

Congestive heart failure is a chronic condition in which the heart is unable to pump a sufficient quantity of blood to meet the needs of peripheral tissues.[39,59] Essentially, the pumping ability of the heart has been compromised by some form of myocardial disease or dysfunction. The congestive aspect of heart failure arises from the tendency for fluid to accumulate in the lungs and peripheral tissues because of the inability of the heart to maintain proper circulation. The pathophysiology of congestive heart failure is fairly complex; the possible causes and mechanisms of heart failure are addressed in more detail in "Pathophysiology of Congestive Heart Failure."

The primary symptoms associated with congestive heart failure are peripheral edema and a decreased tolerance for physical activity.[39] Dyspnea and shortness of breath are also common, especially if the left heart is failing and pulmonary congestion is present (see the next section). In severe cases, cyanosis develops because the heart cannot deliver oxygen to peripheral tissues.

Congestive heart failure represents one of the major illnesses present in industrialized nations.[33,81] In the United States, approximately 3 to 4 million people have been diagnosed with this disease, and the incidence of heart failure (number of new cases each year) is currently 400,000.[40] The prevalence of heart failure also increases in the elderly, and the number of people with heart failure will undoubtedly increase as a larger percentage of our population reaches advanced age.[65] This disease is likewise associated with serious consequences, and the prognosis for congestive heart failure is often poor.[78] Approximately 82 percent of patients die within 6 years after they are diagnosed with heart failure.[44]

Consequently, the effective treatment of congestive heart failure is a critical and challenging task. Pharmacotherapy represents one of the primary methods of treating congestive heart failure, and the drugs discussed in this chapter play a vital role in the optimal management of this disease. As with other cardiac problems, the prevalence of congestive heart failure necessitates that members of the health-care community be aware of the pharmacologic management of this disease. Rehabilitation specialists will often treat patients with heart failure, and therapists should be cognizant of the drugs used to treat this problem.

PATHOPHYSIOLOGY OF CONGESTIVE HEART FAILURE

Vicious Cycle of Heart Failure

The mechanisms underlying chronic heart failure are complex and may include biochemical disturbances in the cardiac cell, altered genetic expression of myocardial proteins, and systemic changes in hemodynamic and neurohormonal factors.[55,68] Heart failure also tends to be self-perpetuating because an aberration in cardiac function often initiates a vicious cycle that leads to further decrements in cardiac function.[48,58,80] Figure 24–1 illustrates the way in which such a vicious cycle might be generated by the interaction of cardiac and neurohumoral factors. The sequence of events depicted in Figure 24–1 is discussed briefly here.

1. *Decreased cardiac performance:* Any number of factors that affect cardiac pumping ability may be responsible for initiating a change in myocardial performance. Factors such as ischemic heart disease, myocardial infarction, valve dysfunction, and hyper-

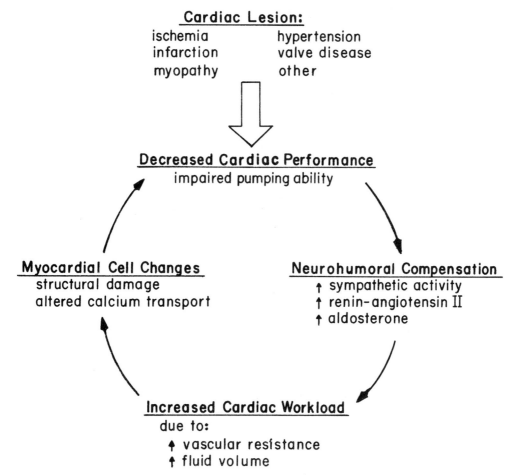

FIGURE 24–1. Vicious cycle of congestive heart failure. An initial cardiac lesion begins a self-perpetuating decrease in myocardial performance.

tension may all compromise the pumping ability of the heart.[11,35,72] Also, cardiomy-opathy may result from other diseases and infections.[40]

2. *Neurohumoral compensations:* The body responds to the decreased cardiac pumping ability in a number of ways. In the early stages of failure, cardiac output decreases, and the delivery of oxygen and nutrients to tissues and organs is diminished. To compensate for this initial decrease in cardiac output, several neural and humoral changes occur that increase cardiac contractility and help maintain blood pressure. In particular, the sympathetic nervous system and renin-angiotensin system are acti-vated, and secretion of aldosterone and antidiuretic hormone increases.[53,61,68,72] Al-though these compensations are initially helpful in maintaining cardiac function, they actually place more stress on the failing heart.[48,61] This increased stress also ini-tiates a vicious cycle because it causes more damage to the myocardium, which fur-ther compromises cardiac pumping ability, which causes more neurohumoral acti-vation, which causes more stress to the heart, and so on (see Fig. 24–1).

3. *Increased cardiac workload:* The neurohumoral changes described previously con-tribute to peripheral vasoconstriction, as well as a general increase in sodium and wa-ter retention.[58] These effects place additional strain on the heart by increasing cardiac preload (the volume of blood returning to the heart) and cardiac afterload (the pres-sure that the heart must pump against).[59,62]

4. *Changes in myocardial cell function:* The increased workload on the heart leads to or ex-aggerates alterations in cell function. Increased cardiac workload may lead to further structural damage to the already compromised myocardial cell.[48,72,80] Also, studies on the molecular basis of heart failure have suggested that alterations in calcium transport, en-ergy production and utilization, free-radical production, and beta-receptor density may occur.[23,63,68] Continued stress on the heart may exacerbate these changes, leading to more cellular dysfunction and inappropriate adaptive changes in myocardial cell structure and function (cardiac remodeling).[62,68] Increased dysfunction on the cellular level results in a further decrease in cardiac performance, thus completing the cycle shown in Figure 24–1.

The changes in cardiac function described previously represent a simplification of the interaction of central and peripheral factors in congestive heart failure. This de-scription does, however, illustrate the primary problems that occur in this disease, as well as the manner in which heart failure tends to be self-perpetuating.

Congestion in Left and Right Heart Failure

The primary problem in heart failure is that the heart is unable to push blood for-ward through the circulatory system, thus causing pressure to build up in the veins that return blood to the heart. In effect, blood begins to back up in the venous system, in-creasing the pressure gradient for fluid to move out of the capillary beds. The net move-ment of fluid out of the capillaries causes the edema or congestion typically found in ad-vanced stages of heart failure.

Although heart disease commonly affects the entire myocardium, congestive heart failure is sometimes divided into left and right heart failure (Fig. 24–2). In *left heart fail-ure,* the left atrium and ventricle are unable to adequately handle the blood returning from the lungs. This causes pressure to build up in the pulmonary veins, and fluid ac-cumulates in the lungs. Consequently, left heart failure is associated with pulmonary edema (see Fig. 24–2A). In *right heart failure,* the right atrium and ventricle are unable to handle blood returning from the systemic circulation. This causes fluid to accumulate in the peripheral tissues, and ankle edema and organ congestion (liver, spleen) are typical

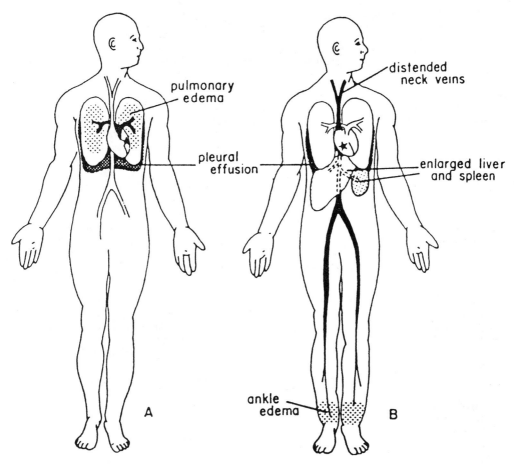

FIGURE 24–2. Effects of congestive heart failure. (*A*) Left-sided heart failure results primarily in pulmonary edema. (*B*) Right-sided heart failure results in peripheral edema (swollen ankles, enlarged organs). (From Kent, TH and Hart, MN: Introduction to Human Disease, ed 2. Appleton-Century-Crofts, Norwalk, CT, 1987, p 141, with permission.)

manifestations of right heart failure (see Fig. 24–2*B*). If both left and right heart failure occur simultaneously, congestion is found in the lungs as well as the periphery.

PHARMACOTHERAPY

One of the basic goals in congestive heart failure is to improve the pumping ability of the heart. Drug administration should selectively increase cardiac contractile performance and produce what is referred to as a *positive inotropic effect.* "Inotropic" refers to the force of muscular contraction, and the primary drugs used to exert a positive inotropic effect are the cardiac glycosides such as digitalis. In addition to increasing cardiac contractility, drugs that decrease cardiac workload through an effect on the heart or the peripheral vasculature or by controlling fluid volume are recognized as beneficial in congestive heart failure. Included in this group are the angiotensin-converting enzyme inhibitors, beta blockers, diuretics, and vasodilators.

The primary drug groups used to treat congestive heart failure are listed in Table 24–1. These drugs are described here according to their primary goal in treating heart failure—

TABLE 24–1 Primary Drugs Used in Congestive Heart Failure

Drug Group	Primary Effect
Agents That Increase Myocardial Contraction Force (Positive Inotropic Agents)	
Digitalis Glycosides	
Digoxin (Lanoxin)	Increase myocardial contractility by elevating
Digitoxin (Digitaline)	intracellular calcium levels and facilitating
	actin-myosin interaction in cardiac cells; may also
	help normalize autonomic effects on the heart
Other Positive Inotropes	
Amrinone (Inocor)	Enhance myocardial contractility by
Milrinone (Primacor)	prolonging effects of cAMP, which increases
	intracellular calcium levels and promotes
	stronger actin-myosin interaction in cardiac cells
Dopamine (Intropin)	Stimulate cardiac beta-1 adrenergic receptors, which
Dobutamine (Dobutrex)	selectively increases myocardial contraction force
Agents That Decrease Cardiac Workload	
Angiotensin-Converting Enzyme Inhibitors	Reduce peripheral vascular resistance by
Captopril (Capoten)	preventing angiotensin II–induced vasocon-
Enalapril (Vasotec)	striction and vascular hypertrophy; also help
Fosinopril (Monopril)	prevent sodium and water retention by
Lisinopril (Prinivil)	limiting aldosterone secretion
(Others, see Table 21–5)	
Beta Adrenergic Blockers	Prevent sympathetic-induced overload on
Acebutolol (Sectral)	the heart by blocking the effects of epinephrine
Carteolol (Cartrol)	and norepinephrine on the myocardium
Labetalol (Normodyne, Trandate)	
Metoprolol (Lopressor)	
(Others, see Table 20–2)	
Diuretics*	Decrease the volume of fluid the heart must
	pump by promoting the excretion of excess
	sodium and water
Vasodilators	Promote dilation in the peripheral vasculature,
Hydralazine (Apresoline)	which decreases the amount of blood returning
Minoxidil (Loniten)	to the heart (cardiac preload) and decreases the
Nitrates (nitroglycerin, others)	pressure against which the heart must pump
Prazosin (Minipress)	(cardiac preload)

*Various thiazide, loop, or potassium-sparing diuretics can be used, depending on the needs of each patient; see Table 21–3 for specific diuretic agents.

that is, drugs that improve myocardial contraction force (positive inotropic agents) and agents that decrease cardiac workload. The mechanism of action and specific agents within each group are presented here.

DRUGS THAT INCREASE MYOCARDIAL CONTRACTION FORCE (POSITIVE INOTROPIC AGENTS)

Digitalis

The cardiac glycosides are digoxin, digitoxin, and similar agents (Table 24–1). For simplicity, the term "digitalis" is often used to represent these drugs. Although the widespread use of digitalis has been questioned, it continues to be one of the primary drugs used to treat congestive heart failure.[31,36,47,88] There is little doubt that digitalis improves cardiac pumping ability and therefore improves the primary symptoms of congestive heart failure.[19,30] Digitalis typically increases cardiac output at rest and during exercise, and exercise tolerance often increases because the heart is able to pump blood more effectively.[30,64] There is little evidence, however, that digitalis prolongs life expectancy in people with heart failure.[20,30,64,73] Also, the use of digitalis is limited to some extent by the toxic effects of this drug (see "Adverse Side Effects").

Nonetheless, the consensus is that digitalis is a useful drug because it can decrease the symptoms of heart failure and decrease the number of hospitalizations and other aspects of morbidity associated with this disease.[19,20,64,73,88] Digitalis must, however, be used cautiously and specifically in certain cases of congestive heart failure, rather than as a panacea for all forms of this disease.[34,88] Also, other agents including diuretics, angiotensin-converting enzyme (ACE) inhibitors, beta blockers, and vasodilators (see the respective headings later in this chapter) are often used in combination with digitalis to provide better clinical effects than can be achieved by using digitalis alone.[30,34,88]

EFFECTS AND MECHANISM OF ACTION

Mechanical Effects

Digitalis and the other cardiac glycosides increase the mechanical pumping ability of the heart by bringing about an increase in intracellular calcium concentration. Increased intracellular calcium enhances contractility by facilitating the interaction between thick (myosin) and thin (actin) filaments in the myocardial cell.[43] Digitalis probably increases intracellular calcium concentration by several mechanisms that are illustrated in Figure 24–3. Digitalis exerts its primary effect on calcium concentration by inhibiting the sodium-potassium pump on the myocardial cell membrane.[37,43] The sodium-potassium pump is an active transport system that normally transports sodium out of the cell and potassium into it. Inhibition of the sodium-potassium pump causes sodium to accumulate within the cell, which then facilitates an increase in intracellular calcium through an effect on the sodium-calcium exchange mechanism (part 1a of Fig. 24–3).[43] Although the details of this exchange mechanism are complex, increased intracellular sodium basically causes intracellular calcium to increase by directly enhancing calcium entry into the cardiac cell and/or by decreasing calcium extrusion from the cardiac cell.[43] Digitalis may also increase intracellular calcium concentration by increasing calcium entry through membrane calcium channels (Fig. 24–3, part 2) and by increasing calcium release from the sarcoplasmic reticulum (Fig. 24–3, part 3).[42]

Autonomic and Electrophysiologic Effects

In addition to its effects on cardiac contractility, digitalis has a direct inhibitory effect on sympathetic nervous system activity.[30,37] This effect is beneficial because it decreases stress on the failing heart by decreasing excessive sympathetic stimulation of the heart and peripheral vasculature.[43] Therapeutic levels of digitalis likewise stabilize heart rate and slow impulse conduction through the myocardium. In fact, digitalis is used to prevent and treat certain arrhythmias such as atrial tachycardia and atrial fibrillation.[43] Some of these electrical properties may be caused by the direct effect of digitalis on the sodium-potassium pump and can be attributed to alterations in sodium, potassium, and calcium fluxes. As indicated, digitalis also decreases excessive sympathetic stimulation of the heart, and this effect helps normalize cardiac excitation and conduction. Digitalis likewise causes reflex stimulation of the vagus nerve, thus further slowing heart rate and conduction.[43] The autonomic and electrical properties of digitalis therefore improve car-

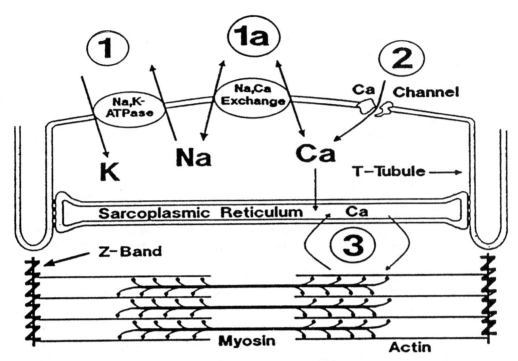

FIGURE 24–3. Proposed mechanism of digitalis action on the sarcomere located within the myocardial cell. Digitalis inhibits the Na$^+$, K$^+$-ATPase (*1*) resulting in increased intracellular sodium (Na$^+$). Increased intracellular sodium alters the Na$^+$, Ca^{++} exchange mechanism (*1a*) so that intracellular Ca^{++} also increases. Digitalis may also directly increase intracellular calcium by opening membrane Ca^{++} channels (*2*) and by increasing Ca^{++} release from the sarcoplasmic reticulum (*3*). The combined effects of these actions causes increased intracellular Ca^{++}, which facilitates contractile protein binding, resulting in increased myocardial contractility. (From Katzung, BG and Parmley, WW: Cardiac glycosides and other drugs used in congestive heart failure. In Katzung, BG (ed): Basic and Clinical Pharmacology, ed 5. Appleton & Lange, Norwalk, CT, 1992, p 179, with permission.)

diac excitation and function, and these effects generally complement the mechanical effects of this drug in treating congestive heart failure.

ADVERSE SIDE EFFECTS

Digitalis toxicity is a fairly common and potentially fatal side effect.[37] Common signs of toxicity include gastrointestinal distress (nausea, vomiting, diarrhea) and CNS disturbances (drowsiness, fatigue, confusion, visual disturbances) (Table 24–2). Because digitalis alters the electrophysiologic properties of the heart, abnormalities in cardiac function are also common during digitalis toxicity. Common adverse cardiac effects include arrhythmias such as premature atrial and ventricular contractions, paroxysmal atrial tachycardia, ventricular tachycardia, and high degrees of atrioventricular block. As toxicity increases, severe arrhythmias such as ventricular fibrillation can occur and may result in death.

To prevent digitalis toxicity, drug dosage should be maintained as low as possible. Plasma levels of digitalis should be monitored in suspected cases of toxicity to determine an appropriate decrease in dosage.[34,84] Health-care personnel should also be encouraged to look for early signs of toxicity so that digitalis can be discontinued before these effects become life-threatening.

TABLE 24–2 Signs and Symptoms of Digitalis Toxicity*

Gastrointestinal Symptoms

Anorexia
Nausea
Vomiting
Abdominal pain

Visual Disturbances

Halos
Photophobia
Problems with color perception
Scotomata

CNS Effects

Headache
Dizziness
Delirium
Confusion
Psychosis
Fatigue
Weakness

Cardiac Effects[†]

Ventricular arrhythmias
Premature ventricular depolarizations, bigeminy, trigeminy,
    ventricular tachycardia, ventricular fibrillation
Atrioventricular (A-V) block
First-degree, second-degree (Mobitz type I), third-degree block
A-V junctional escape rhythms, junctional tachycardia
Atrial rhythms with slowed A-V conduction or A-V block
Particularly paroxysmal atrial tachycardia with A-V block
Sinus bradycardia

*Some adverse effects may be difficult to distinguish from the signs and symptoms of heart failure.
†Digitalis toxicity has been associated with almost every rhythm abnormality; only the more common manifestations are listed.
Source: Adapted from Johnson, Parker, and Geraci,[40] p 177, with permission.

Other Positive Inotropic Agents

AMRINONE AND MILRINONE

These drugs are classified as positive inotropic agents because they increase myocardial contractility in a relatively selective manner.[40] Amrinone and milrinone exert their effects by inhibiting the phosphodiesterase enzyme that breaks down cyclic adenosine monophosphate (cAMP) in cardiac cells. This cAMP is a common second messenger in many cells (see Chap. 4), and drugs that inhibit the phosphodiesterase enzyme allow cAMP concentrations to increase in the cell.[7,38] In cardiac cells, cAMP acts on membrane calcium channels to allow more calcium to enter the cell.[16,38] Thus, amrinone and milrinone cause a cAMP-mediated increase in intracellular calcium that subsequently increases the force of contraction within the myocardial cell. These drugs also have some vasodilating properties, and some of their beneficial effects in congestive heart failure may be due to their ability to decrease cardiac preload and afterload.[16,38,40]

Amrinone and milrinone must be administered parenterally by intravenous infusion; hence, they are usually limited to the short-term treatment of patients with severe congestive heart failure.[1] There is little evidence, however, that these drugs are more effective than digitalis in producing positive inotropic effects, and there is concern that these agents may actually result in more serious side effects, including an increase in patient mortality compared with digitalis.[27,49] Therefore, amrinone and milrinone have limited use in treating heart failure and are usually administered in severe cases that have failed to respond to more traditional drug therapy with digitalis.[40]

DOPAMINE AND DOBUTAMINE

Dopamine and dobutamine are sometimes used to stimulate the heart in cases of acute heart failure (see Chap. 20). These drugs have also been used on a limited basis to treat congestive heart failure. Dopamine and dobutamine exert a fairly specific positive inotropic effect, presumably through their ability to stimulate beta-1 receptors on the myocardium.[40] Other beta-1 agonists (epinephrine, prenalterol, etc.) will also increase myocardial contractility, but most of these other beta-1 agonists also increase heart rate or have other side effects that prevent their use in congestive heart failure. Dopamine and dobutamine are usually reserved for patients with advanced cases of congestive heart failure who fail to respond to more conventional drugs (e.g., digitalis and diuretics).

AGENTS THAT DECREASE CARDIAC WORKLOAD

Angiotensin-Converting Enzyme Inhibitors

Angiotensin-converting enzyme (ACE) inhibitors have been used successfully to treat hypertension (see Chap. 21) and are now recognized as critical in treating congestive heart failure.[8] As discussed previously in this chapter, the renin-angiotensin system is often activated in congestive heart failure. ACE inhibitors interrupt this system and help decrease morbidity and mortality in patients with congestive heart failure by improving the patient's neurohormonal and hemodynamic function.[29,74,75,79] The ACE inhibitors commonly used in congestive heart failure include captopril (Capoten), enalapril (Vasotec), and several similar drugs listed in Table 24–1. In severe congestive heart failure, these drugs are often given in combination with diuretics and digitalis.

ACE inhibitors are now considered one of the mainstays of treatment in congestive heart failure. These drugs are the first agents that have been shown to prolong the life-span of people with this disease[10]; that is, digitalis, diuretics, and other drugs commonly used to treat heart failure may all produce symptomatic improvements, but use of ACE inhibitors alone or in combination with these other drugs actually results in decreased mortality.[2] The use of ACE inhibitors in treating heart failure has increased dramatically over the last several years.[8,70] There is some concern, however, that they should be used even more extensively and in higher doses, especially in the early stages of this disease.[2,51,67] By reducing the detrimental effects of angiotensin II on the vascular system, early use of ACE inhibitors may prevent or delay the progression of this disease (see the next section, "Effects and Mechanism of Action").

EFFECTS AND MECHANISM OF ACTION

As discussed in Chapter 21, ACE inhibitors suppress the enzyme that converts angiotensin I to angiotensin II in the bloodstream. Angiotensin II is a potent vasoconstrictor. By inhibiting the formation of angiotensin II, ACE inhibitors limit peripheral vaso-constriction. This effect results in a decrease in cardiac workload primarily by decreasing the pressure against which the heart must pump (cardiac afterload).[5,10,32] Decreased cardiac afterload eases the strain on the failing heart, resulting in improved cardiac performance and increased exercise tolerance.[32,66] Angiotensin II also stimulates growth and hypertrophy of vascular tissues, which results in thickening of the walls of peripheral blood vessels.[71] This thickening reduces the size of the vessel lumen, which further increases cardiac afterload because the heart must force blood into these narrowed vessels. ACE inhibitors therefore prevent angiotensin I–induced vascular hypertrophy, which helps reduce the workload on the heart and prevent progression of heart failure.[8]

By directly inhibiting angiotensin II formation, ACE inhibitors also inhibit aldosterone secretion.[8] Angiotensin II stimulates aldosterone secretion from the adrenal cortex (actually it is probably a by-product of angiotensin II—that is, angiotensin III, which directly stimulates aldosterone secretion). Aldosterone increases renal sodium reabsorption, with a subsequent increase in water reabsorption (i.e., the exact opposite effect produced by a diuretic). Inhibition of aldosterone secretion is beneficial in congestive heart failure because vascular fluid volume does not increase and overtax the failing heart. Consequently, ACE inhibitors may help decrease cardiac workload in congestive heart failure by both hemodynamic mechanisms (prevention of vasoconstriction by angiotensin II) and fluid-electrolyte mechanisms (inhibition of aldosterone secretion).

Recently, drugs known as angiotensin II receptor blockers have also been introduced for treating disorders associated with the renin-angiotensin system.[85] These drugs include agents such as losartan and valsartan. As indicated in Chapter 21, these drugs prevent angiotensin II from binding to receptors on vascular tissues, thus inhibiting angiotensin II–induced damage of the cardiovascular system. The use of angiotensin II receptor blockers in heart failure remains fairly experimental at this time, but these drugs certainly provide a useful alternative for people who are unable to tolerate traditional ACE inhibitors.[18,52] Clinical studies that compare ACE inhibitors with these newer angiotensin II receptor blockers should help clarify which type of drug—or perhaps a combination of the two—provides optimal treatment in heart failure.[71,87]

ADVERSE SIDE EFFECTS

Serious adverse effects with ACE inhibitors are relatively rare. In fact, one of the primary advantages of these drugs over more toxic compounds such as digitalis is the low incidence of serious adverse effects. ACE inhibitors are occasionally associated with bothersome side effects such as skin rashes, gastrointestinal discomfort, dizziness, and a persistent dry cough, but these effects are often transient or can be resolved with an adjustment in dosage. Likewise, the newer angiotensin II receptor blockers can be used as an alternative to ACE inhibitors if patients are not able to tolerate ACE inhibitor–induced side effects.

Beta Blockers

In the past, beta blockers were considered detrimental in patients with heart failure.[9,83,89] As indicated in Chapter 20, these drugs decrease heart rate and myocardial contraction force by blocking the effects of epinephrine and norepinephrine on the heart. Common sense dictated that a decrease in myocardial contractility would be counterproductive in heart failure, and beta blockers were therefore contraindicated in heart failure.[23,24,83,89] It is now recognized that beta blockers are actually beneficial in people with heart failure because these drugs attenuate the excessive sympathetic activity associated with this disease.[56] As indicated earlier in this chapter, increased sympathetic activity and other neurohumoral changes often contribute to the vicious cycle associated with heart failure, and excessive sympathetic stimulation can accelerate the pathologic changes in the failing heart.[13,57,60,69] Beta blockers reduce the harmful effects of excessive sympathetic stimulation, and use of these drugs has been shown to reduce morbidity and mortality associated with heart failure.[4,12,22,69] Hence, beta blockers are now considered one of the principal treatments of this disease, and use of these drugs along with ACE inhibitors and traditional agents (digitalis, diuretics, and so forth) is advocated as state-of-the-art therapy for providing optimal treatment in heart failure.[9,83]

EFFECTS AND MECHANISM OF ACTION

Beta blockers bind to beta-1 receptors on the myocardium and block the effects of norepinephrine and epinephrine (see Chap. 20). These drugs therefore normalize sympathetic stimulation of the heart and help reduce heart rate (negative chronotropic effect) and myocardial contraction force (negative inotropic effect). Beta blockers may also prevent angina by stabilizing cardiac workload, and they may prevent certain arrhythmias by stabilizing heart rate.[41] These additional properties may be useful to patients with heart failure who also have other cardiac symptoms. Finally, it has been suggested that some of the newer "third-generation" beta blockers may be especially useful in heart failure because these drugs block beta-1 receptors on the heart while also blocking alpha-1 receptors on the vasculature, thus causing peripheral vasodilation.[6,17,46,57] Vasodilation of peripheral vessels could further reduce myocardial stress by decreasing the pressure that the heart must work against in the peripheral vessels (cardiac afterload).

ADVERSE SIDE EFFECTS

The side effects and problems associated with beta blockers were addressed in Chapter 20. The primary problem associated with these drugs is that they may cause excessive inhibition of the heart, resulting in an abnormally slow heart rate and reduced contraction force. This effect is especially problematic in heart failure because the heart is already losing its ability to pump blood. Nonetheless, the risk of this effect and other side effects is acceptable in most people with heart failure, and this risk is minimized by adjusting the dosage so that sympathetic activity is normalized rather than reduced to unacceptably low levels.

Diuretics

Diuretics increase the excretion of sodium and water (see Chap. 21). These agents are useful in congestive heart failure primarily because of their ability to reduce congestion in the lungs and peripheral tissues by excreting excess fluid retained in these tissues.[21,28] Diuretics also decrease the amount of fluid the heart must pump (cardiac preload), thereby reducing the workload on the failing heart.[54,63] Diuretics are often very successful in improving the symptoms of heart failure, and they can be used alone in the early stages of this disease or combined with other drugs such as digitalis or an ACE inhibitor.[54,82] Diuretic drugs, which are also used to treat hypertension, are discussed in more detail in Chapter 21. Diuretics that can be used in the treatment of congestive heart failure and hypertension are listed in Table 21–3.

EFFECTS AND MECHANISM OF ACTION

Diuretics all work by inhibiting the reabsorption of sodium from the nephron, which, in turn, decreases the amount of water that is normally reabsorbed with sodium, thus increasing water excretion. This effect reduces congestion caused by fluids retained in the body and decreases cardiac preload by excreting excess fluid in the vascular system. Chapter 21 provides a more detailed discussion on the mechanism of action of diuretic drugs.

ADVERSE SIDE EFFECTS

By the very nature of their action, diuretics are often associated with disturbances in fluid and electrolyte balance. Volume depletion, hyponatremia, hypokalemia, and altered pH balance are among the most frequently seen problems.[3,76] These electrolyte and pH changes can produce serious consequences by affecting cardiac excitability and precipitating arrhythmias. Patients on diuretics should be monitored closely for symptoms such as fatigue, confusion, and nausea, which may indicate the presence of drug-induced disturbances in fluid-electrolyte balance. Some patients may also become resistant to diuretic drugs; the effectiveness of the diuretic is diminished primarily because the kidneys adapt to the drug-induced sodium excretion.[21,26,45] Resistance can often be prevented, however, by altering the dose and type of the diuretic or by adding a second diuretic.[21,26,77]

Vasodilators

Various drugs that vasodilate peripheral vessels have been used successfully in cases of severe congestive heart failure.[15,25,40] By reducing peripheral vascular resistance, these agents decrease the amount of blood returning to the heart (cardiac preload) and reduce the pressure that the heart must pump against (cardiac afterload). Reduced cardiac preload and afterload helps alleviate some of the stress on the failing heart, thus slowing the progression of this disease. Vasodilators commonly used in heart failure include prazosin, hydralazine, minoxidil, and organic nitrates (e.g., nitroglycerin, sodium nitroprusside) (see Table 24–1).

EFFECTS AND MECHANISM OF ACTION

Prazosin produces vasodilation by blocking alpha-1 receptors on vascular smooth muscle (see Chap. 20), and hydralazine, minoxidil, and organic nitrates produce vasodilation by a direct effect on the vascular smooth-muscle cells (see Chaps. 21 and 22). Although these vasodilators work by different mechanisms, all can decrease cardiac workload by decreasing peripheral vascular resistance. These drugs may be combined with other agents (digoxin, ACE inhibitors) to provide optimal benefits in patients with varying degrees of congestive heart failure.[14,50,79,86]

ADVERSE SIDE EFFECTS

The primary side effects associated with vasodilators include headache, dizziness, hypotension, and orthostatic hypotension. These effects are all related to the tendency of these drugs to increase peripheral blood flow and decrease peripheral vascular resistance. Vasodilators may also cause reflex tachycardia in certain patients if the baroreceptor reflex increases heart rate in an attempt to maintain adequate blood pressure.

SUMMARY OF DRUG THERAPY

Digitalis remains a mainstay in the treatment of congestive heart failure. Digitalis, however, is associated with a number of serious side effects, and there is considerable doubt as to whether digitalis actually increases the rate of survival of patients with congestive heart failure.[31] The use of digitalis in the early stages of failure has been replaced to some extent by drugs that decrease cardiac workload, such as the diuretics, ACE inhibitors, and beta blockers. Digitalis can be added to these other agents as heart failure becomes more pronounced. Vasodilators (prazosin, hydralazine, organic nitrates) have also been used to decrease the workload on the failing heart, especially in the advanced stages of failure. Regardless of which drugs are used, there is consensus that early intervention in the treatment of congestive heart failure is crucial in providing the best outcome in this disease.[40,78]

SPECIAL CONCERNS IN REHABILITATION PATIENTS

Therapists should be aware of the potential for drugs used to treat congestive heart failure to affect the patient's welfare and response to rehabilitation. Acute congestive heart failure may occur in patients with myocardial disease because of a lack of therapeutic drug effects or because of the toxic effects of some cardiac drugs. Therapists should be alert for signs of acute congestive heart failure such as increased cough, difficulty in breathing (dyspnea), abnormal respiratory sounds (rales), and frothy sputum. Therapists should also be alert for signs of digitalis toxicity such as dizziness, confusion, nausea, and arrhythmias. Early recognition by the therapist may prevent serious or even fatal consequences. Likewise, patients taking diuretics sometimes exhibit excessive fatigue and weakness as early signs of fluid and electrolyte depletion. Therapists may help detect serious metabolic and electrolyte imbalances that result from problems with diuretic drugs. Finally, use of vasodilators often causes hypotension and postural hypotension. Therapists must use caution when patients sit up or stand up suddenly. Also, therapeutic techniques that produce systemic vasodilation (whirlpool, exercise) may produce profound hypotension in patients taking vasodilators, and these modalities should therefore be used cautiously.

CASE STUDY

CONGESTIVE HEART FAILURE

Brief History. D.S. is a 67-year-old woman with a long history of congestive heart failure caused by myocarditis. She has been treated successfully with digitalis glycosides (digoxin, 0.5 mg/day) for several years. Despite some swelling in her ankles and feet and a tendency to become winded, she has maintained a fairly active lifestyle and enjoys gardening and other hobbies. Recently, she developed some weakness and incoordination that primarily affected her right side. Subsequent testing revealed that she had suffered a cerebral vascular accident. She was not admitted to the hospital but remained living at home with her husband. Physical therapy, however, was provided in the home to facilitate optimal recovery from her stroke. The therapist began seeing her three times each week for a program of therapeutic exercise and functional training.

Problem/Influence of Medication. The therapist initially found this patient to be alert, coherent, and eager to begin therapy. Although there was some residual weakness and decreased motor skills, the prognosis for a full recovery appeared good. The therapist was impressed by the patient's enthusiasm and pleasant nature during the first two sessions. By the end of the first week, however, the therapist noted a distinct change in the patient's demeanor. She was confused and quite lethargic. The therapist initially suspected that she might have had another stroke. Physical examination did not reveal any dramatic decrease in strength or coordination, however. Realizing that the patient was still taking digitalis for the treatment of heart failure, the therapist began to suspect the possibility of digitalis toxicity.

Decision/Solution. The therapist immediately notified the physician about the change in the patient's status. The patient was admitted to the hospital, where a blood test confirmed the presence of digitalis toxicity (i.e., blood levels of digitalis were well above the therapeutic range). Apparently, the stroke had sufficiently altered the metabolism and excretion of the digitalis so that the dose that was therapeutic prior to the stroke was now accumulating in the patient's body. The altered pharmacokinetic profile was probably caused in part by the decrease in the patient's mobility and level of activity that occurred after the stroke. The digitalis dosage was reduced, and a diuretic was added to provide management of the congestive heart failure. The patient was soon discharged from the hospital and resumed physical therapy at home. Her rehabilitation progressed without further incident.

SUMMARY

Congestive heart failure is a serious cardiac condition in which the ability of the heart to pump blood becomes progressively worse. Decreased myocardial performance leads to a number of deleterious changes including peripheral edema (i.e., congestion) and increased fatigue during physical activity. Treatment of congestive heart failure consists primarily of drug therapy. Certain drugs such as digitalis and other positive inotropic agents attempt to directly increase cardiac pumping ability. Other drugs such as diuretics and vasodilators decrease cardiac workload by decreasing vascular fluid volume or dilating peripheral blood vessels, respectively. More important, ACE inhibitors and beta blockers have gained widespread acceptance in treating heart failure because these drugs decrease the abnormal neurohumoral changes associated with this disease. Specifically, ACE inhibitors decrease activity in the renin-angiotenisn system, and beta blockers prevent excessive cardiovascular stimulation from the sympathetic nervous system. These effects help prevent abnormal stimulation of the heart and vasculature, and early treatment with ACE inhibitors and beta blockers is now recognized as critical in delaying the progression of this disease and decreasing mortality in people with heart failure. Even with optimal treatment, however, the prognosis for patients with congestive heart failure is often poor. Therapists should be aware of the drugs used to treat this disorder and that certain side effects may adversely affect rehabilitation or signal a problem with drug treatment.

REFERENCES

1. Anderson, JL: Hemodynamic and clinical benefits with intravenous milrinone in severe congestive heart failure: Results of a multicenter study in the United States. Am Heart J 121:1956, 1991.
2. Andersson, F, et al: Angiotensin converting enzyme (ACE) inhibitors and heart failure. The consequences of underprescribing. Pharmacoeconomics 15:535, 1999.
3. Antes, LM and Fernandez, PC: Principles of diuretic therapy. Dis Mon 44:254, 1998.
4. Avezum, A, et al: Beta-blocker therapy for congestive heart failure: A systematic overview and critical appraisal of the published trials. Can J Cardiol 14:1045, 1998.
5. Batin, P, et al: Cardiac hemodynamic effects of the non-peptide, angiotensin II–receptor antagonist, DuP-753, in conscious Long Evans and Brattleboro rats. Br J Pharmacol 103:1585, 1991.
6. Bristow, MR, et al: The role of third-generation beta-blocking agents in chronic heart failure. Clin Cardiol 21(Suppl 1):I3, 1998.
7. Brown, L, Nabauer, M, and Erdmann, E: The positive inotropic response to milrinone in isolated human and guinea pig myocardium. Naunyn-Schmiedebergs Arch Pharmacol 334:196, 1986.
8. Brown, NJ and Vaughan, DE: Angiotensin-converting enzyme inhibitors. Circulation 97:1411, 1998.
9. Carson, PE: Beta blocker treatment in heart failure. Prog Cardiovasc Dis 41:301, 1999.
10. Ciccone, CD: Current trends in cardiovascular pharmacology. Phys Ther 76:481, 1996.
11. Cleland, JG and McGowan, J: Heart failure due to ischaemic heart disease: Epidemiology, pathophysiology, and progression. J Cardiovasc Pharmacol 33(Suppl 3):S17, 1999.
12. Cleland, JG, McGowan, J, and Cowburn, PJ: Beta-blockers for chronic heart failure: From prejudice to enlightenment. J Cardiovasc Pharmacol 32(Suppl 1):S52, 1998.
13. Cohn, JN: Beta-blockers in heart failure. Eur Heart J 19(Suppl F):F52, 1998.
14. Cohn, JN, et al: A comparison of enalapril with hydralazine–isosorbide dinitrate in the treatment of congestive heart failure. N Engl J Med 325:303, 1991.
15. Cohn, JN, et al: Effect of vasodilator therapy on mortality in chronic congestive heart failure: Results of a Veteran's Administration cooperative study. N Engl J Med 314:1547, 1986.
16. Colucci, WS: Cardiovascular effects of milrinone. Am Heart J 121:1945, 1991.
17. Constant, J: A review of why and how we may use beta-blockers in congestive heart failure. Chest 113:800, 1998.
18. Coodley, E: Newer drug therapy for congestive heart failure. Arch Intern Med 159:1177, 1999.
19. Demers, C, McKelvie, RS, and Yusuf, S: The role of digitalis in the treatment of heart failure. Coron Artery Dis 10:353, 1999.
20. Digitalis Investigation Group: The effect of digitalis on mortality and morbidity in patients with heart failure. N Engl J Med 336:525, 1997.
21. Dormans, TP, et al: Combination diuretic therapy in severe congestive heart failure. Drugs 55:165, 1998.
22. Eichhorn, EJ: Experience with beta blockers in heart failure mortality trials. Clin Cardiol 22(Suppl 5):V21, 1999.
23. Eichhorn, EJ: Medical therapy of chronic heart failure. Role of ACE inhibitors and beta-blockers. Cardiol Clin 16:711, 1998.
24. Eichhorn, EJ: Restoring function in failing hearts: The effects of beta blockers. Am J Med 104:163, 1998.
25. Elkayam, U, et al: The role of organic nitrates in the treatment of heart failure. Prog Cardiovasc Dis 41:255, 1999.
26. Ellison, DH: Diuretic resistance: Physiology and therapeutics. Semin Nephrol 19:581, 1999.
27. Fisher, TA, Erbel, R, and Tresse, N: Current status of phosphodiesterase inhibitors in the treatment of congestive heart failure. Drugs 44:928, 1992.
28. Follath, F: Do diuretics differ in terms of clinical outcome in congestive heart failure? Eur Heart J 19(Suppl P):P5, 1998.
29. Francis, GS, Cohn, JN, and Johnson, G: Plasma norepinephrine, plasma renin activity, and congestive heart failure: Relations to survival and effects of therapy in V-HeFT II. Circulation 87(Suppl 6):VI-40, 1993.
30. Gheorghiade, M: Digoxin therapy in chronic heart failure. Cardiovasc Drugs Ther 11(Suppl 1):279, 1997.
31. Gheorghiade, M and Zarowitz, BJ: Review of randomized trials of digoxin therapy in patients with chronic heart failure. Am J Cardiol 69:G48, 1992.
32. Giles, T: Enalapril in the treatment of congestive heart failure. J Cardiovasc Pharmacol 15(Suppl 3):S6, 1990.
33. Goldman, L: Cost-effectiveness perspectives in congestive heart disease. Am Heart J 119:733, 1990.
34. Haas, GJ and Young, JB: Inappropriate use of digoxin in the elderly: How widespread is the problem and how can it be solved? Drug Saf 20:223, 1999.
35. Hansson, L: Hypertension-induced congestive heart failure. Scand Cardiovasc J Suppl 47:5, 1998.
36. Hauptman, PJ, Garg, R, and Kelly, RA: Cardiac glycosides in the next millennium. Prog Cardiovasc Dis 41:247, 1999.

37. Hauptman, PJ and Kelly, RA: Digitalis. Circulation 99:1265, 1999.
38. Honerjager, P: Pharmacology of bipyridine phosphodiesterase III inhibitors. Am Heart J 121:1939, 1991.
39. Jennings, RB and Steenbergen, C: The heart. In Rubin, E and Farber, JL (eds): Pathology, ed 3. Lippincott-Raven, Philadelphia, 1999.
40. Johnson, JA, Parker, RB, and Geraci, SA: Heart failure. In DiPiro, JT, et al (eds): Pharmacotherapy: A Pathophysiologic Approach, ed 4. Appleton & Lange, Stamford, CT, 1999.
41. Joseph, J and Gilbert, EM: The sympathetic nervous system in chronic heart failure. Prog Cardiovasc Dis 41(Suppl 1):9, 1998.
42. Katzung, BG and Parmley, WW: Cardiac glycosides and other drugs used in congestive heart failure. In Katzung, BG (ed): Basic and Clinical Pharmacology, ed 7. Appleton & Lange, Stamford, CT, 1998.
43. Kelly, RA and Smith, TW: Pharmacological treatment of heart failure. In Hardman, JG, et al (eds): The Pharmacological Basis of Therapeutics, ed 9. McGraw-Hill, New York, 1996.
44. Konstam, MA and Remme, WJ: Treatment guidelines in heart failure. Prog Cardiovasc Dis 41(Suppl 1):65, 1998.
45. Kramer, BK, Schweda, F, and Riegger, GA: Diuretic treatment and diuretic resistance in heart failure. Am J Med 106:90, 1999.
46. Krum, H: Beta-blockers in heart failure. The "new wave" of clinical trials. Drugs 58:203, 1999.
47. Kulick, DL and Rahimtoola, SH: Current role of digitalis therapy in patients with congestive heart failure. JAMA 265:2995, 1991.
48. Lechat, P: Prevention of heart failure progression: Current approaches. Eur Heart J 19(Suppl B):B12, 1998.
49. Leier, CV: Current status of non-digitalis positive inotropic drugs. Am J Cardiol 69(Suppl 7):120G, 1992.
50. Lewis, BS, et al: Effect of isosorbide-5-mononitrate on exercise performance and clinical status in patients with congestive heart failure. Results of the Nitrates in Congestive Heart Failure (NICE) Study. Cardiology 91:1, 1999.
51. Luzier, AB and DiTusa, L: Underutilization of ACE inhibitors in heart failure. Pharmacotherapy 19:1296, 1999.
52. McAlister, FA and Teo, KK: Recent advances in the drug treatment of heart failure. Postgrad Med J 74:658, 1998.
53. Middlekauff, HR and Mark, AL: The treatment of heart failure: The role of neurohumoral activation. Intern Med 37:112, 1998.
54. Moser, M: Diuretics in the prevention and treatment of congestive heart failure. Cardiovasc Drugs Ther 11(Suppl 1):273, 1997.
55. Olivetti, G, et al: The failing heart. Adv Clin Path 1:137, 1997.
56. Packer, M: Beta-adrenergic blockade in chronic heart failure: Principles, progress, and practice. Prog Cardiovasc Dis 41(Suppl 1):39, 1998.
57. Packer, M: Effects of beta-adrenergic blockade on survival of patients with chronic heart failure. Am J Cardiol 80(Suppl 11A):46L, 1997.
58. Packer, M: New concepts in the pathophysiology of heart failure: Beneficial and deleterious interaction of endogenous haemodynamic and neurohormonal mechanisms. J Intern Med 239:327, 1996.
59. Patterson, JH and Adams, KF: Pathophysiology of heart failure: Changing perceptions. Pharmacotherapy 16(Part 2):27S, 1996.
60. Pepper, GS and Lee, RW: Sympathetic activation in heart failure and its treatment with beta-blockade. Arch Intern Med 159:225, 1999.
61. Pool, PE: Neurohormonal activation in the treatment of congestive heart failure: Basis for new treatments? Cardiology 90:1, 1998.
62. Pool, PE: The clinical significance of neurohormonal activation. Clin Ther 19(Suppl A):53, 1997.
63. Remme, WJ: Congestive heart failure: Pathophysiology and medical treatment. J Cardiovasc Pharmacol 8(Suppl 1):S36, 1986.
64. Riaz, K and Forker, AD: Digoxin in congestive heart failure. Current status. Drugs 55:747, 1998.
65. Rich, MW: Heart failure. Cardiol Clin 17:123, 1999.
66. Riegger, GAJ: The effects of ACE inhibitors on exercise capacity in the treatment of congestive heart failure. J Cardiovasc Pharmacol 15(Suppl 2):S41, 1990.
67. Roe, CM, et al: Angiotensin-converting enzyme inhibitor compliance and dosing among patients with heart failure. Am Heart J 138(Part 1):818, 1999.
68. Ruffolo, RR and Feuerstein, GZ: Neurohormonal activation, oxygen free radicals, and apoptosis in the pathogenesis of congestive heart failure. J Cardiovasc Pharmacol 32(Suppl 1):S22, 1998.
69. Sabbah, HN: The cellular and physiologic effects of beta blockers in heart failure. Clin Cardiol 22(Suppl 5):V16, 1999.
70. Sami, M: Angiotensin-converting enzyme inhibitors and end-organ damage in heart failure. Can J Cardiol 15(Suppl C):19C, 1999.
71. Sander, GE, et al: Angiotensin-converting enzyme inhibitors and angiotensin II receptor antagonists in the treatment of heart failure caused by left ventricular systolic dysfunction. Prog Cardiovasc Dis 41:265, 1999.
72. Sigurdsson, A and Swedberg, K: The role of neurohormonal activation in chronic heart failure and post-myocardial infarction. Am Heart J 132(Part 2 Suppl):229, 1996.
73. Soler-Soler, J and Permanyer-Miralda, G: Should we still prescribe digoxin in mild-to-moderate heart failure? Is quality of life the issue rather than quantity? Eur Heart J 19(Suppl P):P26, 1998.

74. SOLVD Investigators: Effect of enalapril on mortality and the development of heart failure in asymptomatic patients with reduced left ventricular ejection fractions. N Engl J Med 327:685, 1992.
75. SOLVD Investigators: Effect of enalapril on survival in patients with reduced left ventricular ejection fractions and congestive heart failure. N Engl J Med 325:293, 1991.
76. Sonnenblick, M, Friedlander, Y, and Rosin, AJ: Diuretic-induced severe hyponatremia: Review and analysis of 129 reported patients. Chest 103:601, 1993.
77. Suki, WN: Diuretic resistance. Miner Electrolyte Metab 25:28, 1999.
78. Swan, HJC: Can heart failure be prevented, delayed, or reversed? Am Heart J 120:1540, 1990.
79. Swedberg, K: Reduction in mortality by pharmacological therapy in congestive heart failure. Circulation 87(Suppl 4):126, 1993.
80. Symposium (various authors): Heart failure: Adaptive and maladaptive processes. Circulation 87(Suppl 7):1, 1993.
81. Symposium (various authors): The costs and benefits of congestive heart disease risk factor reduction. Am Heart J 119:711, 1990.
82. Taylor, SH: Refocus on diuretics in the treatment of heart failure. Eur Heart J 16(Suppl F):7, 1995.
83. Teerlink, JR and Massie, BM: Beta-adrenergic blocker mortality trials in congestive heart failure. Am J Cardiol 84(Suppl 9A):94R, 1999.
84. Terra, SG, et al: Therapeutic range of digoxin's efficacy in heart failure: What is the evidence? Pharmacotherapy 19:1123, 1999.
85. Timmermans, PB: Angiotensin II receptor antagonists: An emerging new class of cardiovascular therapeutics. Hypertens Res 22:147, 1999.
86. Tisdale, JE and Gheorghiade, M: Acute hemodynamic effects of digoxin alone or in combination with other vasoactive agents in patients with congestive heart failure. Am J Cardiol 69:34G, 1992.
87. Tsuyuki, RT, et al: Combination neurohormonal blockade with ACE inhibitors, angiotensin II antagonists and beta-blockers in patients with congestive heart failure: Design of the Randomized Evaluation of Strategies for Left Ventricular Dysfunction (RESOLVD) pilot study. Can J Cardiol 13:1166, 1997.
88. Van Veldhuisen, DJ, et al: Value of digoxin in heart failure and sinus rhythm: New features of an old drug? J Am Coll Cardiol 28:813, 1996.
89. Zannad, F: Over 20 years' experience of beta-blockade in heart failure. Prog Cardiovasc Dis 41(Suppl 1):31, 1998.

CHAPTER 25

Treatment of Coagulation Disorders and Hyperlipidemia

Blood coagulation, or *hemostasis,* is necessary to prevent excessive hemorrhage from damaged blood vessels. Under normal conditions, clotting factors in the bloodstream spontaneously interact with damaged vessels to create a blood clot that plugs the leaking vessel. Obviously, inadequate blood clotting is harmful in that even minor vessel damage can lead to excessive blood loss. Overactive clotting is also detrimental because it will lead to *thrombogenesis* (i.e., the abnormal formation of blood clots, or thrombi).[34] Thrombus formation may lead directly to vessel occlusion and tissue infarction. Also, a piece of a thrombus may dislodge, creating an embolism that causes infarction elsewhere in the body, for example, in the lungs or brain.

Consequently, normal hemostasis can be regarded as a balance between too much and too little blood coagulation.[34] This balance is often disrupted by a number of factors. Inadequate clotting typically occurs because of insufficient levels of blood clotting factors, as in patients with hemophilia. Excessive clotting often occurs during prolonged bed rest or when blood flow through vessels is partially obstructed, as in coronary atherosclerosis.

Restoration of normal hemostasis is accomplished through pharmacologic methods. Excessive clotting and thrombus formation are rectified by drugs that prevent clot formation (anticoagulants, antithrombotics) or facilitate the removal of previously formed clots (*thrombolytics*). Inadequate clotting is resolved by replacing the missing clotting factors or by drugs that facilitate the synthesis of specific clotting factors.

Hemostasis can also be influenced by *hyperlipidemia,* which is a chronic and excessive increase in plasma lipids. Hyperlipidemia causes cholesterol and other lipids to be progressively deposited onto arterial walls, forming plaquelike lesions indicative of atherosclerosis. These atherosclerotic lesions progressively occlude the arterial lumen, thus leading to thrombosis and infarction. Atherosclerotic heart disease is one of the leading causes of morbidity and mortality in the United States, and pharmacologic methods to lower plasma lipids are often used in conjunction with dietary and lifestyle modifications to treat hyperlipidemia and prevent atherosclerosis.

Drugs used to normalize blood clotting or reduce hyperlipidemia are among the most common medications used clinically, and rehabilitation specialists will deal with many patients taking these agents. Many patients, in fact, will be treated in therapy for problems relating directly to thrombus formation (e.g., ischemic stroke, myocardial infarction, pulmonary embolism). Individuals with inadequate clotting, such as patients with hemophilia, are also seen routinely in rehabilitation because of the intrajoint hemorrhaging and other problems associated with this disease. Consequently, the purpose of this chapter is to acquaint therapists with several common and important groups of drugs used to treat coagulation disorders and hyperlipidemia.

NORMAL MECHANISM OF BLOOD COAGULATION

To understand how various drugs affect hemostasis, a review of the normal way in which blood clots are formed and broken down is necessary. The physiologic mechanisms involved in hemostasis are outlined in Figure 25–1, with clot formation and breakdown illustrated in the upper and lower parts of this figure, respectively.

Clot Formation

Clot formation involves the activation of various clotting factors that are circulating in the bloodstream.[17,25] These clotting factors are proteolytic enzymes synthesized in the liver that remain in an inactive form until there is some injury to a blood vessel. Blood vessel damage begins a cascade effect, whereby the activation of one of the clotting factors leads to the activation of the next factor, and so forth.[17,25] As shown in Figure 25–1, clot formation occurs through two systems, an intrinsic system and an extrinsic system. In the intrinsic system, the direct contact of the first clotting factor (factor XII) with the damaged vessel wall activates the clotting factor and initiates the cascade. In the extrinsic system, a substance known as *tissue thromboplastin* is released from the damaged vascular cell. Tissue thromboplastin directly activates clotting factor VII, which then activates subsequent factors in the clotting mechanism. For optimal coagulation to occur in vivo, both the intrinsic and extrinsic systems must be present.

Both the intrinsic and extrinsic systems ultimately lead to the conversion of prothrombin to thrombin. *Thrombin* is an enzyme that quickly converts the inactive fibrinogen molecule to *fibrin*. Individual strands of fibrin bind together to form a meshlike structure, which ultimately forms the framework for the blood clot. Other cellular components, especially platelets, help reinforce the clot by sticking to the fibrin mesh.

Clot Breakdown

The breakdown of blood clots is illustrated in the lower part of Figure 25–1. *Tissue plasminogen activator* (t-PA) converts plasminogen to plasmin. *Plasmin,* also known as fibrinolysin, is an enzyme that directly breaks down the fibrin mesh, thus destroying the clot.

The balance between clot formation and breakdown is crucial in maintaining normal hemostasis. Obviously, clots should not be broken down as quickly as they are formed because then no coagulation will occur. Likewise, a lack of breakdown would enable clots to proliferate at an excessive rate, leading to thrombus formation.

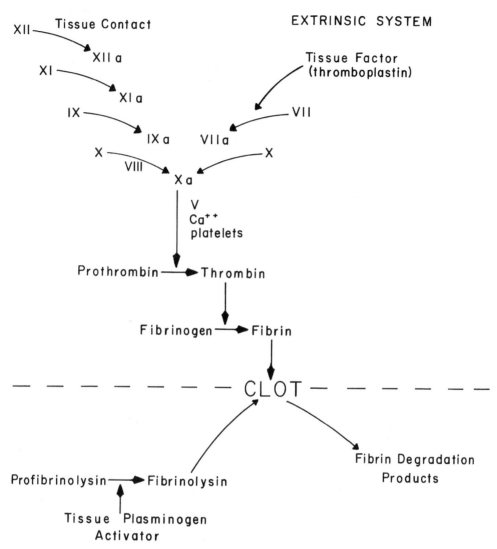

INTRINSIC SYSTEM

FIGURE 25–1. Mechanism of blood coagulation. Factors involved in clot formation are shown above the dashed line; factors involved in clot breakdown are shown below the dashed line. See text for further discussion.

DRUGS USED TO TREAT OVERACTIVE CLOTTING

Drugs used to treat excessive clot formation can be grouped into three primary categories: anticoagulant, antithrombotic, and thrombolytic agents (Table 25–1). Anticoagulants exert their effect by controlling the function and synthesis of clotting factors, and these drugs are used primarily to prevent clot formation in the venous system—that is, venous thrombosis. Antithrombotic drugs act primarily by inhibiting platelet function, and these drugs primarily prevent thrombus formation in arteries. Thrombolytic drugs facilitate the destruction of blood clots, and these drugs are used to re-establish blood

TABLE 25–1 Drugs Used to Treat Overactive Clotting

Drug Category	Primary Effect and Indication
Anticoagulants	

Heparins
  Unfractionated heparin (Calciparine, Liquaemin, others)
  Low-molecular-weight heparins
    Dalteparin (Fragmin)
    Enoxaparin (Lovenox)
Oral anticoagulants
  Anisindione (Miradon)
  Dicumarol (generic)
  Warfarin (Coumadin)
	Inhibit synthesis and function of clotting factors; used primarily to prevent and treat venous thromboembolism

Antithrombotics	

Aspirin
Other platelet aggregation inhibitors
  Clopidogrel (Plavix)
  Dipyridamole (Dipridacot, Persantine)
  Ticlopidine (Ticlid)
  Abciximab (ReoPro)
  Eptifibatide (Integrilin)
  Sulfinpyrazone (Anturane)
  Tirofiban (Aggrastat)
	Inhibit platelet aggregation and platelet-induced clotting; used primarily to prevent arterial thrombus formation

Thrombolytics	
Anistreplase (Eminase) Streptokinase (Streptase) Recombinant tissue plasminogen activator (rt-PA) (Alteplase) Urokinase (Abbokinase)	Facilitate clot dissolution; used to reopen occluded vessels in arterial and venous thrombosis

flow through vessels that have been occluded by thrombi. Specific agents discussed here are listed in Table 25–1.

Anticoagulants

The primary anticoagulants are heparin and a group of orally acting agents including warfarin (Coumadin) and other coumarin derivatives. These drugs are used primarily in the treatment of abnormal clot formation in the venous system. Venous clots typically form in the deep veins of the legs because of the relatively sluggish blood flow through those vessels. Hence, deep vein thrombosis is a primary indication for anticoagulant therapy.[21] Deep vein thrombosis results in thromboembolism when a piece of the clot breaks off and travels through the circulation to lodge elsewhere in the vascular system. Emboli originating in the venous system typically follow the venous flow back to the right side of the heart, where they are then pumped to the lungs. They finally lodge in the smaller vessels within the lungs, thus creating a pulmonary embolism.[21] Consequently, pulmonary embolism secondary to venous thrombosis is often the pathologic condition that initiates anticoagulant therapy.

Anticoagulant drugs are administered for the acute treatment of venous thrombosis and thromboembolism, or they may be given prophylactically to individuals who are at high risk to develop venous thrombosis. For instance, these drugs are often adminis-tered after surgical procedures (joint replacement, mechanical heart valve replacement, and so forth) and during medical conditions when patients will be relatively inactive for extended periods of time.[67,79]

HEPARIN

Heparin is usually the primary drug used in the initial treatment of venous throm-bosis.[39,43] The anticoagulant effects of heparin are seen almost instantly after adminis-tration. Heparin works by potentiating the activity of a circulating protein known as *an-tithrombin III*.[60] Antithrombin III binds to several of the active clotting factors (including thrombin) and renders the clotting factors inactive. Heparin accelerates the antithrom-bin III–induced inactivation of these clotting factors, thus reducing the tendency for clot-ting and thrombogenesis.

Heparin is a large, sugarlike molecule that is poorly absorbed from the gastroin-testinal tract. Consequently, heparin must be administered parenterally. Heparin was traditionally administered by intravenous infusion or by repeated IV injection through a rubber-capped indwelling needle called a *heparin lock*. Heparin preparations used in the past were also somewhat heterogeneous and contained various forms of compounds with heparin-like activity. In recent years, efforts have been made to chemically extract certain types of heparin from the more general (unfractionated) forms of this com-pound.[101] These efforts have led to the extraction and clinical use of specific forms of he-parin known as *low-molecular-weight heparins* (LMWH). These agents are enoxaparin, dalteparin, ardeparin, and other drugs identified by the "-parin" suffix.

The LMWHs seem to be as effective as unfractionated (mixed) heparins, but the LMWHs offer certain advantages. The LMWHs can, for example, be administered by subcutaneous injection into fat tissues, thereby decreasing the need for repeated intra-venous administration. Subcutaneous administration offers an easier and more conve-nient route, especially for people who are being treated at home or as outpatients.[1,82] The anticoagulant effects of the LMWHs are also more predictable, and these agents tend to normalize clotting with less risk of excessive bleeding. The more predictable response to LMWHs also decreases or eliminates the need for repeated laboratory monitoring of par-tial thromboplastin time, international normalized ratio (INR), or other indicators of clotting time.[45,85,93]

The use of traditional (unfractionated) heparin has therefore been replaced to a large extent by LMWHs. It appears, however, that the LMWHs are not all the same and that these agents cannot be used interchangeably.[9,46] Research is currently helping to de-fine and differentiate the advantages and disadvantages of specific agents within this group of LMWHs. Nonetheless, LMWHs seem to be a safer and more convenient alter-native to their unfractionated counterparts, and it appears that these drugs have become the primary method of treating acute venous thrombosis. The use of LMWHs in treat-ing other thrombotic syndromes including ischemic stroke and acute coronary infarc-tion is also being investigated, and it seems likely that these LMWHs will continue to gain widespread acceptance in the future.[43,55]

ORAL ANTICOAGULANTS

Drugs that are structurally and functionally similar to dicumarol constitute a group of orally active anticoagulant agents (see Table 25–1). The primary drug in this group is warfarin. These drugs exert their anticoagulant effects by impairing the hepatic synthesis of several clotting factors.[60] The specific mechanism of coumarin drugs is illustrated in Figure 25–2. In the liver, vitamin K acts as a catalyst in the final step of the synthesis of clotting factors II, VII, IX, and X. In the process, vitamin K is oxidized to an altered form known as vitamin K epoxide. For the process to continue, vitamin K epoxide must be reduced to its original form. As shown in Figure 25–2, coumarin drugs block the conversion of vitamin K epoxide to vitamin K, thus impairing the synthesis of several clotting factors. With time, a decrease in the level of circulating clotting factors results in a decrease in blood coagulation and in thrombogenesis.

Unlike heparin, the primary advantage of coumarin drugs is that they are administered orally.[57] However, because of the nature of their action, there is often a lag time of several days before the decreased production of clotting factors is sufficient to interrupt the clotting cascade and an anticoagulant effect is appreciated.[42] Consequently, anticoagulant therapy often begins with parenteral administration of heparin, followed by oral administration of coumarin drugs.[4,56] Heparin is administered for the first few days to achieve an immediate effect. Coumarin drugs are then initiated, and heparin is discontinued after the coumarin drugs have had time to exert their anticoagulant effect. Oral administration of coumarin drugs may then be continued for several weeks to several months following an incident of thrombosis.

OTHER ANTICOAGULANTS

In addition to heparin and the oral anticoagulants, drugs have been developed that inhibit specific components in the clotting mechanism. In particular, hirudin (Refludan) and similar agents have been used to directly inhibit thrombin, thus targeting a specific step in the clotting process.[78] Likewise, agents that inhibit clotting factor Xa (see Fig. 25–1) have been used on a limited basis to normalize clotting time.[20] Thus, agents that inhibit specific clotting components such as thrombin and factor Xa are currently being investigated, and future research should determine optimal use of these agents either alone or in combination with existing anticoagulants.

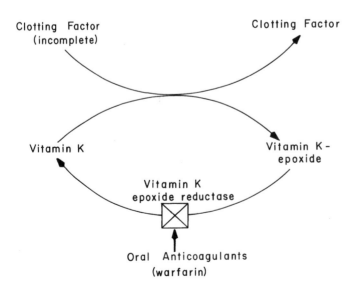

FIGURE 25–2. Role of vitamin K in the synthesis of vitamin K–dependent clotting factors (II, VII, IX, and X). Vitamin K catalyzes the reaction necessary for completion of clotting factor synthesis, but it is oxidized in the process to vitamin K epoxide. Regeneration of vitamin K occurs via vitamin K epoxide reductase. Oral anticoagulants such as warfarin (Coumadin) block the regeneration of the vitamin K, thus halting the further synthesis of the vitamin K–dependent factors.

ADVERSE EFFECTS OF ANTICOAGULANT DRUGS

Predictably, hemorrhage is the primary and most serious problem with drugs used to decrease blood clotting.[33,54,77] Increased bleeding may occur with heparin, warfarin, and other anticoagulants, and this bleeding may be quite severe in some patients. Any unusual bleeding such as blood in the urine or stools, unexplained nosebleeds, or an unusually heavy menstrual flow may indicate a problem. Also, back pain or joint pain may be an indication of abdominal or intrajoint hemorrhage, respectively. To prevent excessive bleeding, laboratory tests that measure hemostasis are sometimes used to monitor patients taking anticoagulant drugs. Tests such as partial thromboplastin time and prothrombin time can indicate the effectiveness of drugs that alter blood coagulation, and adjustments in drug dosage are based on whether coagulation time falls within an acceptable range.[48]

Heparin may also produce a decrease in platelets (thrombocytopenia) in some patients.[22,47,81] Heparin-induced thrombocytopenia (HIT) can be asymptomatic and resolve spontaneously (type I HIT), or it can be severe (type II HIT). Type II HIT is mediated by an immune reaction, and this reaction can lead to serious complications including *increased* thrombosis in vascular tissues throughout the body.[22,81] Development of type II HIT is therefore an emergency situation that is typically resolved by discontinuing heparin and substituting an alternative type of anticoagulant.

Finally, oral anticoagulants may produce some gastrointestinal distress (nausea, stomach cramps, diarrhea), and these side effects are more common with dicumarol than with the other oral anticoagulants.

Antithrombotic Drugs

Whereas anticoagulants affect the synthesis and function of clotting factors, antithrombotics primarily inhibit the function of platelets.[74] In the bloodstream, platelets respond to vascular injury by changing their shape and adhering to one another (aggregation) at the site of clot formation. Platelets may sometimes aggregate inappropriately, however, thus forming a thrombus and occluding certain blood vessels. In particular, arterial thrombi are often formed by abnormal platelet aggregation. Hence, the antithrombotic drugs are used primarily to prevent the formation of arterial clots, such as those that cause coronary artery occlusion or cerebral infarction.

ASPIRIN

Aspirin suppresses platelet aggregation by inhibiting the synthesis of prostaglandins and thromboxanes.[64] As discussed in Chapter 15, aspirin exerts virtually all of its effects by inhibiting the cyclooxygenase enzyme that initiates the synthesis of lipidlike hormones known as prostaglandins and thromboxanes. Certain prostaglandins and thromboxanes, especially thromboxane A_2, have a potent ability to induce platelet aggregation. By inhibiting the synthesis of these proaggregation substances, aspirin prevents platelet-induced thrombus formation. Although the exact dose may vary in specific clinical situations, patients typically experience a meaningful antithrombotic effect at very low aspirin doses. For example, many antithrombotic regimens consist of taking one aspirin tablet (325 mg) each day, or even one pediatric ("baby") aspirin tablet (160 mg) each day.[99]

Because of its antithrombotic effects, aspirin has received a great deal of attention regarding its use in treating and preventing myocardial infarction. During the acute phase of an infarction, aspirin is critical in helping to limit the progression of platelet-induced occlusion, thereby reducing the extent of damage to the myocardium.[26] Following the acute phase, aspirin is often administered for prolonged periods to maintain coronary artery patency and prevent reinfarction.[5,26] Also, low doses of aspirin may decrease the incidence of an initial infarction in susceptible individuals—that is, people who have not yet sustained an infarction but have one or more risk factors for coronary artery disease.[97,104]

These rather remarkable findings have prompted a great deal of debate about the chronic use of aspirin and possible side effects such as increased hemorrhage. In particular, the incidence of intracranial hemorrhage (hemorrhagic stroke) may be increased when aspirin is administered to decrease thrombosis.[97,104] Nonetheless, aspirin is considered standard therapy during the acute phase of myocardial infarction, and prolonged use of aspirin is one of the primary pharmacologic methods used to prevent reinfarction in susceptible individuals.

Although increasing the risk of hemorrhagic stroke, aspirin may help prevent the type of stroke caused by cerebral ischemia and infarction.[2,18,19] The rationale is that aspirin will prevent infarction in cerebral vessels in the same manner that it prevents coronary infarction in heart attacks. The benefits of aspirin in stroke remain somewhat controversial, however. Clearly, the use of aspirin must be limited to only the types of stroke that result from insufficient blood flow, as opposed to hemorrhagic stroke. Even so, the antithrombotic benefits of aspirin in some cerebral vessels must be weighed against possible side effects such as increased bleeding in other vessels. Long-term aspirin therapy is probably beneficial to a certain percentage of stroke patients, but this drug must be used selectively.[2,19]

Consequently, the role of chronic aspirin administration in helping to prevent myocardial and possibly cerebral infarction remains an area of intense investigation. There seems to be little doubt that aspirin can be a very cost-effective method for decreasing the morbidity and mortality associated with these types of infarction. Nonetheless, the long-term effects of aspirin on other organs such as the liver, kidneys, and gastrointestinal tract must be considered. Likewise, men appear to benefit more than women from aspirin's antithrombotic effects, and the reasons for this gender-related difference need to be determined.[62,96] Hence, continued analysis of this topic promises to be an exciting and productive area of pharmacologic research.

Finally, aspirin has also been used to prevent thrombus formation in peripheral veins (deep vein thrombosis or DVT), and aspirin can serve as an adjunct or alternative to anticoagulants (heparin, warfarin) that are routinely used to treat DVTs.[21] Aspirin can likewise be administered to prevent thromboembolism following surgical procedures such as coronary artery bypass, arterial grafts, endarterectomy, and valve replacement.[11,66] By preventing platelet-induced thrombogenesis, aspirin helps maintain patency and prevent reocclusion of vessels following these procedures.

OTHER ANTITHROMBOTIC DRUGS

Although aspirin remains the primary antithombotic agent, this drug is actually only a weak inhibitor of platelet activity.[13] As indicated, aspirin may also increase the risk of intracranial hemorrhage, and aspirin may be poorly tolerated in some patients because of gastric irritation, an allergic response, and so forth.[111] Efforts have therefore been made to develop stronger and safer antiplatelet drugs.

One antiplatelet strategy that has shown considerable promise is the use of drugs that inhibit the ability of fibrinogen to activate platelets.[40,88] These drugs are known as glycoprotein (GP) IIb-IIIa inhibitors because they block (antagonize) the GP receptor on the platelet membrane that is stimulated by fibrinogen.[49,88,111] Fibrinogen is unable to bind to the platelet, thereby decreasing platelet activation and reducing platelet-induced clotting.[35,64] GP IIb-IIIa inhibitors that are currently available include abciximab (Reo-Pro), eptifibatide (Integrilin), and tirofiban (Aggrastat) (see Table 25–1).[106] These drugs are reported to be potent inhibitors of platelet function,[15,64] and future clinical research should determine how these drugs can be used most effectively alone or with other antithrombotics (including aspirin) to decrease and prevent myocardial infarction and similar thrombotic events.[86,111]

Another antiplatelet strategy involves drugs that inhibit the adenosine diphosphate (ADP) receptor on the platelet membrane.[89,102] ADP is another compound that increases platelet activity, and platelet-induced clotting is reduced by drugs that inhibit the receptor for this compound.[40,41] Such drugs include clopidogrel (Plavix) and ticlopidine (Ticlid) (see Table 25–1). These agents produce moderate inhibition of platelet activity, making them somewhat more effective than aspirin but not as strong as the GP IIb-IIIa inhibitors.[12] Likewise, these ADP receptor inhibitors seem to be tolerated fairly well, and they therefore provide an option for decreasing platelet-induced clotting in patients who cannot tolerate other antiplatelet drugs.[89,102,104]

Dipyridamole (Dipridacot, Persantine) has been used alone or in combination with aspirin to decrease platelet-induced clotting. This drug may affect platelet function by impairing adenosine metabolism and/or by increasing the concentration of cyclic adenosine monophosphate within the platelet.[29] The exact mechanism of dipyridamole, however, is poorly understood. It is also not clear if dipyridamole offers distinct advantages over aspirin and the newer antiplatelet drugs. One recent study suggested that combining dipyridamole with aspirin provided substantial benefits over using either drug alone.[38,113] These results are controversial, however, because other studies failed to find any advantage of using dipyridamole or combining this drug with aspirin.[18] Consequently, future use of dipyridamole remains uncertain, and it seems possible that newer agents (GP IIb-IIIa inhibitors, ADP receptor inhibitors) may supplant dipyridamole in treating thrombosis.

Finally, sulfinpyrazone (Anturane) is usually administered to treat gouty arthritis but has also shown some antithrombotic properties because of an ability to decrease platelet function. Sulfinpyrazone decreases platelet aggregation by inhibiting prostaglandin synthesis in a manner similar to aspirin. Sulfinpyrazone can be used as an alternative to aspirin in preventing reinfarction after a heart attack, especially in patients who are not able to tolerate aspirin or other antithrombotic drugs.

ADVERSE EFFECTS OF ANTITHROMBOTIC DRUGS

Increased risk of bleeding is the primary concern with aspirin and other antithrombotic drugs. Patients taking these agents should be especially alert for any unexplained or heavy bleeding or any other symptoms that might indicate hemorrhage (sudden increases in joint or back pain, severe headaches, and so forth). Aspirin can likewise cause gastric irritation, and high doses of aspirin may be toxic to the liver and kidneys (see Chap. 15). However, the likelihood of severe gastric disturbances and liver or renal toxicity is relatively low at the doses needed to create an antithrombotic effect. Other potential side effects of the nonaspirin antithrombotics include hypotension for the GP IIb-IIIa inhibitors (abciximab, eptifibatide), gastrointestinal distress for clopidogrel and dipyridamole, blood dyscrasias (neutropenia, agranulocytosis, thrombocytopenia) for ticlopidine, and formation of kidney stones for sulfinpyrazone.

Thrombolytic Drugs

Thrombolytics facilitate the breakdown and dissolution of clots that have already formed. These drugs work by converting plasminogen (profibrinolysin) to plasmin (fibrinolysin).[7] As shown in Figure 25–1, plasmin is the active form of an endogenous enzyme that breaks down fibrin clots. Drugs that activate this enzyme by various mechanisms can be used to dissolve clots that have already formed, thus reopening occluded blood vessels.

Thrombolytic drugs are extremely valuable in treating acute myocardial infarction.[7,24,37,71] When administered at the onset of infarction, these drugs can actually reestablish blood flow through occluded coronary vessels, often preventing or reversing myocardial damage, thus decreasing the morbidity and mortality normally associated with a heart attack.[8,32] These drugs can help reopen occluded coronary vessels when administered within 12 hours after symptom onset.[37,71] Thrombolytics seem to produce the best results, however, when they are administered fairly soon after the onset of symptoms. Administration within 1 hour after symptom onset, for example, can result in a 50 percent reduction in mortality in patients with acute myocardial infarction.[71]

Consequently, thrombolytic agents are administered whenever possible during the first few hours after an acute myocardial infarction. It was originally thought that these drugs had to be administered directly into the coronary arteries to reopen occluded coronary vessels.[3] It is now realized that these drugs will produce beneficial effects when injected intravenously into the systemic circulation; that is, the drug can be injected into any accessible vein and eventually reach the coronary clot through the general circulation.[99] The intravenous route is a much more practical method of administration because it is easier, faster, and safer than the intracoronary route.

Thrombolytic drugs therefore offer an attractive method of preventing—or even reversing—myocardial damage during acute myocardial infarction. Because these drugs can also stimulate clot breakdown in other vessels including the cerebral vasculature, intracranial hemorrhage and other bleeding problems are the primary drawbacks to thrombolytic treatment.[51,73] Thrombolytics are therefore contraindicated in certain situations, including patients with a history of hemorrhagic stroke, intracranial neoplasm, active internal bleeding, possible aortic dissection, and several other factors that represent increased risk of hemorrhage.[99] Also, thrombolytic therapy may not be curative, and reocclusion will occur in certain patients.

Although thrombolytic drugs are helpful in acute myocardial infarction, their benefits in other types of vascular occlusion are less obvious. For example, it is possible that these drugs could also help resolve thrombus formation in the large veins (deep vein thrombosis or DVT) and in the treatment of pulmonary embolism (PE). These drugs have, in fact, been used to treat these disorders, but they do not seem to produce substantial long-term clinical benefits in DVT or PE.[87] Still, thrombolytics may play a role in treating acute DVT or PE, especially in severe, life-threatening situations. Other possible indications for thrombolytic therapy include atherosclerotic occlusion in peripheral arteries (femoral, popliteal, and so forth).[65,108] Bypass grafts and shunts that have become occluded because of clot formation may also be cleaned out with the use of thrombolytic drugs.[83] Because of the risk of increased intracranial hemorrhage, these drugs are generally *not* used to treat stroke resulting from acute cerebral infarction.[72]

Listed here are the most common thrombolytic agents. Although these drugs differ chemically, they all ultimately activate fibrinolysis in some way. There has likewise been considerable debate about which agent provides optimal long-term benefits following myocardial infarction. Current consensus is that the choice of a specific agent is less important than simply making sure that one of these agents is used in a timely fashion; that is, the time elapsed before beginning treatment is probably more important than the actual type of thrombolytic agent that is administered.[10] Nonetheless, the relative benefits and unique aspects of each agent are presented here.

STREPTOKINASE AND UROKINASE

Although they work by somewhat different methods, these agents both bring about the activation of plasmin. Streptokinase indirectly activates plasmin (fibrinolysin) by binding to the precursor molecule plasminogen (profibrinolysin) and facilitating activation by endogenous mechanisms. Urokinase directly converts plasminogen to plasmin by enzymatically cleaving a peptide bond within the plasminogen molecule. Both agents have been used successfully to resolve acute clot formation in coronary arteries and peripheral vessels. Streptokinase, however, tends to be the most commonly used type of thrombolytic because this drug is relatively inexpensive and because the incidence of intracranial hemorrhage may be somewhat lower with streptokinase than with other thrombolytics.[94,112]

TISSUE PLASMINOGEN ACTIVATOR

In the endogenous control of hemostasis, plasminogen is activated by an intrinsic substance known as *tissue plasminogen activator* (t-PA) (see Fig. 25–1). Intravenous administration of t-PA rapidly and effectively initiates clot breakdown by directly activating plasmin (fibrinolysin). Although extraction of t-PA from human blood is costly and impractical, the commercial synthesis of t-PA has been made possible through the use of recombinant DNA techniques. Consequently, t-PA (known also by the generic name alteplase) is now available in commercial forms (Activase), and this agent joins streptokinase as one of the primary thrombolytic agents.

Tissue plasminogen activator has been used successfully to treat acute myocardial infarction, and the benefits of this treatment have been documented in clinical trials.[14,27,103,109] Preliminary findings suggested that t-PA may also be more effective than streptokinase in its ability to initially reopen coronary arteries in acute myocardial infarction and that t-PA may have a greater ability to dissolve only the harmful clot without impairing normal clot formation elsewhere in the body.[103,109] More recent studies, however, suggest that the thrombolytic effects of t-PA and streptokinase are basically similar[10,32] and that t-PA may actually be associated with a slightly higher incidence of hemorrhagic side effects, including stroke.[59,94] Hence, t-PA does not seem to offer any long-term clinical advantages over streptokinase, and streptokinase may be a more cost-effective method of treatment in the majority of people needing thrombolytic therapy.[94]

ANISTREPLASE

Anistreplase (Eminase) is a new thrombolytic that is also known as anisoylated plasminogen-streptokinase activator complex (APSAC). This compound is formed by combining plasminogen with streptokinase and then chemically altering (anisoylating) the catalytic site on this complex so that plasminogen remains inactive until it is administered. When administered systemically, anistreplase binds to fibrin, where it is then chemically activated so that streptokinase can modify plasminogen and initiate clot breakdown. The supposed advantage of using anistreplase is that this compound will be more selective for clots that have already formed and have less effect on systemic fibrinolysis. Anistreplase does cause considerable systemic fibrinolysis, however, and the advantages of this compound over streptokinase alone remain to be determined.

RETEPLASE

Reteplase (Retevase) is one of the newest thrombolytics. This agent is derived of human tissue plasminogen activator, and reteplase therefore has actions similar to t-PA (alteplase).[115] Reteplase is somewhat easier to administer than other thrombolytics, and there is some evidence that this drug may be able to reopen coronary arteries to a greater extent during the acute phase of infarction than more traditional agents, including t-PA.[58,115] Reteplase therefore offers another therapeutic option, and future studies should help determine if this drug provides better long-term benefits in terms of reduced morbidity and mortality than more traditional thrombolytic treatments.

ADVERSE EFFECTS OF THROMBOLYTIC DRUGS

Hemorrhage is the major adverse effect associated with thrombolytic agents. As indicated, intracranial hemorrhage may occur following thrombolytic therapy, especially in patients who have predisposing risk factors such as advanced age, severe or untreated hypertension, or a history of hemorrhagic stroke.[73] Excessive bleeding may also occur during dressing changes, wound care, and other invasive procedures following thrombolytic treatment. Thrombolytic drugs may cause fever and an allergic reaction (itching, nausea, headache, other symptoms). The risk and severity of fever and allergic responses seems greatest for streptokinase, but all the thrombolytics can potentially cause these reactions.

TREATMENT OF CLOTTING DEFICIENCIES

Hemophilia

Hemophilia is a hereditary disease in which an individual is unable to synthesize adequate amounts of a specific clotting factor. The two most common forms of hemophilia are hemophilia A, which is caused by deficiency of clotting factor VIII, and hemophilia B, which is a deficit in clotting factor IX.[17] In either form of this disease, patients are missing a key clotting factor and have problems maintaining normal hemostasis. Even trivial injuries can produce serious or fatal hemorrhage. Also, patients with hemophilia often develop joint problems because of intra-articular hemorrhage (hemarthrosis).

Treatment of hemophilia consists of replacing the missing clotting factor. Although this treatment seems relatively simple, obtaining sufficient amounts of the missing factor is a very costly procedure. At the present time, the primary source of clotting factors VIII and IX is human blood extract. Obtaining an adequate supply from this source can cost more than $25,000 per patient per year.

A more serious problem is the potential for clotting factor extract to contain viruses such as hepatitis B, or HIV, which causes AIDS. The lack of proper blood screening has resulted in tragic consequences; for example, clotting factors extracted from patients infected with HIV have served as a vehicle for viral transmission to patients with hemophilia. More stringent screening procedures and other techniques such as heat treatment of clotting factor extracts have decreased the risk of AIDS transmission, but patients with hemophilia receiving exogenous factors remain at risk for viral infection. New methods of drug production, such as genetic engineering and recombinant DNA techniques, are currently being used to manufacture specific clotting factors such as factor VIII.[90] It is hoped that these techniques will provide a safer, cheaper source of missing clotting factors for patients with hemophilia.

Deficiencies of Vitamin K–Dependent Clotting Factors

As indicated earlier in this chapter, the liver needs adequate amounts of vitamin K to synthesize clotting factors II, VII, IX, and X. As shown in Figure 25–2, vitamin K catalyzes the final steps in the synthesis of these factors. Normally, vitamin K is supplied through the diet or synthesized by intestinal bacteria and subsequently absorbed from the gastrointestinal tract into the body. However, any defect in vitamin K ingestion, synthesis, or absorption may result in vitamin K deficiency. Insufficient vitamin K in the body results in an inadequate hepatic synthesis of the clotting factors listed previously, thus resulting in poor hemostasis and excessive bleeding.

Deficiencies in vitamin K and the related synthesis of the vitamin K–dependent clotting factors are treated by administering exogenous vitamin K.[17] Various commercial forms of this vitamin are available for oral or parenteral (intramuscular or subcutaneous) administration. Specifically, individuals with a poor diet, intestinal disease, or impaired intestinal absorption may require vitamin K to maintain proper hemostasis. Also, vitamin K is routinely administered to newborn infants to prevent hemorrhage. For the first 5 to 8 days following birth, newborns lack the intestinal bacteria necessary to help synthesize vitamin K. Vitamin K is administered to facilitate clotting factor synthesis until the newborn is able to produce sufficient endogenous vitamin K.

Antifibrinolytics

The excessive bleeding that sometimes occurs following surgery or trauma may be caused by an overactive fibrinolytic system—that is, *hyperfibrinolysis*. Hyperfibrinolysis results in excessive clot destruction and ineffective hemostasis. Likewise, patients with hemophilia who undergo surgery, including dental procedures (tooth extractions, restorations, etc.), will benefit if clot breakdown is inhibited because hemorrhage and the need for additional clotting factors will be reduced. Antifibrinolytic agents such as aminocaproic acid (Amicar) and tranexamic acid (Cyklokapron) are often used in these situations. These drugs appear to inhibit activation of plasminogen (profibrinolysin) to plasmin (fibrinolysin). Plasmin is the enzyme responsible for breaking down fibrin clots (see Fig. 25–1). Antifibrinolytics prevent the activation of this enzyme, thus preserving clot formation.

Aminocaproic acid and tranexamic acid are administered either orally or intravenously for the acute treatment of hyperfibrinolysis or to prevent clot breakdown in patients with hemophilia who are undergoing surgery. Some adverse effects such as nausea, diarrhea, dizziness, and headache may occur when these drugs are administered, but these problems are relatively minor and usually disappear when the drug is discontinued.

AGENTS USED TO TREAT HYPERLIPIDEMIA

Hyperlipidemia, an abnormally high concentration of lipids in the bloodstream, is one of the primary causes of cardiovascular disease in industrialized nations. This condition typically causes deposition of fatty plaquelike lesions on the walls of large and medium-sized arteries (*atherosclerosis*), which can lead to thrombosis and infarction. Hence, elevated plasma lipids are related to some of the events discussed previously in this chapter because atherosclerosis can precipitate increased clotting and thromboembolic disease.

Hyperlipidemia is often caused by poor diet and lifestyle, as well as by several genetic conditions that cause disorders in lipid metabolism.[8,61] It is not possible to review here the endogenous control of lipid metabolism or the various pathologic processes involved in hyperlipidemia, and these topics are addressed in other sources.[61,100,114] It should be realized, however, that lipids such as cholesterol are transported in the bloodstream as part of a lipid-protein complex known as a *lipoprotein*. Certain lipoproteins are considered beneficial because they may decrease the formation of atherosclerotic plaques by removing cholesterol from the arterial wall. These beneficial complexes are known as high-density lipoproteins (HDLs) because of the relatively large amount of protein in the complex. Other lipoproteins are considered harmful because they transport and deposit cholesterol onto the arterial wall. These atherogenic lipoproteins include intermediate-density lipoproteins (IDLs), low-density lipoproteins (LDLs), and very-low-density lipoproteins (VLDLs). Pharmacologic and nonpharmacologic strategies to reduce hyperlipidemia typically focus on reducing these atherogenic lipoproteins and increasing the beneficial HDLs.

Drugs that can be used to treat hyperlipidemia are summarized in Table 25–2 and are discussed briefly here. These agents are typically used when plasma lipid levels are not successfully controlled by nonpharmacologic methods such as low-fat diets, weight reduction, regular exercise, and smoking cessation.[31,75] Likewise, these drugs should be used in conjunction with nonpharmacologic methods, and optimal results are often realized through a combination of drug therapy and various dietary and lifestyle modifications.[53,92]

HMG-CoA Reductase Inhibitors (Statins)

This category includes fluvastatin (Lescol), lovastatin (Mevacor), pravastatin (Pravachol), and simvastatin (Zocor) (Table 25–2). These drugs are characterized by their ability to inhibit an enzyme known as 3-hydroxy-3-methylglutaryl coenzyme A (HMG-CoA) reductase.[63,69] This enzyme catalyzes one of the early steps of cholesterol synthesis, and drugs that inhibit HMG-CoA reductase decrease cholesterol production, especially in liver cells. Decreased hepatic cholesterol biosynthesis also causes more surface receptors for LDL cholesterol to be synthesized, and this increase in surface receptors triggers an increase in the breakdown of LDL cholesterol and a decrease in the synthesis of VLDL, which serves as a precursor for LDL synthesis.[28] HMG-CoA reductase inhibitors can also decrease triglyceride levels[28,98] and produce a modest increase in HDL levels.[30] The exact reasons for the beneficial effects on triglycerides and HDL levels, however, are not entirely clear.

The HMG-CoA reductase inhibitors therefore improve several aspects of the plasma lipid profile. These agents, known also as "statins," may in addition produce several favorable effects that are independent of their ability to affect lipid metabolism.[63] These drugs may, for example, produce direct beneficial effects on the vascular endothelium so that atherosclerotic plaque formation is reduced.[16,23,91,107] These drugs may likewise have antioxidant and antithrombotic effects that contribute to their ability to improve function of the vascular wall.[52,75,107] Statins therefore seem to exert several

TABLE 25–2 Drugs Used to Treat Hyperlipidemia

Generic Name	Trade Name(s)	Dosage*	Primary Effect
Cholestyramine	Questran	4 g 1–6 times each day before meals and at bedtime	Decreases plasma LDL cholesterol levels
Clofibrate	Abitrate, Atromid-S	1.5–2.0 g each day in 2–4 divided doses	Lowers plasma triglycerides by decreasing LDL and IDL levels
Fluvastatin	Lescol	20–40 mg once each day in the evening	Decreases plasma LDL cholesterol and VLDL cholesterol levels; may also decrease triglycerides and increase HDL somewhat
Gemfibrozil	Lopid	1.2 g each day in 2 divided doses 30 min before morning and evening meals	Similar to clofibrate
Lovastatin	Mevacor	20–80 mg each day as a single dose or in divided doses with meals	Similar to fluvastatin
Niacin	Nicobid, others	1–2 g 3 times each day	Lowers plasma triglycerides by decreasing VLDL levels
Pravastatin	Pravachol	10–40 mg once each day at bedtime	Similar to fluvastatin
Probucol	Lorelco	500 mg 2 times each day with morning and evening meals	Decreases LDL and HDL cholesterol; may also inhibit deposition of fat into arterial wall
Simvastatin	Zocor	5–40 mg once each day in the evening	Similar to fluvastatin

*Doses represent typical adult oral maintenance dose.
    HDL = high-density lipoproteins; IDL = intermediate-density lipoproteins; LDL = low-density lipoproteins; VLDL = very-low-density lipoproteins.

complex effects, and their ability to reduce the risk of cardiovascular disease is probably the result of their favorable effects on plasma lipids, combined with their ability to improve the function of the vascular endothelium.

Statins are therefore helpful in decreasing morbidity and mortality in people with high cholesterol, as well as individuals with normal cholesterol but other risk factors for cardiovascular disease.[63,105] It is estimated, for example, that these drugs decrease the risk of a major cardiac event by approximately 30 to 35 percent, although benefits depend on the extent that cholesterol is reduced and the influence of other risk factors.[6,63,84,91] Nonetheless, statins are now regarded as a mainstay in treating cardiovascular disease, and efforts are underway to expand the use of these medications and explore the optimal use of these drugs with other pharmacologic and nonpharmacologic interventions in cardiovascular disease.[53,63]

Fibric Acids

Fibric acids or "fibrates" include clofibrate (Abitrate, Atromid) and gemfibrozil (Lopid). The exact mechanism of these drugs is unclear, but they probably work by increasing the activity of the lipoprotein lipase enzyme in hepatic and peripheral tissues.[44,68,110] Hence, these drugs decrease triglyceride levels and increase the breakdown of triglyceride-rich lipoproteins such as VLDL.[44] Fibrates are therefore most helpful in hyperlipidemias characterized by increased triglycerides and increased VLDLs.[68,95] It is not exactly clear how much these agents can reduce the risk of a major cardiac event (infarction, stroke), but these drugs will probably remain the first choice for people with certain hyperlipidemias (e.g., increased triglycerides), and fibrates can be used with other drugs such as statins to provide more comprehensive pharmacologic control of certain lipid disorders.[80]

Other Lipid-Lowering Agents

Several other agents have beneficial effects on plasma lipid profiles that occur through various cellular mechanisms.[100] Cholestyramine (Questran) attaches to bile acids within the gastrointestinal lumen and increases fecal excretion of these acids. This action leads to decreased plasma cholesterol concentrations because cholesterol breakdown is accelerated to replace the bile acids that are lost in the feces. Niacin (nicotinic acid, vitamin B_3, Nicobid, other names) decreases LDL synthesis by inhibiting the production of VLDL, which serves as a precursor for LDL. This effect reduces the primary lipoproteins used to transport cholesterol in the bloodstream. Probucol (Lorelco) increases LDL breakdown somewhat, and this drug may also directly inhibit the deposition of cholesterol into arterial walls. This latter effect has received considerable attention recently because this drug may directly reduce atherosclerotic plaque formation in certain individuals.

Adverse Effects of Antihyperlipidemia Agents

Most of the drugs used to treat hyperlipidemia are fairly well tolerated. Some gastrointestinal distress (nausea, diarrhea) is fairly common with most of these drugs, but these problems are usually minor and do not require that drug therapy be discontinued. Other bothersome side effects are related to specific agents. Niacin, for instance, is often associated with cutaneous vasodilation and a sensation of warmth when doses are administered, but these sensations are not usually a problem. Some fairly serious problems, including liver dysfunction, gallstones, and pancreatitis, can occur with many antihyperlipidemia drugs, but the incidence of these side effects is relatively rare. Neuromuscular problems have been noted with certain agents. Paresthesias, for example, may occur with probucol. Other neuromuscular side effects such as myalgia, myositis, and fatigue and weakness have been occasionally noted with the HMG-CoA reductase inhibitors (lovastatin, other "statins") and with the fibric acids (clofibrate, gemfibrozil). It has also been suggested that the risk of muscular toxicity (myopathy that may be accompanied by rhabdomyolysis) is increased when a statin is combined with a fibrate.[69,70] Cardiovascular problems such as arrhythmias, blood dyscrasias, and angioneurotic syndrome may also occur with the fibric acids and probucol.

SPECIAL CONCERNS IN REHABILITATION PATIENTS

Therapists will frequently encounter patients taking drugs to alter hemostasis. Many patients on prolonged bed rest have a tendency for increased thrombus formation and are particularly susceptible to deep vein thrombosis. These patients will often be given anticoagulant drugs. Heparin followed by warfarin may be administered prophylactically or in response to the symptoms of thrombophlebitis in patients who have undergone hip surgery, heart valve replacement, and other surgical procedures. Therapists should be aware that the primary problem associated with anticoagulant drugs is an increased tendency for bleeding. Any rehabilitation procedures that deal with open wounds (dressing changes, debridement, etc.) should be carefully administered. Rigorous manual techniques such as deep tissue massage or chest percussion must also be used with caution because these procedures may directly traumatize tissues and induce bleeding in patients taking anticoagulant drugs. Certain manual techniques such as upper cervical manipulation should be avoided or used very cautiously because of increased risk of damage to the vertebral artery in patients taking anticlotting drugs.

Anticoagulants and antithrombotic drugs (e.g., aspirin) may also be given to rehabilitation patients to prevent the recurrence of myocardial infarction. As discussed previously, aspirin appears to be especially attractive in preventing an initial incident or the recurrence of infarction. Aspirin is relatively free from any serious side effects that may influence the rehabilitation session. Long-term anticoagulant and antithrombotic therapy is also frequently employed in specific cases of cerebrovascular accidents (strokes) that are due to recurrent cerebral embolism and occlusion. Obviously, giving anticoagulant and antithrombotic drugs to patients with a tendency toward the hemorrhagic type of stroke is counterproductive, because these drugs would only exacerbate this condition. However, stroke cases in which hemorrhage has been ruled out may benefit from prolonged anticoagulant or antithrombotic therapy. Again, therapists should be cognizant of the tendency for increased bleeding with these agents. However, the long-term use of these agents, especially aspirin, usually does not create any significant problems in the course of rehabilitation.

Thrombolytic drugs (streptokinase, t-PA, others) usually do not have a direct impact on physical therapy or occupational therapy. Thrombolytics are typically given in acute situations, immediately following myocardial infarction. Therapists may, however, benefit indirectly from the effects of these drugs because patients may recover faster and more completely from heart attacks. Thrombolytics may also help reopen occluded peripheral vessels, thus improving tissue perfusion and wound healing in rehabilitation patients.

Therapists will often work with individuals who have chronic clotting deficiencies, such as patients with hemophilia. Intrajoint hemorrhage (*hemarthrosis*) with subsequent arthropathy is one of the primary problems associated with hemophilia.[17,50] The joints most often affected are the knees, ankles, and elbows.[36] Hemarthrosis is usually treated by replacing the missing clotting factor and by rehabilitating the affected joints. Therapists often employ a judicious program of exercise and cryotherapy to help improve joint function following hemarthrosis.[36,76] Consequently, the therapist often works in conjunction with pharmacologic management to help improve function in hemophilia-related joint disorders.

Finally, therapists may encourage patients to comply with pharmacologic and non-pharmacologic methods used to lower plasma lipids. Drugs used to treat hyperlipidemia are typically used in conjunction with diet, exercise, and other lifestyle changes that reduce fat intake and improve plasma lipid profiles. Therapists can help design and implement exercise programs that enable patients to lose weight and increase plasma levels of antiatherogenic components such as HDL, thus maximizing the effects of drug therapy.

CASE STUDY

CLOTTING DISORDERS

Brief History. C.W. is an obese, 47-year-old woman who sustained a compression fracture of the L-1 and L-2 vertebrae during a fall from a second-story window. (There was some suggestion that she may have been pushed during an argument with her husband, but the details remain unclear.) She was admitted to the hospital, where her medical condition was stabilized, and surgical procedures were performed to treat her vertebral fracture. Her injuries ultimately resulted in a partial transection of the spinal cord, with diminished motor and sensory function in both lower extremities. She began an extensive rehabilitation program, including physical therapy and occupational therapy. She was progressing well when she developed shortness of breath and an acute pain in her right thorax. A diagnosis of massive pulmonary embolism was made. Evidently she had developed deep vein thrombosis in both lower extremities, and a large embolism from the venous clots had lodged in her lungs, producing a pulmonary infarction.

Drug Treatment. Because of the extensive nature of the pulmonary infarction, a thrombolytic agent was used to attempt to resolve the clot. An initial dosage of 250,000 units of streptokinase was administered intravenously within 2 hours after the onset of symptoms. Streptokinase was continued via intravenous infusion at a rate of 100,000 units/hour for 24 hours after the initial dose.

To prevent further thromboembolism, streptokinase infusion was followed by heparin. Heparin was administered intravenously, 5000 units every 4 hours. Clotting time was monitored closely by periodic blood tests during the heparin treatment. After 3 days of heparin therapy, C.W. was switched to warfarin. Warfarin was administered orally, and the dosage was adjusted until she was ultimately receiving 5 mg/day. Oral warfarin was continued throughout the remainder of the patient's hospital stay, as well as after discharge.

Impact on Rehabilitation. The drugs used to resolve the thromboembolic episode greatly facilitated the patient's recovery from that incident. The use of a thrombolytic agent (streptokinase) enabled the patient to resume her normal course of rehabilitation within 2 days of the pulmonary embolism. Thus, the use of these drugs directly facilitated physical therapy and occupational therapy by allowing the patient to resume therapy much sooner than if the embolism had been treated more conservatively (i.e., rest and anticoagulants) or more radically (i.e., surgery). Because the patient remained on anticoagulant drugs for an extended period of time, the therapists dealing with the patient routinely looked for signs of excessive bleeding such as skin bruising and hematuria. The patient remained free from any further thromboembolic episodes, however, and was eventually discharged to an extended-care rehabilitation facility to continue her progress.

SUMMARY

Normal hemostasis is a balance between excessive and inadequate blood clotting. Overactive blood clotting is harmful because of the tendency for thrombus formation and occlusion of arteries and veins. Vessels may become directly blocked by the thrombus, or a portion of the thrombus may break off and create an embolism that lodges elsewhere in the vascular system. The tendency for excessive thrombus formation in the venous system is usually treated with anticoagulant drugs such as heparin and warfarin. Prevention of arterial thrombogenesis is often accomplished by platelet inhibitors such as aspirin. Vessels that have suddenly become occluded because of acute thrombus formation may be successfully reopened by thrombolytic drugs (streptokinase, t-PA) that facilitate the dissolution of the harmful clot.

The inadequate blood clotting and excessive bleeding that occur in patients with hemophilia are treated by replacing the missing clotting factor. Other conditions associated with inadequate coagulation may be treated by administering either vitamin K, which helps improve the synthesis of certain clotting factors, or antifibrinolytic agents (aminocaproic acid, tranexamic acid), which inhibit clot breakdown.

Hyperlipidemia can lead to atherosclerosis and subsequent cardiovascular incidents such as thrombosis and infarction. This condition is often treated by a combination of drug therapy and diet and lifestyle modifications. Pharmacologic interventions are typically targeted toward decreasing the synthesis of harmful (atherogenic) plasma components, including certain lipoproteins (IDL, LDL, VLDL) that are associated with atherosclerotic plaque formation.

REFERENCES

1. Agnelli, G, Taliani, MR, and Verso, M: Building effective prophylaxis of deep vein thrombosis in the outpatient setting. Blood Coagul Fibrinolysis 10(Suppl 2):S29, 1999.
2. Albers, GW and Tijssen, JG: Antiplatelet therapy: New foundations for optimal treatment decisions. Neurology 53(Suppl 4):S25, 1999.
3. Anderson, JL, et al: A randomized trial of intracoronary streptokinase in the treatment of acute myocardial infarction. N Engl J Med 308:1312, 1983.
4. Ansell, JE: Oral anticoagulants for the treatment of venous thromboembolism. Baillieres Clin Haematol 11:639, 1998.
5. Antiplatelet Trialists' Collaboration: Secondary prevention of vascular disease by prolonged antiplatelet therapy. BMJ 296:320, 1988.
6. Arntz, HR: Evidence for the benefit of early intervention with pravastatin for secondary prevention of cardiovascular events. Atherosclerosis 147(Suppl 1):S17, 1999.
7. Bell, WR: Evaluation of thrombolytic agents. Drugs 54(Suppl 3):11, 1997.
8. Bell, WR: Thrombolytic therapy: Agents, indications, and laboratory monitoring. Med Clin (Barc) 78:745, 1994.
9. Bick, RL: Low molecular weight heparins in the outpatient management of venous thromboembolism. Semin Thromb Hemost 25(Suppl 3):97, 1999.
10. Bizjak, ED and Mauro, VF: Thrombolytic therapy: A review of its use in acute myocardial infarction. Ann Pharmacother 32:769, 1998.
11. Bollinger, A and Brunner, U: Antiplatelet drugs improve the patency rates after femoro-popliteal endarterectomy. Vasa 14:272, 1985.
12. Boysen, G: Bleeding complications in secondary stroke prevention by antiplatelet therapy: A benefit-risk analysis. J Intern Med 246:239, 1999.
13. Bungard, TJ: An overview of commonly used antiplatelet agents. Can J Cardiovasc Nurs 9:38, 1998.
14. Califf, RM, Topol, EJ, and George, BS: One-year outcome after therapy with tissue plasminogen activator: Report from the thrombolysis and angioplasty in myocardial infarction trial. Am Heart J 119:777, 1990.
15. Cantor, WJ and Ohman, EM: Results of recent large myocardial infarction trials, adjunctive therapies, and acute myocardial infarction: Improving outcomes. Cardiol Rev 7:232, 1999.
16. Corsini, A, et al: New insights into the pharmacodynamic and pharmacokinetic properties of statins. Pharmacol Ther 84:413, 1999.
17. Diaz-Linares, M and Rodvold, KA: Coagulation disorders. In DiPiro, JT, et al (eds): Pharmacotherapy: A Pathophysiologic Approach, ed 4. Appleton & Lange, Stamford, CT, 1999.
18. Dyken, ML: Antiplatelet agents and stroke prevention. Semin Neurol 18:441, 1998.
19. Easton, JD, et al: Antiplatelet therapy: Views from the experts. Neurology 53(Suppl 4):S32, 1999.
20. Eisenberg, PR and Ghigliotti, G: Platelet-dependent and procoagulant mechanisms in arterial thrombosis. Int J Cardiol 68(Suppl 1):S3, 1999.
21. Erdman, SM, Chuck, SK, and Rodvold, KA: Thromboembolic disorders. In DiPiro, JT, et al (eds): Pharmacotherapy: A Pathophysiologic Approach, ed 4. Appleton & Lange, Stamford, CT, 1999.

22. Fabris, F, et al: Heparin-induced thrombocytopenia. Haematologica 85:72, 2000.
23. Farnier, M and Davignon, J: Current and future treatment of hyperlipidemia: The role of statins. Am J Cardiol 82(Suppl 4B):3J, 1998.
24. Fox, KA: Have we reached the limit with thrombolytic therapy? Cardiovasc Drugs Ther 13:211, 1999.
25. Furie, B and Furie, BC: Molecular and cellular biology of blood coagulation. N Engl J Med 326:800, 1992.
26. Gensini, GF, Comeglio, M, and Falai, M: Advances in antithrombotic therapy of acute myocardial infarction. Am Heart J 138(Part 2):171, 1999.
27. Gersh, BJ: Current issues in reperfusion therapy. Am J Cardiol 82(Suppl 8B):3P, 1998.
28. Ginsberg, HN: Effects of statins on triglyceride metabolism. Am J Cardiol 81(Suppl 4A):32B, 1998.
29. Gresele, P, et al: Mechanism of the antiplatelet action of dipyridamole in whole blood: Modulation of adenosine concentration and activity. Thromb Haemost 55:12, 1986.
30. Grover, SA, et al: Cost-effectiveness of 3-hydroxy-3-methylglutaryl-coenzyme A reductase inhibitors in the secondary prevention of cardiovascular disease: Forecasting the incremental benefits of preventing coronary and cerebrovascular events. Arch Intern Med 159:593, 1999.
31. Grundy, SM: Cholesterol management in high-risk patients without heart disease. When is lipid-lowering medication warranted for primary prevention? Postgrad Med 104:117, 1998.
32. GUSTO Angiographic Investigators: The effects of tissue plasminogen activator, streptokinase, or both on coronary artery patency, ventricular function, and survival after acute myocardial infarction. N Engl J Med 329:1615, 1993.
33. Haas, S: Limitations of established antithrombotic strategies. Blood Coagul Fibrinolysis 10(Suppl 2):S11, 1999.
34. Haines, ST and Bussey, HI: Thrombosis and the pharmacology of antithrombotic agents. Ann Pharmacother 29:892, 1995.
35. Harrington, RA: Overview of clinical trials of glycoprotein IIb-IIIa inhibitors in acute coronary syndromes. Am Heart J 138(Part 2):276, 1999.
36. Helske, T, et al: Joint involvement in patients with severe haemophilia A in 1957–59 and 1978–79. Br J Haematol 51:643, 1982.
37. Hennekens, C: The need for wider utilization of thrombolytic therapy. Clin Cardiol 20(Suppl 3):III 26, 1997.
38. Hervey, PS and Goa, KL: Extended-release dipyridamole/aspirin. Drugs 58:469, 1999.
39. Hirsh, J: Drug therapy: Heparin. N Engl J Med 324:1565, 1991.
40. Hirsh, J and Weitz, JI: New antithrombotic agents. Lancet 353:1431, 1999.
41. Hirsh, J and Weitz, JI: Thrombosis and anticoagulation. Semin Hematol 36(Suppl 7):118, 1999.
42. Horton, JD and Bushwick, BM: Warfarin therapy: Evolving strategies in anticoagulation. Am Fam Physician 59:635, 1999.
43. Hovanessian, HC: New-generation anticoagulants: The low molecular weight heparins. Ann Emerg Med 34:768, 1999.
44. Hunninghake, DB: Pharmacologic management of triglycerides. Clin Cardiol 22(Suppl):II 44, 1999.
45. Iobst, CA and Friedman, RJ: The role of low molecular weight heparin in total knee arthroplasty. Am J Knee Surg 12:55, 1999.
46. Kaiser, B, et al: Preclinical biochemistry and pharmacology of low molecular weight heparins in vivo: Studies of venous and arterial thrombosis. Semin Thromb Hemost 25(Suppl 3):35, 1999.
47. Kaplan, KL and Francis, CW: Heparin-induced thrombocytopenia. Blood Rev 13:1, 1999.
48. Kitchen, S and Preston, FE: Standardization of prothrombin time for laboratory control of oral anticoagulant therapy. Semin Thromb Hemost 25:17, 1999.
49. Kleiman, NS: Pharmacokinetics and pharmacodynamics of glycoprotein IIb-IIIa inhibitors. Am Heart J 138(Part 2):263, 1999.
50. Koch, B, et al: Hemophiliac knee: Rehabilitation techniques. Arch Phys Med Rehabil 63:379, 1982.
51. Lagares, A, et al: Cerebral aneurysm rupture after r-TPA thrombolysis for acute myocardial infarction. Surg Neurol 52:623, 1999.
52. Langtry, HD and Markham, A: Fluvastatin: A review of its use in lipid disorders. Drugs 57:583, 1999.
53. LaRosa, JC: The role of diet and exercise in the statin era. Prog Cardiovasc Dis 41:137, 1998.
54. Leizorovicz, A: Long-term consequences of deep vein thrombosis. Haemostasis 28(Suppl 3):1, 1998.
55. Lensing, AW: Anticoagulation in acute ischaemic stroke: Deep vein thrombosis prevention and long-term stroke outcomes. Blood Coagul Fibrinolysis 10(Suppl 2):S123, 1999.
56. Lensing, AW, et al: Deep-vein thrombosis. Lancet 353:479, 1999.
57. Lieberman, JR: Warfarin prophylaxis after total knee arthroplasty. Am J Knee Surg 12:49, 1999.
58. Lopez, LM: Clinical trials in thrombolytic therapy, Part 2: The open-artery hypothesis and RAPID-1 and RAPID-2. Am J Health Syst Pharm 54(Suppl 1):S27, 1997.
59. Maggioni, AP, et al: The risk of stroke in patients with acute myocardial infarction after thrombolytic and antithrombotic treatment. N Engl J Med 327:1, 1992.
60. Majerus, PW, et al: Anticoagulant, thrombolytic, and antiplatelet drugs. In Hardman, JG, et al (eds): The Pharmacological Basis of Therapeutics, ed 9. McGraw-Hill, New York, 1996.
61. Malloy, MJ and Kane, JP: Agents used in hyperlipidemia. In Katzung, BG (ed): Basic and Clinical Pharmacology, ed 7. Appleton & Lange, Stamford, CT, 1998.
62. Manson, JE, et al: A prospective study of aspirin use and primary prevention of cardiovascular disease in women. JAMA 266:521, 1991.

63. Maron, DJ, Fazio, S, and Linton, MF: Current perspectives on statins. Circulation 101:207, 2000.
64. Mazur, W, Kaluza, G, and Kleiman, NS: Antiplatelet therapy for treatment of acute coronary syndromes. Cardiol Clin 17:345, 1999.
65. McNamara, TO: Role of thrombolysis in peripheral arterial occlusion. Am J Med 83(Suppl 2a):6, 1987.
66. Meister, W, et al: Low-dose acetylsalicylic acid (100 mg/day) after aortocoronary bypass surgery: A placebo-controlled trial. Br J Clin Pharmacol 17:703, 1984.
67. Merli, GJ: Deep vein thrombosis and pulmonary embolism prophylaxis in joint replacement surgery. Rheum Dis Clin North Am 25:639, 1999.
68. Miller, DB and Spence, JD: Clinical pharmacokinetics of fibric acid derivatives (fibrates). Clin Pharmacokinet 34:155, 1998.
69. Moghadasian, MH: Clinical pharmacology of 3-hydroxy-3-methylglutaryl coenzyme A reductase inhibitors. Life Sci 65:1329, 1999.
70. Murdock, DK, et al: Long-term safety and efficacy of combination gemfibrozil and HMG-CoA reductase inhibitors for the treatment of mixed lipid disorders. Am Heart J 138(Part 1):151, 1999.
71. Nee, PA: Thrombolysis after acute myocardial infarction. J Accid Emerg Med 14:2, 1997.
72. O'Connor, CM, et al: Stroke and acute myocardial infarction in the thrombolytic era: Clinical correlates and long-term prognosis. J Am Coll Cardiol 16:533, 1990.
73. Patel, SC and Mody, A: Cerebral hemorrhagic complications of thrombolytic therapy. Prog Cardiovasc Dis 42:217, 1999.
74. Patrono, C: Drug therapy: Aspirin as an antiplatelet drug. N Engl J Med 330:1287, 1994.
75. Pauciullo, P and Mancini, M: Treatment challenges in hypercholesterolemia. Cardiovasc Drugs Ther 12:325, 1998.
76. Pelletier, JR, Findlay, TW, and Gemma, SA: Isometric exercise for an individual with hemophiliac arthropathy. Phys Ther 67:1359, 1987.
77. Pindur, G and Morsdorf, S: The use of prothrombin complex concentrates in the treatment of hemorrhages induced by oral anticoagulation. Thromb Res 95(Suppl 1):S57, 1999.
78. Pineo, GF and Hull, RD: Thrombin inhibitors as anticoagulant agents. Curr Opin Hematol 6:298, 1999.
79. Planes, A, Vochelle, N, and Fafola, M: Venous thromboembolic prophylaxis in orthopedic surgery: Knee surgery. Semin Thromb Hemost 25(Suppl 3):73, 1999.
80. Rader, DJ and Haffner, SM: Role of fibrates in the management of hypertriglyceridemia. Am J Cardiol 83(Suppl 9B):30F, 1999.
81. Raible, MD: Hematologic complications of heparin-induced thrombocytopenia. Semin Thromb Hemost 25(Suppl 1):17, 1999.
82. Raskob, GE: Heparin and low molecular weight heparin for treatment of acute pulmonary embolism. Curr Opin Pulm Med 5:216, 1999.
83. Risius, B, et al: Recombinant human tissue-type plasminogen activator for thrombolysis in peripheral arteries and bypass grafts. Radiology 160:183, 1986.
84. Ross, SD, et al: Clinical outcomes in statin treatment trials: A meta-analysis. Arch Intern Med 159:1793, 1999.
85. Rydberg, EJ, Westfall, JM, and Nicholas, RA: Low-molecular-weight heparin in preventing and treating DVT. Am Fam Physician 59:1607, 1999.
86. Salame, M, et al: GPIIbIIIa inhibitors as adjunctive therapy in acute myocardial infarction. Int J Cardiol 69:231, 1999.
87. Sanson, BJ and Buller, H: Is there a role for thrombolytic therapy in venous thromboembolism? Haemostasis 29(Suppl S1):81, 1999.
88. Schafer, AI: Antiplatelet therapy with glycoprotein IIb/IIIa receptor inhibitors and other novel agents. Tex Heart Inst J 24:90, 1997.
89. Schror, K: Clinical pharmacology of the adenosine diphosphate (ADP) receptor antagonist, clopidogrel. Vasc Med 3:247, 1998.
90. Schwartz, RS, et al: Human recombinant DNA-derived antihemophiliac factor (factor VIII) in the treatment of hemophilia A. N Engl J Med 323:1800, 1990.
91. Scott, R: Lipid modifying agents: Mechanisms of action and reduction of cardiovascular disease. Clin Exp Pharmacol Physiol 24:A26, 1997.
92. Sikand, G, Kashyap, ML, and Yang, I: Medical nutrition therapy lowers serum cholesterol and saves medication costs in men with hypercholesterolemia. J Am Diet Assoc 98:889, 1998.
93. Simonneau, G: New perspectives for treatment of pulmonary embolism. Haemostasis 28(Suppl 3):95, 1998.
94. Smith, BJ: Thrombolysis in acute myocardial infarction: Analysis of studies comparing accelerated t-PA and streptokinase. J Accid Emerg Med 16:407, 1999.
95. Spencer, CM and Barradell, LB: Gemfibrozil. A reappraisal of its pharmacological properties and place in the management of dyslipidaemia. Drugs 51:982, 1996.
96. Spranger, M, Aspey, BS, and Harrison, MJG: Sex differences in antithrombotic effect of aspirin. Stroke 20:34, 1989.
97. Steering Committee of the Physicians' Health Study Research Group: Preliminary report: Findings from the aspirin component of the on-going physicians' health study. N Engl J Med 318:262, 1988.
98. Stein, EA, Lane, M, and Laskarzewski, P: Comparison of statins in hypertriglyceridemia. Am J Cardiol 81(Suppl 4A):66B, 1998.

99. Stringer, KA and Lopez, LM: Myocardial infarction. In DiPiro, JT, et al (eds): Pharmacotherapy: A Pathophysiologic Approach, ed 4. Appleton & Lange, Stamford, CT, 1999.

100. Talbert, RL: Hyperlipidemia. In DiPiro, JT, et al (eds): Pharmacotherapy: A Pathophysiologic Approach, ed 4. Appleton & Lange, Stamford, CT, 1999.

101. Ten Cate, JW: Evolution of therapies in deep vein thrombosis management. Blood Coagul Fibrinolysis 10(Suppl 2):S5, 1999.

102. Thizon-de-Gaulle, I: Antiplatelet drugs in secondary prevention after acute myocardial infarction. Rev Port Cardiol 17:993, 1998.

103. TIMI Study Group: The thrombolysis in myocardial infarction (TIMI) trial. N Engl J Med 312:932, 1985.

104. Tisdale, JE: Antiplatelet therapy in coronary artery disease: Review and update of efficacy studies. Am J Health Syst Pharm 55(Suppl 1):S8, 1998.

105. Tonkin, AM and Ryan, EW: Prevention of mortality from coronary heart disease with pravastatin. Biomed Pharmacother 53:405, 1999.

106. Topol, EJ, Byzova, TV, and Plow, EF: Platelet GPIIb-IIIa blockers. Lancet 353:227, 1999.

107. Vaughan, CJ, Gotto, AM, and Basson, CT: The evolving role of statins in the management of atherosclerosis. J Am Coll Cardiol 35:1, 2000.

108. Verhaeghe, R, Wilms, G, and Vermylen, J: Local low-dose thrombolysis in arterial disease of the limbs. Semin Thromb Hemost 13:206, 1987.

109. Verstraete, M, et al: Randomized trial of intravenous recombinant tissue-type plasminogen activator versus intravenous streptokinase in acute myocardial infarction. Lancet I:842, 1985.

110. Watts, GF and Dimmitt, SB: Fibrates, dyslipoproteinaemia and cardiovascular disease. Curr Opin Lipidol 10:561, 1999.

111. White, HD: Newer antiplatelet agents in acute coronary syndromes. Am Heart J 138(Part 2):S570, 1999.

112. White, HD: Direct thrombin inhibition and thrombolytic therapy: Rationale for the Hirulog and Early Reperfusion/Occlusion (HERO-2) trial. Am J Cardiol 82(Suppl 8B):57P, 1998.

113. Wilterdink, JL and Easton, JD: Dipyridamole plus aspirin in cerebrovascular disease. Arch Neurol 56:1087, 1999.

114. Witztum, JL: Drugs used in the treatment of hyperlipoproteinemias. In Hardman, JG, et al (eds): The Pharmacological Basis of Therapeutics, ed 9. McGraw-Hill, New York, 1996.

115. Wooster, MB and Luzier, AB: Reteplase: A new thrombolytic for the treatment of acute myocardial infarction. Ann Pharmacother 33:318, 1999.

Respiratory and Gastrointestinal Pharmacology

CHAPTER 26

Respiratory Drugs

The respiratory system is responsible for mediating gas exchange between the external environment and the bloodstream. The upper respiratory tract conducts air to the lower respiratory passages and ultimately to the lungs. The upper respiratory tract also humidifies and conditions inspired air and serves to protect the lungs from harmful substances. In the lungs, gas exchange takes place between the alveoli and the pulmonary circulation.

The drugs discussed in this chapter are directed primarily at maintaining proper airflow through the respiratory passages. Agents that treat specific problems in the lungs themselves are not discussed here but are covered in other areas of this text. For instance, drugs used to treat infectious diseases of the lower respiratory tract and lungs are presented in Section VIII (Chaps. 33 to 35).

The respiratory agents presented here are divided into two primary categories. The first group includes drugs that treat acute and relatively minor problems, such as nasal congestion, coughing, and seasonal **allergies.** The second category includes drugs that treat more chronic and serious airway obstructions, such as bronchial asthma, chronic bronchitis, and emphysema. Physical therapists and occupational therapists will frequently treat patients with both acute and chronic respiratory conditions. Consequently, the overview of the drugs presented in this chapter interest rehabilitation specialists.

DRUGS USED TO TREAT RESPIRATORY TRACT IRRITATION AND CONTROL RESPIRATORY SECRETIONS

The drugs presented here are used to treat symptomatic coughing and irritation resulting from problems such as the common cold, seasonal allergies, and upper respiratory tract infections. Many of these drugs are found in over-the-counter preparations. Often, several different agents are combined in the same commercial preparation; for example, a decongestant, an antitussive, and an expectorant may be combined and identified by a specific trade name. Also, agents within a specific category may have some properties that overlap into other drug categories. Certain antihistamines, for instance, may also have antitussive properties.

Antitussives

Antitussive drugs are used to suppress coughing that is associated with the common cold and other minor throat irritations. When used to treat cold and flu symptoms, these drugs are often combined with aspirin or acetaminophen, as well as with other respiratory tract agents.[1] Antitussives are usually recommended only for short-term use in relieving symptomatic coughing. The extensive use of antitussives in our society has been questioned. Coughing is a type of defense mechanism that can help expel mucus and foreign material from the upper respiratory tract.[48] By inhibiting this mechanism, antitussives may reduce the ability of coughing to raise secretions. Hence, antitussives may be helpful in treating an annoying dry cough, but use of these drugs to treat an active and productive cough may not be justified.[48,72]

Some of the commonly used antitussives are listed in Table 26–1. As shown in the table, codeine and similar opiate derivatives suppress the cough reflex by a central inhibitory effect.[87] Other nonopioid antitussives work by inhibiting the irritant effects of histamine on the respiratory mucosa or by a local anesthetic action on the respiratory epithelium. The primary adverse effect associated with most antitussives is sedation. Dizziness and gastrointestinal upset may also occur with antitussive use.

Decongestants

Congestion within and mucous discharge from the upper respiratory tract are familiar symptoms of many conditions. Allergies, the common cold, and various respiratory infections often produce a runny nose and a stuffy head sensation. Decongestants used to treat these symptoms are usually alpha-1–adrenergic agonists (see Chap. 20).[53,65] These agents bind to alpha-1 receptors located on the blood vessels of the nasal mucosa and stimulate vasoconstriction, thus effectively drying up the mucosal vasculature and decreasing local congestion in the nasal passages.[51]

Alpha-1 agonists used as decongestants are listed in Table 26–2. Depending on the preparation, these agents may be taken systemically or applied locally to the nasal mucosa via aerosol sprays. The primary adverse effects associated with decongestants are headache, dizziness, nervousness, nausea, and cardiovascular irregularities (increased blood pressure, palpitations). These adverse effects become more apparent at higher doses and during prolonged or excessive use of these drugs.[39,65]

TABLE 26–1 Common Antitussive Agents

Generic Name	Trade Name(s)*	Method of Action
Benzonatate	Tessalon	Local anesthetic effect on respiratory mucosa
Codeine	Many trade names	Inhibits cough reflex by direct effect on brainstem cough center
Dextromethorphan	Many trade names	Similar to codeine
Diphenhydramine	Benadryl (others)	Antihistamine
Hydrocodone	Detussin, Hycodan, Hycomine, many others	Similar to codeine
Hydromorphone	Dilaudid Cough	Similar to codeine

*Trade names often reflect combination of the antitussive with other agents (i.e., expectorants, decongestants).

TABLE 26–2 Common Nasal Decongestants

Generic Name	Trade Name(s)*	Dosage Forms
Ephedrine	Rynatuss, others	Oral
Oxymetazoline	Afrin, Neo-Synephrine 12 hour, others	Nasal spray
Phenylephrine	Neo-Synephrine, others	Nasal spray
Phenylpropanolamine	Propagest, Triaminic, others	Oral
Pseudoephedrine	Actifed, Sudafed, many others	Oral
Xylometazoline	Otrivin	Nasal spray

*Trade names often reflect combination of the decongestant with other ingredients.

Antihistamines

Antihistamines are used for reasons ranging from sedation to the treatment of parkinsonism. One of the most common applications of antihistamines, however, is the treatment of the respiratory allergic response to seasonal allergies (hay fever and so forth) and other allergens[45,116] (hence their inclusion in this chapter).

Histamine is an endogenous chemical that is involved in the normal regulation of certain physiologic functions (gastric secretion, CNS neural modulation), as well as various hypersensitivity (allergic) reactions.[4,107] Histamine exerts its effects on various cells through two primary receptor subtypes: the H_1 and H_2 receptors.[4] H_1 receptors are located on several tissues, including vascular, respiratory, and gastrointestinal smooth muscle. H_2 receptors are involved primarily in the regulation of gastric acid secretion. By definition, antihistamines are drugs that specifically block the H_1 subtype of histamine receptors. Drugs that selectively block the H_2 receptor (referred to simply as H_2 antagonists) may help control gastric secretion in conditions such as peptic ulcer; these drugs are discussed in Chapter 27. A third receptor subtype, the H_3 receptor, has also been identified, and this subtype may be involved in the local regulation of histamine release from CNS nerve terminals.[2] The clinical and pharmacologic significance of H_3 receptors remains to be fully determined, however.[4]

Antihistamines used in the symptomatic treatment of hay fever and similar allergies are listed in Table 26–3. By blocking the effects of histamine on the upper respiratory tissues, these drugs help decrease the nasal congestion, mucosal irritation and discharge (rhinitis, sinusitis), and conjunctivitis caused by inhaled allergens.[34,45] Similarly, antihistamines may decrease the coughing and sneezing associated with the common cold. In general, these drugs do not prevent the inflammation-induced bronchospasm associated with asthma (see "Treatment of Bronchial Asthma"). Antihistamines may, however, be used occasionally as an adjunct in patients with asthma to help control rhinitis and sinusitis.[93]

The primary adverse effects associated with antihistamines are sedation, fatigue, dizziness, blurred vision, and incoordination. Gastrointestinal distress (nausea, vomiting) is also quite common. Certain side effects, however, are related directly to each drug's ability to cross the blood-brain barrier (see Chap. 5 for a description of the blood-brain barrier). The original or "first-generation" antihistamines readily cross the blood-brain barrier and enter the brain, thus causing CNS-related side effects such as sedation and psychomotor slowing.[55,90] Newer "second-generation" antihistamines, however, do not easily cross the blood-brain barrier, and the risk of sedation and other CNS side effects is reduced substantially.[74,104] These newer agents, also known as nonsedating antihistamines, include astemizole (Hismanal), loratadine (Claritin), and terfenadine

TABLE 26–3 Antihistamines

Generic Name	Trade Name(s)*	Dosage†	Sedation Potential‡
Astemizole	Hismanal	10 mg once a day	Very low
Azatadine	Optimine	1–2 mg every 8–12 hr	Low
Brompheniramine	Bromphen, Dimetapp, others	4 mg every 4–6 hr	Low
Carbinoxamine	Cardec, Rondec, others	4–8 mg every 6–8 hr	Low to moderate
Cetirizine	Zyrtec	5–10 mg once a day	Very low
Chlorpheniramine	Chlor-Trimeton, Telachlor, others	4 mg every 4–6 hr	Low
Clemastine	Tavist	1.34 mg twice daily or 2.68 mg 1–3 times daily	Low
Cyproheptadine	Periactin	4 mg every 6–8 hr	Moderate
Dexchlorpheniramine	Polaramine	2 mg every 4–6 hr	Low
Dimenhydrinate	Dramamine, others	50–100 mg every 4 hr	High
Diphenhydramine	Benadryl, others	25–50 mg every 4–6 hr	High
Doxylamine	Unisom Nighttime Sleep-Aid	12.5–25 mg every 4–6 hr	High
Hydroxyzine	Atarax, Vistaril	25–100 mg 3–4 times a day	Moderate
Loratadine	Claritin	10 mg once a day	Very low
Phenindamine	Nolahist	25 mg every 4–6 hr	Low
Pyrilamine	Codimal, others	25–50 mg every 8 hr	Moderate
Terfenadine	Seldane	60 mg every 12 hr	Very low
Tripelennamine	PBZ	25–50 mg every 4–6 hr	Moderate
Triprolidine	Actifed, others	2.5 mg every 6–8 hr	Low

*Some trade names reflect the combination of the antihistamine with other agents (decongestants, antitussives, and so forth).

†Normal adult dosage when taken orally for antihistamine effects.

‡Sedation potential is based on comparison with other antihistamines and may vary considerably from person to person.

(Seldane) (see Table 26–3). These drugs, however, are not devoid of side effects. For example, certain nonsedating antihistamines such as astemizole and terfenadine may be cardiotoxic, and problems such as severe ventricular arrhythmias (torsades de pointes) have occurred when these drugs are taken in high doses or taken by individuals with pre-existing cardiac and liver problems.[27,101,116] Nonetheless, the newer nonsedating agents have become the agent of choice for many people because they decrease histamine-related symptoms without producing excessive sedation and other neuropsychiatric effects.

Mucolytics and Expectorants

Mucolytic drugs attempt to decrease the viscosity of respiratory secretions. **Expectorant** drugs facilitate the production and ejection of mucus. These drugs are used to prevent the accumulation of thick, viscous secretions that can clog respiratory passages and lead to pulmonary problems. Expectorants and mucolytics are used in acute disorders ranging from the common cold to pneumonia, as well as in chronic disorders such as emphysema and chronic bronchitis.[26] These drugs are often used in combination with other agents (e.g., antitussives, decongestants, bronchodilators). Although mucolytics and expectorants are widely used, there is some question about whether these drugs actually produce beneficial effects in various types of respiratory disease.[26] Some studies have documented that these drugs can improve the ability to expel mucus and increase pulmonary function, but the extent of these benefits may vary widely according to the specific patient and type of respiratory illness.[21,32,59,69]

The primary mucolytic drug currently in use is acetylcysteine (Mucomyst, Mucosil).[32,38] This drug is thought to work by splitting the disulfide bonds of respiratory mucoproteins, thus forming a less viscous secretion. There is, however, some evidence that this drug also has antioxidant effects, and some of acetylcysteine's benefits may be due to its ability to decrease free-radical damage in the respiratory tissues.[56,100] Acetylcysteine is usually administered directly to the respiratory mucosa by inhalation or by intratracheal instillation (through a tracheostomy). The primary adverse effects associated with this drug include nausea, vomiting, inflammation of the oral mucosa (stomatitis), and rhinorrhea. Serious adverse effects are relatively rare, however.

Several expectorant agents have been used in the past, but only guaifenesin is currently acknowledged by the FDA to have evidence of therapeutic effects.[61] This drug is administered to increase the production of respiratory secretions, thus encouraging ejection of phlegm and sputum. Exactly how guaifenesin exerts this effect, however, is not fully understood. Guaifenesin, which is usually administered orally in some form of syrup or elixir, is often combined with other agents in over-the-counter preparations, which are known by many different trade names. The primary adverse effect associated with guaifenesin is gastrointestinal upset, which is exacerbated if excessive doses are taken or if this drug is taken on an empty stomach.

DRUGS USED TO MAINTAIN AIRWAY PATENCY IN OBSTRUCTIVE PULMONARY DISEASE

Airway obstruction is a major problem in respiratory disorders such as bronchial asthma, chronic bronchitis, and emphysema. The latter two disorders are usually grouped under the heading of *chronic obstructive pulmonary disease* (COPD).[43] Asthma and COPD are characterized by bronchospasm, airway inflammation, and mucous plugging of the airways.[35,43] One of the primary goals of drug treatment is to prevent or reverse the bronchial constriction and subsequent obstruction of the airways in these disorders by using bronchodilators (beta-adrenergic agonists, xanthine derivatives, anticholinergics) and anti-inflammatory agents (glucocorticoids, others). These agents are discussed in the next section.

Beta-Adrenergic Agonists

RATIONALE FOR USE AND MECHANISM OF ACTION

Respiratory smooth-muscle cells contain the beta-2 subtype of adrenergic receptors.[80] (See Chapter 18 for a discussion of adrenergic receptor classifications.) Stimulation of these beta-2 receptors results in relaxation of bronchiole smooth muscle. Hence, drugs that stimulate these beta-2 adrenergic receptors (i.e., beta-adrenergic agonists) produce bronchodilation and can be used to prevent or inhibit airway obstruction in bronchospastic diseases.[35,89]

Beta-adrenergic agonists are believed to induce smooth-muscle relaxation by the mechanism illustrated in Figure 26–1. As shown in the figure, stimulation of the beta-2 receptor increases activity of the adenyl cyclase enzyme. This enzyme increases the production of intracellular cyclic adenosine monophosphate (cAMP). The cAMP acts as an

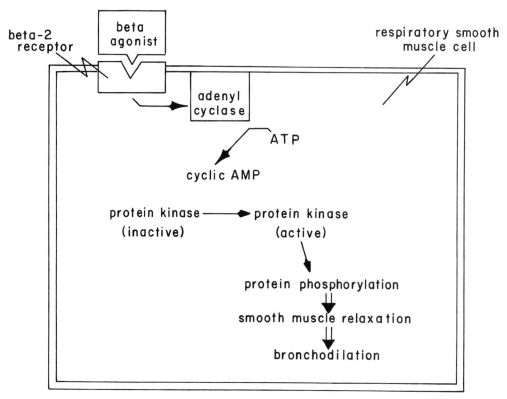

FIGURE 26–1. Mechanism of action of beta agonists on respiratory smooth muscle. Beta agonists facilitate bronchodilation by stimulating adenyl cyclase activity, which in turn increases intracellular cyclic AMP production. Cyclic AMP activates protein kinase, which appears to add an inhibitory phosphate group to contractile proteins, thus causing muscle relaxation and bronchodilation.

intracellular second messenger, which then increases the activity of other enzymes such as protein kinase. The increased protein kinase activity ultimately inhibits smooth-muscle contraction, probably by adding a phosphate group to specific contractile proteins.

SPECIFIC AGENTS AND METHOD OF ADMINISTRATION

Beta-adrenergic agonists that are used to induce bronchodilation are listed in Table 26–4. As shown in Table 26–4, some drugs are nonselective and stimulate alpha and beta receptors fairly equally. Other agonists are more selective and preferentially stimulate the beta-adrenergic receptors. Finally, the beta-2–specific agents are the most selective and tend to bind preferentially to beta-2 receptors. These beta-2–selective agonists offer an advantage when administered systemically because there is less chance of side effects caused by stimulation of other adrenergic receptors located on other tissues (e.g., beta-1 receptors on the myocardium).[54] When administered via inhalation, however, the issue of adrenergic receptor selectivity becomes less important because the drug is applied directly to the respiratory tissues that primarily contain the beta-2 subtype.[80] These agents also have different durations of action, with some of the newer drugs (formoterol, salmeterol) considered to be long-acting beta-adrenergic agonists.[13,54,77] These long-acting agents may provide more stable and sustained bronchodilation in conditions such as asthma.[8,77]

TABLE 26–4 Beta-Adrenergic Bronchodilators

Drug	Primary Receptor	Route of Administration	Onset of Action (min)	Time to Peak Effect (hr)	Duration of Action (hr)
Albuterol	Beta-2	Inhalation	5–15	1–1.5	3–6
		Oral	15–30	2–3	8 or more
Bitolterol	Beta-2	Inhalation	3–4	0.5–1	5–8
Epinephrine	Alpha, beta-1, 2	Inhalation	3–5	—	1–3
		Intramuscular	Variable	—	<1–4
		Subcutaneous	6–15	0.3	<1–4
Fenoterol	Beta-2	Inhalation	5	0.5–1	2–3
		Oral	30–60	2–3	6–8
Isoetharine	Beta-2	Inhalation	1–6	0.25–1	1–4
Isoproterenol	Beta-1, 2	Inhalation	2–5	—	0.5–2
		Intravenous	Immediate	—	<1
		Sublingual	15–30	—	1–2
Metaproterenol	Beta-2	Inhalation (aerosol)	Within 1	1	1–5
		Oral	Within 15–30	Within 1	Up to 4
Pirbuterol	Beta-2	Inhalation	Within 5	0.5–1	5
Procaterol	Beta-2	Inhalation	Within 5	1.5	6–8
Salmeterol	Beta-2	Inhalation	10–20	3–4	12
Terbutaline	Beta-2	Inhalation	15–30	1–2	3–6
		Oral	Within 60–120	Within 2–3	4–8
		Parenteral	Within 15	Within 0.5–1	1.5–4

Beta-adrenergic drugs can be administered orally, subcutaneously, or by inhalation. Inhalation of these drugs is often the preferred method of administration in treating respiratory disorders. Inhalation allows the drug to be delivered directly to the respiratory tissues, with a minimum of systemic side effects because of absorption into the systemic circulation. The onset of action is also more rapid with inhalation. Oral or subcutaneous administration is usually associated with more side effects. Beta agonists, however, may reach the more distal branches of the airway to a greater extent when administered orally or subcutaneously rather than by inhalation. The bronchioles are usually constricted during an asthmatic attack, and the drug may simply not reach the distal respiratory passages when administered by inhalation.

When given by inhalation, several beta agonists are available in metered-dose inhalers (MDIs). MDIs contain the drug in a small aerosol canister, and a specific amount of the drug is dispensed each time the patient depresses the canister.[57] Although MDIs are convenient because of their small size and portability, there is a certain amount of coordination required on the part of the patient to ensure adequate delivery of the drug. Some patients (e.g., young children) may have trouble timing the inhaled dose with a proper inspiratory effort. In these patients, drug delivery can be facilitated by using a spacer or reservoir-like attachment that sequesters the drug between the MDI and the patient's mouth.[57] The patient can first dispense the drug into the reservoir and then take a deep breath, thus improving delivery to the respiratory tissues. The other primary method of inhaling beta agonists is through a *nebulizer*. These devices are not portable and must be used in the home. They are much easier to use, however, and administer the drug over a more prolonged period of time (10 minutes), which allows better delivery to the more distal bronchioles.

ADVERSE SIDE EFFECTS

With prolonged or excessive use, inhaled adrenergic agonists may actually *increase* bronchial responses to allergens and other irritants.[19,89] Hence, the regular and repeated use of adrenergic agonists has been questioned somewhat in recent years (see "Treatment of Bronchial Asthma"). Other side effects depend on the relative selectivity and route of administration of specific agents. Adrenergic agonists that also stimulate beta-1 receptors may cause cardiac irregularities if they reach the myocardium through the systemic circulation. Similarly, stimulation of CNS adrenergic receptors may produce symptoms of nervousness, restlessness, and tremor. Severe adverse effects are relatively infrequent, however, when beta-adrenergic agonists are used as directed and administered locally via inhalation.

Xanthine Derivatives

RATIONALE FOR USE AND MECHANISM OF ACTION

The xanthine derivatives are a group of chemically similar compounds that exert a variety of pharmacologic effects. Common xanthine derivatives include theophylline, caffeine, and theobromine (Fig. 26–2), and these compounds are frequently found in various foods and beverages (tea, coffee, soft drinks). In addition, theophylline and several theophylline derivatives are administered therapeutically to produce bronchodilation in asthma and other forms of reversible airway obstruction (bronchitis, emphysema).[83,96,103] Theophylline and caffeine are also potent CNS stimulants, and some of the more common side effects of these drugs are related to this CNS excitation (see the next "Adverse Side Effects" later in this chapter).

Although the ability of xanthine derivatives to produce bronchodilation has been recognized for some time, the exact mechanism of action of theophylline and similar agents has been the subject of much debate. These drugs may enhance bronchodilation by inhibiting the phosphodiesterase (PDE) enzyme located in bronchial smooth-muscle cells.[96,108] PDE breaks down cAMP. Inhibiting this enzyme results in higher intracellular cAMP concentrations. As discussed previously in this section (see "Beta-Adrenergic Agonists"), cAMP is the second messenger that brings about respiratory smooth-muscle relaxation and subsequent bronchodilation. By inhibiting PDE, theophylline can prolong the effects of this second messenger and increase bronchodilation. More important, PDE inhibition may decrease the function of inflammatory cells and inhibit the production of inflammatory mediators, thus accounting for theophylline's anti-inflammatory properties.[23,96] There is, in fact, considerable evidence that much of theophylline's beneficial effects are related to this drug's anti-inflammatory properties rather than to a direct bronchodilating effect.[85,86] The importance of controlling airway inflammation is addressed in more detail later in this chapter.

Theophylline may also act as an adenosine antagonist.[23,108] Adenosine is thought to bind to specific receptors on the smooth-muscle cells and to stimulate contraction. By blocking this effect, theophylline would facilitate smooth-muscle relaxation. Theophylline may likewise help produce bronchodilation by other mechanisms, such as inhibition of intracellular calcium release and stimulation of catecholamine release.[23,108] In reality, theophylline and similar drugs may induce bronchodilation and help protect the airways through a combination of several mechanisms, but the relative importance of each cellular effect remains to be determined.

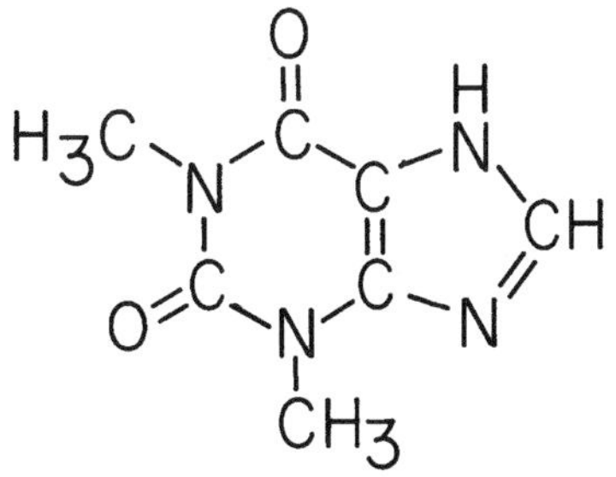

theophylline

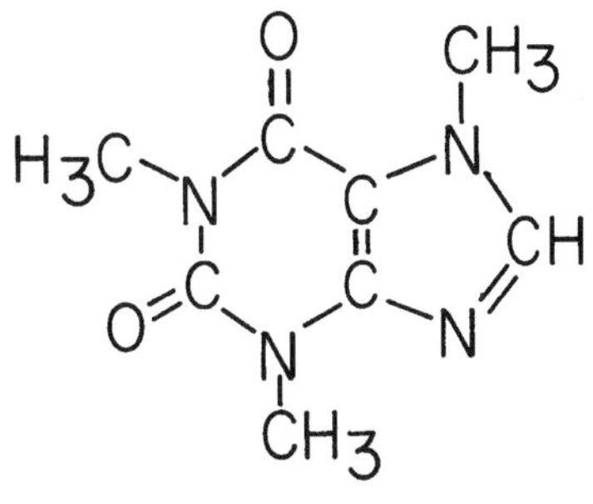

caffeine

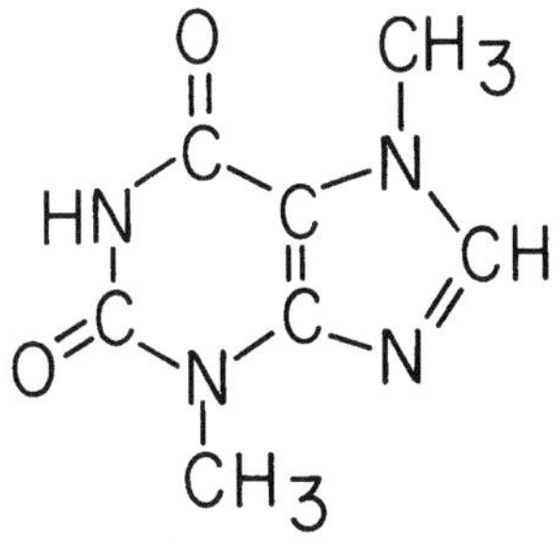

theobromine

FIGURE 26–2. Common xanthine derivatives. Theophylline is often administered therapeutically to reduce bronchoconstriction.

SPECIFIC AGENTS AND METHOD OF ADMINISTRATION

Xanthine derivatives used in the treatment of bronchospastic disease are listed in Table 26–5. In general, these drugs are administered orally, although certain drugs may be given rectally or by injection if the oral route is not tolerated. When the oral route is used, sustained-release preparations of theophylline are available (see Table 26–5). These preparations enable the patient to take the drug just once or twice each day, thus often improving patient compliance.

TABLE 26–5 Xanthine Derivative Bronchodilators

Drug	Common Trade Names	Dosage Forms
Aminophylline	Phyllocontin	Oral, extended-release oral, rectal, injection
Dyphylline	Dilor, Lufyllin	Oral, injection
Oxtriphylline	Choledyl	Oral, extended-release oral
Theophylline	Aerolate, Lanophyllin, Theo-Dur, many others	Oral, extended-release oral, injection

ADVERSE SIDE EFFECTS

The most serious limitation in the use of xanthine bronchodilators is the possibility of toxicity.[83] Toxicity may appear when plasma levels are between 15 and 20 μg/mL. Because the recommended levels are between 10 and 20 μg/mL, signs of toxicity may occur in some patients even when blood levels are in the therapeutic range. Early signs of toxicity include nausea, confusion, irritability, and restlessness. When blood levels exceed 20 μg/mL, serious toxic effects such as cardiac arrhythmias and seizures may occur. In some patients, the serious toxic effects may be the first indication that there is a problem, because these serious effects are not always preceded by the more innocuous signs of toxicity. Theophylline-induced seizures are a life-threatening phenomenon, with fatalities reported in 50 percent of the patients exhibiting such seizures.[22]

Consequently, during long-term use, care should be taken to avoid a toxic accumulation of theophylline. Patients in whom the metabolism of this drug is altered are especially prone to toxicity. In particular, factors such as liver disease, heart failure, alcohol consumption, cigarette smoking, concomitant use of other drugs (e.g., cimetidine), and patient age (older than 55) have all been identified as possible predisposing factors in theophylline toxicity.[22,52,78] To prevent toxicity, the dosage should be individualized for each patient, and the lowest possible dose should be used (see "Treatment of Bronchial Asthma").

Anticholinergic Drugs

RATIONALE FOR USE AND MECHANISM OF ACTION

The lungs receive extensive parasympathetic innervation via the vagus nerve.[9,57] The efferent fibers of the vagus nerve release acetylcholine onto respiratory smooth-muscle cells, which contain muscarinic cholinergic receptors. When stimulated, these receptors mediate bronchoconstriction. Consequently, drugs that block muscarinic cholinergic receptors prevent acetylcholine-induced bronchoconstriction, thus improving airflow in asthma and COPD. Anticholinergics are usually not the first choice as bronchodilators in obstructive pulmonary disease, but these drugs may be useful in certain patients with COPD or in patients who are unable to tolerate other bronchodilator drugs.[28,35,41]

SPECIFIC AGENTS AND ROUTE OF ADMINISTRATION

The anticholinergic bronchodilators include atropine and similar muscarinic receptor blockers. Although atropine is the prototypical muscarinic antagonist, its use in respiratory conditions is somewhat limited because it must be administered through a nebulizer. Atropine is also absorbed easily into the systemic circulation and tends to cause side effects fairly frequently. A newer drug, ipratropium (Atrovent), appears to be more advantageous for several reasons.[40,41,114] Ipratropium can be administered by an aerosol inhaler, and it is poorly absorbed into the systemic circulation. Thus, inhaled ipratropium is associated with substantially fewer systemic side effects. This drug is often equal to, or slightly more potent than, beta-2 agonists in producing bronchodilation in patients with COPD, but ipratropium is somewhat less effective than other bronchodilators in patients with asthma.[41] Ipratropium, however, can be combined with beta-agonist therapy to provide optimal treatment of acute asthma attacks.[88,99]

ADVERSE SIDE EFFECTS

Systemic side effects associated with atropine include dry mouth, constipation, urinary retention, tachycardia, blurred vision, and confusion. As stated previously, these effects appear to occur much less often with inhaled anticholinergics like ipratropium, which are not absorbed as readily into the systemic circulation.

Glucocorticoids

RATIONALE FOR USE AND MECHANISM OF ACTION

Inflammation appears to be a key underlying factor in the exaggerated responsiveness of the respiratory passages in asthma and other obstructive pulmonary disorders.[5,15] Because of their powerful anti-inflammatory effects, glucocorticoids are used to control inflammation-mediated bronchospasm and are undoubtedly the most effective agents for controlling asthma.[6,58,106]

Glucocorticoids (known also as corticosteroids) inhibit the inflammatory response in several important ways.[106] These drugs directly affect the genes and transcription factors that produce inflammatory components.[106] As a result, these drugs inhibit the production of proinflammatory products (cytokines, prostaglandins, leukotrienes, and so forth) while increasing the production of anti-inflammatory proteins. Glucocorticoids also reverse increases in vascular permeability and inhibit the migration of neutrophils and monocytes that typically occurs during the inflammatory response. The mechanism of action of glucocorticoids and cellular responses mediated by the glucocorticoids is discussed in more detail in Chapter 29.

SPECIFIC AGENTS AND ROUTES OF ADMINISTRATION

Glucocorticoids used to treat asthma are listed in Table 26–6. During severe, acute episodes of bronchoconstriction (e.g., *status asthmaticus*), glucocorticoids are usually administered intravenously. For more prolonged use, glucocorticoids are given orally or by inhalation. As with the beta agonists, the inhaled route is preferable because of the decreased chance of systemic side effects.[18,68] Glucocorticoids that are currently available via inhalation include beclomethasone, budesonide, flunisolide, and triamcinolone (see Table 26–6). Inhalation of a glucocorticoid allows the drug to be applied directly to the respiratory mucosa, and any glucocorticoid that does happen to be absorbed into the systemic circulation is rapidly metabolized. When these drugs are administered appropriately by the inhalation route, the chance of severe adverse effects is greatly reduced, compared with the possible effects associated with systemic administration (see the next section).[18,68] Patients should rinse their mouth cavities with water after using oral glucocorticoid inhalers, however, to prevent local irritation of the oral mucosa.

TABLE 26–6 Corticosteroids Used in Obstructive Pulmonary Disease

Generic Name	Trade Name(s)	Dosage Forms*
Beclomethasone	Beclovent, Vanceril	Inhalation
Betamethasone	Celestone	Oral; intravenous or intramuscular injection
Budesonide	Pulmicort	Inhalation
Cortisone	Cortone	Oral; intramuscular injection
Dexamethasone	Decadron	Oral; intravenous or intramuscular injection
Flunisolide	Aerobid	Inhalation
Hydrocortisone	Cortef	Oral; intravenous or intramuscular injection
Methylprednisolone	Medrol	Oral; intravenous injection
Prednisolone	Hydeltrasol	Oral
Prednisone	Deltasone, others	Oral
Triamcinolone	Azmacort	Inhalation; oral; intramuscular injection

*Dosage forms that use the inhalation route are often preferred in asthma and other obstructive pulmonary diseases. Systemic administration by the oral route or by injection is typically reserved for acute or severe bronchoconstrictive disease (see text for details).

ADVERSE SIDE EFFECTS

The major limitation of the glucocorticoids in any disease is the risk of serious adverse effects. Because of the general catabolic effect of these drugs on supporting tissues, problems with osteoporosis, skin breakdown, and muscle wasting can occur during prolonged systemic administration.[33,42,115] Other possible systemic effects include retardation of growth in children, cataracts, glaucoma, hyperglycemia, aggravation of diabetes mellitus, and hypertension.[16] Prolonged or excessive use can also have a negative feedback effect on the adrenal gland, resulting in loss of adrenal function (adrenal suppression) while these drugs are being administered.[30,42]

Fortunately, the risk of these adverse effects is minimal when these drugs are administered by inhalation. Inhalation provides a more direct and topical application of the glucocorticoid to the respiratory tissues, with fairly limited absorption of the drug into the systemic circulation. The risk of adverse effects is also minimized when the total dose of the glucocorticoid is kept below certain levels.[49,50,67] Consequently, prolonged systemic administration of these drugs should be avoided, and glucocorticoids should be administered by inhalation, using the lowest effective dose. It is also prudent to periodically examine patients for bone mineral loss and other side effects when these drugs are used for prolonged periods.[82,95] Nonetheless, these drugs are extremely effective in treating various types of bronchoconstriction, and they should be used judiciously whenever possible.[94,115]

Cromones

RATIONALE FOR USE AND MECHANISM OF ACTION

Cromones such as cromolyn sodium and nedocromil sodium can help prevent bronchospasm in people with asthma. These drugs are not bronchodilators and will not reverse bronchoconstriction during an asthmatic attack. Hence, these agents must be taken prior to the onset of bronchoconstriction, and they must typically be administered prophylactically to prevent asthma attacks that are initiated by specific, well-defined activities (e.g., exercise, exposure to a friend's pet, pollen).[57] Likewise, the regular use of these drugs several times each day for several months may decrease airway hyperresponsiveness so that the incidence of asthmatic attacks is decreased.[79]

Although the exact mechanism of cromolyn and nedocromil is not known, these drugs are believed to prevent bronchoconstriction by inhibiting the release of inflammatory mediators such as histamine and leukotrienes from pulmonary mast cells.[57] Both agents can be administered by MDI, and cromolyn can also be administered through a nebulizer. In addition, cromolyn is available in a nonprescription nasal spray (Nasalcrom) that can be helpful in preventing allergic rhinitis associated with seasonal allergies such as hay fever.

ADVERSE SIDE EFFECTS

Some irritation of the nasal and upper respiratory passages may occur following inhalation, but these drugs are remarkably free of severe adverse reactions. Hence, cromolyn and nedocromil are often used preferentially to treat mild persistent asthma, especially in children or in individuals who are unable to tolerate the side effects of other antiasthma drugs.[57,109]

Leukotriene Inhibitors

RATIONALE FOR USE AND MECHANISM OF ACTION

Leukotrienes are inflammatory compounds that are especially important in mediating the airway inflammation that underlies bronchoconstrictive disease.[29,64,112] As indicated in Chapter 15, leukotrienes are 20-carbon fatty acids (eicosanoids) that are similar in structure and function to prostaglandins. Leukotrienes are actually derived from the same precursor as prostaglandins (arachidonic acid), but leukotrienes are synthesized by the lipoxygenase enzyme rather than by the cyclooxygenase enzyme (see Fig. 15–2). Recently, strategies have been developed to selectively decrease the effects or synthesis of leukotrienes. For example, zileuton (Zyflo) inhibits the lipoxygenase enzyme, thereby reducing the production of leukotrienes.[112] Other drugs such as montelukast (Singulair) and zafirlukast (Accolate) block the receptor for leukotrienes on respiratory tissues.[112] These drugs therefore offer a fairly selective method for controlling a specific aspect of inflammation in bronchoconstrictive disease.[113] Preliminary evidence suggests that these drugs can be combined with other drugs (glucocorticoids, beta agonists) to provide optimal management in specific patients with asthma and COPD.[31,112]

ADVERSE SIDE EFFECTS

Leukotriene inhibitors are safer than other anti-inflammatory agents such as the glucocorticoids. Some hepatic impairment has been reported with these drugs, but cases of severe toxicity are relatively rare.

TREATMENT OF BRONCHIAL ASTHMA

Pathophysiology of Bronchial Asthma

Asthma is a disease of the respiratory system characterized by bronchial smooth-muscle spasm, airway inflammation, and mucous plugging of the airways.[70,98] Patients with asthma have an exaggerated bronchoconstrictor response of the airways to various stimuli.[14,57] In some patients, the stimuli that trigger an asthmatic attack are well defined (e.g., allergens like dust, pollen, chemicals, or certain drugs). Other factors such as exercise, cold, psychologic stress, and viral infections may trigger an asthmatic attack in some individuals. In other patients, the initiating factor may be unknown.

Although the exact cause of asthma remains to be determined, the basis for the increased airway reactivity in asthma has been elucidated somewhat. Airway inflammation is the critical factor in initiating the exaggerated bronchial reactions associated with this disease.[15,66,102] In asthmatic airways, there seems to be a complex interaction between several different cells including macrophages, neutrophils, eosinophils, platelets, and the airway epithelial cells themselves.[12,14,62] These cells release proinflammatory chemical mediators such as prostaglandins, leukotrienes, bradykinin, histamine, and platelet activating factor.[14,57] These chemicals irritate the respiratory epithelium, as well as stimulate contraction of bronchiole smooth muscle. Thus, the localized inflammation appears to sensitize airway structures to asthmatic triggers, and the bronchoconstriction and other features of asthma seem to be related directly to the inflammatory response underlying this disease.

Long-Term Management of Asthma

The primary focus of treating asthma has undergone a shift within the past few years. In the past, treatment consisted primarily of bronchodilators such as the beta-adrenergic agonists and the xanthine derivatives, with systemic anti-inflammatory steroids (glucocorticoids) added only in more advanced and severe cases. The use of glucocorticoids has increased, however, and these drugs are now used as first-line agents in most patients, including cases of newly detected, mild asthma.[5,20,92,102,111] The increased use of glucocorticoids is largely due to the fact that certain types of glucocorticoids can now be administered by inhalation. As indicated previously, inhaled glucocorticoids are not absorbed readily into the systemic circulation, and the risk of serious systemic side effects is therefore substantially reduced. Another reason for the shift toward increased glucocorticoid use is the recognition that these drugs directly reduce the inflammation that underlies asthmatic disease, whereas bronchodilators merely treat the secondary manifestations of this disease.[58,75] Put more simply, glucocorticoids directly affect the underlying disease process by decreasing the inflammation that causes airway hyperresponsiveness.

Glucocorticoids have therefore assumed the leading role in treating asthma. Beta-2 agonists are still used extensively, however, and these drugs remain the primary method of *symptomatically* treating asthma attacks. Many patients, for example, inhale beta-2 agonists through MDIs as "rescue" therapy at the onset of a bronchospastic attack, and this technique is a mainstay in managing acute episodes of asthma.[89] Nonetheless, the use of beta-2 agonists as long-term maintenance therapy for asthma has been questioned. Prolonged and excessive use of beta-2 agonists may actually *increase* airway hyperresponsiveness, thus increasing the risk of bronchoconstrictive attacks.[19,83,97]

The current philosophy is that beta-2 agonists still serve an important role in the treatment of periodic or acute bronchospasm[57]; that is, the intermittent use of a short-acting form of a beta-2 agonist can help decrease the severity of an acute asthma attack. The role of beta-2 agonists in the long-term treatment of asthma is less obvious. These drugs are clearly not the primary form of treatment, but long-acting beta-2 agonists such as salmeterol and formoterol can be combined with glucocorticoids to provide optimal results in certain patients.[8,84,89] Long-acting beta-2 agonists are therefore considered a supplement to glucocorticoid therapy, and addition of these beta agonists should be considered if glucocorticoid treatment alone is not successful in the long-term management of asthma.[8,77,89] Combining a long-acting beta-2 drug with a glucocorticoid can also reduce the dosage of the glucocorticoid, thus reducing the risk of side effects associated with high doses of glucocorticoids.[81]

The role of theophylline in treating asthma has also been re-examined. Once considered the foundation for drug therapy, theophylline has assumed a secondary role to glucocorticoids. Theophylline is a powerful bronchodilator, but problems with toxicity often limited its use in the long-term management of asthma.[83] Currently, low doses of theophylline are sometimes added to the drug regimen of patients who are resistant to treatment using glucocorticoids and beta agonists.[103,108] The combination of theophylline with a glucocorticoid may likewise provide optimal effects at lower doses of glucocorticoid.[73] As indicated earlier, it is also recognized that theophylline may have anti-inflammatory effects, and some of the renewed interest in using low-dose theophylline therapy is based on this drug's ability to control airway inflammation rather than actually produce bronchodilation.[86] Hence, theophylline remains an important adjunct in treating certain patients with asthma, and this drug may be used more extensively as more is learned about the synergistic effects of theophylline and glucocorticoids.

Inhaled glucocorticoids are therefore the cornerstone of drug therapy for patients with asthma. Beta agonists, theophylline, and other agents (cromolyn, nedocromil, ipratropium) can be used to supplement glucocorticoids as needed, with the specific drug regimen determined on a patient-by-patient basis. The drug regimen must be reviewed constantly and adjusted in response to the patient's needs and the clinical course of the asthmatic disease.

Along with drug therapy, several nonpharmacologic interventions should be employed. Efforts should be made to determine the initiating factors of an asthmatic attack, and patients should be taught how to avoid these factors whenever possible. Also, considerable evidence exists that aerobic conditioning may help decrease the incidence of asthmatic attacks and the concomitant need for antiasthmatic drugs in certain patients.[44] Of course, exercise itself may be an asthmatic trigger in some individuals.[76] However, certain forms of aerobic exercise such as swimming may be an excellent way to improve the cardiorespiratory status of patients with asthma without causing excessive risk of bronchospastic attacks in these individuals.[36]

TREATMENT OF REVERSIBLE BRONCHOSPASM IN COPD

As indicated previously, bronchospasm is often present in COPD—that is, in chronic bronchitis and emphysema.[63,71] *Chronic bronchitis* is a clinical diagnosis applied to a long-standing inflammation of the bronchial tree. *Emphysema* is a pathologic condition marked by destruction of alveolar walls and enlargement of the terminal air spaces.

Drug therapy for COPD is directed primarily toward maintaining airway patency and preventing airflow restriction.[35,71] Thus, bronchodilators such as inhaled beta-2 agonists or anticholinergics (ipratropium) are typically the first drugs used, followed by oral theophylline.[35,37,71,85] Glucocorticoids have also been used to treat airway inflammation in COPD, but their use in these situations remains controversial. In contrast to their beneficial effects in asthma, glucocorticoids have not always produced clear therapeutic benefits in patients in the long-term treatment of COPD.[10,110] Hence, these drugs are not typically prescribed on a routine basis but are usually reserved for the more severe cases or acute exacerbations of COPD-related bronchospasm.[35,47]

TREATMENT OF RESPIRATORY PROBLEMS IN CYSTIC FIBROSIS

Cystic fibrosis is one of the most common hereditary diseases in white populations. This autosomal-recessive trait is found in approximately 1 of every 2000 live white births.[11] Cystic fibrosis essentially affects all the major exocrine glands, resulting in very thick, viscous secretions. These thickened secretions often form mucous plugs, which obstruct major ducts in various glands and organs.[11,110] For instance, the pancreatic and bile ducts are often obstructed, resulting in problems with nutrient digestion and absorption. Mucous plugging of the bronchioles occurs quite frequently, leading to pulmonary problems such as pneumonia, bronchiectasis, pulmonary fibrosis, and various pulmonary infections (especially *Staphylococcus*). These respiratory problems are usually the primary health threat to individuals with cystic fibrosis.[11,110]

Pharmacologic management of respiratory problems in cystic fibrosis is focused on maintaining airway patency as much as possible. Bronchodilators and mucolytic and/or expectorant drugs may help limit the formation of mucous plugs. Systemic glucocorticoids (e.g., prednisone) may also be beneficial in some patients in limiting airway inflammation and improving pulmonary function.[3] The side effects and risks of systemic glucocorticoids, however, may outweigh any benefits, especially in children.[11] Respiratory infections are treated with appropriate antibiotic agents.[11,110] In addition to drug therapy, daily maintenance of respiratory hygiene (postural drainage, breathing exercises, etc.) is essential in sustaining pulmonary function.[25] Even with optimal medical care, however, the prognosis for this disease remains poor. Individuals with cystic fibrosis often succumb to respiratory-related problems within their second or third decade of life.

Although there is still no cure for cystic fibrosis, several pharmacologic techniques have been developed recently that may help decrease the viscosity of respiratory secretions in patients with this disease. One technique uses aerosol preparations that contain enzymes known as *deoxyribonucleases*. These enzymes can be inhaled to break down the large quantities of DNA that are present in respiratory secretions of patients with cystic fibrosis.[7,46] Respiratory secretions in these patients often contain large amounts of DNA because the genetic material contained in airway inflammatory cells is deposited into the airway lumen when these cells are destroyed. DNA increases the viscosity and thickness of the respiratory secretions, and preparations that contain recombinant human deoxyribonuclease (rhDNAse) can lyse this DNA, thus decreasing the viscosity of these secretions and reducing the chance of lung collapse (atelectasis) and infection.[7,91] The response of individual patients to this treatment may vary, however, and it is not clear if deoxyribonuclease therapy provides substantial long-term benefits in people with cystic fibrosis.[24,91] Further research is needed to clarify the clinical outcomes associated with deoxyribonuclease therapy and determine if these drugs are cost effective in treating cystic fibrosis.[17]

Several other new therapies are being evaluated for treating cystic fibrosis. For example, nucleotide compounds such as adenosine triphosphate and uridine triphosphate can be administered by inhalation to stimulate chloride secretion from airway epithelial cells.[60] The increased chloride secretion creates an osmotic force that draws water into the airway, thus hydrating respiratory secretions and decreasing the viscosity of these secretions. Efforts are also being made to correct the defective gene that causes cystic fibrosis. This so-called gene therapy may someday provide an effective long-term treatment by replacing the defective gene with a functionally correct gene.[11] These strategies and other new techniques are still experimental at the present time, but there is hope that these interventions may someday provide a means to alleviate the primary respiratory complications that often lead to illness and death in patients with cystic fibrosis.

SPECIAL CONCERNS IN REHABILITATION PATIENTS

Proper respiratory hygiene is crucial in preventing the serious adverse effects of respiratory infection and obstructive pulmonary disease. The accumulation of bronchial secretions can lead to decreased gas exchange, atelectasis, and additional infection. Rehabilitation specialists often play a critical role in preventing pulmonary mucus accumulation.[105] Therapists can facilitate the pharmacotherapeutic effects of mucolytic and expectorant drugs by performing postural drainage and breathing exercises. Even if patients are not being treated directly with chest physical therapy and respiratory hygiene, rehabilitation specialists should always encourage patients to cough and raise secretions for expectoration. Physical therapists and occupational therapists should also coordinate their treatments with respiratory therapy. Often, mucolytic and expectorant drugs are administered by the respiratory therapist through a nebulizer or positive-pressure ventilator. A program of chest physical therapy may be most effective when administered 30 minutes to 1 hour after these agents are administered (i.e, after these drugs have had some time to exert an effect on respiratory secretions).

Therapists should be aware of which patients are prone to bronchospastic attacks. If patients use some sort of portable aerosol bronchodilator, they should be encouraged to bring their medication to therapy. Rehabilitation procedures that involve exercise may trigger a bronchospastic attack in some individuals, so the medication should be close at hand.

Therapists should also be aware of the potential side effects of bronchodilator drugs. In particular, the cardiac side effects of the beta-adrenergic agonists and xanthine derivatives (theophylline, others) should be considered. Therapists may notice cardiac arrhythmias while monitoring the ECG or taking the patient's pulse, and these cardiac abnormalities may indicate a problem with bronchodilator medications. Noncardiac symptoms such as nervousness, confusion, and tremors may also indicate bronchodilator toxicity and should be brought to the physician's attention. Early recognition of toxicity may be lifesaving, especially when xanthine derivatives such as theophylline are used. Finally, patients receiving systemic glucocorticoid treatment may be prone to the well-known catabolic effects of these drugs. Therapists should be especially alert for skin breakdown, and care should be taken not to overstress bones and musculotendinous structures that may be weakened by the prolonged use of glucocorticoids.

CASE STUDY

RESPIRATORY DRUGS

Brief History. V.C., a 63-year-old man, has a long history of COPD and hypertension. Twelve years ago, he was diagnosed with emphysema. During the past 5 years, his symptoms of shortness of breath, wheezing, and bronchospasm have become progressively worse. He is also a chronic cigarette smoker and has had a cough for many years, which produces large amounts of sputum daily. Although his physician advised him repeatedly to quit smoking, the patient was unable to kick the habit. To control his bronchospasm, the patient self-administers a beta-2 agonist (albuterol) via an MDI. He is also taking a diuretic and beta-1 blocker to control his hypertension. Two days ago, he was admitted to the hospital with weakness and incoordination in his left arm and leg. Subsequent medical tests indicated that he had suffered a cerebral vascular accident. Physical therapy was ordered to begin at the patient's bedside to facilitate optimal recovery from the stroke. The physical therapist began treating the patient with passive and active exercises to encourage motor return. The patient was also being seen by a respiratory therapist. The respiratory therapy treatments included administration of the mucolytic drug acetylcysteine via a nebulizer three times daily. The patient continued to self-administer the beta-2 agonist at the onset of bronchospasms.

Problem/Influence of Medication. Despite the program of respiratory therapy, bronchial secretions began to accumulate in the patient's airways. The patient had also been instructed in deep-breathing and coughing exercises, and he was told by the respiratory therapist to perform these exercises periodically throughout the day. However, no postural drainage was being performed to encourage ejection of sputum.

Decision/Solution. In addition to the neuromuscular facilitation activities, the physical therapist initiated a program of chest physical therapy including postural drainage and deep-breathing exercises. The physical therapist coordinated these activities with the respiratory therapist so that the patient first received a treatment of the mucolytic agent. Also, the physical therapist had the patient self-administer a dose of the inhaled beta-2 bronchodilator approximately 1 hour prior to the chest therapy session, thus allowing the bronchodilator to produce maximal airway dilation and permit optimal clearance of bronchial secretions.

SUMMARY

The drugs discussed in this chapter are used to control irritation and maintain airflow through the respiratory passages. Drugs such as the antitussives, decongestants, antihistamines, mucolytics, and expectorants are used primarily for the temporary relief of cold, flu, and seasonal allergy symptoms. These agents are frequently found in over-the-counter preparations, and several different agents are often combined in the same commercial product. Airway obstruction in chronic disorders such as bronchial asthma, chronic bronchitis, and emphysema is treated primarily with bronchodilator agents (beta-adrenergic agonists, xanthine derivatives, anticholinergics) and anti-inflammatory drugs (glucocorticoids, cromones, leukotriene inhibitors). Rehabilitation specialists should also be cognizant of which patients suffer from bronchospastic disorders (e.g., asthma) and of what medications are being used to control airway obstruction in each patient. Therapists can help facilitate the pharmacotherapeutic goals in patients with obstructive pulmonary disease by encouraging proper respiratory hygiene and breathing exercises and by helping improve overall cardiorespiratory endurance whenever possible.

REFERENCES

1. Agrawal M: OTC cold, cough, and allergy products: More choice or more confusion? J Hosp Mark 13:79, 1999.
2. Arrang, J-M, et al: Highly potent and selective ligands for histamine H_3-receptors. Nature 327:117, 1987.
3. Auerbach, HS, et al: Alternate-day prednisone reduces morbidity and improves pulmonary function in cystic fibrosis. Lancet 2:686, 1985.

4. Babe, KS and Serafin, WE: Histamine, bradykinin, and their antagonists. In Hardman, JG, et al (eds): The Pharmacological Basis of Therapeutics, ed 9. McGraw-Hill, New York, 1996.
5. Barnes, PJ: Current issues for establishing inhaled corticosteroids as the antiinflammatory agents of choice in asthma. J Allergy Clin Immunol 101(Part 2):S427, 1998.
6. Barnes, PJ: Efficacy of inhaled corticosteroids in asthma. J Allergy Clin Immunol 102(Part 1):531, 1998.
7. Bates, RD and Nahata, MC: Aerosolized dornase alpha (rhDNAase) in cystic fibrosis. J Clin Pharm Ther 20:313, 1995.
8. Bjermer, L and Larsson, L: Long-acting beta(2)-agonists: How are they used in an optimal way? Respir Med 91:587, 1997.
9. Bleecker, ER: Cholinergic and neurogenic mechanisms in obstructive airway disease. Am J Med 81(Suppl 5a):93, 1986.
10. Borron, W and deBoisblanc, BP: Steroid therapy for chronic obstructive pulmonary disease. Curr Opin Pulm Med 4:61, 1998.
11. Bosso, JA: Cystic fibrosis. In DiPiro, JT, et al (eds): Pharmacotherapy: A Pathophysiologic Approach, ed 4. Appleton & Lange, Stamford, CT, 1999.
12. Boushey, HA: Effects of inhaled corticosteroids on the consequences of asthma. J Allergy Clin Immunol 102(Part 2):S5, 1998.
13. Buchwald, A and Hochhaus, G: Pharmacokinetic and pharmacodynamic aspects of salmeterol therapy. Int J Clin Pharmacol Ther 36:652, 1998.
14. Busse, WW: Inflammation in asthma: The cornerstone of the disease and the target of therapy. J Allergy Clin Immunol 102(Part 2):S17, 1998.
15. Busse, WW, Calhun, CF, and Segwick, JD: Mechanism of airway inflammation in asthma. Am Rev Resp Dis 147(Suppl 6):S20, 1993.
16. Cave, A, Arlett, P, and Lee, E: Inhaled and nasal corticosteroids: Factors affecting the risks of systemic adverse effects. Pharmacol Ther 83:153, 1999.
17. Christopher, F, et al: rhDNAase therapy for the treatment of cystic fibrosis patients with mild to moderate lung disease. J Clin Pharm Ther 24:415, 1999.
18. Chrousos, GP and Harris, AG: Hypothalamic-pituitary-adrenal axis suppression and inhaled corticosteroid therapy. 2. Review of the literature. Neuroimmunomodulation 5:288, 1998.
19. Cockcroft, DW: Inhaled beta2-agonists and airway responses to allergen. J Allergy Clin Immunol 102:S96, 1998.
20. Connolly, CK, Alcock, SM, and Prescott, RJ: Management and control of asthma as assessed by actual/best function and corticosteroid used 1980–1993/4. Eur Respir J 12:859, 1998.
21. Connolly, MA: Mucolytics and the critically ill patient: Help or hindrance? AACN Clin Issues 6:307, 1995.
22. Covelli, HD, Knodel, AR, and Heppner, BT: Predisposing factors to apparent theophylline-induced seizures. Ann Allergy 54:411, 1985.
23. Coward, WR, Sagara, H, and Church, MK: Asthma, adenosine, mast cells, and theophylline. Clin Exp Allergy 28(Suppl 3):42, 1998.
24. Davies, J, et al: Retrospective review of the effects of rhDNAase in children with cystic fibrosis. Pediatr Pulmonol 23:243, 1997.
25. DeCesare, JA and Graybill, CA: Physical therapy for the child with respiratory dysfunction. In Irwin, S and Tecklin, JS (eds): Cardiopulmonary Physical Therapy, ed 2. CV Mosby, St Louis, 1990.
26. Del Donno, M and Olivieri, D: Mucoactive drugs in the management of chronic obstructive pulmonary disease. Monaldi Arch Chest Dis 53:714, 1998.
27. Delpon, E, Valenzuela, C, and Tamargo, J: Blockade of cardiac potassium and other channels by antihistamines. Drug Saf 21(Suppl 1):11, 1999.
28. Demirkan, K, et al: Can we justify ipratropium therapy as initial management of acute exacerbations of COPD? Pharmacotherapy 19:838, 1999.
29. Diamant, Z, Bel, EH, and Dekhuijzen, PN: Anti-leukotriene therapy in asthma. Neth J Med 53:176, 1998.
30. Dluhy, RG: Clinical relevance of inhaled corticosteroids and HPA axis suppression. J Allergy Clin Immunol 101(Part 2):S447, 1998.
31. Drazen, J: Clinical pharmacology of leukotriene receptor antagonists and 5-lipoxygenase inhibitors. Am J Respir Crit Care Med 157(Part 2):S233, 1998.
32. Duijvestijn, YC and Brand, PL: Systematic review of N-acetylcysteine in cystic fibrosis. Acta Paediatr 88:38, 1999.
33. Efthimiou, J and Barnes, PJ: Effect of inhaled corticosteroids on bones and growth. Eur Respir J 11:1167, 1998.
34. Ferguson, BJ: Cost-effective pharmacotherapy for allergic rhinitis. Otolaryngol Clin North Am 31:91, 1998.
35. Ferguson, GT and Cherniak, RM: Current concepts: Management of COPD. N Engl J Med 328:1017, 1993.
36. Fitch, KD, Morton, AR, and Blanksby, BA: Effect of swimming training on children with asthma. Arch Dis Child 51:190, 1976.
37. Fragoso, CAV and Miller, MA: Review of the clinical efficacy of theophylline in the treatment of chronic obstructive pulmonary disease. Am Rev Resp Dis 147(Suppl 6):S40, 1993.
38. Gallon, AM: Evaluation of nebulised acetylcysteine and normal saline in the treatment of sputum retention following thoracotomy. Thorax 51:429, 1996.
39. Graf, P, et al: Effects of sustained-release oral phenylpropanolamine on the nasal mucosa of healthy subjects. Acta Otolaryngol 119:837, 1999.

40. Gross, NJ: Ipratropium bromide. N Engl J Med 319:486, 1988.

41. Gross, NJ and Skorodin, MS: Anticholinergic, antimuscarinic bronchodilators. Am Rev Respir Dis 129:856, 1984.

42. Grossman, A: Steroid safety: The endocrinologist's view. Int J Clin Pract Suppl 96:33, 1998.

43. Hansen, M: Pathophysiology: Foundations of Disease and Clinical Intervention. WB Saunders, Philadelphia, 1998.

44. Henriksen, JM and Nielsen, TT: Effect of physical training on exercise-induced bronchoconstriction. Acta Paediatr Scand 72:31, 1983.

45. Howarth, PH: Assessment of antihistamine efficacy and potency. Clin Exp Allergy 29(Suppl 3):87, 1999.

46. Hubbard, RC, et al: A preliminary study of aerosolized recombinant human deoxyribonuclease I in the treatment of cystic fibrosis. N Engl J Med 326:812, 1992.

47. Ikeda, A, Nishimura, K, and Izumi, T: Pharmacological treatment in acute exacerbations of chronic obstructive pulmonary disease. Drugs Aging 12:129, 1998.

48. Irwin, RS, et al: Managing cough as a defense mechanism and as a symptom. A consensus panel report of the American College of Chest Physicians. Chest 114(Suppl):133S, 1998.

49. Jackson, LD, et al: Comparative efficacy and safety of inhaled corticosteroids in asthma. Can J Clin Pharmacol 6:26, 1999.

50. Jarvis, B and Faulds, D: Inhaled fluticasone propionate: A review of its therapeutic efficacy at dosages < or = 500 microg/day in adults and adolescents with mild to moderate asthma. Drugs 57:769, 1999.

51. Jawad, SS and Eccles, R: Effect of pseudoephedrine on nasal airflow in patients with nasal congestion associated with common cold. Rhinology 36:73, 1998.

52. Jenne, JW: Effect of disease states on theophylline elimination. J Allergy Clin Immunol 78:727, 1986.

53. Johannssen, V, et al: Alpha 1-receptors at pre-capillary resistance vessels of the human nasal mucosa. Rhinology 35:161, 1997.

54. Johnson, M: Pharmacology of long-acting beta-agonists. Ann Allergy Asthma Immunol 75:177, 1995.

55. Kay, GG and Harris, AG: Loratadine: A non-sedating antihistamine. Review of its effects on cognition, psychomotor performance, mood, and sedation. Clin Exp Allergy 29(Suppl 3):147, 1999.

56. Kelly, GS: Clinical applications of N-acetylcysteine. Altern Med Rev 3:114, 1998.

57. Kelly, HW and Kamada, AK: Asthma. In DiPiro, JT, et al (eds): Pharmacotherapy: A Pathophysiologic Approach, ed 4. Appleton & Lange, Stamford, CT, 1999.

58. Kemp, JP: Approaches to asthma management: Realities and recommendations. Arch Intern Med 153:805, 1993.

59. King, M and Rubin, BK: Mucus-controlling agents: Past and present. Respir Care Clin N Am 5:575, 1999.

60. Knowles, MR, Clarke, LL, and Boucher, RC: Activation of extracellular nucleotides of chloride secretion in the airway epithelia of patients with cystic fibrosis. N Engl J Med 325:533, 1991.

61. Koda-Kimple, MA: Therapeutic and toxic potential of over-the-counter agents. In Katzung, BG (ed): Basic and Clinical Pharmacology, ed 7. Appleton & Lange, Stamford, CT, 1998.

62. Kon, OM and Kay, AB: T cells and chronic asthma. Int Arch Allergy Immunol 118:133, 1999.

63. Konzem, SL and Stratton, MA: Chronic obstructive lung disease. In DiPiro, JT, et al (eds): Pharmacotherapy: A Pathophysiologic Approach, ed 4. Appleton & Lange, Stamford, CT, 1999.

64. Kraft, M: Corticosteroids and leukotrienes: Chronobiology and chronotherapy. Chronobiol Int 16:683, 1999.

65. Krause, HF: Antihistamines and decongestants. Otolaryngol Head Neck Surg 107:835, 1992.

66. Lazarus, SC: Inflammation, inflammatory mediators, and mediator antagonists in asthma. J Clin Pharmacol 38:577, 1998.

67. Ledford, D, et al: Osteoporosis in the corticosteroid-treated patient with asthma. J Allergy Clin Immunol 102:353, 1998.

68. Lipworth, BJ: Systemic adverse effects of inhaled corticosteroid therapy: A systematic review and meta-analysis. Arch Intern Med 159:941, 1999.

69. Livingstone, CR, et al: Model systems for the evaluation of mucolytic drugs: Acetylcysteine and S-carboxymethylcysteine. J Pharm Pharmacol 42:73, 1990.

70. Lowhagen, O: Asthma and asthma-like disorders. Respir Med 93:851, 1999.

71. Lu, CC: Bronchodilator therapy for chronic obstructive pulmonary disease. Respirology 2:317, 1997.

72. MacRedmond, R and O'Connell, F: Treatment of persistent dry cough: If possible, treat the cause; if not, treat the cough. Monaldi Arch Chest Dis 54:269, 1999.

73. Markham, A and Faulds, D: Theophylline. A review of its potential steroid sparing effects in asthma. Drugs 56:1081, 1998.

74. Mattila, MJ and Paakkari, I: Variations among non-sedating antihistamines: Are there real differences? Eur J Clin Pharmacol 55:85, 1999.

75. McDonald, C and Lipp, J: Pharmacological management of asthma. Aust Fam Physician 27:64, 1998.

76. McFadden, ER and Gilbert, IA: Current concepts: Exercise-induced asthma. N Engl J Med 330:1362, 1994.

77. Moore, RH, Khan, A, and Dickey, BF: Long-acting inhaled beta2-agonists in asthma therapy. Chest 113:1095, 1998.

78. Muhlberg, W, et al: Pharmacokinetics and pharmacodynamics of theophylline in geriatric patients with multiple diseases. Klin Wochenschr 65:551, 1987.

79. Murphy, S and Kelly, HW: Cromolyn sodium: A review of mechanisms and clinical use in asthma. Drug Intell Clin Pharm 21:22, 1987.
80. Nadel, JA and Barnes, PJ: Autonomic regulation of the airways. Annu Rev Med 35:451, 1984.
81. Nielsen, LP, et al: Salmeterol reduces the need for inhaled corticosteroid in steroid-dependent asthmatics. Respir Med 93:863, 1999.
82. Niewoehner, CB and Niewoehner, DE: Steroid-induced osteoporosis. Are your asthmatic patients at risk? Postgrad Med 105:79, 1999.
83. Page, CP: Recent advances in our understanding of the use of theophylline in the treatment of asthma. J Clin Pharmacol 39:237, 1999.
84. Pearlman, DS, et al: Inhaled salmeterol and fluticasone: A study comparing monotherapy and combination therapy in asthma. Ann Allergy Asthma Immunol 82:257, 1999.
85. Peleman, RA, Kips, JC, and Pauwels, RA: Therapeutic activities of theophylline in chronic obstructive pulmonary disease. Clin Exp Allergy 28(Suppl 3):53, 1998.
86. Rabe, KF and Dent, G: Theophylline and airway inflammation. Clin Exp Allergy 28(Suppl 3):35, 1998.
87. Reisine, T and Pasternak, G: Opioid analgesics and antagonists. In Hardman, JG, et al (eds): The Pharmacological Basis of Therapeutics, ed 9. McGraw-Hill, New York, 1996.
88. Rodrigo, G, Rodrigo, C, and Burschtin, O: A meta-analysis of the effects of ipratropium bromide in adults with acute asthma. Am J Med 107:363, 1999.
89. Sears, MR: Asthma treatment: Inhaled beta-agonists. Can Respir J 5(Suppl A):54A, 1998.
90. Settipane, RA: Complications of allergic rhinitis. Allergy Asthma Proc 20:209, 1999.
91. Shah, PL and Hodson, ME: The overuse or underuse of dornase alpha. Curr Opin Pulm Med 3:410, 1997.
92. Simon, RA: Update on inhaled corticosteroids: Safety, compliance, and new delivery systems. Allergy Asthma Proc 20:161, 1999.
93. Simons, FE: Is antihistamine (H1-receptor antagonist) therapy useful in clinical asthma? Clin Exp Allergy 29(Suppl 3):98, 1999.
94. Simons, FE: Benefits and risks of inhaled glucocorticoids in children with persistent asthma. J Allergy Clin Immunol 102:S77, 1998.
95. Sorkness, CA: Establishing a therapeutic index for the inhaled corticosteroids: Part II. Comparisons of systemic activity and safety among different inhaled corticosteroids. J Allergy Clin Immunol 102(Part 2):S52, 1998.
96. Spina, D, Landells, LJ, and Page, CP: The role of theophylline and phosphodiesterase 4 isoenzyme inhibitors as anti-inflammatory drugs. Clin Exp Allergy 28(Suppl 3):24, 1998.
97. Spitzer, WO, et al: The use of beta-agonists and the risk of death and near death from asthma. N Engl J Med 326:501, 1992.
98. Stoloff, SW: Pharmacologic therapy for asthma. Clin Cornerstone 1:17, 1998.
99. Stoodley, RG, Aaron, SD, and Dales, RE: The role of ipratropium bromide in the emergency management of acute asthma exacerbation: A metaanalysis of randomized clinical trials. Ann Emerg Med 34:8, 1999.
100. Strapkova, A, Nosal'ova, G, and Franova, S: Mucolytics and antioxidant activity. Life Sci 65:1923, 1999.
101. Taglialatela, M, et al: Cardiac ion channels and antihistamines: Possible mechanisms of cardiotoxicity. Clin Exp Allergy 29(Suppl 3):182, 1999.
102. Tavakkoli, A and Rees, PJ: Drug treatment of asthma in the 1990s: Achievements and new strategies. Drugs 57:1, 1999.
103. Thomson, NC: Asthma therapy: Theophylline. Can Respir J 5(Suppl A):60A, 1998.
104. Timmerman, H: Why are non-sedating antihistamines non-sedating? Clin Exp Allergy 29(Suppl 3):13, 1999.
105. Van der Schans, CP, et al: Physiotherapy and bronchial mucus transport. Eur Respir J 13:1477, 1999.
106. Van der Velden, VH: Glucocorticoids: Mechanisms of action and anti-inflammatory potential in asthma. Mediators Inflamm 7:229, 1998.
107. Van Dyke, K and Head, RJ: Histamine and histamine antagonists. In Craig, CR and Stitzel, RE (eds): Modern Pharmacology with Clinical Applications, ed 5. Little, Brown, Boston, 1997.
108. Vassallo, R and Lipsky, JJ: Theophylline: Recent advances in the understanding of its mode of action and uses in clinical practice. Mayo Clin Proc 73:346, 1998.
109. Volcheck, GW and O'Connell, EJ: Anti-inflammatory drugs for controlling asthma. Postgrad Med 104:127, 1998.
110. Weinberger, SE: Medical progress: Recent advances in pulmonary medicine. N Engl J Med 328:1389, 1993.
111. Weltman, JK: The use of inhaled corticosteroids in asthma. Allergy Asthma Proc 20:255, 1999.
112. Wenzel, SE: Leukotriene receptor antagonists and related compounds. Can Respir J 6:189, 1999.
113. Wenzel, SE: New approaches to anti-inflammatory therapy for asthma. Am J Med 104:287, 1998.
114. Witek, TJ: Anticholinergic bronchodilators. Respir Care Clin N Am 5:521, 1999.
115. Woodcock, A: Effects of inhaled corticosteroids on bone density and metabolism. J Allergy Clin Immunol 101(Part 2):S456, 1998.
116. Yap, YG and Camm, AJ: Arrhythmogenic mechanisms of non-sedating antihistamines. Clin Exp Allergy 29(Suppl 3):174, 1999.

CHAPTER 27

Gastrointestinal Drugs

This chapter discusses drugs that are used to treat specific problems in the gastrointestinal (GI) system. The GI tract is responsible for the digestion of food and the absorption of nutrients and water. Dietary constituents normally undergo a series of digestive processes as they progress through the GI system. Under normal conditions, the transit time of food and water is adequate to allow the processes of digestion and absorption to take place. Indigestible and nonabsorbable products are eliminated by defecation.

The primary disorders that occur in the GI tract are related to damage from gastric acid secretion and abnormal movement of food through the GI tract. Problems may develop if digestive secretions in the stomach begin to damage the upper GI mucosa and cause a peptic ulcer. Certain drugs attempt to prevent or heal peptic ulcers by controlling gastric acid secretion and protecting the mucosal lining. Problems with gastrointestinal motility may also respond to pharmacologic management. Excessive motility (*diarrhea*) and inadequate bowel evacuation (*constipation*) are treated with various agents that normalize peristalsis and facilitate normal bowel movements. Drugs are also available to treat other problems with digestion and vomiting (*emesis*). The GI system is also susceptible to various infectious and parasitic invasions. The drugs used to treat these disorders are presented in Chapters 33 through 35, which deal with the chemotherapy of infectious diseases.

Rehabilitation specialists will often treat patients taking some form of GI agent. These medications are commonly used by the general public, as well as by hospitalized individuals and outpatients receiving physical therapy and occupational therapy. Although the direct impact of most GI drugs on physical rehabilitation is relatively small, an understanding of how these drugs are used will help therapists recognize their role in the patient's pharmacotherapeutic regimen.

DRUGS USED TO CONTROL GASTRIC ACIDITY AND SECRETION

The acidic nature of the gastric juices is essential for activating digestive protease activity and controlling intestinal bacteria. The gastric acids, however, can cause severe ulceration and hemorrhage of the stomach lining if excessive amounts of acid are produced or if the normal protection of the stomach mucosa is disturbed by irritants, drugs, or bacterial infection.[16,51] Consequently, several different types of drugs are available that attempt to control or prevent the detrimental effects of gastric acid. These agents are used to treat *peptic ulcers*—that is, ulcerations of the mucosal lining of the esophagus, stomach, and duodenum.[12,51] These drugs may also be helpful in treating general problems related to indigestion and epigastric pain (dyspepsia) and to the heartburn sensations caused by leakage of gastric acid into the distal esophagus, called *gastroesophageal reflux*.[31] Agents used to control gastric acidity and secretion are presented here.

Antacids

RATIONALE FOR USE AND MECHANISM OF ACTION

Antacids attempt to chemically neutralize stomach acids. These drugs typically contain a base such as carbonate or hydroxide combined with aluminum, magnesium, or calcium.[1,33] In the stomach, the base combines with excess hydrogen ions (H^+) to increase intragastric pH. The basic strategy of this chemical neutralization is illustrated in Figure 27–1.

Antacids are frequently used to treat the episodic minor gastric discomfort (indigestion, heartburn) that often accompanies overeating or indulging in certain incompatible foods. One concern regarding antacids is that they may be abused in this respect. The public has come to regard antacids as a panacea for poor eating habits. Antacids can also be used in the more serious and chronic conditions of peptic ulcer and chronic gastroesophageal reflux, but large amounts of antacids must be used for prolonged periods.[5] Hence, the use of antacids in these more serious conditions has been replaced to a large extent by other drugs such as H_2 receptor blockers and proton pump inhibitors (see later).[18,33] Consequently, antacids are used primarily to treat fairly minor and transient dyspepsia that occurs from eating spicy foods, overeating, and so forth.[33]

Basic Strategy:

antacid + hydrochloric acid ---> salt + water

Examples:

aluminum hydroxide
$$Al(OH)_3 + 3\ HCl \longrightarrow AlCl_3 + 3\ H_2O$$

magnesium hydroxide
$$Mg(OH)_2 + 2\ HCl \longrightarrow MgCl_2 + 2\ H_2O$$

calcium carbonate
$$CaCO_3 + 2\ HCl \longrightarrow CaCl_2 + H_2O + CO_2$$

sodium bicarbonate
$$NaHCO_3 + HCl \longrightarrow NaCl + H_2O + CO_2$$

FIGURE 27–1. Neutralization of hydrochloric acid (HCl) by the primary forms of antacids. In each reaction, the antacid combines with HCl to form a salt and water. Carbon dioxide (CO_2) is also produced by calcium carbonate and sodium bicarbonate antacids.

SPECIFIC AGENTS

Antacids are identified by many trade names and frequently appear in over-the-counter products. There is such a plethora of antacids on the market that even a partial listing of commercial preparations is difficult. The primary antacids are classified as aluminum-containing, magnesium-containing, calcium carbonate–containing, sodium bicarbonate–containing, or virtually any combination of these classifications. These drugs are typically taken orally, either as tablets or as a liquid oral suspension.

ADVERSE SIDE EFFECTS

Constipation is the most common side effect associated with the aluminum-containing antacids, whereas diarrhea often occurs with magnesium-containing preparations. A common problem with all antacids is the acid-rebound phenomenon.[24] Antacids increase the pH of the gastric fluids, which serves as the normal stimulus for increased acid secretion. This situation does not present a problem while the antacid is in the stomach, because most of the excess acid will be neutralized. Gastric secretion may remain elevated, however, even after the antacid effects diminish and stomach pH returns to normal levels. The unopposed rebound of acid secretion may then cause increased gastric distress. Finally, excessive use of antacids can alter the absorption of electrolytes (especially phosphate) and other drugs from the GI tract, and antacids can cause changes in urinary pH that affect drug elimination. Electrolyte imbalances and altered pharmacokinetics can therefore occur if antacids are used in high doses for prolonged periods.[33]

H_2 Receptor Blockers

RATIONALE FOR USE AND MECHANISM OF ACTION

The regulation of gastric acid secretion involves the complex interaction of many endogenous chemicals, including histamine.[3,10] Histamine stimulates specific receptors on stomach parietal cells to increase gastric acid secretion. These histamine receptors are classified as H_2 receptors to differentiate them from the H_1 receptors located on vascular, respiratory, and gastrointestinal smooth muscle.[10] Drugs have been developed that selectively bind to H_2 receptors without activating the receptor. These H_2 antagonists or blockers prevent the histamine-activated release of gastric acid under basal conditions and during stimulation by food and other factors.[10]

The H_2 blockers are therefore used for both acute and long-term management of peptic ulcer and other problems such as dyspepsia and gastroesophageal reflux disease.[6,18] These drugs also have a remarkably good safety profile, and many of the H_2 blockers that were introduced originally as prescription agents are now available as over-the-counter preparations.

SPECIFIC AGENTS

The primary H_2 blockers used to control gastric secretions are listed in Table 27–1. Cimetidine was the first H_2 blocker to be widely used as an antiulcer agent. Newer drugs such as famotidine, nizatidine, and ranitidine appear to be at least as effective as cimetidine, but they are more potent and may be better tolerated than cimetidine in some patients.[22,42] Likewise, some of the newer agents—famotidine and nizatidine in particular—appear to have a lower potential for interacting with other drugs, hence their preferential use in patients taking several different types of medications.[19]

TABLE 27–1 H_2 Receptor Blockers

Generic Name	Trade Name	Adult Oral Dosage*
Cimetidine	Tagamet	300 mg 4 times each day with meals and at bedtime, 400 or 600 mg in the morning and at bedtime, or 800 mg at bedtime
Famotidine	Pepcid	40 mg once daily at bedtime or 20 mg BID
Nizatidine	Axid	300 mg once daily at bedtime or 150 mg BID
Ranitidine	Zantac	150 mg twice daily or 300 mg at bedtime

*Represents typical dose for treatment of gastric or duodenal ulcers. Doses for treating gastroesophageal reflux disease (heartburn) may be somewhat lower.

ADVERSE SIDE EFFECTS

These drugs are generally well tolerated in most patients, and serious adverse effects are rare during short-term or periodic use. Problems that may occur include headache and dizziness. Mild, transient GI problems (nausea, diarrhea, constipation) may also occur with the H_2 blockers, and arthralgia and myalgia have been reported with cimetidine use. Tolerance may also occur during long-term use, and acid rebound can occur when these drugs are discontinued after prolonged use.[18,46]

Proton Pump Inhibitors

RATIONALE FOR USE AND MECHANISM OF ACTION

These drugs inhibit the H^+, K^+ -ATPase enzyme that is ultimately responsible for secreting acid from gastric parietal cells into the lumen of the stomach.[41,45] This enzyme is also known as the "proton pump"; hence these drugs are often referred to as proton pump inhibitors (PPIs). PPIs are extremely effective at inhibiting the proton pump, and therapeutic doses can virtually eliminate gastric acid secretion.[1,41] There is some evidence that PPIs also have antibacterial effects against *Helicobacter pylori* infection and that these drugs may have some anti-inflammatory properties that help decrease gastric irritation.[13] Evidence suggests that PPIs are more effective in controlling acid secretion and that they promote healing of ulcers better than H_2 blockers and antacids.[25,41] These agents have therefore gained acceptance in treating gastric problems, and PPIs are often the drug of choice in the long-term treatment of patients with gastric and duodenal ulcers and gastroesophageal reflux disease.[61]

SPECIFIC AGENTS

Omeprazole (Prilosec) was the original PPI, and this drug is now joined by lansoprazole (Prevacid) and pantoprazole (Pantoloc). These drugs are all fairly similar, with selection of a specific agent based on the cost, availability, and potential for drug interactions of each agent for each patient.[61]

ADVERSE SIDE EFFECTS

These drugs are usually tolerated very well. As with antacids and H_2 blockers, increased secretion of gastric acid (acid rebound) can occur when PPIs are discontinued after prolonged use.[58] Nonetheless, PPIs are relatively safe, and these drugs do not usually produce any major adverse effects during the long-term treatment of peptic ulcer and gastrointestinal reflux disease.[21,40]

Treatment of *H. Pylori* Infection in Gastric Ulcer Disease

Helicobacter pylori (*H. pylori*) is a gram-negative bacterium that is often present in the upper GI tract in people with gastric ulcer disease.[63] It has therefore been suggested that this bacterium may cause or potentiate gastroduodenal ulcers and that treatment of *H. pylori* infection is essential in the treatment of these ulcers.[20,30] Use of antibiotics has indeed resulted in an increased healing rate and decreased recurrence of gastric ulcers in many people who test positive for *H. pylori* infection.[26,57] The fact that *H. pylori* is present in certain patients should not eliminate the possibility that other factors (stress, diet, and so forth) may also be contributing to gastric ulcer disease.[28,54] There are likewise people who are infected with *H. pylori* who do *not* develop gastric ulcers.[6] Hence, the exact role of this bacterium as a causative factor in gastric ulcers remains uncertain. Nonetheless, *H. pylori* may contribute to the development of gastric ulcers in susceptible individuals, and antibacterial drugs should be considered in patients with ulcers who are infected with this bacterium.

Treatment of *H. pylori* infection typically consists of combination therapy, using several drugs simultaneously.[9] For example, one common form of "triple therapy" consists of two antibacterials (amoxicillin and clarithromycin) and one of the PPIs described earlier in this chapter.[20,37,41] Alternatively, bismuth compound (described later in the section on "Treatment of Diarrhea") could be combined with a PPI, tetracycline, and metronidazole.[15,20,55] These drug regimens are typically administered for 1 to 2 weeks, after which time the antibacterial drugs are discontinued. Some patients, however, may need to remain on maintenance doses of the PPI or other antiulcer drugs to facilitate ulcer healing and prevent recurrence.[52,56]

Consequently, treatment of *H. pylori* infection may improve the prognosis of people with gastric ulcers and other forms of upper GI distress (dyspepsia, gastroesophageal reflux disease). Patients with clinical signs of ulcers who also test positive for this infection should receive a treatment regimen that attempts to eradicate the infection. Successful treatment of *H. pylori* infection may reduce or eliminate the need for subsequent antiulcer medications in patients with gastric ulcer disease.[17]

Other Agents Used to Control and Treat Gastric Ulcers

Several other agents besides the antacids, H_2 blockers, and PPIs have proved successful in preventing or treating problems associated with gastric acidity and mucosal breakdown. Some of the more frequently used agents are discussed here.

Anticholinergics. The role of muscarinic cholinergic antagonists in treating peptic ulcers was discussed in Chapter 19. Cholinergic stimulation of the gut via vagal efferent fibers produces a general increase in GI motility and secretion. Drugs that block the effects of acetylcholine on stomach parietal cells will decrease the release of gastric acid. Atropine and similar anticholinergics are only occasionally used to control gastric acid secretion because most cholinergic muscarinic inhibitors cause many side effects, such as dry mouth, constipation, urinary retention, and confusion.[10] One notable exception is the antimuscarinic drug pirenzepine (Gastrozepin). Pirenzepine, which is fairly selective for muscarinic receptors located on the stomach mucosa, effectively decreases gastric secretion at a dose that does not cause excessive side effects.[10] Hence, this drug may be a viable alternative to the other agents currently available to treat excessive gastric secretions.

Metoclopramide (Octamide, Reglan, others). This drug is officially classified as a dopamine receptor antagonist but also appears to enhance the peripheral effects of acetylcholine. Primarily because of this latter effect, metoclopramide stimulates motility in the upper GI tract, which may be useful in moving the stomach contents toward the small intestine, thus decreasing the risk of gastric acid moving backward into the esophagus. This drug may therefore be helpful in treating gastroesophageal reflux disease.[39] The primary side effects associated with metoclopramide are related to its antagonistic effects on CNS dopamine receptors. Restlessness, drowsiness, and fatigue are fairly common. Some extrapyramidal symptoms (i.e., parkinsonism-like tremor and rigidity) may also occur because of the central antidopamine effects.

Prostaglandins. There is little doubt that certain prostaglandins such as PGE_2 and PGI_2 inhibit gastric secretion and help protect the stomach mucosa by stimulating gastric mucus secretion.[2,36,43] The problem has been determining exactly how the prostaglandins are involved and whether exogenous prostaglandin analogs can be used to help treat peptic ulcer. Two prostaglandin analogs, enprostil and misoprostol, have been studied as possible treatments for peptic ulcer.[4,23,49,60] The general consensus from clinical trials has been that these drugs are successful in treating ulcers, but they do not seem to offer any advantages over the more traditional antiulcer drugs such as cimetidine.[49,62] Also, prostaglandin analogs may be effective only at doses that also cause other GI effects, such as diarrhea.[49,62]

Consequently, prostaglandin analogs have not gained overwhelming acceptance as antiulcer drugs. Currently, only misoprostol (Cytotec) is available for clinical use, and this drug is typically reserved for the treatment of gastric damage caused by aspirin and similar nonsteroidal anti-inflammatory drugs (NSAIDs).[10,14,27,59] The use of misoprostol to reduce or prevent NSAID-induced gastropathy is discussed in more detail in Chapter 15.

Sucralfate (Carafate, Sulcrate). Sucralfate is a disaccharide that exerts a cytoprotective effect on the stomach mucosa.[6,27,44] Although the exact mechanism is unclear, sucralfate may form a protective gel within the stomach that adheres to ulcers and shields them from the stomach contents. The protective barrier formed by the drug prevents further erosion and permits healing of duodenal and gastric ulcers. Sucralfate is fairly well tolerated, although constipation may occur in some patients.

ANTIDIARRHEAL AGENTS

Normal propulsion of food through the GI tract is crucial for proper absorption of nutrients and water. If transit time is too fast, diarrhea occurs, resulting in poor food absorption and dehydration. Diarrhea is often a temporary symptom of many relatively minor GI disorders. Diarrhea may also occur with more serious conditions such as **dysentery,** ulcerative colitis, and cholera. If diarrhea is sustained for even a few days, the resulting dehydration can be a serious problem, especially in infants or debilitated patients. Consequently, efforts should be made to control diarrhea as soon as possible. Antidiarrheal agents are listed in Table 27–2, and their pharmacology is discussed in the following sections.

Opioid Derivatives

RATIONALE FOR USE AND MECHANISM OF ACTION

The constipating effects of morphine and certain other opioid derivatives have been recognized for some time. These drugs produce a general decrease in GI motility, and they may also reduce fluid loss by increasing the absorption of salt and water or by de-

TABLE 27–2 Antidiarrheal Agents

Generic Name	Trade Names	Dosage
Adsorbents		
Kaolin	Kaopectate, Kao-Spen,	60–120 mL regular-strength suspension
Pectin	Kapectolin*	after each loose bowel movement
Bismuth salicylate	Pepto-Bismol, others	525 mg every half hour to 1 hour or 1050 mg every hour if needed
Opioid derivatives		
Diphenoxylate	Lomotil, others†	5 mg 3 or 4 times daily
Loperamide	Imodium, others	4 mg initially, 2 mg after each unformed stool
Opium tincture	—	0.3–1.0 mL 1–4 times daily
Paregoric	—	5–10 mL 1–4 times daily

*Commercial products typically contain both kaolin and pectin.
†Commercial products often combine diphenoxylate (an opioid) with atropine (an anticholinergic).

creasing fluid and electrolyte excretion from the GI tract.[11,29] The exact manner in which opioids exert these effects, however, is not known. Effects on GI motility (antiperistalsis) and absorption may occur because opioids bind to neuronal receptors on the enteric nerve plexus within the gut wall or by a direct effect of opioids on GI epithelial and smooth muscle cells.[7,11] Some of the antidiarrheal effects may likewise be caused by a central inhibitory effect of opioids on the brain.[8,32]

SPECIFIC AGENTS

Opioid derivatives used to treat diarrhea are listed in Table 27–2. Opium tincture (laudanum) and camphorated opium tincture (paregoric) are naturally occurring opiates that are very potent inhibitors of peristalsis. These natural agents are still available for treating diarrhea, but they have essentially been replaced by newer opioids such as diphenoxylate and loperamide. These newer opioids are somewhat less potent but may produce fewer side effects.

ADVERSE SIDE EFFECTS

The primary side effects with these drugs are nausea, abdominal discomfort, constipation, and other GI disturbances. Drowsiness, fatigue, and dizziness have also been reported. Although addiction is a potential problem when opioids are administered, the risk of tolerance and physical dependence is fairly small when these drugs are used in recommended dosages for the short-term treatment of diarrhea.

Adsorbents

RATIONALE FOR TREATMENT AND MECHANISM OF ACTION

Adsorbents are administered to take up and hold harmful substances such as bacteria and toxins in the intestinal lumen.[29] Theoretically, these adsorbents sequester the harmful products causing the diarrhea. These products are used frequently in minor diarrhea, although there is some doubt as to whether they really help decrease stool production and water loss.

SPECIFIC AGENTS

Adsorbents used to treat diarrhea are listed in Table 27–2. These agents frequently appear as the active ingredients in over-the-counter products and may be combined with each other or with other drugs such as antacids.

ADVERSE SIDE EFFECTS

Adsorbents are essentially free from side effects, although constipation may follow prolonged or excessive use.

Bismuth Salicylate

RATIONALE FOR TREATMENT AND MECHANISM OF ACTION

Bismuth salicylate has a number of properties that contribute to its antidiarrheal effects. This drug may stimulate water and electrolyte absorption from the lower GI tract, thus decreasing fecal fluid loss. In addition, the bismuth component of this compound may have antibacterial effects, and the salicylate component may inhibit the production of prostaglandins that irritate the intestinal lining. The combination of these properties makes this drug fairly effective in treating mild-to-moderate diarrhea.[11] Bismuth salicylate also decreases gastric acid secretion and exerts antacid effects, hence its use in stomach upset and minor gastric irritation.

SPECIFIC AGENTS

Bismuth salicylate is the active ingredient in Pepto-Bismol, a fairly inexpensive and readily available over-the-counter commercial product.

ADVERSE SIDE EFFECTS

This drug is relatively free from serious side effects. Problems with salicylate intoxication may occur during overdose or in people who are sensitive to aspirin and other salicylates.

LAXATIVES AND CATHARTICS

Rationale for Use

Laxatives are used to promote evacuation of the bowel and defecation. **Cathartics,** or purgatives, are also used to promote lower GI evacuation, but in a somewhat more rapid fashion than with typical laxatives. For this discussion, the term "laxative" will be used to include both the relatively slow-acting and fast-acting agents.

Laxatives are typically used whenever normal bowel movements have been impaired but no obstruction exists in the GI system. For instance, laxatives may benefit patients on prolonged bed rest, patients with infrequent or painful bowel movements, individuals with spinal cord injuries, or patients who should avoid straining during defecation (e.g., postpartum patients and those recovering from surgical procedures). Laxatives are also indicated for bowel evacuation prior to surgical or diagnostic procedures.

The problem with laxatives is that they are frequently abused. The long-term, chronic use of laxatives is usually unnecessary and often unhealthy. These agents are often self-administered by individuals who are obsessed with maintaining daily bowel movements. Such individuals may have the misconception that daily bowel evacuation is needed to maintain normal GI function. Also, laxatives are often relied upon instead of other factors that promote normal bowel evacuation, such as a high-fiber diet, adequate hydration, and physical activity.[47,50] Consequently, laxatives serve an important but finite role in GI function, and their role in helping maintain routine daily evacuation should be de-emphasized.

Specific Agents and Mechanism of Action

The many different available types of laxatives are usually classified by their apparent mode of action.[34,48,53] Often, two different laxatives, either from the same class or from two different classes, are combined in the same commercial preparation. Some of the more common laxatives are listed in Table 27–3 according to their apparent mechanisms of action. The major laxative classes and the rationale for their use are also outlined in the next few sections.

Bulk-Forming Laxatives. These agents absorb water and swell within the lower GI tract. The increased size of the water-laden laxative stretches the bowel, thus stimulating intestinal movements (peristalsis). Bulk laxatives commonly contain natural and semisynthetic dietary fiber such as bran, psyllium, and methylcellulose.

Stimulant Laxatives. The precise mechanism of stimulant laxatives is not known. They may activate peristalsis by a direct irritant effect on the intestinal mucosa or by stimulating the nerve plexus within the gut wall. Some evidence suggests that they may work by increasing fluid accumulation within the small intestine. Common stimulant laxatives are castor oil, bisacodyl, polyethylene glycol, and phenolphthalein.

Hyperosmotic Laxatives. Administration of osmotically active substances pro-

TABLE 27–3 Laxatives*

Generic Name	Common Trade Name(s)
Bulk-forming	
Methylcellulose	Citrucel, Cologel
Psyllium	Fiberall, Metamucil
Stimulants	
Bisacodyl	Correctol, Dulcolax, Feen-A-Mint
Castor oil	Purge
Phenolphthalein	Ex-Lax
Senna	Senokot
Hyperosmotic	
Glycerin	Sani-Supp
Lactulose	Chronulac, Heptalac
Magnesium hydroxide	Phillips Milk of Magnesia, Haley's MO
Magnesium sulfate	Epsom salts
Sodium phosphate	Fleet Phospho-Soda
Lubricants and stool softeners	
Docusate	Colace, Doxidan
Mineral oil	Agoral, Nujol

*Some of the more common agents are listed as examples in each laxative category. Many other preparations are available that combine two or more laxatives in the same commercial product.

duces a gradient that draws water into the bowel and small intestine. This gradient increases stool fluid content and stimulates peristalsis. A variety of hyperosmotic substances, including magnesium salts, sodium salts, potassium salts, lactulose, and glycerin, can be used to achieve this effect.

Lubricants and Stool Softeners. Agents like mineral oil and docusate facilitate entry of water into the fecal mass, thus softening the stool and permitting easier defecation. These agents may also exert a laxative effect because of the increased pressure in the bowel secondary to the increased stool size.

Adverse Effects

Disturbances in the GI system, such as nausea and cramps, may occur with laxative use. With prolonged use, serious lower GI irritation, including spastic colitis, may occur. Fluid and electrolyte abnormalities are also a potential problem. Excessive loss of water and the concomitant loss of electrolytes may transpire, resulting in dehydration and possible acid-base imbalances.[35] These fluid and electrolyte abnormalities are especially significant in older or debilitated patients. Finally, chronic administration may result in a laxative dependence when bowel evacuation has become so subservient to laxative use that the normal mechanisms governing evacuation and defecation are impaired.

MISCELLANEOUS GASTROINTESTINAL DRUGS

Several other types of drugs are administered for specific purposes in controlling GI function. These other drugs are introduced here only to alert the reader to their existence. For a more detailed description of the use of any of these agents, one of the drug indexes such as the *Physician's Desk Reference* (PDR) should be consulted.

Digestants

These agents are administered to aid in the digestion of food. The primary digestant preparations contain pancreatic enzymes or bile salts. Pancreatic enzymes such as amylase, trypsin, and lipase are responsible for digestion of carbohydrates, proteins, and lipids, respectively. These enzymes are normally synthesized in the pancreas and secreted into the duodenum via the pancreatic duct. Bile salts are synthesized in the liver, stored in the gallbladder, and released into the duodenum via the common bile duct. Bile salts serve to emulsify lipids in the intestinal tract and are important in lipid digestion and absorption.

Digestant preparations are used to replace digestive constituents in the stomach and upper small intestine whenever the endogenous production of these constituents is impaired. In particular, digestants are often administered to individuals with cystic fibrosis.[11] As discussed in Chapter 26, cystic fibrosis is a hereditary disease that affects all the major exocrine glands, resulting in thick, viscous secretions. These thickened secretions may form mucous plugs that obstruct certain ducts such as the pancreatic and bile ducts. This condition leads to a chronic deficiency of pancreatic enzymes and bile salts, and, as a result, patients cannot digest and absorb nutrients from the GI tract. Preparations containing these digestants may be administered orally to replace these missing compounds, thus improving digestion and nutrient absorption.

Emetics

Emetics are used to induce vomiting and are frequently administered to help empty the stomach of poisons or ingested toxins. The two primary emetics are apomorphine and ipecac. Both agents seem to work by stimulating the medullary emetic center, and ipecac also exerts a direct emetic effect on the stomach.

Antiemetics

Antiemetics are used to decrease the nausea and vomiting that are associated with motion sickness and recovery from surgery or that develop in response to other medical treatments, such as cancer chemotherapy and radiation treatments.[11] Antiemetic agents include antihistamines (dimenhydrinate, meclizine, others), anticholinergics (scopolamine), drugs that block specific CNS dopamine (D_2) and serotonin (5-HT_3) receptors, and several other drugs that act at various sites in the CNS to suppress nausea and vomiting. Other antiemetic drugs such as antacids and adsorbents act locally to soothe the gastric mucosa and decrease the irritation that may cause vomiting.

Cholelitholytic Agents

Certain types of gallstones can be dissolved by drugs like chenodiol. This drug decreases the cholesterol content of bile and may help dissolve the types of gallstones that are supersaturated with cholesterol, but chenodiol does not appear effective in the treatment of calcified gallstones.[11]

SPECIAL CONCERNS IN REHABILITATION PATIENTS

Drugs affecting the GI system are important in rehabilitation patients by virtue of their frequent use. About 60 to 100 percent of critically ill patients will suffer some degree of stress-related damage to the stomach mucosa.[38] This stress ulceration syndrome appears to be especially prevalent in patients with burns, multiple traumas, renal failure, and CNS trauma. Drugs such as the PPIs (omeprazole, others) and H_2 receptor blockers (cimetidine, ranitidine, others) are often helpful in controlling gastric acid secretions, thus preventing damage to the mucosal lining in these patients. Patients seen in rehabilitation are often relatively inactive and suffer from many adverse effects of prolonged bed rest, including constipation. Constipation and fecal impaction may also be a recurrent and serious problem in patients with spinal cord injuries. Laxatives are used routinely in these patients to facilitate adequate bowel evacuation. Patients receiving cancer chemotherapy often have problems with nausea and vomiting, and antiemetic drugs may be helpful to these individuals. Various other GI disorders, including diarrhea and chronic indigestion, occur frequently in many rehabilitation patients and are often treated effectively with the appropriate agents.

Despite their frequent use, most GI drugs do not produce any significant side effects that will impair rehabilitation procedures. Some dizziness and fatigue may occur with agents such as the opiates used to treat diarrhea or the antiulcer H_2 blockers, but these effects are fairly mild. Other problems with GI drugs are generally related to transient GI disturbances. In general, GI drugs are well tolerated and fairly safe in most patients.

In effect, these drugs indirectly facilitate physical rehabilitation by resolving annoying and uncomfortable GI symptoms, thus allowing the patient to participate more readily in the rehabilitation program.

CASE STUDY

GASTROINTESTINAL DRUGS

Brief History. M.B. is a 48-year-old insurance sales representative with a long history of back pain. He has had recurrent episodes of sciatica because of a herniated disk at the L5-S1 interspace. Currently, he is being seen as an outpatient in a private physical therapy practice. Despite several treatments, his back pain did not improve. In fact, his pain was recently exacerbated when he was straining to pass a stool during a period of constipation. Evidently, this occurrence had been repeated often, and the patient's back problems had been increased by bowel-related problems causing straining during defecation.

Decision/Solution. The physical therapist consulted with the patient's physician and recommended that a brief trial with a bulk-forming laxative might be helpful during the acute episode of back pain in this patient. The therapist also explained to the patient that straining during defecation exacerbated his back problems. To prevent the recurrence of this problem, the patient was encouraged to ingest a high-fiber diet and adequate amounts of water to prevent constipation. M.B. was also informed that the short-term use of a laxative might be necessary to avoid constipation and straining. The therapist warned the patient, however, about the laxative dependence that can occur during chronic laxative use.

SUMMARY

A variety of pharmacologic agents are used to maintain proper function in the GI system. Drugs such as antacids and H_2 receptor antagonists help control gastric acid secretion and protect the stomach mucosa. These agents are widely used to prevent and treat peptic ulcer. Specific drugs are used to control GI motility. Drugs that inhibit excessive peristalsis (i.e., diarrhea) include the opiate derivatives, adsorbents, and bismuth salicylate. Decreased motility (constipation) is usually treated with various laxatives. Other GI agents attempt to treat specific problems such as poor digestion, emesis, or gallstones. GI drugs are used frequently in rehabilitation patients and, it is hoped, will produce beneficial effects that will allow the patient to participate more actively in the rehabilitation program.

REFERENCES

1. Altman, DF: Drugs used in gastrointestinal diseases. In Katzung, BG (ed): Basic and Clinical Pharmacology, ed 7. Appleton & Lange, Stamford, CT, 1998.
2. Arakawa, T, et al: Prostaglandins in the stomach: An update. J Clin Gastroenterol 27(Suppl 1):S1, 1998.
3. Babe, KS and Serafin, WE: Histamine, bradykinin, and their antagonists. In Hardman, JG, et al (eds): The Pharmacological Basis of Therapeutics, ed 9. McGraw-Hill, New York, 1996.
4. Bader, JP (ed): Symposium: Advances in prostaglandins and gastroenterology: Focus on misoprostol. Am J Med 83(Suppl 1a):1, 1987.

5. Becker, U, et al: Antacid treatment of duodenal ulcer. Acta Med Scand 221:95, 1987.
6. Berardi, RR: Peptic ulcer disease. In DiPiro, JT, et al (eds): Pharmacotherapy: A Pathophysiologic Approach, ed 4. Appleton & Lange, Stamford, CT, 1999.
7. Bianchi, G, et al: Morphine tissue levels and reduction of gastrointestinal transit in rats: Correlation supports primary action site in gut. Gastroenterology 85:852, 1983.
8. Borody, TJ and Quigley, EMM: Effects of morphine and atropine on motility and transit in the human ileum. Gastroenterology 89:522, 1985.
9. Borody, TJ, Shortis, NP, and Reyes, E: Eradication therapies for *Helicobacter pylori.* J Gastroenterol 33(Suppl 10):53, 1998.
10. Brunton, LL: Agents for control of gastric acidity and treatment of peptic ulcers. In Hardman, JG, et al (eds): The Pharmacological Basis of Therapeutics, ed 9. McGraw-Hill, New York, 1996.
12. Brunton, LL: Agents affecting gastrointestinal water flux and motility; emesis and antiemetics; bile acids and pancreatic enzymes. In Hardman, JG, et al (eds): The Pharmacological Basis of Therapeutics, ed 9. McGraw-Hill, New York, 1996.
12. Burt, MJ: The management of peptic ulceration. N Z Med J 106:107, 1993.
13. Dattilo, M and Figura, N: *Helicobacter pylori* infection, chronic gastritis, and proton pump inhibitors. J Clin Gastroenterol 27(Suppl 1):S163, 1998.
14. Day, RO, et al: Non-steroidal anti-inflammatory induced upper gastrointestinal haemorrhage and bleeding. Med J Aust 157:810, 1992.
15. De Boer, WA: Bismuth triple therapy: Still a very important drug regimen for curing *Helicobacter pylori* infection. Eur J Gastroenterol Hepatol 11:697, 1999.
16. Desai, JK, Goyal, RK, and Parmar, NS: Pathogenesis of peptic ulcer disease and current trends in therapy. Indian J Physiol Pharmacol 41:3, 1997.
17. De Wit, NJ, Quartero, AO, and Numans, ME: *Helicobacter pylori* treatment instead of maintenance therapy for peptic ulcer disease: The effectiveness of case-finding in general practice. Aliment Pharmacol Ther 13:1317, 1999.
18. Earnest, DL and Robinson, M: Treatment advances in acid secretory disorders: The promise of rapid symptom relief with disease resolution. Am J Gastroenterol 94(Suppl):S17, 1999.
19. Feldman, M and Burton, ME: Drug therapy: Histamine$_2$-receptor antagonists: Standard therapy for acid-peptic diseases. N Engl J Med 323:1672, 1990.
20. Freston, JW: Management of peptic ulcers: Emerging issues. World J Surg 24:250, 2000.
21. Garnett, WR: Considerations for long-term use of proton-pump inhibitors. Am J Health Syst Pharm 55:2268, 1998.
22. Gough, KR, et al: Ranitidine and cimetidine in prevention of duodenal ulcer relapse: A double-blind, randomized, multicenter, comparative trial. Lancet 2:659, 1984.
23. Herting, RL and Nissen, CH: Overview of misoprostol clinical experience. Dig Dis Sci 31(Suppl):47S, 1986.
24. Holtermuller, KH and Dehdaschti, M: Antacids and hormones. Scand J Gastroenterol 17(Suppl 75):24, 1982.
25. Howden, CW: Use of proton-pump inhibitors in complicated ulcer disease and upper gastrointestinal bleeding. Am J Health Syst Pharm 56(Suppl 4):S5, 1999.
26. Konturek, PC, et al: *Helicobacter pylori* associated gastric pathology. J Physiol Pharmacol 50:695, 1999.
27. Lazzaroni, M, Sainaghi, M, and Bianchi Porro, G: Non-steroidal anti-inflammatory drug gastropathy: Clinical results with antacids and sucralfate. Ital J Gastroenterol Hepatol 31(Suppl 1):S48, 1999.
28. Levenstein, S: Peptic ulcer at the end of the 20th century: Biological and psychological risk factors. Can J Gastroenterol 13:753, 1999.
29. Longe, RL and DiPiro, JT: Diarrhea and constipation. In DiPiro, JT, et al (eds): Pharmacotherapy: A Pathophysiologic Approach, ed 4. Appleton & Lange, Stamford, CT, 1999.
30. Louw, JA and Marks, IN: *Helicobacter pylori:* Therapeutic targets. Yale J Biol Med 71:113, 1998.
31. Malfertheiner, P: Current concepts in dyspepsia: A world perspective. Eur J Gastroenterol Hepatol 11(Suppl 1):S25, 1999.
32. Manara, L and Bianchetti, A: The central and peripheral influences of opioids on gastrointestinal propulsion. Annu Rev Pharmacol Toxicol 25:249, 1985.
33. Maton, PN and Burton, ME: Antacids revisited: A review of their clinical pharmacology and recommended therapeutic use. Drugs 57:855, 1999.
34. Muller-Lissner, S: Classification, pharmacology, and side-effects of common laxatives. Ital J Gastroenterol Hepatol 31(Suppl 3):S234, 1999.
35. Muller-Lissner, SA: Adverse effects of laxatives: Fact or fiction. Pharmacology 47(Suppl 1):138, 1993.
36. Peskar, BM and Maricic, N: Role of prostaglandins in gastroprotection. Dig Dis Sci 43(Suppl):23S, 1998.
37. Peura, D: *Helicobacter pylori:* Rational management options. Am J Med 105:424, 1998.
38. Peura, DA and Freston, JW: Introduction: Evolving perspectives on parenteral H$_2$-receptor antagonist therapy. Am J Med 83(Suppl 6a):1, 1987.
39. Ramirez, B and Richter, JE: Review article: Promotility drugs and the treatment of gastro-esophogeal reflux disease. Aliment Pharmacol Ther 7:5, 1993.
40. Reilly, JP: Safety profile of the proton-pump inhibitors. Am J Health Syst Pharm 56(Suppl 4):S11, 1999.
41. Richardson, P, Hawkey, CJ, and Stack, WA: Proton pump inhibitors. Pharmacology and rationale for use in gastrointestinal disorders. Drugs 56:307, 1998.

42. Rohner, H-G and Gugler, R: Treatment of active duodenal ulcers with famotidine: A double-blind comparison with ranitidine. Am J Med 81(Suppl 4b):13, 1986.
43. Russel, RI: Protective effects of the prostaglandins on the gastric mucosa. Am J Med 81(Suppl 2a):2, 1986.
44. Sabesin, SM and Lam, SK (eds): Symposium: International sucralfate research conference. Am J Med 83(Suppl 3b):1, 1987.
45. Sachs, G, et al: Gastric H$^+$, K$^+$-ATPase as a therapeutic target. Annu Rev Pharmacol Toxicol 28:269, 1988.
46. Sandvik, AK, Brenna, E, and Waldrum, HL: Review article: The pharmacological inhibition of gastric acid secretion—tolerance and rebound. Aliment Pharmacol Ther 11:1013, 1997.
47. Schaefer, DC and Cheskin, LJ: Constipation in the elderly. Am Fam Physician 58:907, 1998.
48. Schiller, LR: Clinical pharmacology and use of laxatives and lavage solutions. J Clin Gastroenterol 28:11, 1999.
49. Shield, MJ: Interim results of a multicenter international comparison of misoprostol and cimetidine in the treatment of out-patients with benign gastric ulcers. Dig Dis Sci 30(Suppl):178S, 1985.
50. Soffer, EE: Constipation: An approach to diagnosis, treatment, referral. Cleve Clin J Med 66:41, 1999.
51. Soll, AH: Peptic ulcer and dyspepsia. Clin Cornerstone 1:29, 1999.
52. Tan, AC, Hartog, GD, and Mulder, CJ: Eradication of *Helicobacter pylori* does not decrease the long-term use of acid-suppression medication. Aliment Pharmacol Ther 13:1519, 1999.
53. Tedesco, FJ: Laxative use in constipation. Am J Gastroenterol 80:303, 1985.
54. Tovey, FI and Hobsley, M: Is *Helicobacter pylori* the primary cause of duodenal ulceration? J Gastroenterol Hepatol 14:1053, 1999.
55. Tytgat, GN: Ulcers and gastritis. Endoscopy 32:108, 2000.
56. Tytgat, GN: Treatment of peptic ulcer. Digestion 59:446, 1998.
57. Vakil, N: Treatment of *Helicobacter pylori* infection. Am J Ther 5:197, 1998.
58. Waldrum, HL and Brenna, E: Personal review: Is profound acid inhibition safe? Aliment Pharmacol Ther 14:15, 2000.
59. Walt, RP: Drug therapy: Misoprostol for the treatment of peptic ulcer and anti-inflammatory-drug induced gastroduodenal ulceration. N Engl J Med 327:1575, 1992.
60. Waterbury, LD, Mahoney, JM, and Peak, TM: Stimulatory effect of enprostil, an anti-ulcer prostaglandin, on gastric mucus secretion. Am J Med 81(Suppl 2a):30, 1986.
61. Welage, LS and Berardi, RR: Evaluation of omeprazole, lansoprazole, pantoprazole, and rabeprazole in the treatment of acid-related diseases. J Am Pharm Assoc (Wash) 40:52, 2000.
62. Winters, L: Comparison of enprostil and cimetidine in active duodenal ulcer disease: Summary of pooled European studies. Am J Med 81(Suppl 2a):69, 1986.
63. Wood, DW and Block, KP: *Helicobacter pylori*: A review. Am J Ther 5:253, 1998.

Endocrine Pharmacology

CHAPTER 28

Introduction to Endocrine Pharmacology

The endocrine system helps maintain internal homeostasis through the use of endogenous chemicals known as hormones. A *hormone* is typically regarded as a chemical messenger that is released into the bloodstream to exert an effect on target cells located some distance from the site of hormonal release.[8] Various endocrine glands manufacture and release specific hormones that help regulate such physiologic processes as reproduction, growth and development, energy metabolism, fluid and electrolyte balance, and response to stress and injury.[8,25]

The use of drugs to help regulate and control endocrine function is an important area of pharmacology. In one sense, hormones can be considered drugs that are manufactured by the patient's body. This situation presents an obvious opportunity to use exogenous chemicals to either mimic or attenuate the effects of specific hormones during endocrine dysfunction.

Drugs can be used as replacement therapy during hormonal deficiency, for example, insulin administration in diabetes mellitus. Likewise, exogenous hormone analogs can be administered to accentuate the effects of their endogenous counterparts, such as using glucocorticoids to help treat inflammation. Conversely, drugs can be administered to treat endocrine hyperactivity, for example, the use of antithyroid drugs in treating hyperthyroidism. Finally, drugs can be used to regulate normal endocrine function to achieve a desired effect, as is done through inhibition of ovulation by oral contraceptives.

The purpose of this chapter is to review the basic aspects of endocrine function, including the primary hormones and their effects. The factors regulating hormonal release and cellular mechanisms of hormone action are also briefly discussed. Finally, the basic ways in which drugs can be used to alter endocrine function are presented. This overview is intended to provide rehabilitation specialists with a general review of endocrine and hormone activity, with subsequent chapters dealing with specific endocrine drugs and the problems they are used to treat.

PRIMARY ENDOCRINE GLANDS AND THEIR HORMONES

The primary endocrine glands and the hormones they produce are briefly discussed here. These glands and the physiologic effects of their hormones are also summarized in Tables 28–1 and 28–2. For the purpose of this chapter, only the primary endocrine glands and their respective hormones are discussed. Substances such as prostaglandins and kinins, which are produced locally by a variety of different cells, are not discussed here, but are referred to elsewhere in this text (e.g., see Chap. 15). Also, chemicals such as norepinephrine, which serve a dual purpose as hormones and neurotransmitters, are discussed in this chapter only with regard to their endocrine function.

Hypothalamus and Pituitary Gland

The pituitary gland is a small, pea-shaped structure located within the sella turcica at the base of the brain. The pituitary lies inferior to the hypothalamus and is attached to the hypothalamus by a thin stalk of tissue known as the *infundibulum*. The structural and functional relationships between the hypothalamus and pituitary gland are briefly discussed later in this section. A more detailed presentation of the anatomic and physiologic functions of the hypothalamus and pituitary gland can be found in several sources listed at the end of this chapter.[2,6,14]

The pituitary can be subdivided into an anterior, an intermediate, and a posterior lobe. These subdivisions and their respective hormones are listed in Table 28–1 and are briefly discussed here.

TABLE 28–1 Hypothalamic and Pituitary Hormones

Hypothalamic Hormones and Releasing Factors	Effect
Growth hormone–releasing hormone (GHRH)	↑ GH release
Growth hormone–inhibitory hormone (GHIH)	↓ GH release
Gonadotropin-releasing hormone (GnRH)	↑ LH and FSH release
Thyrotropin-releasing hormone (TRH)	↑ TSH release
Corticotropin-releasing hormone (CRH)	↑ ACTH release
Prolactin-inhibitory factor (PIF)	↓ Pr release

Pituitary Hormones	Principal Effects
Anterior lobe	
Growth hormone (GH)	↑ Tissue growth and development
Luteinizing hormone (LH)	*Female:* ↑ ovulation; ↑ estrogen and progesterone synthesis from corpus luteum *Male:* ↑ spermatogenesis
Follicle-stimulating hormone (FSH)	*Female:* ↑ follicular development and estrogen synthesis *Male:* Enhance spermatogenesis
Thyroid-stimulating hormone (TSH)	↑ synthesis of thyroid hormones (T_3, T_4)
Adrenocorticotropic hormone (ACTH)	↑ adrenal steroid synthesis (e.g., cortisol)
Prolactin (Pr)	Initiates lactation
Posterior lobe	
Antidiuretic hormone (ADH)	↑ Renal reabsorption of water
Oxytocin	↑ Uterine contraction; ↑ milk ejection during lactation

TABLE 28–2 Other Primary Endocrine Glands

Gland	Hormone(s)	Principal Effects
Thyroid	Thyroxine (T_4), triiodothyronine (T_3)	Increase cellular metabolism; facilitate normal growth and development
Parathyroids	Parathormone (PTH)	Increase blood calcium
Pancreas	Glucagon	Increase blood glucose
	Insulin	Decrease blood glucose; increase carbohydrate, protein, and fat storage
Adrenal cortex	Glucocorticoids	Regulate glucose metabolism; enhance response to stress
	Mineralocorticoids	Regulate fluid and electrolyte levels
Adrenal medulla	Epinephrine, norepinephrine	Vascular and metabolic effects that facilitate increased physical activity
Testes	Testosterone	Spermatogenesis; male sexual characteristics
Ovaries	Estrogens, progesterone	Female reproductive cycle and sexual characteristics

Anterior Lobe. The anterior pituitary, or adenohypophysis, secretes six important peptide hormones. Hormones released from the anterior pituitary are growth hormone (GH), luteinizing hormone (LH), follicle-stimulating hormone (FSH), thyroid-stimulating hormone (TSH), adrenocorticotropic hormone (ACTH), and prolactin (Pr). The physiologic effects of these hormones are listed in Table 28–1.

Hormonal release from the anterior pituitary is controlled by specific hormones or releasing factors from the hypothalamus.[2,21] Basically, a releasing factor is sent from the hypothalamus to the anterior pituitary via local vascular structures known as the hypothalamic-hypophysial portal vessels. For example, to increase the secretion of growth hormone, the hypothalamus first secretes growth hormone–releasing hormone (GHRH) into the portal vessels. The GHRH travels the short distance to the anterior pituitary via the hypothalamic-hypophysial portal system. Upon arriving at the pituitary, the GHRH causes the anterior pituitary to release growth hormone into the systemic circulation, where it can then travel to various target tissues in the periphery. Other hypothalamic-releasing factors that have been identified are listed in Table 28–1. Specific releasing factors are still being investigated, and the identification of additional releasing factors (including factors that inhibit anterior pituitary hormone release) will undoubtedly be forthcoming.

Intermediate Lobe. In mammals, there is a small intermediate lobe of the pituitary that may secrete melanocyte-stimulating hormone (MSH). Although it can influence skin pigmentation in lower vertebrates, MSH is not produced in meaningful amounts in humans, and human skin does not have receptors that mediate MSH responses similar to those seen in other animals.[2] Hence, MSH does not have any apparent physiologic or pharmacologic significance in humans.

Posterior Lobe. The posterior pituitary, or neurohypophysis, secretes two hormones: antidiuretic hormone (ADH) and oxytocin.[16] ADH exerts its effect primarily on the kidney, where it increases the reabsorption of water from the distal renal tubules. Oxytocin, which is important in parturition, stimulates the uterus to contract. It also promotes lactation by stimulating the ejection of milk from the mammary glands.

The hypothalamic control of the posterior pituitary is quite different than that of the anterior and intermediate lobes. Specific neurons have their cell bodies in certain hypothalamic nuclei. Cell bodies in the paraventricular nuclei manufacture oxytocin, whereas the supraoptic nuclei contain cell bodies that synthesize ADH. The axons from these cells extend downward through the infundibulum to terminate in the posterior pituitary. The hormones synthesized in the hypothalamic cell bodies are transported down the axon to be stored in neurosecretory granules in their respective nerve terminals located in the posterior pituitary. When an appropriate stimulus is present, these neurons fire an action potential, which causes the hormones to be released from their pituitary nerve terminals. The hormones are ultimately picked up by the systemic circulation and transported to their target tissues.

Thyroid Gland

The thyroid gland is located in the anterior neck region, approximately at the level of the fifth cervical to first thoracic vertebrae.[13] This gland consists of bilateral lobes that lie on either side of the trachea and are connected by a thin piece of the gland known as the isthmus. The thyroid synthesizes and secretes two hormones: thyroxine (T_4) and tri-iodothyronine (T_3). The synthesis of these hormones is controlled by the hypothalamic-pituitary system via thyroid-releasing hormone from the hypothalamus, which causes thyroid-stimulating hormone release from the anterior pituitary. Thyroid-stimulating hormone increases T_3 and T_4 synthesis and release from the thyroid gland.

The primary effect of the thyroid hormones is to increase cellular metabolism in most body tissues.[5,13] These hormones stimulate virtually all aspects of cellular function, including protein, fat, and carbohydrate metabolism. By exerting a stimulatory effect on the cellular level, the thyroid hormones play a crucial role in helping maintain and regulate body heat (*thermogenesis*) in the whole organism. T_3 and T_4 also play an important role in growth and development, especially in the growth and maturation of normal bone. Finally, thyroid hormones play a permissive role in allowing other hormones such as steroids to exert their effects. The physiology and pharmacology of the thyroid hormones are further discussed in Chapter 31.

Parathyroid Gland

The parathyroid glands are small, egg-shaped structures embedded in the posterior surface of the thyroid gland. There are usually four parathyroid glands, with two glands located on each half of the thyroid gland. The parathyroids synthesize and release parathyroid hormone (PTH). PTH is essential in maintaining normal calcium homeostasis in the body, and the primary effect of PTH is to increase the concentration of calcium in the bloodstream.[3] PTH increases circulating calcium levels primarily by mobilizing calcium from storage sites in bone.

The primary factor regulating PTH release is the level of calcium in the bloodstream.[7] Parathyroid gland cells appear to act as calcium sensors that monitor circulating calcium levels. As circulating calcium levels fall below a certain point, PTH secretion is increased. Conversely, elevated plasma calcium titers inhibit PTH secretion. The ability of PTH to control plasma calcium levels and regulate bone mineral metabolism is discussed in more detail in Chapter 31.

Pancreas

The pancreas is located behind the stomach in the lower left area of the abdomen. This gland is unique in that it serves both endocrine and exocrine functions.[11] The exocrine aspect of this gland involves digestive enzymes that are excreted into the duodenum. As an endocrine gland, the pancreas primarily secretes two peptide hormones: insulin and glucagon. These hormones are synthesized and secreted by cells located in specialized clusters known as the *islets of Langerhans*. In the islets of Langerhans, glucagon and insulin are synthesized by alpha and beta cells, respectively.

Pancreatic hormones are involved in the regulation of blood glucose, and the glucose concentration in the blood serves as the primary stimulus for the release of these hormones. As blood glucose levels fall—for example, following a fast—glucagon is released from pancreatic alpha cells. Glucagon mobilizes the release of glucose from storage sites in the liver, thus bringing blood glucose levels back to normal. An increase in blood glucose after eating a meal stimulates insulin release from the beta cells. Insulin facilitates the storage of glucose in the liver and muscle, thus removing glucose from the bloodstream and returning blood glucose to normal levels. Insulin also exerts a number of other effects on protein and lipid metabolism. The effects of insulin and the pharmacologic replacement of insulin in diabetes mellitus are discussed in more detail in Chapter 32.

Adrenal Gland

The adrenal glands are located at the superior poles of each kidney. Each adrenal gland is composed of an outer cortex and an inner medulla. The hormones associated with the adrenal cortex and adrenal medulla are described in the following sections.

Hormones of the Adrenal Cortex. The adrenal cortex synthesizes and secretes two primary groups of steroidal hormones: the **glucocorticoids** and the **mineralocorticoids**.[15] Small amounts of sex steroids (estrogens, androgens, progesterone) are also produced, but these amounts are essentially insignificant during normal adrenal function.

Glucocorticoids such as cortisol have a number of physiologic effects.[17] Glucocorticoids are involved in the regulation of glucose metabolism and are important in enhancing the body's ability to handle stress. Glucocorticoids also have significant anti-inflammatory and immunosuppressive properties and are often used therapeutically to control inflammation or suppress the immune response in various clinical situations. Glucocorticoid synthesis is controlled by the hypothalamic-pituitary system. Corticotropin-releasing hormone (CRH) from the hypothalamus stimulates ACTH release from the anterior pituitary, which in turn stimulates the synthesis of glucocorticoids.

Mineralocorticoids are involved in controlling electrolyte and fluid levels.[1] The primary mineralocorticoid produced by the adrenal cortex is *aldosterone*. Aldosterone increases the reabsorption of sodium from the renal tubules. By increasing sodium reabsorption, aldosterone facilitates the reabsorption of water. Aldosterone also inhibits the renal reabsorption of potassium, thus increasing potassium excretion. Mineralocorticoid release is regulated by fluid and electrolyte levels in the body and by other hormones, such as the renin-angiotensin system.

The pharmacologic aspects of the glucocorticoids and mineralocorticoids are discussed in more detail in Chapter 29.

Hormones of the Adrenal Medulla. The adrenal medulla synthesizes and secretes epinephrine and norepinephrine.[26] These hormones have a number of physiologic effects, which are discussed in Chapters 18 and 20. Small amounts of epinephrine and norepinephrine are released under resting, basal conditions. The primary significance of these hormones, however, seems to be in helping prepare the body for sudden physical activity. The classic function of the adrenal medulla is illustrated by the fight-or-flight reaction, in which a stressful challenge is presented to the individual and interpreted as requiring either defense or a need to flee from the challenge.

The release of epinephrine and norepinephrine from the adrenal medulla is controlled by the sympathetic division of the autonomic nervous system. As discussed in Chapter 18, sympathetic cholinergic preganglionic neurons directly innervate this gland. An increase in sympathetic activity causes increased firing in these neurons, which in turn stimulates the release of epinephrine and norepinephrine from the adrenal medulla.

Gonads

The reproductive organs are the primary source of the steroid hormones that influence sexual and reproductive functions. In men, the testes produce *testosterone* and similar **androgens** that are responsible for spermatogenesis and the secondary sexual characteristics of adult males.[24] In women, sexual maturation and reproductive function are governed by the production of **estrogens** and **progestins** from the ovaries.[23] The release of male and female sex steroids is controlled by hormones from the hypothalamus and anterior pituitary.[23,24] The control of male and female hormone activity and the pharmacologic implications of these hormones are discussed in Chapter 30.

ENDOCRINE PHYSIOLOGY AND PHARMACOLOGY

Hormone Chemistry

Hormones can be divided into several primary categories according to their basic chemical structure. *Steroid hormones* share a common chemical framework that is derived from lipids such as cholesterol.[17] Examples of steroids include the sex hormones (androgens, estrogens, progesterone), the glucocorticoids, and the mineralocorticoids. *Peptide hormones* consist of amino acids linked together in a specific sequence. These peptide chains can range in length from 3 to 180 amino acids. Primary examples of peptide hormones are the hypothalamic releasing factors and the pituitary hormones. Finally, several hormones are modified from a single amino acid. For instance, the thyroid hormones (T_3 and T_4) are manufactured from the amino acid tyrosine. Also, hormones from the adrenal medulla (epinephrine, norepinephrine) are synthesized from either phenylalanine or tyrosine.

The basic chemical structure of various hormones is significant in determining how the hormone will exert its effects on target tissues (see "Hormone Effects on the Target Cell"). Also, different hormones that are fairly similar in structure can often have similar physiologic and pharmacologic effects. This is especially true for the steroids, in which one category of steroidal agents may have some of the properties of a different category.[17] For instance, the endogenous glucocorticoids—for example, cortisol—also exert some mineralocorticoid effects, presumably because of their similar chemical structure. These overlapping effects and their consequences are discussed in more detail in Chapters 29 through 32, which deal with specific endocrine systems.

Synthesis and Release of Hormones

Hormones are typically synthesized within the cells of their respective endocrine glands. Most hormones are synthesized and packaged in storage granules within the gland. When the gland is stimulated, the storage granule fuses with the cell membrane, and the hormone is released by exocytosis. Notable exceptions to this are the steroid hormones, which are not stored to any great extent but are synthesized on demand when an appropriate stimulus is present.[8]

Hormone synthesis and release can be initiated by both extrinsic and intrinsic factors.[8] Extrinsic factors include various environmental stimuli such as pain, temperature, light, and smell. Intrinsic stimuli include various humoral and neural factors. For instance, release of a hormone can be initiated by other hormones. These occurrences are particularly typical of the anterior pituitary hormones, which are controlled by releasing hormones from the hypothalamus. Hormonal release can be influenced by neural input; a primary example is the sympathetic neural control of epinephrine and norepinephrine release from the adrenal medulla. Other intrinsic factors that affect hormone release are the levels of ions and metabolites within the body. For instance, parathyroid hormone release is directly governed by the calcium concentration in the bloodstream, and the release of glucagon from pancreatic alpha cells is dependent on blood glucose levels.

Feedback Control Mechanisms in Endocrine Function

As mentioned previously, the endocrine system is concerned with maintaining homeostasis within the body. When a disturbance in physiologic function occurs, hormones are released to rectify the disturbance. As function returns to normal, hormone release is attenuated and homeostasis is resumed. For example, an increase in the blood glucose level initiates the release of insulin from pancreatic beta cells. Insulin increases the incorporation into and storage of glucose in liver, skeletal muscle, and other tissues. Blood glucose levels then return to normal, and insulin release is terminated.

Hormonal release is also frequently regulated by some form of negative feedback system.[8] In these feedback systems, increased release of a specific hormone ultimately serves to inhibit its own release, thus preventing the amount of the released hormone from becoming excessive. An example of a negative feedback system involving the hypothalamic-pituitary axis is illustrated in Figure 28–1. The endocrine hormone ultimately inhibits its own release by inhibiting the secretion of specific hypothalamic releasing factors and pituitary hormones. Numerous examples of such negative feedback loops are present in various endocrine pathways.

There are also a few examples of positive feedback mechanisms in the endocrine system.[8] In a positive feedback loop, rising concentrations of one hormone cause an increase in other hormones, which, in turn, facilitates increased production of the first hormone. The primary example of this type of feedback occurs in the female reproductive system, where low levels of estrogen production increase the release of pituitary hormones (LH, FSH).[12] Increased LH and FSH then facilitate further estrogen production, which further increases pituitary hormone secretion and so on (see Chap. 30). Positive feedback mechanisms are relatively rare, however, compared with negative feedback controls in the endocrine system.

The presence of feedback systems in endocrine function is important from a pharmacologic perspective. Drugs can be administered that act through the intrinsic feedback loops to control endogenous hormone production. A primary example is the use of oral contraceptives, when exogenous estrogen and progesterone are administered in controlled amounts to inhibit ovulation (see Chap. 30). Therapeutic administration of hormonal agents may create problems, however, because of these negative feedback

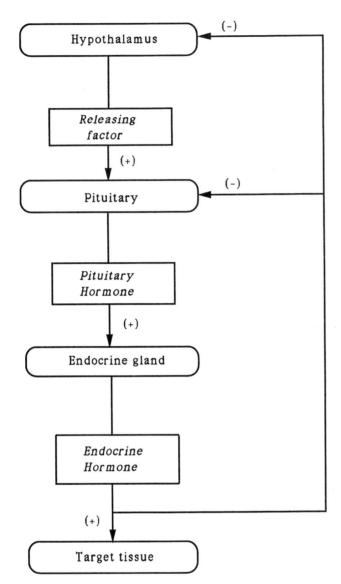

FIGURE 28–1. Negative feedback control in the hypothalamic–pituitary–endocrine pathways. Excitatory and inhibitory effects are indicated by (+) and (−), respectively. Negative feedback loops occur owing to inhibition of the endocrine hormone on the pituitary and hypothalamus.

effects. For instance, glucocorticoid administration may act as negative feedback to suppress the normal endogenous production of adrenal steroids.[18] If the body is unable to produce its own supply of adrenal steroids, abrupt withdrawal of the exogenous compounds can result in severe or even fatal consequences. Adrenocortical suppression is discussed in more detail in Chapter 29.

Hormone Transport

Hormones are usually carried from their site of origin to the target cell via the systemic circulation.[8] During transport in the bloodstream, certain hormones such as steroids are bound to specific plasma proteins. These protein carriers appear to help prolong the half-life of the hormone and prevent premature degradation. Other protein carriers may be important in the local effects of hormone function. For instance, the testes produce androgen-binding protein, which helps transport and concentrate testosterone within the seminiferous tubules of the testes (see Chap. 30).

Hormone Effects on the Target Cell

Most hormones affect their target cell by interacting with a specific receptor. Hormone receptors are usually located at one of the three locations shown in Figure 28–2. These primary locations are on the surface membrane of the cell, within the cytosol of the cell, or within the cell's nucleus.[8] Receptors at each location tend to be specific for different types of hormones and also tend to affect cell function in a specific manner. Each type of receptor is briefly discussed here.

Surface Membrane Receptors. These receptors are located on the outer surface of the plasma membrane (see Fig. 28–2).[10] Surface receptors tend to recognize the peptide hormones and some amino acid derivatives (e.g., pituitary hormones, catecholamines). Surface receptors are typically linked to specific intracellular enzymes. When stimulated by a peptidelike hormone, the receptor initiates some change in the enzymatic machinery located within the cell. This event usually results in a change in the production of some intracellular chemical second messenger such as cyclic adenosine monophosphate (cAMP).[8]

An example of a hormone that exerts its effects through a surface receptor–second messenger system is ACTH.[9] ACTH is a polypeptide that binds to a surface receptor on adrenal cortex cells. The surface receptor then stimulates the adenylate cyclase enzyme to increase production of cAMP. The cAMP acts as a second messenger (the hormone

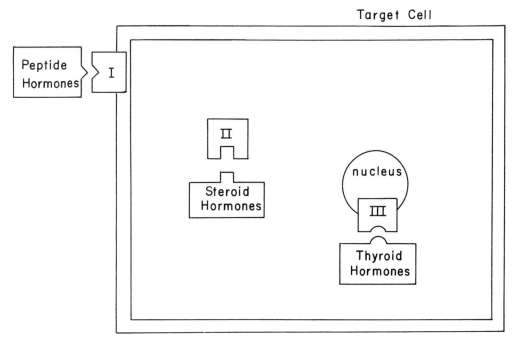

FIGURE 28–2. Primary cellular locations of hormone receptors. Peptide hormones tend to bind to surface membrane receptors (site I); steroid hormones bind to cytosolic receptors (site II); and thyroid hormones bind to receptors in the cell nucleus (site III).

was the first messenger), which then increases the activity of other enzymes within the cell to synthesize adrenal steroids such as cortisol. For a more detailed description of surface receptor–second messenger systems, see Chapter 4.

Cytosolic Hormone Receptors. The steroid hormones typically bind to protein receptors, which are located directly within the cytosol (see Fig. 28–2).[22] Of course, this means that the hormone must first enter the cell, which is easily accomplished by the steroid hormones because they are highly lipid soluble. After entering the cell, the hormone initiates a series of events that are depicted in Figure 28–3. Basically, the hormone and receptor form a large activated steroid-receptor complex.[22] This complex then trav-

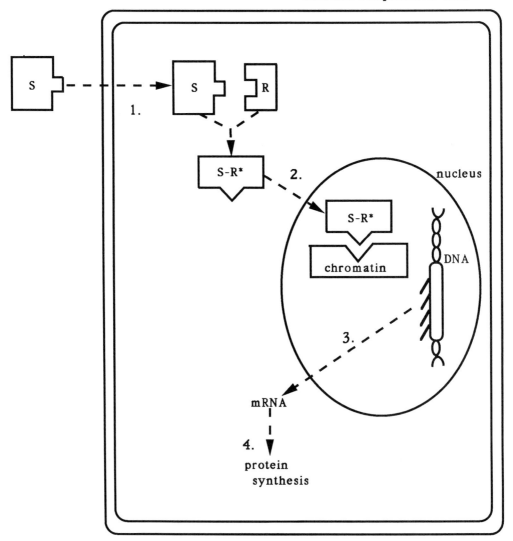

FIGURE 28–3. Sequence of events of steroid hormone action. (1) Steroid hormone enters the cell, binds to a cytosolic receptor, and creates an activated steroid-receptor complex (S-R). (2) S-R complex travels to the cell's nucleus, where it binds to specific gene segments on nuclear chromatin. (3) DNA undergoes transcription into messenger RNA (mRNA) units. (4) mRNA undergoes translation in the cytosol into specific proteins that alter cell function.

els to the cell's nucleus, where it binds to specific genes located within the DNA sequence.[4,22] This process initiates gene expression and transcription of messenger RNA units, which go back to the cytosol and are translated into specific proteins by the endoplasmic reticulum.[4] These newly manufactured proteins are usually enzymes or structural proteins that change cell function in a specific manner. For instance, **anabolic steroids** increase muscle size by facilitating the production of more contractile proteins. Thus, steroids tend to exert their effects on target cells by directly affecting the cell's nucleus and subsequently altering the production of certain cellular proteins.

Nuclear Hormone Receptors. Receptors located directly on the chromatin within the cell nucleus are specific for the thyroid hormones (see Fig. 28–2).[20] Thyroid hormones (T_3 and T_4) that reach these nuclear receptors invoke a series of changes similar to those caused by the steroid–cytosolic receptor complex; that is, the nucleus begins to transcribe messenger RNA, which ultimately is translated into specific proteins. In the case of the thyroid hormones, these new proteins usually alter the cell's metabolism. The thyroid hormones are discussed in more detail in Chapter 31.

Hormone receptors have some obvious and important pharmacologic distinctions. Drugs that can bind to and activate specific hormonal receptors (agonists) will mimic the effects of the endogenous compounds. Drugs that block the receptors (antagonists) will attenuate any unwanted hormonal effects. In fact, drugs may be produced that are even more specific for hormonal receptors than their endogenous counterparts. For instance, synthetic glucocorticoids, such as dexamethasone, exert anti-inflammatory effects in a manner similar to that of endogenous glucocorticoids, but with diminished mineralocorticoid-like side effects such as water and sodium retention. This increased specificity is presumably brought about by a more precise action of the synthetic compound on the glucocorticoid receptors rather than the mineralocorticoid receptors.

CLINICAL USE OF ENDOCRINE DRUGS

The general ways in which pharmacologic agents can be used to alter endocrine activity are as follows.

Replacement Therapy. If the endogenous production of a hormone is deficient or absent, therapeutic administration of the hormone can be used to restore normal endocrine function.[19] The exogenous hormone can be obtained from natural sources, such as extracts from animal tissues, or from chemical synthesis. In addition, new recombinant DNA techniques are being used to produce hormones from cell cultures, and these techniques have shown great promise in being able to generate hormones like human insulin.

Hormone substitution is sometimes referred to as simple replacement therapy. The use of exogenous hormones to replace normal endocrine function is sometimes a complicated task, however. Problems such as regulation of optimal dosage, interaction of the exogenous drug with other endogenous hormone systems, and drug-induced side effects are frequently encountered.

Diagnosis of Endocrine Disorders. Hormones or their antagonists can be administered to determine the presence of excess endocrine function or endocrine hypofunction. For example, hormones or their synthetic analogs can be administered that either increase or decrease pituitary secretion to determine if pituitary function is normal. Likewise, antagonists to specific hormones can be administered to see if symptoms are caused by excessive production of these hormones. Specific examples of how hormones are used to diagnose endocrine abnormalities are presented in subsequent chapters.

Treatment of Excessive Endocrine Function. Hyperactive or inappropriate endocrine function is often treated pharmacologically. Inhibition of hormone function can occur at several levels. For instance, drugs may be administered that directly inhibit the synthesis of the hormone or inhibit its release through various negative feedback mechanisms (see "Feedback Control Mechanisms in Endocrine Function"). Also, hormone antagonists, drugs that block hormone receptors, may be used for prolonged periods to attenuate the effects of excessive hormone production.

Exploitation of Beneficial Hormone Effects. Hormones and their synthetic analogs are often administered to exaggerate the beneficial effects of their endogenous counterparts. The classic example is the use of glucocorticoids to treat inflammation. Doses of glucocorticoids that are much higher than the physiologic levels produced by the body can be very effective in decreasing inflammation in a variety of clinical conditions (e.g., rheumatoid arthritis, allergic reactions). Of course, the use of high doses of hormones to accentuate beneficial effects may also cause some adverse side effects and impair various aspects of endocrine function. The short-term use of hormones in this capacity is often a useful therapeutic intervention, however.

Use of Hormones to Alter Normal Endocrine Function. Because of the intrinsic control mechanisms in the endocrine system, administration of exogenous hormones can often affect the normal release of hormones. This fact can be exploited in certain situations to cause a desired change in normal endocrine function. For instance, oral contraceptives containing estrogen and progesterone inhibit ovulation by inhibiting the release of LH and FSH from the anterior pituitary.

Use of Hormones in Nonendocrine Disease. There are many examples of how various hormones and hormone-related drugs can be used to treat conditions that are not directly related to the endocrine system. For instance, certain forms of cancer respond to treatment with glucocorticoids (see Chap. 36). Drugs that block the cardiac beta-1 receptors may help control angina and hypertension by preventing excessive stimulation from adrenal medulla hormones (epinephrine, norepinephrine) (see Chaps. 21 and 22).

SUMMARY

The endocrine glands regulate a variety of physiologic processes through the release of specific hormones. Hormones are the equivalent of endogenously produced drugs that usually travel through the bloodstream to exert an effect on specific target tissues. Hormones typically alter cell function by binding to receptors located at specific sites on or within the target cell. Pharmacologic agents can be administered to mimic or exaggerate hormonal effects, inhibit excessive hormonal activity, and produce other desirable changes in endocrine activity. The use of hormones and hormone-related substances in the pharmacologic management of specific disorders is discussed in Chapters 29 through 32.

REFERENCES

1. Agarwal, MK and Mirshahi, M: General overview of mineralocorticoid hormone action. Pharmacol Ther 84:273, 1999.
2. Ascoli, M and Segaloff, DL: Adenohypophyseal hormones and their hypothalamic releasing factors. In Hardman, JG, et al (eds): The Pharmacological Basis of Therapeutics, ed 9. McGraw-Hill, New York, 1996.
3. Bringhurst, FR, Demay, MB, and Kronenberg, HM: Hormones and disorders of mineral metabolism. In Wilson, JD, et al (eds): Textbook of Endocrinology, ed 9. WB Saunders, Philadelphia, 1998.

4. Burnstein, KL and Cidlowski, JA: Regulation of gene expression by glucocorticoids. Annu Rev Physiol 51:683, 1989.
5. Farwell, AP and Braverman, LE: Thyroid and antithyroid drugs. In Hardman, JG, et al (eds): The Pharmacological Basis of Therapeutics, ed 9. McGraw-Hill, New York, 1996.
6. Fitzgerald, PA and Klonoff, DC: Hypothalamic and pituitary hormones. In Katzung, BG (ed): Basic and Clinical Pharmacology, ed 7. Appleton & Lange, Stamford, CT, 1998.
7. Genuth, SM: Endocrine regulation of the metabolism of calcium and phosphate. In Berne, RM and Levy, MN (eds): Physiology, ed 3. Mosby Year Book, St Louis, 2000.
8. Genuth, SM: General principles of endocrine physiology. In Berne, RM and Levy, MN (eds): Physiology, ed 3. Mosby Year Book, St Louis, 2000.
9. Goldfien, A: Adrenocorticosteroids and adrenocortical antagonists. In Katzung, BG (ed): Basic and Clinical Pharmacology, ed 7. Appleton & Lange, Stamford, CT, 1998.
10. Kahn, CR, Smith, RJ, and Chin, WW: Mechanism of action of hormones that act at the cell surface. In Wilson, JD, et al (eds): Textbook of Endocrinology, ed 9. WB Saunders, Philadelphia, 1998.
11. Kang, SY and Go, VL: Pancreatic exocrine-endocrine interrelationship. Clinical implications. Gastroenterol Clin North Am 28:551, 1999.
12. Karsch, FJ: Central actions of ovarian steroids in the feedback regulation of pulsatile secretion of luteinizing hormone. Annu Rev Physiol 49:365, 1990.
13. Larsen, PR, Davies, TF, and Hay, ID: The thyroid gland. In Wilson, JD, et al (eds): Williams Textbook of Endocrinology, ed 9. WB Saunders, Philadelphia, 1998.
14. Norman, AW and Litwack, G: Hormones, ed 2. Academic Press, San Diego, 1997.
15. Orth, DN and Kovacs, WJ: The adrenal cortex. In Wilson, JD and Foster, DW (eds): Textbook of Endocrinology, ed 9. WB Saunders, Philadelphia, 1998.
16. Reeves, WB, Bichet, DG, and Andreoli, TE: Posterior pituitary and water metabolism. In Wilson, JD, et al (eds): Textbook of Endocrinology, ed 9. WB Saunders, Philadelphia, 1998.
17. Schimmer, BP and Parker, KL: Adrenocorticotropic hormone; adrenocortical steroids and their synthetic analogs; inhibitors of the synthesis and actions of adrenocortical hormones. In Hardman, JG, et al (eds): The Pharmacological Basis of Therapeutics, ed 9. McGraw-Hill, New York, 1996.
18. Schlaghecke, R, et al: The effect of long-term glucocorticoid therapy on pituitary-adrenal responses to exogenous corticotropin-releasing hormone. N Engl J Med 326:226, 1992.
19. Symposium (various authors): Hormone replacement therapy. Br Med Bull 48:249, 1992.
20. Tenbaum, S and Baniahmad, A: Nuclear receptors: Structure, function, and involvement in disease. Int J Biochem Cell Biol 29:1325, 1997.
21. Thorner, MO, et al: The anterior pituitary. In Wilson, JD and Foster, DW (eds): Textbook of Endocrinology, ed 9. WB Saunders, Philadelphia, 1998.
22. Tsai, M-J, et al: Mechanisms of action of hormones that act as transcription-regulatory factors. In Wilson, JD, et al (eds): Textbook of Endocrinology, ed 9. WB Saunders, Philadelphia, 1998.
23. Williams, CL and Stancel, GM: Estrogens and progestins. In Hardman, JG, et al (eds): The Pharmacological Basis of Therapeutics, ed 9. McGraw-Hill, New York, 1996.
24. Wilson, JD: Androgens. In Hardman, JG, et al (eds): The Pharmacological Basis of Therapeutics, ed 9. McGraw-Hill, New York, 1996.
25. Wilson, JD, et al: Principles of endocrinology. In Wilson, JD and Foster, DW (eds): Textbook of Endocrinology, ed 9. WB Saunders, Philadelphia, 1998.
26. Young, JB and Landsberg, L: Catecholamines and the adrenal medulla. In Wilson, JD, et al (eds): Textbook of Endocrinology, ed 9. WB Saunders, Philadelphia, 1998.

CHAPTER 29

Adrenocorticosteroids

This chapter discusses the pharmacology of the steroid hormones produced by the adrenal cortex. The two primary types of adrenal steroids are the glucocorticoids and mineralocorticoids. Small amounts of other steroids such as the sex hormones (androgens, estrogens, and progestins) are also produced by the adrenal cortex. These steroids are discussed in Chapter 30.

The **adrenocorticosteroids** have several important physiologic and pharmacologic functions. The **glucocorticoids** (cortisol, corticosterone) are primarily involved in the control of glucose metabolism and the body's ability to deal with stress. Glucocorticoids have other attributes, such as their ability to decrease inflammation and suppress the immune system. **Mineralocorticoids** such as aldosterone are involved in maintaining fluid and electrolyte balance in the body.

Adrenal steroids and their synthetic analogs can be administered pharmacologically to mimic the effects of their endogenous counterparts. This approach is frequently undertaken as replacement therapy in various hormonal deficiencies. The quantity administered during hormonal replacement is roughly equivalent to the normal endogenous production and is often referred to as a **physiologic dose.** In higher doses, adrenal steroids can be used to capitalize on a particular beneficial effect, such as using glucocorticoids as anti-inflammatory agents. The larger quantity used to obtain a particular effect is typically referred to as a **pharmacologic dose** to differentiate it from the amount used to maintain normal endocrine function.

Physical therapists and occupational therapists will encounter many patients who are receiving adrenal steroids for replacement of missing hormones or for various other therapeutic reasons. This chapter first discusses the biosynthesis of the adrenal steroids in an effort to show some of the structural and functional similarities between various steroid groups. The basic physiologic and pharmacologic properties of the glucocorticoids are then addressed, followed by a description of mineralocorticoid function. This discussion should provide therapists with a better understanding of the pharmacotherapeutic and toxic characteristics of these compounds.

STEROID SYNTHESIS

The primary pathways involved in steroid biosynthesis are shown in Figure 29–1. These hormones are manufactured by enzymes located in the cytosol of adrenocortical

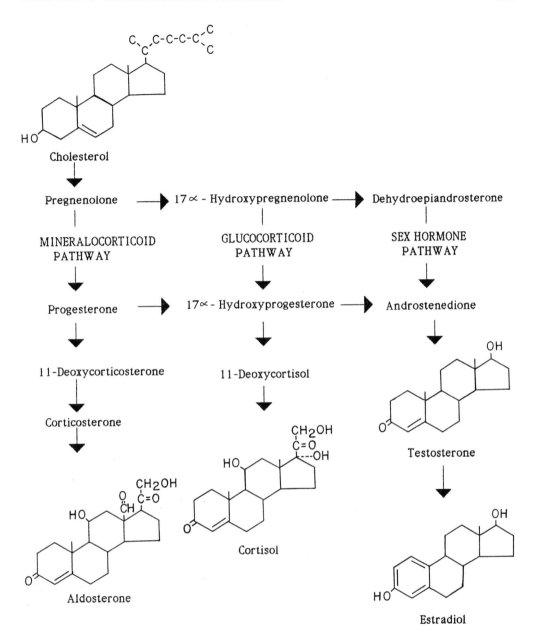

FIGURE 29–1. Pathways of adrenal steroid biosynthesis. Cholesterol is the precursor for the three steroid hormone pathways. Note the similarity between the structures of the primary mineralocorticoid (aldosterone), the primary glucocorticoid (cortisol), and the sex hormones (testosterone, estradiol). See text for further discussion.

cells. As shown in Figure 29–1, there are three primary pathways, each leading to one of the major types of steroid hormone.[27,44] The mineralocorticoid pathway synthesizes aldosterone, the glucocorticoid pathway synthesizes cortisol, and the androgen/estrogen pathway leads to synthesis of the sex hormones. Although all three pathways are present in the adrenal cortex, the mineralocorticoid and glucocorticoid pathways predominate. The appropriate enzymes for sex hormone biosynthesis are also present in the gonads, and the primary site for synthesis of these hormones is in the testes (men) or ovaries (women).

The steroid hormones bear a remarkable structural similarity to one another (see Fig. 29–1). The precursor for steroid biosynthesis is cholesterol. Consequently, all of the steroid hormones share the same basic chemical configuration as their parent compound. This fact has several important physiologic and pharmacologic implications. First, even relatively minor changes in the side chains of the parent compound create steroids with dramatically different physiologic effects. For instance, the addition of only one hydrogen atom in the sex steroid pathway changes testosterone (the primary male hormone) to estradiol (one of the primary female hormones). Second, the structural similarity between different types of steroids helps explain why there is often some crossover in the physiologic effects of each major category. One can readily understand how aldosterone has some glucocorticoid-like activity and cortisol has some mineralocorticoid-like effects when one considers the similarity in their organic configuration. Corticosterone (a glucocorticoid) is even the precursor to aldosterone (a mineralocorticoid).

Steroid structure and biosynthesis have been used from a pharmacologic standpoint. Pharmacologists have tried to develop more effective and less toxic synthetic steroids by manipulating the chemical side groups of these compounds. An example is the synthetic glucocorticoid prednisolone, which is four times more potent than cortisol in reducing inflammation but has less of a tendency to cause sodium retention than the naturally occurring glucocorticoid.[54] Also, excessive steroid synthesis can be rectified in certain situations by using drugs that inhibit specific enzymes shown in the biosynthetic pathways.

GLUCOCORTICOIDS

Role of Glucocorticoids in Normal Function

The primary glucocorticoid released in humans is *cortisol* (also known as hydrocortisone). Cortisol synthesis and secretion are under the control of specific hypothalamic and pituitary hormones.[21,27,51,58,62] Corticotropin-releasing hormone (CRH) from the hypothalamus stimulates the release of adrenocorticotropic hormone (ACTH) from the anterior pituitary. ACTH travels in the systemic circulation to reach the adrenal cortex, where it stimulates cortisol synthesis. Cortisol then travels in the bloodstream to various target tissues to exert a number of physiologic effects (see "Physiologic Effects of Glucocorticoids").

Cortisol also plays a role in controlling the release of CRH and ACTH from the hypothalamus and pituitary, respectively. As illustrated in Figure 29–2, the relationship between plasma cortisol and CRH and ACTH release is a classic example of a negative feedback control system. Increased plasma cortisol levels serve to inhibit subsequent release of CRH and ACTH, thus helping to maintain homeostasis by moderating glucocorticoid activity.

Under normal conditions, cortisol release occurs on a cyclic basis, as shown in Figure 29–3. In an unstressed human, plasma cortisol levels rise slowly throughout the early morning hours and peak at approximately 8 AM. This type of physiologic event is often referred to as a *circadian rhythm,* indicating that the cycle is repeated over a 24-hour period. The fact that plasma cortisol levels progressively increase as the individual is preparing to arise suggests that cortisol helps prepare the organism for increased activity. Indeed, this belief is supported by the observation that in the rat, plasma gluco-

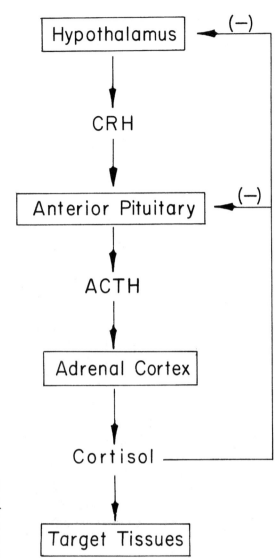

FIGURE 29–2. Negative feedback control of glucocorticoid synthesis. Cortisol limits its own synthesis by inhibiting the release of corticotropin-releasing hormone (CRH) from the hypothalamus and adrenocorticotropic hormone (ACTH) from the anterior pituitary.

corticoid levels peak at around midnight, which corresponds to the time when nocturnal animals are becoming active.

In addition to their normal circadian release, glucocorticoids are also released in response to virtually any stressful stimulus. For instance, trauma, infection, hemorrhage, temperature extremes, food and water deprivation, and any perceived psychologic stress can increase cortisol release.[54] Various stressful events generate afferent input to the hypothalamus, thus evoking CRH and ACTH release from the hypothalamus and anterior pituitary, respectively.

Mechanism of Action of Glucocorticoids

Glucocorticoids affect various cells in a manner characteristic of steroid hormones (see Chap. 28, Fig. 28–3). In general, steroids alter protein synthesis in responsive cells

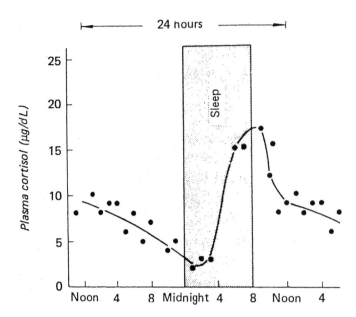

FIGURE 29–3. Circadian rhythm of cortisol production in humans. Peak plasma cortisol levels normally occur at approximately the time an individual awakens (6 to 8 AM). (Reproduced, with permission, from Katzung, BG: Basic and Clinical Pharmacology, ed 2, Lange Medical Publications, 1984, p 454; after Liddle, 1966. Reproduced with permission of the McGraw-Hill Companies.)

through a direct effect on the cell's nucleus. These hormones alter the transcription of specific DNA genes, which results in subsequent changes in RNA synthesis and the translation of RNA into cellular proteins.[48,64]

Specifically, glucocorticoids exert their classic cellular effects by first entering the target cell and binding to a receptor located in the cytosol.[41,48,59] Binding the glucocorticoid to the receptor creates an activated hormone-receptor complex. This activated complex then travels to the nucleus of the cell, where it binds directly to specific DNA gene segments.[9,54] The activated hormone-receptor complex basically acts as a "transcription factor" because it modulates the transcription of DNA into messenger RNA (mRNA) units.[13,61,65] The activated hormone-receptor complex can also inhibit other transcription factors, thereby indirectly altering mRNA transcription.[8,65] Changes in mRNA transcription ultimately lead to a change in protein synthesis in the cell.[2] For example, glucocorticoids exert their anti-inflammatory effects by increasing the transcription of proteins that decrease inflammation while decreasing the transcription of inflammatory cytokines, enzymes, and other inflammatory proteins (see "Anti-Inflammatory Effects").[6,8] Other physiologic and therapeutic effects of glucocorticoids are likewise mediated by altering the expression of proteins that act as cellular enzymes, membrane carriers, receptors, structural proteins, and so on.

Consequently, glucocorticoids induce their primary effects by binding to specific genes and acting as transcription factors that ultimately alter protein synthesis and lead to a change in the physiologic status of the cell. This genomic effect often takes several hours or days to occur because of the time required to alter protein synthesis and create new proteins that reach meaningful concentrations in the cell. However, glucocorticoids may also have a more immediate effect on cell function that is independent of hormonal action at the cell's nucleus.[56] This more rapid effect is probably mediated through a different set of glucocorticoid receptors that are located on the cell membrane.[7,71] By binding to these surface receptors, glucocorticoids could induce rapid changes in cell function by altering membrane permeability, enzyme activity, and other factors.[56] Hence, glucocorticoids may actually affect cell function through two mechanisms: a rapid effect that is mediated by surface receptors and a delayed but more prolonged effect that is mediated by intracellular receptors that affect transcription at the genomic level.[3] Future research should lend insight to the importance of the rapid effects and increase our understanding of how these two effects may interact in producing glucocorticoid-related responses.

Physiologic Effects of Glucocorticoids

Glucocorticoids exert a number of diverse physiologic effects, which are briefly discussed here.

EFFECTS ON GLUCOSE, PROTEIN, AND LIPID METABOLISM

Cortisol and other glucocorticoids increase blood glucose and liver glycogen.[54] This fact is something of a metabolic paradox because circulating levels of glucose are increased at the same time that glucose storage is enhanced. This situation is analogous to being able to draw money out of a savings account while increasing the amount of money in the savings account. The withdrawn money is available to be spent (i.e., the increased blood glucose is readily available as an energy source) while the savings account accrues additional funds (i.e., liver glycogen is increased).

Glucocorticoids accomplish this paradox by affecting the metabolism of glucose, fat, and protein, as shown in Figure 29–4. Cortisol facilitates the breakdown of muscle into

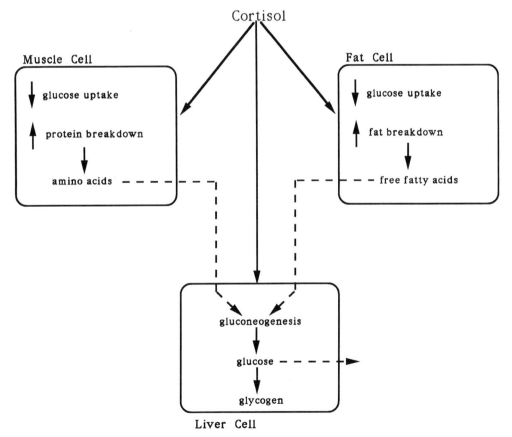

FIGURE 29–4. Effects of cortisol on muscle, fat, and liver cells. Cortisol causes breakdown of muscle and fat into amino acids and free fatty acids, which can be used by the liver to produce glucose.

amino acids and of lipids into free fatty acids, which can be transported to the liver to form glucose (gluconeogenesis). Glucose that is synthesized in the liver can be either stored as glycogen or released back into the bloodstream to increase blood glucose levels. Cortisol also inhibits the uptake of glucose into muscle and fat cells, thus allowing more glucose to remain available in the bloodstream.

Consequently, one of the primary effects of glucocorticoids is to maintain blood glucose and liver glycogen levels to enable a supply of this energy substrate to be readily available for increased activity. This effect occurs during the daily basal release of cortisol and to even a greater extent when high levels of cortisol are released in response to stress. The beneficial effects on glucose titers occur largely at the expense of muscle breakdown, however. This muscle catabolism is one of the primary problems that occurs when glucocorticoids are administered for long periods as a therapeutic agent (see "Adverse Effects of Glucocorticoids").

ANTI-INFLAMMATORY EFFECTS

Glucocorticoids are effective and potent anti-inflammatory agents. Regardless of the cause of the inflammation, glucocorticoids attenuate the heat, erythema, swelling, and tenderness of the affected area. The exact way that these agents intervene in the inflammatory process is complex and not completely understood. Some of the primary anti-inflammatory mechanisms are addressed here.

As indicated earlier, glucocorticoids often inhibit transcription factors that normally stimulate genes within specific cells to express inflammatory components.[8,65] Glucocorticoids, for example, act on macrophages, lymphocytes, and endothelial cells to inhibit the expression of inflammatory proteins (cytokines) such as interleukin-1, interleukin-6, tissue necrosis factor alpha, interferon gamma, and similar inflammatory cytokines.[54] These cytokines are the primary chemical signal for activating various inflammatory cells such as T lymphocytes, fibroblasts, and natural killer cells.[54] By inhibiting the production and release of these inflammatory cytokines, glucocorticoids inhibit the function of key cells that comprise the inflammatory response.

Glucocorticoids also inhibit the transcription and expression of adhesion molecules such as endothelial leukocyte adhesion molecule-1 and intracellular adhesion molecule-1.[8,65] These adhesion molecules are responsible for attracting leukocytes in the bloodstream to endothelial cells at the site of inflammation.[34] Glucocorticoids inhibit the production of these adhesion molecules, thereby diminishing the ability of leukocytes to find and enter the tissues that are inflamed. Glucocorticoids likewise inhibit the production of other chemoattractive chemicals, such as platelet-activating factor and interleukin-1.[54] By limiting the production of factors that attract leukocytes to the site of inflammation, glucocorticoids inhibit a critical step in the initiation of the inflammatory process.[24]

Glucocorticoids inhibit the production of other pro-inflammatory substances such as prostaglandins and leukotrienes.[40,52] The role of these substances in mediating the inflammatory response was discussed in Chapter 15. Glucocorticoids activate specific genes that promote the synthesis of a family of proteins known as *lipocortins*.[17,30,54] Lipocortins inhibit the phospholipase A_2 enzyme, which is the enzyme responsible for liberating phospholipids from cell membranes so that they can be transformed into prostaglandins and leukotrienes (see Chap. 15, Fig. 15–1). By inhibiting this enzyme, glucocorticoids eliminate the precursor for prostaglandin and leukotriene biosynthesis, thus preventing the production of these pro-inflammatory substances.

Finally, high doses of glucocorticoids appear to stabilize lysosomal membranes, thereby making them less fragile and susceptible to rupture.[24] Lysosomes are subcellu-

lar organelles that contain a variety of degradative enzymes. When lysosomes are ruptured, these enzymes begin to digest cellular components, thus contributing to the local
damage present at a site of inflammation. Glucocorticoids may help prevent lysosomal
rupture and the subsequent damage that contributes to the inflammatory response. Glucocorticoids also decrease vascular permeability either by directly causing vasoconstriction or by suppressing the local release of vasoactive substances such as histamine,
kinins, and other chemicals that cause increased capillary permeability.[24] This reduction
in vascular permeability helps control swelling and erythema at the site of inflammation.

IMMUNOSUPPRESSION

Glucocorticoids have long been recognized for their ability to inhibit hypersensitivity reactions, especially the delayed or cell-mediated allergic reactions. The exact way in
which this immunosuppression occurs is unclear, but many of the immunosuppressive
effects are mediated by the same actions that explain the anti-inflammatory effects of
these drugs. As indicated previously, glucocorticoids inhibit the transcription of various
factors that signal and direct other cells in the inflammatory and immune responses.
Loss of these key signals results in decreased migration of leukocytes and macrophages
to the location of a foreign tissue or antigen.[54] These drugs also suppress the ability of
immune cells to synthesize or respond to chemical mediators such as interleukins and
interferons.[3,38,39] Chemicals such as interleukin-1, gamma interferon, and related substances normally mediate the communication between immune system cells such as T
cells, B cells, and other lymphocytes.[18] By suppressing the synthesis and effects of these
mediators, glucocorticoids interrupt cellular interaction and inhibit activation of key
cellular components that cause the immune response. The effects of glucocorticoids on
the immune response and the clinical applications of glucocorticoid-induced immunosuppression are discussed further in Chapter 37.

OTHER EFFECTS OF GLUCOCORTICOIDS

Cortisol and similar glucocorticoids affect a variety of other tissues.[54] These hormones
affect renal function by enhancing sodium and water reabsorption and by impairing the
ability of the kidneys to excrete a water load. They alter CNS function, with abnormal glucocorticoid levels (either too high or too low) producing changes in behavior and mood.
Glucocorticoids alter the formed elements in the blood by facilitating an increase in erythrocytes, neutrophils, and platelets while decreasing the number of lymphocytes,
eosinophils, monocytes, and basophils. Adequate amounts of glucocorticoids are needed
for normal cardiac and skeletal muscle function. Vascular reactivity diminishes and capillary permeability increases if glucocorticoids are not present. Clearly, these hormones are
involved in regulating a number of diverse and important physiologic functions.

THERAPEUTIC GLUCOCORTICOID AGENTS

The primary glucocorticoids used pharmacologically are listed in Table 29–1. These
drugs are either chemically identical to the naturally occurring hormones, or they are
synthetic analogs of cortisol. The clinical choice of a particular agent depends on the
problem being treated and the desired effect in each patient.

As indicated in Table 29–1, glucocorticoids are available in various preparations
that correspond to specific routes of administration. For instance, systemic preparations

TABLE 29–1 Therapeutic Glucocorticoids

Generic Name	Common Trade Name(s)	Systemic	Topical	Inhalation	Ophthalmic	Otic	Nasal
				Type of Preparation Available			
Alclometasone	Aclovate		X				
Amcinonide	Cyclocort		X				
Beclomethasone	Beclovent, Vanceril, others		X	X			X
Betamethasone	Celestone, Uticort, others	X	X		X	X	X
Budesonide	Pulmicort Turbohaler, Rhinocort			X			X
Clobetasol	Dermovate, Temovate		X				
Clocortolone	Cloderm		X				
Cortisone	Cortone	X					
Desonide	DesOwen, Tridesilon		X				
Desoximetasone	Topicort		X				
Dexamethasone	Decadron, Dexasone, others	X	X	X	X	X	X
Diflorasone	Florone, Maxiflor		X				
Flumethasone	Locacorten		X				
Flunisolide	Aerobid, Nasalide			X			X
Fluocinolone	Flurosyn, Synalar, others		X				
Fluocinonide	Lidex, others		X				
Fluorometholone	FML S.O.P., Fluor-Op, others				X		
Flurandrenolide	Cordran		X				
Fluticasone	Cutivate, Flonase		X				X
Halcinonide	Halog		X				
Halobetasol	Ultravate		X				
Hydrocortisone	Cortaid, Dermacort, Hydrocortone, many others	X	X		X		
Medrysone	HMS Liquifilm				X		
Methylprednisolone	Medrol	X					
Mometasone	Elocon, Nasonex		X				X
Prednisolone	Pediapred, Prelone, others				X		
Prednisone	Deltasone, Meticorten, others	X					
Triamcinolone	Azmacort, Aristocort, Nasacort	X	X	X			X

can be administered either orally or parenterally to treat systemic disorders (such as collagen diseases and adrenocortical insufficiency). In more localized problems, these agents may be applied directly to a specific area using other preparations (e.g., topical, ophthalmic). Glucocorticoids are sometimes injected into a specific tissue or anatomic space to treat a localized problem. For instance, certain types of back and neck pain may be treated by injection into the epidural space,[12,60] and local glucocorticoid injections have been used to treat problems such as carpal tunnel syndrome.[23] Likewise, glucocorticoids may be injected directly into a joint to treat severe acute inflammation that is isolated to that joint. The repeated intra-articular administration of glucocorticoids is not advisable, however, because of the catabolic effect of these hormones on supporting tissues (see "Adverse Effects of Glucocorticoids"). Also, the repeated injection of glucocorticoids in and around tendons is not recommended because glucocorticoids can cause breakdown and rupture of these structures.[16,43] Hence, a general rule of thumb is to limit the number of glucocorticoid injections into a specific joint to four or fewer per year.[49]

CLINICAL USES OF GLUCOCORTICOIDS

Glucocorticoids are used in two primary situations: to evaluate and treat endocrine disorders and to help resolve the symptoms of a variety of nonendocrine problems. These two major applications are discussed here.

Glucocorticoid Use in Endocrine Conditions

REPLACEMENT THERAPY

Glucocorticoids are administered to help restore normal function in conditions of adrenal cortical hypofunction. Glucocorticoid replacement is instituted in both primary and secondary adrenal insufficiency. In primary insufficiency (Addison disease), glucocorticoid production is deficient because of destruction of the adrenal cortex. In secondary insufficiency, adrenal cortex function is diminished because of other factors, such as a lack of adequate ACTH release from the anterior pituitary. Replacement therapy can also be initiated after the removal of the adrenals or pituitary gland because of disease and tumors. For instance, adrenalectomy or destruction of the pituitary to resolve adrenal cortical hypersecretion (Cushing syndrome) is typically followed by long-term glucocorticoid administration. Replacement therapy is needed to maintain optimum health whenever normal physiologic function of the adrenal cortex is disrupted.

EVALUATION OF ENDOCRINE DYSFUNCTION

Glucocorticoids may be given for diagnostic purposes to evaluate hormonal disorders. Exogenous glucocorticoids (especially the synthetic hormones such as dexamethasone) are potent inhibitors of ACTH secretion from the anterior pituitary. By suppressing the secretion of ACTH, glucocorticoids can help determine whether an endocrine imbalance is influenced by ACTH secretion. Favorable changes in the endocrine profile during ACTH suppression indicate that ACTH and ACTH-related hormones have a role in mediating the abnormality.

Use in Nonendocrine Conditions

Glucocorticoids are used primarily for their anti-inflammatory and immunosuppressive effects to treat a long and diverse list of nonendocrine conditions. Some of the approved indications for glucocorticoid administration are listed in Table 29–2. Of particular interest to rehabilitation specialists is the use of these agents in treating collagen diseases and rheumatic disorders, including rheumatoid arthritis.

As indicated in Table 29–2, these drugs are generally used to control inflammation or suppress the immune system for relatively short periods of time, regardless of the underlying pathology. The very fact that these drugs are successful in such a wide range of disorders illustrates that glucocorticoids do not cure the underlying problem. In a sense, they treat only a symptom of the original disease—that is, inflammation. This fact is important because the patient may appear to be improving, with decreased symptoms of inflammation, while the disease continues to worsen. Also, glucocorticoids are often administered in fairly high dosages to capitalize on their anti-inflammatory and im-

TABLE 29–2 Nonendocrine Disorders Treated with Glucocorticoids

General Indication	Principal Desired Effect of Glucocorticoids	Examples of Specific Disorders
Allergic disorders	Decreased inflammation	Anaphylactic reactions, drug-induced allergic reactions, severe hay fever, serum sickness
Collagen disorders	Immunosuppression	Acute rheumatic carditis, dermatomyositis, systemic lupus erythematosus
Dermatologic disorders	Decreased inflammation	Alopecia areata, dermatitis (various forms), keloids, lichens, mycosis fungoides, pemphigus, psoriasis
Gastrointestinal disorders	Decreased inflammation	Crohn disease, ulcerative colitis
Hematologic disorders	Immunosuppression	Autoimmune hemolytic anemia, congenital hypoplastic anemia, erythroblastopenia, thrombocytopenia
Nonrheumatic inflammation	Decreased inflammation	Bursitis, tenosynovitis
Neoplastic disease	Immunosuppression	Leukemias, lymphomas, nasal polyps, cystic tumors
Neurologic disease	Decreased inflammation and immunosuppression	Tuberculous meningitis, multiple sclerosis, myasthenia gravis
Neurotrauma	Decreased edema*	Brain surgery, closed head injury, certain brain tumors
Ophthalmic disorders	Decreased inflammation	Chorioretinitis, conjunctivitis, herpes zoster ophthalmicus, iridocyclitis, keratitis, optic neuritis
Respiratory disorders	Decreased inflammation	Bronchial asthma, berylliosis, aspiration pneumonitis, symptomatic sarcoidosis, pulmonary tuberculosis
Rheumatic disorders	Decreased inflammation and immunosuppression	Ankylosing spondylitis, psoriatic arthritis, rheumatoid arthritis, gouty arthritis, osteoarthritis

*Efficacy of glucocorticoid use in decreasing cerebral edema has not been conclusively proved.

munosuppressive effects. These high dosages may create serious adverse effects when given for prolonged periods (see the next section, "Adverse Effects of Glucocorticoids"). Despite these limitations, glucocorticoids can be extremely helpful and even lifesaving in the short-term control of severe inflammation and various allergic responses.

ADVERSE EFFECTS OF GLUCOCORTICOIDS

The effectiveness and extensive clinical use of natural and synthetic glucocorticoids must be tempered by the serious side effects produced by these agents. Some of the more common problems associated with glucocorticoid use are described here.

Adrenocortical Suppression

Adrenocortical suppression occurs because of the negative feedback effect of the administered glucocorticoids on the hypothalamic–anterior pituitary system and the adrenal glands.[26,55] Basically, the patient's normal production of glucocorticoids is shut down by the exogenous hormones. The magnitude and duration of this suppression are related to the dosage, route of administration, and duration of glucocorticoid therapy.[19,54] Some degree of adrenocortical suppression can occur after even a single large systemic dose.[72] This suppression will become more pronounced as systemic administration is continued for longer periods. Also, topical glucocorticoid administration over an extensive area of the body (especially in infants) may provide enough systemic absorption to suppress adrenocortical function.[22,57] Adrenocortical suppression can be a serious problem when glucocorticoid therapy is terminated. Patients who have experienced complete suppression will not be able to immediately resume production of glucocorticoids. Because abrupt withdrawal can be life-threatening, glucocorticoids must be withdrawn slowly by tapering the dose.[35]

Drug-Induced Cushing Syndrome

In drug-induced Cushing syndrome, patients begin to exhibit many of the symptoms associated with the adrenocortical hypersecretion typical of naturally occurring Cushing syndrome.[27] These patients commonly exhibit symptoms of roundness and puffiness in the face, fat deposition and obesity in the trunk region, muscle wasting in the extremities, hypertension, osteoporosis, increased body hair (*hirsutism*), and glucose intolerance. These changes are all caused by the metabolic effects of the glucocorticoids. These adverse effects can be alleviated somewhat by reducing the glucocorticoid dosage. Some of the Cushing syndrome effects must often be tolerated, however, to allow the glucocorticoids to maintain a therapeutic effect (decreased inflammation or immunosuppression).

Breakdown of Supporting Tissues

Glucocorticoids exert a general catabolic effect not only on muscle (as described previously) but also on other tissues. Bone, ligaments, tendons, and skin are also subject to a wasting effect from prolonged glucocorticoid use. Glucocorticoids weaken these supporting tissues by inhibiting collagen formation. Glucocorticoids appear to bind directly to the genes that are responsible for collagen production and to prevent transcription of these genes.[47] The molecular basis for the effects of glucocorticoids on skeletal muscle is complex and somewhat unclear, but glucocorticoids probably interfere with muscle protein synthesis by altering the muscle's ability to retain and use amino acids.[4,10] Thus, these drugs cause atrophy of skeletal muscle by increasing the rate of protein breakdown and decreasing the rate of protein synthesis.[29] In severe cases, glucocorticoids can induce a steroid myopathy that is characterized by proximal muscle weakness that can affect ambulation and functional ability.[54] This type of myopathy is typically resolved by discontinuing the glucocorticoid, but symptoms may persist long after the drug has been withdrawn.[54]

The magnitude of the wasting effect caused by systemic glucocorticoids is dependent on many factors, including the patient's overall health and the duration and dosage of drug therapy. Although some evidence exists that low doses of these drugs can be given for prolonged periods without excessive bone loss,[45] other sources believe that significant bone and muscle loss can occur in some women even when these drugs are given in low doses.[14,30] Likewise, moderate to high doses will almost certainly cause some degree of muscle and bone loss in all patients when glucocorticoids are administered continuously for more than a few weeks.[37,69,70]

The potential for tissue breakdown must always be considered during rehabilitation of patients taking these drugs, and therapists must be especially careful to avoid overstressing tissues that are weakened by the prolonged use of systemic glucocorticoids. Likewise, bone loss and risk of osteoporosis should be evaluated periodically in patients receiving long-term systemic glucocorticoids.[70] Patients with evidence of excessive bone loss can be treated with drugs such as the bisphosphonates (etidronate, pamidronate) and calcitonin.[20,36] Estrogen replacement may also be helpful in minimizing bone loss in women receiving glucocorticoids.[20,25] The ability of various drugs to stabilize bone and prevent osteoporosis is addressed in Chapter 31.

Other Adverse Effects

Several other problems can occur during prolonged glucocorticoid use. Peptic ulcer may develop because of either the breakdown of supporting proteins in the stomach wall or direct mucosal irritation by the drugs. An increased susceptibility to infection often occurs because of the immunosuppressive effect of glucocorticoids. These drugs may retard growth in children because of their inhibitory effect on bone and muscle growth and because they inhibit growth hormone.[15] Glucocorticoids may cause glaucoma by impairing the normal drainage of aqueous fluid from the eye, and cataract formation is also associated with prolonged use.[63] Mood changes and even psychoses have been reported, but the reasons for these occurrences are not clear.[68] Glucocorticoids with some mineralocorticoid-like activity may cause hypertension because of sodium and water retention. Some of the newer synthetic drugs have fewer mineralocorticoid effects, however, and hypertension occurs less frequently with these. Finally, glucocorticoids alter glucose metabolism, and people with diabetes mellitus will have an increased risk of hyperglycemia, insulin resistance, and decreased control of blood glucose levels.[5,31]

DRUGS THAT INHIBIT ADRENOCORTICAL HORMONE BIOSYNTHESIS

Occasionally, the production of adrenal steroids must be inhibited because of adrenocortical hyperactivity. Several agents are available that block specific enzymes in the glucocorticoid biosynthetic pathway. Aminoglutethimide (Cytadren) inhibits the first step in adrenal corticoid synthesis by blocking the conversion of cholesterol to subsequent hormone precursors (see Fig. 29–1). Metyrapone (Metopirone) inhibits the hydroxylation reaction of several intermediate compounds in the adrenal corticoid pathway. Trilostane (Modrastane) likewise inhibits a key enzyme in steroid biosynthesis, but this drug does not seem as effective as other agents in this category. Finally, mitotane (Lysodren) is an antineoplastic drug used in treating adrenal tumors (see Chap. 36), but mitotane can also be used to reduce hyperactivity of the adrenal gland in endocrine disorders. Mitotane directly suppresses the adrenal gland, although the exact mechanism of this suppression is unclear.

These drugs therefore reduce adrenal corticoid hypersecretion in conditions such as adrenal tumors. Adrenal hypersecretion caused by increased pituitary ACTH release (Cushing syndrome of pituitary origin) may also be resolved temporarily by these drugs. However, a longer term solution to pituitary ACTH hypersecretion, such as pituitary irradiation, is usually desirable.[54] Metyrapone is also used to test hypothalamic–anterior pituitary function. Specifically, this drug is used to evaluate the ability of the anterior pituitary to release ACTH. When this drug attenuates the production of adrenal glucocorticoids, the anterior pituitary should respond by secreting ACTH into the bloodstream. If the ACTH response is too low, pituitary hypofunction is indicated. Pituitary hyperfunction, Cushing syndrome of pituitary origin, is indicated if the ACTH response is exaggerated.

MINERALOCORTICOIDS

Mineralocorticoids are also steroid hormones that are produced by the adrenal cortex. The principal mineralocorticoid in humans is *aldosterone*. Aldosterone is primarily involved in maintaining fluid and electrolyte balance in the body. This hormone works on the kidneys to increase sodium and water reabsorption and potassium excretion.

Regulation of Mineralocorticoid Secretion

Aldosterone release is regulated by several factors that are related to the fluid and electrolyte status in the body.[50] A primary stimulus for aldosterone release is increased levels of *angiotensin II*.[42,46] Angiotensin II is part of the renin-angiotensin system, which is concerned with maintaining blood pressure (see Chap. 21). Basically, a sudden fall in blood pressure initiates a chain of events that generates increased circulating levels of angiotensin II. Angiotensin II helps maintain blood pressure by vasoconstricting peripheral vessels. Angiotensin II (and probably also its metabolic by-product angiotensin III) also helps exert a more prolonged antihypotensive effect by stimulating aldosterone secretion from the adrenal cortex. Aldosterone can then facilitate sodium and water retention, thus maintaining adequate plasma volume.

In addition to the angiotensin II effects, aldosterone secretion is regulated by increased plasma potassium levels.[50] Presumably, elevated plasma potassium serves as a stimulus to increase aldosterone release, thus causing increased potassium excretion and a return to normal plasma levels. Finally, there is evidence that ACTH may also play a role in aldosterone release. Although ACTH is primarily involved in controlling glucocorticoid secretion, this hormone may also stimulate mineralocorticoid release to some extent.[50]

Mechanism of Action and Physiologic Effects of Mineralocorticoids

Aldosterone exerts its effects on the kidneys by binding to specific receptors in epithelial cells that line the distal tubule of the nephron.[56,67] These receptors have a high affinity for mineralocorticoid hormones. They also have a moderate affinity for many of the natural glucocorticoid hormones (e.g., cortisol) and a low affinity for the newer synthetic glucocorticoids, such as dexamethasone. This accounts for the finding that certain glucocorticoids exert some mineralocorticoid-like effects, whereas others have relatively minor effects on electrolyte and fluid balance.[54]

Mineralocorticoids are believed to increase sodium reabsorption by affecting sodium channels and sodium pumps on the epithelial cells that line the renal tubules.[1,11] The ability of mineralocorticoids to increase the expression of sodium channels is illustrated in Figure 29–5. These hormones enter the tubular epithelial cell, bind to receptors in the cell, and create an activated hormone-receptor complex.[56] This complex then travels to the nucleus to initiate transcription of messenger RNA units, which are translated into specific membrane-related proteins.[53] These proteins in some way either create or help open sodium pores on the cell membrane, thus allowing sodium to leave the tubule and enter the epithelial cell by passive diffusion.[67] Sodium is then actively transported out of the cell and reabsorbed into the bloodstream. Water reabsorption is increased as water follows the sodium movement back into the bloodstream. As sodium is reabsorbed, potassium is secreted by a sodium-potassium exchange, thus increasing potassium excretion (see Fig. 29–5).

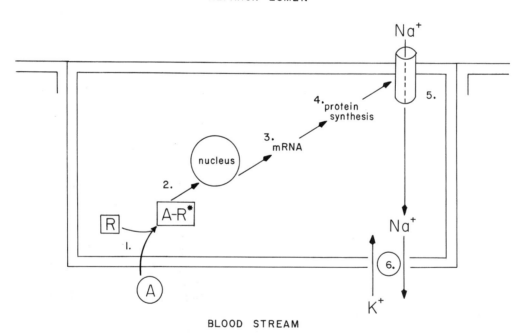

FIGURE 29–5. Effect of aldosterone on renal tubule cells. (*1*) Aldosterone (A) enters the cell and binds to a cytosolic receptor (R), creating an activated hormone-receptor complex (A–R). (*2*) A–R complex travels to the cell's nucleus, where it induces mRNA synthesis. (*3*) mRNA units undergo translation in the cytosol. (*4*) Specific proteins are synthesized that increase membrane permeability to sodium (Na^+). (*5*) Na^+ leaves the nephron lumen and enters the cell down an electrochemical gradient. (*6*) Na^+ is actively reabsorbed into the body, and potassium (K^+) is actively secreted from the bloodstream by the cellular Na^+-K^+ pump.

In addition to their effects on the synthesis of membrane sodium channels, mineralocorticoids also have a more rapid and immediate effect on sodium reabsorption.[11,66] This effect probably occurs because the hormone binds to a different set of receptors on the epithelial cell membrane and increases the activity of existing sodium channels and pumps such as the Na^+-K^+ ATPase.[56] Hence, the effects of mineralocorticoids, like the glucocorticoids discussed earlier, seem to occur in two phases: a rapid phase that is mediated by surface receptors and a delayed but prolonged phase that is mediated by intracellular receptors that bind to the cell's nucleus and increase transcription of specific proteins.[11,56] These two phases of mineralocorticoid action both play a role in the physiologic action of these hormones, and future research should help define how these actions can be affected by various drugs and diseases.

Therapeutic Use of Mineralocorticoid Drugs

Drugs with mineralocorticoid-like activity (aldosterone agonists) are frequently administered as replacement therapy whenever the natural production of mineralocorticoids is impaired. Mineralocorticoid replacement is usually required in patients with chronic adrenocortical insufficiency (Addison disease), following adrenalectomy, and in other forms of adrenal cortex hypofunction. These conditions usually require both mineralocorticoid and glucocorticoid replacement.

Fludrocortisone (Florinef) is the primary aldosterone-like agent that is used in replacement therapy. This compound is chemically classified as a glucocorticoid, but it has high levels of mineralocorticoid activity and is used exclusively as a mineralocorticoid. Fludrocortisone is administered orally.

Adverse Effects of Mineralocorticoid Agonists

The primary problem associated with mineralocorticoid agonists is hypertension. Because these drugs increase sodium and water retention, blood pressure may increase if the dosage is too high. Other adverse effects may include peripheral edema, weight gain, and hypokalemia. These problems are also caused by the effects of these drugs on electrolyte and fluid balance, and they are usually resolved by adjusting the dosage.

Mineralocorticoid Antagonists

Spironolactone (Aldactone) is a competitive antagonist of the aldosterone receptor. This drug binds to the receptor but does not activate it. When bound to the receptor, spironolactone blocks the effects of endogenous mineralocorticoids by preventing them from binding. Consequently, spironolactone antagonizes the normal physiologic effects of aldosterone, resulting in increased sodium and water excretion and decreased potassium excretion.

Spironolactone is used primarily as a diuretic in treating hypertension. This drug is classified as a potassium-sparing diuretic because it helps increase sodium and water excretion without increasing the excretion of potassium (see Chap. 21). Spironolactone is also used to help diagnose hyperaldosteronism. The drug is given for several days to antagonize the effects of excessive aldosterone production. When the drug is discontinued, serum potassium levels will decrease sharply if hyperaldosteronism is present; that is, plasma potassium levels will fall when aldosterone is again permitted to increase potassium excretion.

Mineralocorticoid antagonists such as spironolactone may cause an increase in plasma potassium levels (hyperkalemia), which could be life-threatening if prolonged or severe. This drug can also interfere with the function of the endogenous sex hormones, thereby producing side effects such as increased body hair, deepening of the voice, decreased libido, menstrual irregularities, and breast enlargement in men. Spironolactone is likewise associated with CNS effects (drowsiness, lethargy, confusion, headache) and gastrointestinal disturbances (diarrhea, stomach pain, gastric ulcers).

SPECIAL CONCERNS OF ADRENAL STEROID USE IN REHABILITATION PATIENTS

Adrenal steroids play an important role in the pharmacologic management of many patients seen in rehabilitation. As indicated in Table 29–2, systemic conditions such as rheumatoid arthritis, ankylosing spondylitis, and lupus erythematosus are often treated with glucocorticoid drugs. More localized musculoskeletal conditions, such as acute bursitis and tenosynovitis, may also be treated for short periods with glucocorticoids. Because these problems are often being treated simultaneously in a rehabilitation setting, therapists must be especially cognizant of the effects and implications of glucocorticoids.

The primary aspect of glucocorticoid administration that should concern therapists is the catabolic effect of these hormones on supporting tissues. As discussed previously, glucocorticoids cause a general breakdown in muscle, bone, skin, and other collagenous structures. The glucocorticoid-induced catabolism of these tissues can be even greater than expected in the presence of other contributing factors such as inactivity, poor nutrition, and the effects of aging. For instance, a certain amount of osteoporosis would be expected in an elderly, sedentary woman with rheumatoid arthritis. The use of glucocorticoids, however, may greatly accelerate the bone dissolution in such a patient, even when these drugs are used for relatively limited periods.[45]

Therapists can help attenuate some of the catabolic effects of these drugs. Strengthening activities help maintain muscle mass and prevent severe wasting of the musculotendinous unit.[28,29,32,33] Various strengthening and weight-bearing activities may also reduce bone loss to some extent. In general, any activities that promote mobility and ambulation will be beneficial during and after glucocorticoid therapy. Therapists must use caution, however, to avoid injuring structures that are weakened by glucocorticoid use. The load placed on the musculoskeletal system must be sufficient to evoke a therapeutic response but not so excessive that musculoskeletal structures are damaged. The difference between therapeutic stress and harmful stress may be rather small in some patients taking glucocorticoids. Therapists must use sound clinical judgment when developing and implementing exercise routines for these patients. Because glucocorticoids also cause thinning and wasting of skin, therapists should also ensure that extra efforts are made to prevent skin breakdown in patients on prolonged glucocorticoid therapy.

Other aspects of prolonged adrenocorticoid administration also concern physical therapists and occupational therapists. Therapists should be aware of the sodium- and water-retaining properties of both glucocorticoids and mineralocorticoids. When used in acute situations or in long-term replacement therapy, both groups of adrenal steroids may cause hypertension. Therapists should routinely monitor blood pressure in patients taking either type of agent. Because of their immunosuppressive effects, glucocorticoids increase patients' susceptibility to infection. Therapists must be especially cautious about exposing these patients to any possible sources of infection. Finally, therapists should be alert for any other signs of toxicity to adrenal steroids, such as mood changes or psychoses. Therapists may recognize the early stages of such toxic reactions and prevent serious consequences by alerting the medical staff.

CASE STUDY

ADRENOCORTICOSTEROIDS

Brief History. E.M. is a 58-year-old woman with a history of rheumatoid arthritis. She has involvement of many joints in her body, but her knees are especially affected by this disease. Her symptoms of pain, swelling, and inflammation are controlled fairly well by nonsteroidal anti-inflammatory drugs. She does experience periods of exacerbation and remission, however. During periods of exacerbation, she receives physical therapy as an outpatient at a physical therapy private practice. Physical therapy typically consists of heat, ultrasound, range of motion, and strengthening activities to both knees. During a recent exacerbation, her symptoms were more severe than usual, and the patient began to develop flexion contractures in both knees. The therapist suggested that she consult her physician. Upon noting the severe inflammation, the physician elected to inject both knees with a glucocorticoid agent. Prednisolone (Predicort-RP) was injected into the knee joints. The patient was advised to continue physical therapy on a daily basis.

Problem/Influence of Medication. Glucocorticoid administration produced a dramatic decrease in the swelling and inflammation in both knees. The therapist was tempted to begin aggressive stretching activities to resolve the knee flexion contractures and restore normal range of motion. The therapist was aware, however, that glucocorticoids may weaken ligaments, tendons, and other supporting structures because of an inhibitory effect on collagen formation. The therapist also realized that this effect may be present for some time after glucocorticoid administration. Even though only a single intra-articular injection was used, the drug may be retained locally within fat and other tissues because of the high degree of lipid solubility of steroid agents. Consequently, the injected glucocorticoid may continue to exert a catabolic effect on knee joint structures for some time.

Decision/Solution. The therapist was especially careful to use low-intensity, prolonged-duration stretching forces when trying to resolve the knee flexion contractures. Gentle stretching, massage, and other manual techniques were continued until full active and passive knee extension was achieved.

SUMMARY

The two principal groups of adrenal steroids are the glucocorticoids and mineralocorticoids. These hormones are synthesized from cholesterol within cells of the adrenal cortex. The primary glucocorticoid produced in humans is cortisol (hydrocortisone), and the primary mineralocorticoid is aldosterone. Glucocorticoids exert a number of effects such as regulation of glucose metabolism, attenuation of the inflammatory response, and suppression of the immune system. Mineralocorticoids are involved primarily in the control of fluid and electrolyte balance.

Pharmacologically, natural and synthetic adrenal steroids are often used as replacement therapy to resolve a deficiency in adrenal cortex function. The glucocorticoids are also administered primarily for their anti-inflammatory and immunosuppressive effects in a diverse group of clinical problems. These agents can be extremely beneficial in controlling the symptoms of various rheumatic and allergic disorders. Prolonged glucocorticoid use, however, is limited by a number of serious adverse effects, such as adrenocortical suppression and breakdown of muscle, bone, and other tissues. Physical therapists and occupational therapists should be especially aware of the potential side effects of glucocorticoids, which are used in many disorders that are seen in a rehabilitation setting.

REFERENCES

1. Agarwal, MK and Mirshahi, M: General overview of mineralocorticoid hormone action. Pharmacol Ther 84:273, 1999.
2. Ahluwalia, A: Topical glucocorticoids and the skin—mechanisms of action: An update. Mediators Inflamm 7:183, 1998.
3. Almawi, WY, Hess, DA, and Rieder, MJ: Multiplicity of glucocorticoid action in inhibiting allograft rejection. Cell Transplant 7:511, 1998.
4. Almon, RR and Dubois, DC: Fiber-type discrimination in disease and glucocorticoid-induced atrophy. Med Sci Sports Exerc 22:304, 1990.
5. Andrews, RC and Walker, BR: Glucocorticoids and insulin resistance: Old hormones, new targets. Clin Sci (Colch) 96:513, 1999.
6. Angeli, A, et al: Modulation by cytokines of glucocorticoid action. Ann N Y Acad Sci 876:210, 1999.
7. Barbarino, A and Colasanti, S: Membrane receptors and hormones. Q J Nucl Med 39(Suppl 1):78, 1995.
8. Barnes, PJ: Anti-inflammatory actions of glucocorticoids: Molecular mechanisms. Clin Sci 94:557, 1998.
9. Becker, PB, et al: In vivo protein-DNA interactions in a glucocorticoid response element require the presence of the hormone. Nature 324:686, 1986.
10. Block, KP and Buse, MG: Glucocorticoid regulation of muscle branched-chain amino acid metabolism. Med Sci Sports Exerc 22:316, 1990.
11. Bonvalet, JP: Regulation of sodium transport by steroid hormones. Kidney Int Suppl 65:S49, 1998.
12. Bowman, SJ, et al: Outcome assessment after epidural corticosteroid injection for low back pain and sciatica. Spine 18:1345, 1993.
13. Burnstein, KL and Cidlowski, JA: Regulation of gene expression by glucocorticoids. Annu Rev Physiol 51:683, 1989.
14. Caldwell, JR and Furst, DE: The efficacy and safety of low-dose corticosteroids for rheumatoid arthritis. Semin Arthritis Rheum 21:1, 1991.
15. Cave, A, Arlett, P, and Lee, E: Inhaled and nasal corticosteroids: Factors affecting the risks of systemic adverse effects. Pharmacol Ther 83:153, 1999.
16. Cox, JS: Current concepts in the role of steroids in the treatment of sprains and strains. Med Sci Sports Exerc 16:216, 1984.
17. Davidson, FF and Dennis, EA: Biological relevance of lipocortins and related proteins as inhibitors of phospholipase A_2. Biochem Pharmacol 38:3645, 1989.
18. Dinarello, CA and Mier, JW: Lymphokines. N Engl J Med 317:940, 1987.
19. Dluhy, RG: Clinical relevance of inhaled corticosteroids and HPA axis suppression. J Allergy Clin Immunol 101(Part 2):S447, 1998.
20. Eastell, R, et al: A UK consensus group on management of glucocorticoid-induced osteoporosis: An update. J Intern Med 244:271, 1998.
21. Fitzgerald, PA and Klonoff, DC: Hypothalamic and pituitary hormones. In Katzung, BG (ed): Basic and Clinical Pharmacology, ed 7. Appleton & Lange, Stamford, CT, 1998.
22. Garden, JM and Freinkel, RK: Systemic absorption of topical steroids: Metabolic effects as an index of mild hypercortisolism. Arch Dermatol 122:1007, 1986.
23. Giannini, F, et al: Electrophysiologic evaluation of local steroid injection in carpal tunnel syndrome. Arch Phys Med Rehabil 72:738, 1991.
24. Goldfien, A: Adrenocorticosteroids and adrenocortical antagonists. In Katzung, BG (ed): Basic and Clinical Pharmacology, ed 7. Appleton & Lange, Stamford, CT, 1998.
25. Goldstein, MF, Fallon, JJ, and Harning, R: Chronic glucocorticoid therapy-induced osteoporosis in patients with obstructive lung disease. Chest 116:1733, 1999.
26. Grossman, A: Steroid safety: The endocrinologist's view. Int J Clin Pract Suppl 96:33, 1998.
27. Gums, JG and Smith, JD: Adrenal gland disorders. In DiPiro, JT, et al (eds): Pharmacotherapy: A Pathophysiologic Approach, ed 4. Appleton & Lange, Stamford, CT, 1999.

28. Hickson, RC, et al: Glucocorticoid antagonism by exercise and androgenic-anabolic steroids. Med Sci Sports Exerc 22:331, 1990.
29. Hickson, RC and Marone, JR: Exercise and inhibition of glucocorticoid-induced muscle atrophy. Exerc Sport Sci Rev 21:135, 1993.
30. Hirata, F: Glucocorticoids and head injury: A possible participation of lipocortin (lipomodulin) in actions of steroid hormones. Neurochem Pathol 7:33, 1987.
31. Hoogwerf, B and Danese, RD: Drug selection and the management of corticosteroid-related diabetes mellitus. Rheum Dis Clin North Am 25:489, 1999.
32. Horber, FF, et al: Impact of physical training on the ultrastructure of midthigh muscle in normal subjects and in patients treated with glucocorticoids. J Clin Invest 79:1181, 1987.
33. Horber, FF, et al: Evidence that prednisone-induced myopathy is reversed by physical training. J Clin Endocrinol Metab 61:83, 1985.
34. Insel, PA: Analgesic-antipyretic and antiinflammatory agents and drugs employed in the treatment of gout. In Hardman, JG, et al (eds): The Pharmacological Basis of Therapeutics, ed 9. McGraw-Hill, New York, 1996.
35. Kountz, DS and Clark, CL: Safely withdrawing patients from chronic glucocorticoid therapy. Am Fam Physician 55:521, 1997.
36. Laan, RF, Jansen, TL, and van Riel, PL: Glucocorticoids in the management of rheumatoid arthritis. Rheumatology 38:6, 1999.
37. Lane, NE and Lukert, B: The science and therapy of glucocorticoid-induced bone loss. Endocrinol Metab Clin North Am 27:465, 1998.
38. Lee, SW, et al: Glucocorticoids selectively inhibit the transcription of the interleukin 1-beta gene and decrease stability of interleukin 1-beta messenger RNA. Proc Natl Acad Sci U S A 85:1204, 1988.
39. Lew, W, Oppenheim, JJ, and Matsushima, K: Analysis of the suppression of IL-1 alpha and IL-1 beta products in human peripheral blood mononuclear adherent cells by a glucocorticoid hormone. J Immunol 140:1895, 1988.
40. Lewis, GD, Campbell, WB, and Johnson, AR: Inhibition of prostaglandin synthesis of glucocorticoids in human endothelial cells. Endocrinology 119:62, 1986.
41. Litwack, G, et al: Steroid receptor activation: The glucocorticoid receptor as a model system. In Chrousos, GP, Loriaux, DL, and Lipsett, MD (eds): Steroid Hormone Resistance: Mechanism and Clinical Aspects. Plenum Press, New York, 1986.
42. Lumbers, ER: Angiotensin and aldosterone. Regul Pept 80:91, 1999.
43. Mahler, F and Fritschy, D: Partial and complete ruptures of the Achilles tendon and local corticosteroid injections. Br J Sports Med 26:7, 1992.
44. Milgrom, E: Steroid hormones. In Baulieu, EE and Kelly, PA (eds): Hormones: From Molecules to Disease. Chapman & Hall, New York, 1990.
45. Mitchell, DR and Lyles, KW: Minireview: Glucocorticoid-induced osteoporosis: Mechanisms for bone loss; evaluation of strategies for prevention. J Gerontol 45:M153, 1990.
46. Mulrow, PJ: Angiotensin II and aldosterone regulation. Regul Pept 80:27, 1999.
47. Oikarinen, AI, et al: Modulation of collagen metabolism by glucocorticoids: Receptor-mediated effects of dexamethasone on collagen biosynthesis in chick embryo fibroblasts and chondrocytes. Biochem Pharmacol 37:1451, 1988.
48. O'Malley, BW, Schrader, WT, and Tsai, M-J: Molecular actions of steroid hormones. In Chrousos, GP, Loriaux, DL, and Lipsett, MD (eds): Steroid Hormone Resistance: Mechanism and Clinical Aspects. Plenum Press, New York, 1986.
49. Porter, DR and Sturrock, RD: Fortnightly review: Medical management of rheumatoid arthritis. BMJ 307:425, 1993.
50. Quinn, SJ and Williams, GH: Regulation of aldosterone secretion. Annu Rev Physiol 50:409, 1988.
51. Rivier, CL and Plotsky, PM: Mediation by corticotropin releasing factor (CRF) of adenohypophyseal hormone secretion. Annu Rev Physiol 48:475, 1986.
52. Robinson, DR: Prostaglandins and the mechanism of action of anti-inflammatory drugs. Am J Med 75(Suppl 4b):26, 1983.
53. Rogerson, FM and Fuller, PJ: Mineralocorticoid action. Steroids 65:61, 2000.
54. Schimmer, BP and Parker, KL: Adrenocorticotropic hormone; adrenocortical steroids and their synthetic analogs; inhibitors of the synthesis and actions of adrenocortical hormones. In Hardman, JG, et al (eds): The Pharmacological Basis of Therapeutics, ed 9. McGraw-Hill, New York, 1996.
55. Schlaghecke, R, et al: The effect of long-term glucocorticoid therapy on pituitary-adrenal responses to exogenous corticotropin-releasing hormone. N Engl J Med 326:226, 1992.
56. Schmidt, BM, et al: Nongenomic steroid actions: Completing the puzzle. Aldosterone as an example. Exp Clin Endocrinol Diabetes 106:441, 1998.
57. Shohat, M, et al: Adrenocortical suppression by topical application of glucocorticoids in infants with seborrheic dermatitis. Clin Pediatr (Phila) 25:209, 1986.
58. Simpson, ER and Waterman, MR: Regulation of the synthesis of steroidogenic enzymes in adrenal cortical cells by ACTH. Annu Rev Physiol 50:427, 1988.
59. Slater, EP, et al: Mechanisms of glucocorticoid hormone action. In Chrousos, GP, Loriaux, DL, and Lipsett, MD (eds): Steroid Hormone Resistance: Mechanism and Clinical Aspects. Plenum Press, New York, 1986.

60. Stav, A, et al: Cervical epidural steroid injection for cervicobrachialgia. Acta Anaesthesiol Scand 37:562, 1993.
61. Tenbaum, S and Baniahmad, A: Nuclear receptors: Structure, function, and involvement in disease. Int J Biochem Cell Biol 29:1325, 1997.
62. Thorner, MO, et al: The anterior pituitary. In Wilson, JD, et al (eds): Textbook of Endocrinology, ed 9. WB Saunders, Philadelphia, 1998.
63. Tripathi, RC, et al: Corticosteroids and glaucoma risk. Drugs Aging 15:439, 1999.
64. Tsai, M-J, et al: Mechanisms of action of hormones that act as transcription-regulatory factors. In Wilson, JD, et al (eds): Textbook of Endocrinology, ed 9. WB Saunders, Philadelphia, 1998.
65. Van der Velden, VH: Glucocorticoids: Mechanisms of action and anti-inflammatory potential in asthma. Mediators Inflamm 7:229, 1998.
66. Verrey, F: Early aldosterone action: Toward filling the gap between transcription and transport. Am J Physiol 277:F319, 1999.
67. Verrey, F: Early aldosterone effects. Exp Nephrol 6:294, 1998.
68. Wolkowitz, OM, et al: Glucocorticoid medication, memory, and steroid psychosis in medical illness. Ann N Y Acad Sci 823:81, 1997.
69. Zaqqa, D and Jackson, RD: Diagnosis and treatment of glucocorticoid-induced osteoporosis. Cleve Clin J Med 66:221, 1999.
70. Ziegler, R and Kasperk, C: Glucocorticoid-induced osteoporosis: Prevention and treatment. Steroids 63:344, 1998.
71. Zinder, O and Dar, DE: Neuroactive steroids: their mechanism of action and their function in the stress response. Acta Physiol Scand 167:181, 1999.
72. Zora, JA, et al: Hypothalamic-pituitary axis suppression after short-term, high-dose glucocorticoid therapy in children with asthma. J Allergy Clin Immunol 77:9, 1986.

CHAPTER 30

Male and Female Hormones

In this chapter, the pharmacology of the male and female hormones is discussed. The male hormones such as testosterone are usually referred to collectively as **androgens**. The female hormones consist of two principal groups: the **estrogens,** such as estradiol, and the **progestins,** such as progesterone. Androgens, estrogens, and progestins are classified as **steroid** hormones, and their chemical structure is similar to those of the other primary steroid groups, the glucocorticoids and mineralocorticoids (see Chap. 29). The principal functions, however, of the male and female hormones are control of reproductive function and secondary sexual characteristics in their respective gender groups.

Male and female hormones are produced primarily in the gonads. Androgens are synthesized in the testes in the male. In the female, the ovaries are the principal site of estrogen and progestin production. As discussed in Chapter 29, small amounts of the sex-related hormones are also produced in the adrenal cortex in both sexes, accounting for the fact that small amounts of the opposite sex hormones are seen in females and males; that is, low testosterone levels are seen in females, and males produce small quantities of estrogen. However, under normal conditions, the amounts of sex-related hormones produced by the adrenal cortex are usually too small to produce significant physiologic effects.

This chapter first discusses the physiologic role of the male hormones and the pharmacologic use of natural and synthetic androgens. The physiologic and pharmacologic characteristics of the female hormones are then addressed. As these discussions indicate, there are several aspects of the male and female hormones that should concern physical therapists and occupational therapists. These agents may be used by rehabilitation patients for approved purposes, for example, female hormones as oral contraceptives. These agents may also be used for illicit reasons, such as the use of male hormones to enhance athletic performance. Hence, rehabilitation specialists should be aware of the therapeutic and potential toxic effects of these drugs.

ANDROGENS

Source and Regulation of Androgen Synthesis

In adult males, *testosterone* is the principal androgen produced by the testes.[37,104,107] Testosterone is synthesized by Leydig cells located in the interstitial space between the seminiferous tubules (Fig. 30–1). The *seminiferous tubules* are convoluted ducts within the testes in which sperm production (*spermatogenesis*) takes place. Testosterone produced by the Leydig cells exerts a direct effect on the seminiferous tubules, as well as systemic effects on other physiologic systems (see "Physiologic Effects of Androgens").

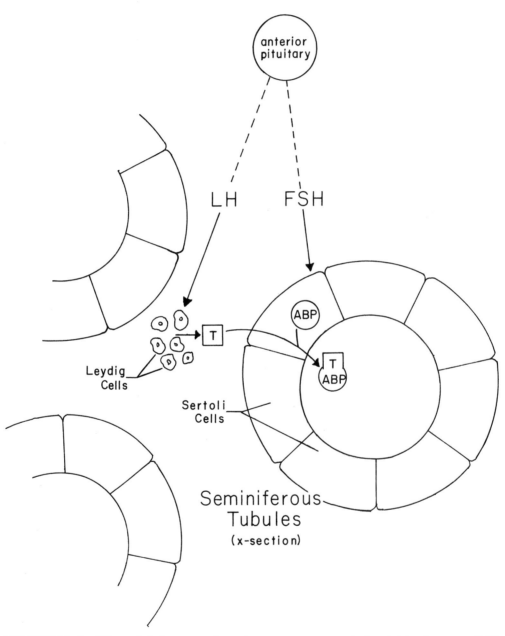

FIGURE 30–1. Effects of pituitary gonadotropins on spermatogenesis. Luteinizing hormone (LH) stimulates testosterone (T) production from Leydig cells. Follicle-stimulating hormone (FSH) acts primarily on Sertoli cells to increase synthesis of androgen-binding protein (ABP). ABP appears to bind with T and facilitate transport into the seminiferous tubule, where spermatogenesis takes place.

Production of testosterone by the Leydig cells is regulated by the pituitary **gonadotropins** *luteinizing hormone* (LH) and *follicle-stimulating hormone* (FSH).[74,107] LH and FSH appear to control spermatogenesis, as shown in Figure 30–1. LH is the primary hormone that stimulates testosterone production. LH released from the anterior pituitary binds to receptors on the surface of Leydig cells and directly stimulates testosterone synthesis.[74] The exact role of FSH is less clear. Although it does not directly increase steroidogenesis, FSH may augment the effects of LH by increasing Leydig cell differentiation and function.[37] For instance, FSH appears to increase the number of LH binding sites on Leydig cells.[104] However, FSH is believed to exert its primary effects on the Sertoli cells, which line the seminiferous tubules and are responsible for the development and maturation of normal sperm (see Fig. 30–1).[107] FSH stimulates the growth and function of Sertoli cells, and this hormone may also induce Sertoli cells to produce a polypeptide known as androgen-binding protein (ABP). ABP helps concentrate testosterone within the seminiferous tubules and helps transport testosterone to the epididymis.[104] Consequently, adequate amounts of FSH, combined with testosterone from Leydig cells, are needed to initiate and maintain normal spermatogenesis within the seminiferous tubules.[107]

Both pituitary gonadotropins are therefore required for optimal androgen function. LH acts on the Leydig cells to stimulate testosterone synthesis, whereas FSH acts on the Sertoli cells to stimulate their function and help testosterone reach target tissues within the seminiferous tissues. Other hormones may also play a synergistic role in steroidogenesis in the male; for instance, growth hormone and prolactin may also increase the effects of LH on testosterone synthesis.[37]

Release of the pituitary gonadotropins (LH, FSH) is regulated by gonadotropin-releasing hormone (GnRH) from the hypothalamus.[30] A classic negative feedback system exists between the GnRH/pituitary gonadotropins and testosterone synthesis. Increased plasma levels of testosterone inhibit the release of GnRH, LH, and FSH, thus maintaining testosterone levels within a relatively finite range. Also, testosterone production is fairly tonic in normal men. Fluctuations may occur in the amount of testosterone produced over a given period of time, and androgen production tends to diminish slowly as part of normal aging.[114] Androgen production, however, does not correspond to a regular monthly cycle similar to hormonal production in women; that is, testosterone is produced more or less constantly, whereas the female hormones are typically produced according to the stages of the menstrual cycle (see "Estrogen and Progesterone").

Physiologic Effects of Androgens

Testosterone and other androgens are involved in the development of the sexual characteristics in males and in the stimulation of spermatogenesis. These two primary effects are described here.

DEVELOPMENT OF MALE CHARACTERISTICS

The influence of testosterone on sexual differentiation begins in utero. In the fetus, the testes produce small amounts of testosterone that affect the development of the male reproductive organs. Androgen production then remains relatively unimportant until puberty. At the onset of puberty, a complex series of hormonal events stimulates the testes to begin to synthesize significant amounts of testosterone. The production of testosterone brings about the development of most of the physical characteristics associated with men. Most notable are increased body hair, increased skeletal muscle mass, voice change, and maturation of the external genitalia.

These changes are all caused by the effect of androgenic steroids on their respective target tissues. Like other steroids, the androgens enter the target cell and bind to a cytoplasmic receptor.[51,56,106] The activated steroid-receptor complex then travels to the cell's nucleus, where it binds to specific chromatin units. Binding of the activated complex to DNA gene segments increases protein synthesis through the transcription/translation of RNA. The proteins produced then cause a change in cellular function, which is reflected as one of the maturational effects of the androgens. For instance, testosterone increases protein synthesis in skeletal muscle, thus increasing muscle mass in certain situations, such as at the onset of puberty. This particular androgenic effect (increased muscle mass) as it relates to androgen abuse in athletes is discussed in more detail under "Androgen Abuse" later in this chapter.

ROLE IN SPERMATOGENESIS

As discussed previously, androgens are essential for the production and development of normal sperm.[104,107] Testosterone is produced by the Leydig cells located in the interstitial space between the seminiferous tubules. LH serves as the primary stimulus to increase androgen production from Leydig cells. Testosterone then enters the tubules to directly stimulate the production of sperm through an effect on protein synthesis within the tubule cells.

PHARMACOLOGIC USE OF ANDROGENS

Clinical Use of Androgens

Androgens and their synthetic derivatives are approved for administration in several clinical situations, which are given here.

Replacement Therapy. Testosterone and other androgens are administered as replacement therapy when the endogenous production of testosterone is impaired. Such conditions include removal of the testes (orchiectomy), various intrinsic forms of testicular failure (cryptorchidism, orchitis), and problems in the endocrine regulation of testosterone production, such as lack of LH production.[125]

Because androgen production also diminishes slowly with aging, relatively small or "physiologic" doses of androgens have been used to replace the age-related decline in endogenous production in some older men.[114] This type of replacement has been reported to produce beneficial effects on body composition, strength, bone mineralization, mood, libido, and other characteristics associated with normal androgen production.[10,116,125] Although androgen replacement is not used routinely in all older men, it appears that androgens can be considered as a therapeutic option in certain men who are experiencing an excessive decline in androgen production during aging.[10,48,68]

Catabolic States. Androgens can be administered for their anabolic properties in conditions in which there is substantial muscle catabolism and protein loss.[17] Such conditions include chronic infections, severe trauma, and recovery from extensive surgery. However, the use of androgens in these situations is somewhat controversial. These agents are not typically used as the primary treatment, but they are used as adjuncts to more conventional treatments such as dietary supplementation and exercise.

Androgens can also be used to increase lean body mass in men who are infected with human immunodeficiency virus (HIV). Men with HIV infection may have muscle wasting because of low testosterone production combined with the catabolic effects of this infection and subsequent anti-HIV therapies (see Chap. 34).[27,36] Physiologic doses of androgens have therefore been used to maintain or increase muscle mass in such individuals. The effects of this treatment, however, have not been overwhelmingly successful, with only modest increases in lean body mass seen in some studies.[36] Still, androgens may be a possible option to help reduce wasting and maintain muscle strength and function in men who experience severe muscle loss during HIV infection and AIDS.[14,27]

Delayed Puberty. In males, androgens may be administered on a limited basis to accelerate the normal onset of puberty.[16] These drugs are typically used when puberty is anticipated to occur spontaneously but at a relatively late date—that is, when puberty is not delayed because of some pathologic condition.

Breast Cancer. Androgens have been used to treat a limited number of hormone-sensitive tumors such as certain cases of breast cancer in women. The use of androgens in such cancers, however, has been largely replaced by other drugs such as the antiestrogens. The role of various hormones in the treatment of cancer is discussed in more detail in Chapter 36.

Anemia. Testosterone and similar compounds are potent stimulators of erythropoietin synthesis from the kidneys and other tissues.[124] Erythropoietin, in turn, stimulates production of red blood cell synthesis in bone marrow. Hence, androgens can be used in certain types of anemia caused by renal failure[58] or in congenital conditions such as aplastic anemia, hypoplastic anemia, and myelofibrotic anemias.[124] Androgens may also be helpful in certain anemias caused by other medications, such as cancer chemotherapy drugs.

Hereditary Angioedema. This hereditary disorder is characterized by a defect in the control of clotting factors that ultimately leads to increased vascular permeability. Loss of vascular fluid from specific capillary beds causes localized edema in various tissues such as the skin, upper respiratory tract, and gastrointestinal tract. Certain androgens act on the liver to restore production of several clotting factors and to increase production of a glycoprotein that inhibits the initial stages of the clotting sequence that leads to increased vascular permeability.[124] Hence, androgens are typically given prophylactically to decrease the frequency and severity of angioedema attacks.

Specific Agents

Androgens that are used clinically are listed in Table 30–1. As indicated, specific agents are usually administered orally or intramuscularly to replace endogenous androgen production or to treat various medical problems. Androgens can also be classified according to their relative androgenic and anabolic properties; that is, certain androgens are given primarily to mimic the male sexual characteristics (androgenic effects), whereas other androgens are given primarily to enhance tissue metabolism (anabolic effects) (see Table 30–1). This distinction is not absolute, however, because all compounds given to produce anabolism will also produce some androgenic effects. Many other androgenic and anabolic steroids exist and can be acquired relatively easily on the black market by individuals engaging in androgen abuse (see "Androgen Abuse"). Nonetheless, the agents listed in Table 30–1 are the principal androgens approved for clinical use, and these drugs are used to treat catabolic states, anemias, and similar conditions.

TABLE 30–1 Clinical Use of Androgens

Generic Name	Trade Name(s)	Primary Indication(s)	Routes of Administration
Fluoxymesterone	Android-F, Halotestin	Androgen deficiency, breast cancer in women, delayed puberty in boys, anemia	Oral
Methyltestosterone	Android, Oreton, Testred, Virilon	Androgen deficiency, breast cancer in women, delayed puberty in boys	Oral
Nandrolone	Durabolin, Deca-Durabolin, others	Anemia, breast cancer in women	Intramuscular
Oxandrolone	Oxandrin	Catabolic states	Oral
Oxymetholone	Anadrol	Anemia, angioedema	Oral
Stanozolol	Winstrol	Angioedema	Oral
Testosterone injectable suspension	Testamone, Testaqua	Androgen deficiency, breast cancer, delayed puberty in boys	Intramuscular
Testosterone cypionate injection	Andronate, Depo-Testosterone, others	Androgen deficiency, breast cancer in women, delayed puberty in boys	Intramuscular
Testosterone enanthate injection	Delatest, Delatestryl, others	Androgen deficiency, breast cancer in women, delayed puberty in males, anemia	Intramuscular
Testosterone propionate injection	Testex	Androgen deficiency, breast cancer in women, delayed puberty in boys	Intramuscular
Testosterone implants	Testopel pellets	Androgen deficiency, delayed puberty in boys	Subcutaneous
Testosterone transdermal systems	Testoderm, Androderm	Androgen deficiency	Transdermal

Adverse Effects of Clinical Androgen Use

The primary problems associated with androgens are related to the masculinizing effects of these drugs.[96] In women, androgen administration can produce hirsutism, hoarseness or deepening of the voice, and changes in the external genitalia (enlarged clitoris). Irregular menstrual periods and acne may also occur in women undergoing androgen therapy. In men, these drugs may produce bladder irritation, breast swelling and soreness, and frequent or prolonged erections. When used in children, androgens may cause accelerated sexual maturation and impairment of normal bone development because of premature closure of epiphyseal plates. Consequently, these drugs are used very cautiously in children.

The adverse effects just described are related to the dose and duration of androgen use, with problems seen more frequently during prolonged androgen administration at relatively high doses. In adults, most of these adverse effects are reversible, and symptoms will diminish with discontinued use. A few effects, however, such as vocal changes in females, may persist even after the drugs are withdrawn. Skeletal changes are irreversible, and permanent growth impairment may occur if these drugs are used in children.

Other serious side effects of long-term, high-dose androgen use include liver damage and hepatic carcinoma. Hypertension may occur because of the salt-retaining and water-retaining effects of these drugs. Although these hepatic and cardiovascular problems may occur during therapeutic androgen use, their incidence is even more prevalent when extremely large doses of androgens are used to enhance athletic performance. The use and abuse of androgens in athletes are discussed in "Androgen Abuse."

Antiandrogens

Antiandrogens are drugs that inhibit the synthesis or effects of endogenous androgen production.[45] These agents can be helpful in conditions such as prostate cancer and other conditions aggravated by excessive androgen production.[75,93] Specific antiandrogens affect endogenous male hormones in several different ways. Finasteride (Proscar) inhibits the conversion of testosterone to dihydrotestosterone. Dihydrotestosterone accelerates the growth and development of the prostate gland, and finasteride may be helpful in attenuating this effect in conditions such as benign prostate hypertrophy. Flutamide (Eulexin), bicalutamide (Casodex), and nilutamide (Nilandron) act as antagonists (blockers) of the cellular androgen receptor, and these drugs are used to decrease hirsutism in women or to help treat prostate cancer.

Advanced prostate cancer is also treated with a number of drugs that mimic the effects of GnRH. These GnRH analogs include buserelin (Suprefact), goserelin (Zoladex), leuprolide (Lupron), and nafarelin (Synarel). When first administered, these agents cause an increase in pituitary LH release, which, in turn, stimulates testicular androgen production. However, continued administration of GnRH analogs desensitizes pituitary GnRH receptors, thus decreasing LH and testosterone production from the pituitary and testes, respectively.[6]

ANDROGEN ABUSE

Nature of Androgen Abuse

The use of androgens or **anabolic steroids** to increase athletic performance is an issue of controversy and concern. The fact that certain athletes self-administer large doses of androgens in an effort to increase muscle size and strength has been known for some time. Typically, androgen use has been associated with athletes involved in strength and power activities such as weight lifting, bodybuilding, shot put, and the like. Androgen abuse, however, has infiltrated many aspects of athletic competition at both the amateur and professional levels.

Individuals who admit to using anabolic steroids or who test positive for androgen abuse represent some of the top performers in their respective sports.[13] Also, the use of anabolic steroids among the general athletic population may be reaching alarming proportions. A comprehensive survey of male high school seniors indicated that almost 7 percent of the athletes were using or had previously used anabolic steroids.[18] Clearly, androgen abuse is one of the major problems affecting the health and welfare of athletes of various ages and athletic pursuits.

Athletes engaging in androgen abuse usually obtain these drugs from various illicit but readily available sources.[4] Some examples of anabolic steroids that are used by athletes are listed in Table 30–2. Several different androgens are often taken simultaneously

TABLE 30–2 Examples of Anabolic Androgens That Are
Abused by Athletes

Generic Name	Trade Name
Orally active androgens	
Ethylestrenol	Maxibolin
Fluoxymesterone	Android-F, Halotestin
Methandrostenolone	Dianabol
Oxandrolone	Anavar, Oxandrin
Oxymetholone	Anadrol-50
Stanozolol	Winstrol
Androgens administered by intramuscular injection	
Nandrolone phenpropionate	Durabolin
Nandrolone decanoate	Deca-Durabolin
Testosterone cypionate	Depo-Testosterone
Testosterone enanthate	Delatestryl

for a combined dose that is 10 to 40 times greater than the therapeutic dose.[63,84,85] This "stacking" of different anabolic steroids often consists of combining oral and injectable forms of these drugs (see Table 30–2). Athletes often self-administer these drugs in cycles that last between 7 and 14 weeks, and the dosage of each drug is progressively increased during the cycle. An example of a dosing cycle using stacked anabolic steroids is shown in Table 30–3.

To help control anabolic steroid abuse, drug testing at the time of a specific competition has been instituted in many sports. To prevent detection, the athlete will also employ a complex pattern of high-dosage androgen administration followed by washout periods. Washouts are scheduled a sufficient period of time prior to the competition, thus allowing the drug to be eliminated from the body prior to testing. The practice of planned schedules can be negated to some extent, however, through randomized drug testing that subjects the athlete to testing at any point in the training period, as well as at the time of the competition.[24]

TABLE 30–3 Example of a Steroid Dosing Cycle Used
during Androgen Abuse*

	Dosage (mg)							
	Week							
Drug Name	1	2	3	4	5	6	7	8
Testosterone cypionate	200	400	600	1200	2400	4200	4200	4200
Nandrolone (Deca-Durabolin)	100	100	100	200	400	600	600	600
Oxymetholone (Anadrol)	100	150	200	250	300	500	750	1000
Methandrostenolone (Dianabol)	25	30	35	50	60	75	100	125
Methandrostenolone (Dianabol injectable)	25	25	50	50	100	100	100	100
Oxandrolone (Anavar)	25	30	35	50	50	50	50	50

*This regimen was used by a bodybuilder who went through three of these cycles each year for 8 years. The subject also reported taking 600 mg of testosterone per week between cycles. This subject ultimately developed avascular necrosis in both femoral heads.

Source: From Pettine,[86] p 96, with permission.

Two primary questions usually arise concerning anabolic steroids: Do these agents really enhance athletic performance, and what are the adverse effects of androgen abuse? Definitive answers to these questions are difficult because of the illicit nature of androgen abuse and because of the ethical and legal problems of administering large doses of androgens to healthy athletes as part of controlled research studies. The effects of androgens on athletic performance and the potential adverse effects of these drugs are discussed briefly here.

Effects of Androgens on Athletic Performance

There is little doubt that androgens can promote skeletal muscle growth and increase strength in people who do not synthesize meaningful amounts of endogenous androgens (women, prepubescent males). The question has often been whether large amounts of exogenous androgens can increase muscle size, strength, and athletic performance in healthy men. For example, certain athletic men taking androgens during strength training may experience greater increments in lean body mass and muscle strength than athletes training without androgens.[2–5,52] Increased muscle strength with steroid use has not been consistently reported in all research studies, however. In one review, approximately half of the investigations observed a significant effect of steroid administration on muscle strength, whereas the other half of the studies were inconclusive.[63] Some of this discrepancy was undoubtedly caused by differences in dosage and types of androgens used.

The magnitude of any strength gains that can be directly attributed to anabolic steroids also remains unclear. For instance, the anabolic effects of the steroids cannot be easily isolated from the other factors that produce increments in strength and muscle size (e.g., weight training). In particular, androgens appear to increase aggressiveness, and individuals taking these drugs may train longer and more intensely than athletes who are not taking anabolic steroids.[3] Consequently, strength increments in the athlete taking androgens may be brought about by the enhanced quality and quantity of training rather than as a direct effect of anabolic steroids on muscle protein synthesis.

Thus, the effects of androgens on athletic performance in men remain unclear. It seems probable that high doses of androgens would increase muscle size and strength, which might ultimately translate into improved athletic performance.[126] Nonetheless, we may never know the exact ergogenic effects of these drugs in men because of the illicit nature of androgen abuse and the ethical problems involved in performing clinical studies of these drugs in humans.[128]

Adverse Effects of Androgen Abuse

Virtually any drugs that are taken at extremely high dosages can be expected to produce some serious side effects. Exactly how harmful androgen abuse is in an athletic population remains somewhat uncertain, however.[128] The illicit nature of androgen abuse and the various dosage regimens have made it difficult to determine the precise incidence and type of adverse effects.[126] Also, the long-term effects of androgen abuse may not be known for some time; that is, pathologies may not be fully realized until several years after the drugs are discontinued.[126,128] Nonetheless, there is considerable evidence, often in the form of individual reports and case studies, that androgen abuse can have severe and possibly fatal consequences. Some of the more common adverse effects associated with androgen administration are presented here. Further discussion of the potential adverse effects in athletes can be found in several reviews listed at the end of this chapter.[3,4,13,61,63,115]

High doses of androgens can produce liver damage, including the formation of hepatic tumors and peliosis hepatis (blood-filled cysts within the liver).[4,20,32] In some individuals, these liver abnormalities have proved fatal. Androgens can also produce detrimental changes in cardiac structure and function that result in cardiomyopathy, ischemic heart disease, arrhythmias, and heart failure.[111,112] Furthermore, these hormones pose additional cardiovascular risks by producing unfavorable changes in blood lipid profiles, such as decreased high-density lipoprotein cholesterol levels.[120] These effects on plasma lipids predispose the athlete to atherosclerotic lesions and subsequent vessel occlusion, and specific cases of stroke and myocardial infarction in athletes using androgens have been attributed to the atherogenic effects of these drugs.[44,71] Androgens also cause hypertension because of direct effects on the myocardium and because of the salt-retaining and water-retaining properties of these drugs.[112] Problems with glucose metabolism brought about by insulin resistance have also been reported.[28]

Androgens can affect bone metabolism, and avascular necrosis of the femoral heads has been documented in a weight lifter using these drugs.[86] Androgens also accelerate closure of epiphyseal plates and can lead to impaired skeletal growth in young children. This effect on skeletal development is important because athletes may begin to self-administer anabolic steroids at a relatively young age (i.e., prior to age 16).[18] As previously mentioned, androgens may produce behavioral changes, including increased aggression, leading to radical mood swings and violent episodes in some individuals.[3,31,87–89]

Androgens can produce changes in reproductive function and secondary sexual characteristics. In males, high levels of androgens act as negative feedback and lead to testicular atrophy and impaired sperm production. Infertility in males may result because of an inability to form sperm (*azoospermia*).[57] In females, androgens produce certain masculinizing effects, such as increased body hair, deepening of the voice, and changes in the external genitalia. Androgens may also impair the normal female reproductive (menstrual) cycle. Some changes in male and female sexual and reproductive function appear to be reversible, but changes such as male infertility and azoospermia may take 4 months or longer to return to normal levels.[57] Other effects, such as vocal changes in females, may be permanent.

In summary, anabolic steroids may produce some ergogenic benefits in a limited subset of athletes, but rather serious consequences may occur. Nonetheless, athletes may be so driven to succeed that the adverse effects are disregarded. Also, athletes may suspect that their competitors are using steroids and feel that they must also take these drugs to remain competitive. Clearly, there is a need for governing agencies to try to eliminate the illicit use of these substances from athletic competition. Health-care professionals can also discourage androgen abuse by informing athletes that the risks of androgen abuse exceed any potential benefits.[115]

ESTROGEN AND PROGESTERONE

In women, the ovaries produce two major categories of steroid hormones: estrogens and progestins. The primary estrogen produced in humans is *estradiol*, and the primary progestin is *progesterone*. For simplicity, the terms *estrogen* and *progesterone* will be used to indicate these two primary forms of female hormones. Small amounts of male hormones (androgens) are also produced by the ovaries, and these androgens may play a role in the development of some secondary sexual characteristics in the female during puberty, for example, increased body hair and growth spurts. Nonetheless, the hormones that exert the major influence on sexual development and reproduction in the female are estrogen and progesterone. The physiologic effects of these hormones are presented here.

Effects of Estrogen and Progesterone on Sexual Maturation

Estrogen and progesterone play a primary role in promoting sexual differentiation in the developing female fetus. These hormones also become important in completing female sexual maturation during puberty. At the onset of puberty, a complex series of hormonal events stimulates the ovaries to begin producing estrogen and progesterone. Ovarian production of these hormones initiates the maturation of reproductive function and development of secondary sexual characteristics in the female.

Estrogen is the primary hormone that initiates the growth and development of the female reproductive system during puberty. Changes in the external genitalia and maturation of the internal reproductive organs (e.g., uterus, oviducts, vagina) are primarily brought about by the influence of estrogen. Estrogen also produces several other characteristic changes of female sexual maturation, such as breast development, deposition of subcutaneous fat stores, and changes in the skeletal system (for example, closure of epiphyseal plates, widening of the pelvic girdle). Progesterone is less important in sexual maturation but is involved to a greater extent in facilitating and maintaining pregnancy.

Regulation and Effects of Hormonal Synthesis during the Menstrual Cycle

In the nonpregnant, postpubescent female, production of estrogen and progesterone is not tonic in nature but follows a pattern or cycle of events commonly referred to as the *menstrual cycle*. The menstrual cycle involves a sequence of events usually occurring over a 28-day period. The primary function of this cycle is to stimulate the ovaries to produce an ovum that is available for fertilization, while simultaneously preparing the endometrium of the uterus for implantation of the ovum, should fertilization occur. The primary events of the menstrual cycle are illustrated in Figure 30–2. This cycle is characterized by several specific phases and events that are briefly outlined here. A more detailed description of the regulation of female reproduction can be found in several sources listed at the end of this chapter.[60,81,94,123,127]

Follicular Phase. The first half of the menstrual cycle is influenced by hormonal release from a developing ovarian follicle, hence the term *follicular phase*. In the follicular phase, FSH is released by the anterior pituitary. As its name implies, FSH stimulates the maturation of several follicles within the ovary. Usually, one such follicle undergoes full maturation and ultimately yields an ovum. Because of the effect of FSH, the developing follicle also begins to secrete increasing amounts of estrogen. Estrogen produced by the ovarian follicle causes proliferation and thickening of the endometrial lining of the uterus. The follicular phase is also referred to as the *proliferative phase*. Endometrial vascularization is also increased, and glandular structures begin to develop in the uterine wall. The uterine glands, however, do not begin to function (secrete mucus) to any great extent during the follicular phase.

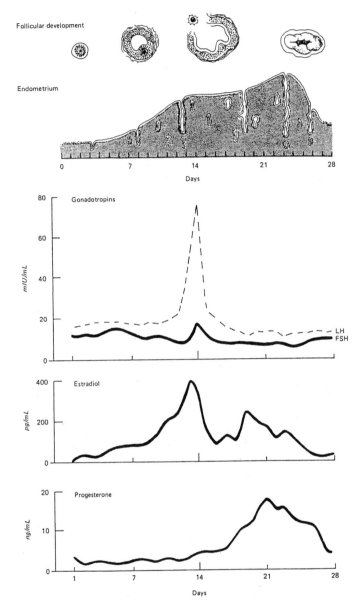

FIGURE 30–2. The menstrual cycle, showing changes in follicular development, uterine endometrium, pituitary gonadotropins (LH, FSH), and ovarian hormones. (Reproduced, with permission, from Katzung, BG: Basic and Clinical Pharmacology, ed 7, Appleton & Lange, 1998, p 654. Reproduced with permission of the McGraw-Hill Companies.)

Ovulation. Just prior to the midpoint of the cycle, the anterior pituitary secretes a sudden, large burst of LH. A smaller burst of FSH secretion also occurs around the midpoint of the cycle, as seen in Figure 30–2. The LH surge is the primary impetus for ovulation. During ovulation, the mature follicle ruptures, releasing the ovum from the ovary. At this point, the ovum should begin to travel toward the uterus via the fallopian tubes. The ruptured follicle remains in the ovary and continues to play a vital role in the reproductive cycle. After releasing the ovum, the follicle becomes infiltrated with lipids and is referred to as the *corpus luteum* (yellow body). The role of the corpus luteum is described here.

Luteal Phase. The *luteal phase* refers to the fact that the corpus luteum governs the events in the second half of the menstrual cycle. In response to the residual effects of the

LH-FSH surge, the corpus luteum continues to grow and develop for approximately 1 week after ovulation. During this time, the corpus luteum secretes both estrogen and progesterone. The combined effects of estrogen and progesterone cause further thickening in the uterine lining, as well as an increase in the vascularization and glandular secretion of the endometrium. During the luteal phase, progesterone is the primary stimulus that causes the uterine glands to fully develop and secrete a mucous substance that provides a favorable environment for implantation of the fertilized egg. Hence, the luteal phase is also referred to as the *secretory phase* because of the enhanced function of the uterine glands.

Corpus Luteum Regression and Termination of the Cycle. If the egg is not fertilized or implantation does not occur, the corpus luteum begins to regress, primarily because of a lack of continued support for the corpus luteum from the pituitary gonadotropins (LH, FSH). Because the corpus luteum regresses, it can no longer produce adequate amounts of estrogen and progesterone to maintain the endometrium of the uterus. Consequently, the endometrium begins to slough off, creating the menstrual bleeding that typifies the female reproductive cycle. The onset of menstrual bleeding marks the end of one reproductive cycle and the beginning of the next.

In summary, the menstrual cycle is primarily regulated by the interaction between pituitary and ovarian hormones. Also, releasing hormones from the hypothalamus play a role in controlling female reproduction through their effects on LH and FSH release from the anterior pituitary.[30] A complex series of positive and negative feedback mechanisms control the cyclic release of various female hormones.[94,127] For instance, increased estrogen secretion in the follicular phase stimulates the LH surge that evokes ovulation. This event is considered an example of positive feedback because low estrogen levels increase LH release, which further increases estrogen secretion, thus further increasing LH release, and so on. Conversely, secretion of the pituitary gonadotropins (LH, FSH) is inhibited toward the latter part of the luteal phase, presumably because of the negative feedback influence of high levels of estrogen and progesterone.

Pharmacologic intervention can take advantage of these complex feedback systems in certain situations. Most notable is the use of estrogen and progesterone as oral contraceptives. By altering the normal control between pituitary and ovarian hormones and uterine function, preparations containing these two steroids are an effective means of birth control. This particular pharmacologic use of female hormones is discussed in more detail in "Pharmacologic Use of Estrogen and Progesterone."

Female Hormones in Pregnancy and Parturition

Estrogen and progesterone also play a significant role in pregnancy and childbirth. For successful implantation and gestation of the fertilized egg, synthesis of these two steroids must be maintained to prevent the onset of menstruation. As just mentioned, menstruation begins when the corpus luteum is no longer able to produce sufficient estrogen and progesterone to sustain the endometrium. When fertilization does occur, however, some hormonal response must transpire to maintain steroid production from the corpus luteum and ensure that the endometrium remains ready for implantation. This response is caused by the release of human chorionic gonadotropin (HCG) from the fertilized ovum. HCG takes over the role of LH and rescues the corpus luteum from destruction.[80,81] The corpus luteum then continues to produce steroids (especially progesterone), which maintain the uterine lining in a suitable state for implantation and gestation of the fertilized egg.

Eventually the corpus luteum does begin to degenerate between the 9th and 14th week of gestation. By that point, the placenta has assumed estrogen and progesterone production. Generally speaking, maternal progesterone helps to maintain the uterus and placenta throughout the rest of the pregnancy. Progesterone also increases the growth and development of the maternal mammary glands in preparation for lactation. Although the role of estrogen is less clear, increased estrogen production may play a pivotal part in setting the stage for parturition. Clearly, both steroids are needed for normal birth and delivery.

PHARMACOLOGIC USE OF ESTROGEN AND PROGESTERONE

The most frequent and prevalent use of the female hormones is in oral contraceptive preparations (see "Oral Contraceptives"). The other primary indications for estrogen and progesterone are replacement of endogenous hormone production and subsequent resolution of symptoms related to hormonal deficiencies. This replacement can be especially important following menopause—that is, when the female reproductive cycle ceases and the associated cyclic production of the ovarian hormones ends. Specific clinical conditions that may be resolved by estrogen and progesterone are listed here.

Conditions Treated with Estrogen and Progesterone

Replacement Therapy. Estrogen and progesterone are often used to replace the endogenous production of these hormones following menopause or in women who have had an ovariectomy. In particular, estrogens are often very effective in reducing some of the severe symptoms associated with menopause.[11,33,59] These include symptoms such as atrophic vaginitis, atrophic dystrophy of the vulva, and vasomotor effects such as hot flashes.

Estrogens are also considered essential in preventing and treating postmenopausal osteoporosis.[29,34,42,101,119] Women receiving hormone replacement with estrogen are able to maintain or increase bone mineral density, and estrogen replacement is often associated with a decreased incidence of vertebral fractures and other osteoporosis-related problems.[92,101] Estrogen can also be combined with other interventions such as calcium supplements and physical activity to provide optimal protection against osteoporosis following menopause.[1,39]

Estrogen replacement may also reduce the risk factors associated with coronary heart disease in postmenopausal women.[72,91,103] Low doses of estrogen cause favorable changes in plasma lipid profiles, including decreased levels of low-density lipoproteins and increased levels of high-density lipoproteins.[50,79,99,117,121] These beneficial effects on plasma lipoproteins decrease the risk of atherosclerotic lesions and should therefore reduce the incidence of coronary heart disease.[98] However, the idea that estrogen replacement offers protection against coronary heart disease was challenged somewhat by a recent study known as the Heart and Estrogen/Progesterone Replacement Study (HERS). According to the HERS findings, estrogen combined with progesterone did not decrease the incidence of infarction and death in postmenopausal women with a history of coronary heart disease.[73] Nonetheless, it is still generally thought that estrogen replacement can play a role in modifying the risk factors associated with coronary heart disease, and continued research in this area should clarify how hormone replacement therapy can help decrease cardiac morbidity and mortality in certain postmenopausal women.[62,98]

Finally, it has been suggested that estrogen replacement may offer some protection against cognitive decline in conditions such as Alzheimer disease and other forms of dementia.[78,108] Estrogen may, for example, have several neuroprotective effects, including the ability to decrease free radical–induced damage, sustain cholinergic function in the brain, and inhibit the neuronal degeneration associated with Alzheimer disease.[76] Conclusive evidence of these beneficial effects, however, is lacking.[108] Estrogen replacement is therefore not currently accepted as standard treatment for Alzheimer disease, and additional studies are needed to determine if hormone replacement therapy has a role in the treatment and prevention of dementia.

Hypogonadism. Estrogens or a combination of estrogen and progesterone may be used to treat abnormally low ovarian function. Appropriate use of these hormones induces the uterine changes and cyclic bleeding associated with the normal female reproductive cycle.

Failure of Ovarian Development. Occasionally, the ovaries fail to undergo normal development because of hypopituitarism or other disorders. Estrogens may be given at the time of puberty to encourage development of secondary sexual characteristics (e.g., breast development).

Menstrual Irregularities. Various problems with normal menstruation are treated by estrogen and progesterone. These hormones are used either separately or in combination to resolve amenorrhea, dysmenorrhea, and other types of functional uterine bleeding that are caused by a hormonal imbalance.

Endometriosis. Endometriosis is a condition characterized by growths of uterine-like tissue that occur at various locations within the pelvic cavity. Progesterone and estrogen-progesterone combinations help suppress bleeding from these tissues and may help regress the size of these growths.

Carcinoma. Estrogen has been used to treat metastatic breast cancer in men and postmenopausal women. Advanced prostate cancer in men may also respond to estrogen treatment. Progesterone is helpful in treating uterine cancer and several other types of metastases, such as breast, renal, and endometrial carcinoma.

Specific Agents

Types of estrogens and progestins that are used therapeutically are listed in Tables 30–4 and 30–5. Both types of hormones can be administered in their natural form (estradiol and progesterone), and several synthetic derivatives of each type are also available. Most of the drugs listed in Tables 30–4 and 30–5 are available as oral preparations, and many conditions can be conveniently treated by oral administration. Estrogens may also be administered transdermally via patches, and the transdermal route may offer certain advantages, such as decreased side effects and liver problems.[25,38,110] Certain progesterone preparations can be administered by vaginal suppositories, and vaginal administration can be helpful in treating dysfunction of the endometrium of the uterus.[26,118] Finally, several preparations are also available for injection, and parenteral routes may be used in some situations, such as severe uterine bleeding.

Adverse Effects of Estrogen and Progesterone

Therapeutic use of estrogen may cause nausea, which is usually transient. Swelling of the feet and ankles may also occur because of sodium and water retention. Higher

TABLE 30–4 Clinical Use of Estrogens

Generic Name	Trade Name(s)	Primary Indication(s)
Dienestrol	Ortho Dienestrol	Estrogen replacement (vaginal)
Diethylstilbestrol	Honvol, Stilphostrol	Antineoplastic
Estradiol	Depo-Estradiol, Estrace, Estraderm, Vivelle, many others	Estrogen replacement, antineoplastic, prevention of osteoporosis
Conjugated estrogens	Premarin	Estrogen replacement, antineoplastic, prevention of osteoporosis, prevention of abnormal uterine bleeding
Esterified estrogens	Estratab, Menest	Estrogen replacement, antineoplastic, prevention of osteoporosis
Estrone	Aquest, Estragyn, Wehgen, many others	Estrogen replacement, antineoplastic, prevention of abnormal uterine bleeding
Estropipate	Ogen, Ortho-Est	Estrogen replacement, prevention of osteoporosis
Ethinyl estradiol	Estinyl	Estrogen replacement, antineoplastic

doses of estrogen have been associated with serious cardiovascular problems, including myocardial infarction and thromboembolism.[82] These problems are significant when relatively large doses are administered to men for the treatment of breast and prostate cancer. Estrogen replacement in postmenopausal women may increase the risk of endometrial and breast cancer, especially if estrogen is given for prolonged periods without concomitant progesterone therapy.[9,12,113] The primary problems associated with progesterone also involve abnormal blood clotting, which may lead to thrombophlebitis, pulmonary embolism, and cerebral infarction.[7] Progesterone may alter the normal menstrual cycle, leading to unpredictable changes in the bleeding pattern.

Selective Estrogen Receptor Modulators

Selective estrogen receptor modulators (SERMs) are so named because they bind to and activate estrogen receptors on certain tissues while blocking the effects of es-

TABLE 30–5 Clinical Use of Progestins

Generic Name	Trade Name(s)	Primary Indication(s)
Hydroxyprogesterone	Hylutin, Prodrox, others	Amenorrhea, dysfunctional uterine bleeding
Levonorgestrel	Norplant	Contraception
Medrogestone	Colprone	Secondary amenorrhea, dysfunctional uterine bleeding
Medroxyprogesterone	Cycrin, Provera, others	Secondary amenorrhea, dysfunctional uterine bleeding, breast or endometrial carcinoma
Megestrol	Megace	Breast or endometrial carcinoma; advanced prostate cancer
Norethindrone	Aygestin, Micronor, others	Secondary amenorrhea, dysfunctional uterine bleeding, endometriosis
Norgestrel	Ovrette	Contraception
Progesterone	Gesterol, Prometrium, others	Secondary amenorrhea, dysfunctional uterine bleeding

trogen on other tissues.[47,53,77] Specifically, these agents activate estrogen receptors on bone and vascular tissues (including plasma lipids) while acting as estrogen antagonists (blockers) on uterine and breast tissues. SERMs therefore have the obvious advantage of producing favorable effects on bone mineralization and cardiovascular function while reducing the potential carcinogenic effects of estrogen on breast and uterine tissues.

Tamoxifen (Nolvadex) was the first SERM developed for clinical use, and this drug is approved for the prevention and treatment of breast cancer because it has strong antiestrogen effects on breast tissues. This anticancer effect is achieved while simultaneously stimulating other estrogen receptors that help maintain bone mineral density and improve cardiovascular function and plasma lipid profiles.[77,83] Tamoxifen, however, does not completely block estrogen receptors on uterine tissues, and this drug may actually stimulate endometrial proliferation and increase the incidence of uterine cancers.[47,122] This drug is generally well tolerated, although symptoms that mimic estrogen withdrawal (hot flashes, vaginitis) may occur when tamoxifen is first administered to women. These symptoms often diminish, however, with continued use of this drug.

More recently, a second SERM known as raloxifene (Evista) was developed. Raloxifene is similar to tamoxifen except that raloxifene blocks estrogen receptors on breast *and* uterine tissues and may therefore produce beneficial effects (inhibit breast cancer, improve bone and cardiovascular function) without increasing the risk of endometrial cancers.[35,46,49,83,122] Raloxifene is currently approved for treating osteoporosis. This drug may cause several bothersome side effects, including hot flashes, joint or muscle pain, depression, insomnia, and gastrointestinal disturbances. More serious problems with raloxifene may be indicated by symptoms such as chest pain, flu-like syndrome, leg cramping, skin rash, and cystitis or urinary tract infections.

Efforts continue to develop other SERMs that will capitalize on the beneficial effects of estrogen while minimizing or even reducing the carcinogenic effects of estrogen on other tissues. As newer agents are developed, SERMs may have an expanded role in the treatment of various diseases and perhaps provide a safer and more effective method of estrogen relacement.[70]

Antiestrogens

In addition to the SERMs, a limited number of drugs directly antagonize all the effects of estrogen and are considered to be true antiestrogens. These antiestrogens appear to bind to estrogen receptors in the cytosol but do not cause any subsequent changes in cellular function. Hence, these drugs block the effects of estrogen by occupying the estrogen receptor and preventing estrogen from exerting a response. The principal antiestrogen used clinically is clomiphene (Clomid, Serophene). Clomiphene is administered to women to treat infertility. The mechanism of clomiphene as a fertility drug is somewhat complex. Relatively high levels of estrogen normally produce an inhibitory or negative feedback effect on the release of pituitary gonadotropins (LH and FSH). As an antiestrogen, clomiphene blocks this inhibitory effect, thus facilitating gonadotropin release.[79] Increased gonadotropins (especially LH) promote ovulation, thus improving the chance of fertilization. The primary adverse effects associated with clomiphene are vascular hot flashes. Enlarged ovaries may also occur because of the stimulatory effect of increased gonadotropin release.

Antiprogestins

Agents that specifically block progesterone receptors were first developed in the early 1980s.[123] The primary clinical application of these drugs is termination of pregnancy; that is, these drugs can be used to induce abortion during the early stages of gestation. Because progesterone is largely responsible for sustaining the placenta and fetus, blockade of progesterone receptors in the uterus negates the effects of this hormone, with subsequent detachment of the placenta and loss of placental hormones such as human chorionic gonadotropin. Detachment of the placenta from the uterine lining results in loss of the fetus and termination of the pregnancy.

The primary antiprogestin is mifepristone, known also as RU486. This drug can be administered orally during the first 7 weeks of pregnancy, with abortion typically occurring within the next 2 to 3 days. To stimulate uterine contraction and ensure complete expulsion of the detached embryo, a prostaglandin analog such as misoprostol or prostaglandin E_1 is typically administered orally or intravaginally 48 hours after mifepristone administration.[19] This regimen of mifepristone followed by a prostaglandin agent is successful in terminating pregnancy in approximately 95 percent of the cases.[90,109]

Mifepristone has been used as an abortive agent in China and parts of Europe for some time, and this drug recently received FDA approval for use in the United States. This drug is marketed in the United States under the trade name Mifeprex. When used to induce abortion, the primary physical side effects of mifepristone are excessive uterine bleeding and cramping, although these side effects may be related more to the use of prostaglandins following mifepristone treatment.[109] The chance of incomplete abortion must also be considered, and a follow-up physician visit approximately 2 weeks after mifepristone administration is needed to ensure that the pregnancy was terminated.

Consequently, the major focus on this drug at the present time is its potential for use in terminating pregnancy. In the future, mifepristone may also be used for other reasons. This drug could, for example, have contraceptive potential because it blocks the effects of progesterone on endometrial proliferation and vascularization, thus rendering the endometrium less favorable for implantation of the fertilized egg. Mifepristone may likewise be useful as a "morning after" pill to prevent conception after unprotected sex (see "Types of Contraceptive Preparations").[102] In addition to its effects on progesterone receptors, mifepristone can also block cellular glucocorticoid receptors, and the clinical significance of this effect remains to be explored.[21] Finally, mifepristone may be useful in treating certain growths and tumors that are exacerbated by progesterone, including endometriosis, leiomyoma, meningioma, and breast cancer.[69] It will be interesting to see how this drug is ultimately used to prevent or terminate pregnancy and perhaps manage progesterone-related diseases as well.

ORAL CONTRACEPTIVES

During the 1960s, oral contraceptives containing estrogens and progestins were approved for use in preventing pregnancy. The introduction of these birth control pills provided a relatively easy and effective method of contraception. Today, oral contraceptives are taken routinely by many women of child-bearing age, and these drugs are among the most commonly prescribed medications in the United States and throughout the world.[123]

Types of Contraceptive Preparations

The most common form of oral contraceptive contains a fixed amount of estrogen and progesterone in the same pill. Examples of some common estrogen-progestin contraceptives are listed in Table 30–6. When taken appropriately, these preparations appear to be 99 to 100 percent effective in preventing pregnancy.[123] Typically, the contraceptive pill is taken each day for 3 weeks, beginning at the onset of menstruation. This intake is followed by 1 week in which either no pill is taken or a "blank" pill that lacks the hormones is taken. For convenience and improved compliance, these preparations are usually packaged in some form of dispenser that encourages the user to remember to take one pill each day.

Other versions of oral contraceptives are available that contain only a progestin (norethindrone, norgestrel) (see Table 30–6). These "minipills" were developed to avoid the adverse effects normally attributed to estrogen. Progestin-only minipills are somewhat less attractive as an oral contraceptive because these preparations are only about 97 to 98 percent effective and because they tend to cause irregular and unpredictable menstrual cycles. An implantable form of a progestin-only preparation (Norplant) has also been developed, whereby small, semipermeable tubes containing levonorgestrel are inserted subcutaneously in the arm.[54] The progestin is delivered in a slow, continuous fashion, allowing effective contraception for up to 5 years. These implants appear to have contraceptive efficacy that is better than progestin-only pills and only slightly less effective than combined estrogen-progestin oral contraceptives. Progestin-only implants can be replaced at the end of 5 years to continue this method of contraception, or they can be removed at any time because of side effects or other reasons. There is likewise a form of progesterone (Depo Provera) that can be administered by deep intramuscular injection every 12 weeks.[15] These implantable and injectable forms of progesterone therefore offer alternatives to women who cannot tolerate estrogen-progesterone pills or who have difficulty adhering to traditional oral contraceptive regimens.

Oral contraceptives that contain various types of estrogen are sometimes used to prevent conception following sexual intercourse, especially in specific situations such as rape or unprotected sex. These postcoital interventions or "morning-after pills" typically consist of a high dose of a natural or synthetic estrogen, or estrogen combined with a progestin (e.g., ethinyl estradiol combined with norgestrel). The exact mechanism of these

TABLE 30–6 Oral Contraceptives

Estrogen Component	Progestin Component	Common Trade Name(s)
Ethinyl estradiol	Desogestrel	Desogen, Mircette, others
Ethinyl estradiol	Ethynodiol diacetate	Demulen, Zovia
Ethinyl estradiol	Levonorgestrel	Levlen, Nordette, Triphasil, others
Ethinyl estradiol	Norethindrone acetate	Loestrin
Ethinyl estradiol	Norethindrone	Brevicon, Genora 1/35, Ortho-Novum 10/11, others
Ethinyl estradiol	Norgestimate	Ortho-Cyclen
Ethinyl estradiol	Norgestrel	Lo/Ovral, Ovral
Mestranol	Norethindrone	Genora 1/50, Norinyl 1+50, Ortho-Novum 1/50, others
NA*	Levonorgestrel	Norplant
NA*	Norethindrone	Micronor, Nor-Q D
NA*	Norgestrel	Ovrette

*NA = Not applicable; these products contain only progesterone.

morning-after pills is not known, but they appear to somehow interfere with ovulation or make the endometrium less favorable to implantation.[54,123] As indicated earlier, mifepristone may also have potential as a morning-after pill because this drug blocks progesterone receptors in the uterus, thereby negating the effects of progesterone on the endometrium and developing placenta.[102] Hence, several options exist for preventing pregnancy after a specific incident of sexual intercourse. These pills can be helpful in emergency situations, but they are not meant to be an alternative to traditional birth control methods.

Mechanism of Contraceptive Action

Oral contraceptives exert their effects primarily by inhibiting ovulation and by impairing the normal development of the uterine endometrium.[64,95] As discussed previously, the normal menstrual cycle is governed by the complex interaction between endogenous ovarian hormones and the pituitary gonadotropins. High levels of estrogen and progesterone in the bloodstream act as negative feedback and inhibit the release of LH and FSH from the anterior pituitary. Oral contraceptives maintain fairly high plasma levels of estrogen and progestin, thus limiting the release of LH and FSH through this negative feedback system. Because ovulation is normally caused by the midcycle LH surge (see Fig. 30–2), inhibition of LH release prevents ovulation. This event prevents an ovum from being made available for fertilization.

The estrogen and progestin supplied by the contraceptive also affect the development of the uterine lining. Oral contraceptives promote a certain amount of growth and proliferation of the uterine endometrium. The endometrium, however, does not develop to quite the same extent or in quite the same manner as it would if controlled by normal endogenous hormonal release. Consequently, the endometrial environment is less than optimal for implantation even if ovulation and fertilization should take place. Also, there is an increase in the thickness and viscosity of the mucous secretions in the uterine cervix, thus impeding the passage of sperm through the cervical region, which adds to the contraceptive efficacy of these preparations.

Through the effects on the endometrium, oral contraceptive administration can be used to mimic a normal menstrual flow. When the contraceptive hormones are withdrawn at the end of the third week, the endometrium undergoes a sloughing similar to that in the normal cycle. Of course, the endometrium is being regulated by the exogenous hormones rather than the estrogen and progesterone normally produced by the ovaries. Still, this method of administration and withdrawal can produce a more or less normal pattern of uterine activity, with the exception that chances of conception are dramatically reduced.

Adverse Effects of Oral Contraceptives

Although oral contraceptives provide an easy and effective means of birth control, their use has been limited somewhat by potentially serious side effects. In particular, the pill has been associated with cardiovascular problems such as thrombophlebitis, stroke, and myocardial infarction.[40] However, the incidence of these side effects may be diminished with the newer forms of oral contraceptives, which contain relatively less estrogen than their predecessors.

Over the years, the amount of estrogen contained in the combined estrogen-progesterone preparations has been reduced without sacrificing the contraceptive efficacy of these drugs.[8,41,55] Evidently, the lower estrogen content reduces the risk of cardiovascular problems.[23] Likewise, the newer oral contraceptives tend to contain progestins that have less androgenic properties, and these newer progestins may help reduce the risk of cardiovascular complications.[54,55] This does not mean that oral contraceptives are devoid of cardiovascular side effects. The pill clearly has the potential to impair normal hemostasis and lead to venous thromboembolism, myocardial infarction, and stroke.[23,40,66] This risk is relatively modest, however, with the current estrogen-progesterone preparations. Still, oral contraceptives should not be used by women with any pre-existing cardiovascular problems (hypertension, recurrent thrombosis) or any conditions or situations that may lead to cardiovascular disease (e.g., cigarette smoking).[23,40,66,100,129]

There has been some indication that oral contraceptives may lead to certain forms of cancer. Some early versions of the pill were believed to cause tumors of the endometrium of the uterus. This effect may have been caused by early forms that were sequential in nature; that is, they provided only estrogen for the first half of the menstrual cycle and estrogen combined with progesterone for the second half. The newer combined forms that supply both hormones throughout the cycle do not appear to increase the risk of uterine cancer, however. In fact, it appears that the form of oral contraceptive commonly used may actually *decrease* the risk of endometrial cancer, as well as prevent other forms of cancer, including ovarian cancer.[8,22,43,65,67,105] The carcinogenic properties of oral contraceptives have not been totally ruled out, however. The effects on breast cancer remain controversial, and the possibility exists that certain subgroups of women may have an increased risk of breast cancer, depending on factors such as how long they used the pill prior to their first full-term pregnancy.[97] There is also considerable evidence that prolonged use of oral contraceptives (more than 8 years) may increase the risk of liver cancer.[8]

There are a number of other less serious but bothersome side effects associated with oral contraceptives. Problems such as nausea, loss of appetite, abdominal cramping, headache, dizziness, weight gain, and fatigue are fairly common. These symptoms are often transient and may diminish following continued use.

Consequently, the serious risks associated with oral contraceptives have diminished somewhat since their initial appearance on the market. These drugs are not without some hazards, however. In general, it is a good policy to reserve this form of birth control for relatively young, healthy women who do not smoke. Avoiding continuous, prolonged administration to diminish the risk of liver cancer may also be prudent. Finally, any increase in the other side effects associated with oral contraceptives, such as headache and abdominal discomfort, should be carefully evaluated to rule out a more serious underlying problem.

SPECIAL CONCERNS OF SEX HORMONE PHARMACOLOGY IN REHABILITATION PATIENTS

Therapists should be cognizant of the adverse effects related to the estrogens, progesterones, and androgens so that they may help recognize problems related to these compounds. For instance, therapists should routinely monitor blood pressure during therapeutic administration of the sex hormones. These compounds tend to promote salt and water retention (mineralocorticoid-like properties), which may promote hypertension. Therapists may also play an important role in educating patients about the dangers of androgen abuse. When dealing with an athletic population, physical therapists may serve as a source of information about anabolic steroids. Therapists should advise athletes about the potential side effects, such as liver, cardiovascular, and reproductive abnormalities. Therapists can also monitor blood pressure in athletes who appear to be using androgenic steroids. This interaction may help prevent a hypertensive crisis, as well as illustrate to the athlete the harmful effects of these drugs.

CASE STUDY

MALE AND FEMALE HORMONES

Brief History. B.P. is a 72-year-old woman who sustained a compression fracture of the L-1 vertebral body. Evidently, the fracture occurred as she twisted sideways and leaned forward to get out of her daughter's car. X-ray films revealed generalized bone demineralization, and the compression fracture was apparently caused by osteoporosis. The patient was admitted to the hospital and confined to bed rest. Physical therapy was ordered, and heat and gentle massage were initiated at the bedside to decrease pain. To help attenuate bone demineralization, the patient was started on oral conjugated estrogen tablets (Premarin), at a dosage of 0.625 mg/day. A calcium supplement of 1500 mg/day was also added to the pharmacotherapeutic regimen.

Problem/Influence of Medication. The therapist realized that a program of exercise and general conditioning would augment the effects of the estrogen and calcium supplements. The combined effects of physical activity with pharmacologic management would offer the best chance at preventing further bone demineralization and osteoporosis.

Decision/Solution. Upon consultation with the referring physician, the physical therapist began a gradual strengthening and conditioning program. After the acute pain subsided, sitting and progressive ambulation activities were instituted at the bedside. Vertebral extension and abdominal strengthening exercises were also initiated as tolerated by the patient. This exercise and conditioning program was continued after the patient was discharged from the hospital, and a home program was supervised by periodic home visits from a physical therapist. Ambulation and exercise activities were gradually increased over the course of the next few weeks. The fracture had fully healed approximately 3 months following the initial incident. By that time, a formal exercise program had been established, consisting of daily ambulation and active range-of-motion activities. The therapist encouraged the patient to continue the exercise program indefinitely to help maintain bone mineral content and prevent subsequent fractures.

SUMMARY

The male hormones are the androgens, and the female hormones are the estrogens and progestins. These steroid hormones are primarily involved in the control of reproduction and sexual maturation. Male and female hormones also serve several important pharmacologic functions. These agents are often used as replacement therapy to resolve deficiencies in endogenous endocrine function. Androgens and estrogens and/or progestins are administered for a variety of other therapeutic reasons, including the control of some neoplastic diseases. Estrogens and progestins can also be administered to women as an effective means of birth control, and these hormones are used extensively as oral contraceptive agents. Finally, androgens are sometimes used in high doses by athletes in an attempt to increase muscle strength and performance. Although these drugs may produce increments in muscle strength in some individuals, the dangers of using high doses of anabolic steroids outweigh any potential ergogenic benefits.

REFERENCES

1. Aisenbrey, JA: Exercise in the prevention and management of osteoporosis. Phys Ther 67:1100, 1987.
2. Alen, M and Hakkinen, K: Androgenic steroid effects on serum hormones and on maximal force development in strength athletes. J Sports Med Phys Fitness 27:38, 1987.
3. American College of Sports Medicine: Position stand on the use of anabolic-androgenic steroids in sports. Med Sci Sports Exerc 19:534, 1987.
4. American Medical Association Council on Scientific Affairs: Medical and nonmedical uses of anabolic-androgenic steroids. JAMA 264:2923, 1990.
5. American Medical Association Council on Scientific Affairs: Drug abuse in athletes: Anabolic steroids and human growth hormone. JAMA 259:1703, 1988.
6. Ascoli, M and Segaloff, DL: Adenohypophyseal hormones and their hypothalamic releasing factors. In Hardman, JG, et al (eds): The Pharmacological Basis of Therapeutics, ed 9. McGraw-Hill, New York, 1996.
7. Badimon, L and Bayes-Genis, A: Effects of progestins on thrombosis and atherosclerosis. Hum Reprod Update 5:191, 1999.
8. Baird, DT and Glasier, AF: Hormonal contraception. N Engl J Med 328:1543, 1993.
9. Barrett-Connor, E: Hormone replacement and cancer. Br Med Bull 48:345, 1992.
10. Basaria, S and Dobs, AS: Risks versus benefits of testosterone therapy in elderly men. Drugs Aging. 15:131, 1999.
11. Belchetz, PE: Drug therapy: Hormonal treatment of post-menopausal women. N Engl J Med 330:1062, 1994.
12. Beral, V, et al: Use of HRT and the subsequent risk of cancer. J Epidemiol Biostat 4:191,1999.
13. Bergman, R and Leach, RE: The use and abuse of anabolic steroids in Olympic-caliber athletes. Clin Orthop 198:169, 1985.
14. Bhasin, S and Javanbakht, M: Can androgen therapy replete lean body mass and improve muscle function in wasting associated with human immunodeficiency virus infection? JPEN J Parenter Enteral Nutr 23(Suppl):S195, 1999.
15. Bigrigg, A, et al: Depo Provera. Position paper on clinical use, effectiveness and side effects. Br J Fam Plann 25:69, 1999.
16. Brook, CG: Treatment of late puberty. Horm Res 51(Suppl 3):101, 1999.
17. Bross, R, et al: Androgen effects on body composition and muscle function: Implications for the use of androgens as anabolic agents in sarcopenic states. Baillieres Clin Endocrinol Metab 12:365, 1998.
18. Buckley, WE, et al: Estimated prevalence of anabolic steroid use among male high school seniors. JAMA 260:3441, 1988.
19. Bygdeman, M, et al: The use of progesterone antagonists in combination with prostaglandin for termination of pregnancy. Hum Reprod 9(Suppl 1):121, 1994.
20. Cabasso, A: Peliosis hepatis in a young adult bodybuilder. Med Sci Sports Exerc 26:2, 1994.
21. Cadepond, F, Ulmann, A, and Baulieu, EE: RU486 (mifepristone): Mechanisms of action and clinical uses. Annu Rev Med 48:129, 1997.
22. Cancer and Steroid Hormone Study of the Center for Disease Control and the National Institute of Child Health and Human Development: Combination oral contraceptive use and the risk of endometrial cancer. JAMA 257:796, 1987.
23. Castelli, WP: Cardiovascular disease: Pathogenesis, epidemiology, and risk among users of oral contraceptives who smoke. Am J Obstet Gynecol 180(Part 2):S349, 1999.
24. Catlin, DH and Murray, TH: Performance-enhancing drugs, fair competition, and Olympic sport. JAMA 276:231, 1996.
25. Chetkowski, RJ, et al: Biologic effects of transdermal estradiol. N Engl J Med 314:1615, 1986.
26. Cicinelli, E, et al: Direct transport of progesterone from vagina to uterus. Obstet Gynecol 95:403, 2000.
27. Cofrancesco, J, Whalen, JJ, and Dobs, AS: Testosterone replacement treatment options for HIV-infected men. J Acquir Immune Defic Syndr Hum Retrovirol 16:254, 1997.
28. Cohen, JC and Hickman, R: Insulin resistance and diminished glucose tolerance in powerlifters ingesting anabolic steroids. J Clin Endocrinol Metab 64:960, 1987.
29. Compston, JE: Hormone replacement therapy and osteoporosis. Br Med Bull 48:309, 1992.
30. Conn, PM, et al: Mechanism of action of gonadotropin releasing hormone. Annu Rev Physiol 48:495, 1986.
31. Corrigan, B: Anabolic steroids and the mind. Med J Aust 165:222, 1996.
32. Creagh, TM, Rubin, A, and Evans, DJ: Hepatic tumors induced by anabolic steroids in an athlete. J Clin Pathol 41:441, 1988.

33. Cutson, TM and Meuleman, E: Managing menopause. Am Fam Physician 61:1391, 2000.
34. Delmas, PD: HRT in the prevention and treatment of osteoporosis. J Epidemiol Biostat 4:155, 1999.
35. Dhingra, K: Antiestrogens: Tamoxifen, SERMs, and beyond. Invest New Drugs 17:285, 1999.
36. Dobs, AS: Androgen therapy in AIDS wasting. Baillieres Clin Endocrinol Metab 12:379, 1998.
37. Dufau, ML: Endocrine regulation and communicating functions of the Leydig cell. Annu Rev Physiol 50:483, 1988.
38. Ellerington, MC, Whitcroft, SIJ, and Whitehead, MI: Hormone replacement therapy: Developments in therapy. Br Med Bull 48:401, 1992.
39. Ettinger, B, Genant, HK, and Cann, CE: Postmenopausal bone loss is prevented by treatment with low-dosage estrogen with calcium. Ann Intern Med 106:40, 1987.
40. Farley, TM, Collins, J, and Schlesselman, JJ: Hormonal contraception and risk of cardiovascular disease. An international perspective. Contraception 57:211, 1998.
41. Farley, TM, Meirik, O, and Collins, J: Cardiovascular disease and combined oral contraceptives: Reviewing the evidence and balancing the risks. Hum Reprod Update 5:721, 1999.
42. Felson, DT, et al: The effect of postmenopausal estrogen therapy on bone density in elderly women. N Engl J Med 329:1141, 1993.
43. Franceschi, S and La Vecchia, C: Oral contraceptives and colorectal tumors. A review of epidemiologic studies. Contraception 58:335, 1998.
44. Frankle, MA, Eichberg, R, and Zachariah, SB: Anabolic androgenic steroids and a stroke in an athlete: Case report. Arch Phys Med Rehabil 69:632, 1988.
45. Goldfien, A: The gonadal hormones and inhibitors. In Katzung, BG: Basic and Clinical Pharmacology, ed 7. Appleton & Lange, Stamford, CT, 1998.
46. Goldfrank, D, et al: Raloxifene, a new selective estrogen receptor modulator. J Clin Pharmacol 39:767, 1999.
47. Goldstein, SR: Selective estrogen receptor modulators: A new category of compounds to extend postmenopausal women's health. Int J Fertil Womens Med 44:221, 1999.
48. Gooren, LJ: Endocrine aspects of aging in the male. Mol Cell Endocrinol 145:153, 1998.
49. Guzzo, JA: Selective estrogen receptor modulators: A new age of estrogens in cardiovascular disease? Clin Cardiol 23:15, 2000.
50. Haddock, BL, et al: The effects of hormone replacement therapy and exercise on cardiovascular disease risk factors in postemenopausal women. Sports Med 29:39, 2000.
51. Hansen, KA and Tho, SP: Androgens and bone health. Semin Reprod Endocrinol 16:129, 1998.
52. Haupt, HA: Anabolic steroids and growth hormone. Am J Sports Med 21:468, 1993.
53. Haynes, B and Dowsett, M: Clinical pharmacology of selective estrogen receptor modulators. Drugs Aging 14:323, 1999.
54. Hewitt, G and Cromer, B: Update on adolescent contraception. Obstet Gynecol Clin North Am 27:143, 2000.
55. Jamin, C, Benifla, JL, and Madelenat, P: The role of selective prescribing in the increased risk of VTA associated with third-generation oral contraceptives. Hum Reprod Update 5:664, 1999.
56. Janne, OA and Bardin, CW: Androgen and antiandrogen receptor binding. Annu Rev Physiol 46:107, 1984.
57. Jarow, JP and Lipshultz, LI: Anabolic steroid-induced hypogonadotropic hypogonadism. Am J Sports Med 18:429, 1990.
58. Johnson, CA: Use of androgens in patients with renal failure. Semin Dial 13:36, 2000.
59. Kenemans, P: Menopause, HRT and menopausal symptoms. J Epidemiol Biostat 4:141, 1999.
60. Keyes, PL and Wiltbank, MC: Endocrine regulation of the corpus luteum. Annu Rev Physiol 50:465, 1988.
61. Kibble, MW and Ross, MB: Adverse effects of anabolic steroids in athletes. Clin Pharm 6:686, 1987.
62. Kuller, LH: Hormone replacement therapy and coronary heart disease. A new debate. Med Clin North Am 84:181, 2000.
63. Lamb, DR: Anabolic steroids in athletes: How well do they work and how dangerous are they? Am J Sports Med 12:31, 1984.
64. Larimore, WL and Stanford, JB: Postfertilization effects of oral contraceptives and their relationship to informed consent. Arch Fam Med 9:126, 2000.
65. La Vecchia, C and Franceschi, S: Oral contraceptives and ovarian cancer. Eur J Cancer Prev 8:297, 1999.
66. Leblanc, ES and Laws, A: Benefits and risks of third-generation oral contraceptives. J Gen Intern Med 14:625, 1999.
67. Lee, NC, et al: The reduction in risk of ovarian cancer associated with oral contraceptive use. N Engl J Med 316:650, 1987.
68. Lund, BC, Bever-Stille, KA, and Perry, PJ: Testosterone and andropause: The feasibility of testosterone replacement therapy in elderly men. Pharmacotherapy 19:951, 1999.
69. Mahajan, DK and London, SN: Mifepristone (RU486): A review. Fertil Steril 68:967, 1997.
70. McDonnell, DP: Selective estrogen replacement modulators (SERMs): A first step in the development of perfect hormone replacement therapy regimen. J Soc Gynecol Investig 7(Suppl):S10, 2000.
71. McNutt, RA, et al: Acute myocardial infarction in a 22-year-old world class weight lifter. Am J Cardiol 62:164, 1988.
72. Meade, TW and Berra, A: Hormone replacement therapy and cardiovascular disease. Br Med Bull 48:276, 1992.
73. Meade, TW and Vickers, MR: HRT and cardiovascular disease. J Epidemiol Biostat 4:165, 1999.

74. Mendis-Handagama, SM: Luteinizing hormone on Leydig cell structure and function. Histol Histopathol 12:869, 1997.
75. Migliara, R, et al: Antiandrogens: A summary review of pharmacodynamic properties and tolerability in prostate cancer therapy. Arch Ital Urol Androl 71:293, 1999.
76. Miller, MM and Franklin, KB: Theoretical basis for the benefit of postmenopausal estrogen substitution. Exp Gerontol 34:587, 1999.
77. Mitlak, BH and Cohen, FJ: Selective estrogen receptor modulators: A look ahead. Drugs 57:653, 1999.
78. Monk, D and Brodaty, H: Use of estrogens for the prevention and treatment of Alzheimer's disease. Dement Geriatr Cogn Disord 11:1, 2000.
79. Nabulsi, AA, et al: Association of hormone replacement therapy with various cardiovascular risk factors in postmenopausal women. N Engl J Med 328:1069, 1993.
80. Nakano, R: Control of the luteal function in humans. Semin Reprod Endocrinol 15:335, 1997.
81. Niswender, GD, et al: Mechanisms controlling the function and life span of the corpus luteum. Physiol Rev 80:1, 2000.
82. Oger, E and Scarabin, PY: Assessment of the risk for venous thromboembolism among users of hormone replacement therapy. Drugs Aging 14:55, 1999.
83. Osborne, MP: Breast cancer prevention by antiestrogens. Ann N Y Acad Sci 889:146, 1999.
84. Perlumutter, G and Lowenthal, DT: Use of anabolic steroids by athletes. Am Fam Physician 32:208, 1985.
85. Perry, PJ, Andersen, KH, and Yates, WR: Illicit anabolic steroid use in athletes: A series of case analyses. Am J Sports Med 18:422, 1990.
86. Pettine, KA: Association of anabolic steroids and avascular necrosis of femoral heads. Am J Sports Med 19:96, 1991.
87. Pope, HG and Katz, DL: Homicide and near-homicide by anabolic steroid users. J Clin Psychiatry 51:28, 1990.
88. Pope, HG and Katz, DL: Affective and psychotic symptoms associated with anabolic steroid abuse. Am J Psychiatry 145:487, 1988.
89. Porcerelli, JH and Sandler, BA: Anabolic-androgenic steroid abuse and psychopathology. Psychiatr Clin North Am 21:829, 1998.
90. Prasad, RN and Choolani, M: Termination of early human pregnancy with either 50 mg or 200 mg single oral dose of mifepristone (RU486) in combination with either 0.5 mg or 1.0 mg vaginal gemeprost. Aust N Z J Obstet Gynaecol 36:20, 1996.
91. Psaty, BM, et al: A review of the association of estrogens and progestins with cardiovascular disease in postmenopausal women. Arch Intern Med 153:1421, 1993.
92. Reid, IR: Pharmacological management of osteoporosis in postmenopausal women: A comparative review. Drugs Aging 15:349, 1999.
93. Reid, P, Kantoff, P, and Oh, W: Antiandrogens in prostate cancer. Invest New Drugs 17:271, 1999.
94. Richards, JS and Hedin, L: Molecular aspects of hormone action in ovarian follicular development, ovulation, and luteinization. Annu Rev Physiol 50:441, 1988.
95. Rivera, R, Yacobson, I, and Grimes, D: The mechanism of action of hormonal contraceptives and intrauterine contraceptive devices. Am J Obstet Gynecol 181(Part 1):1263, 1999.
96. Rolf, C and Nieschlag, E: Potential adverse effects of long-term testosterone therapy. Baillieres Clin Endocrinol Metab 12:521, 1998.
97. Romieu, I, Berlin, JA, and Colditz, G: Oral contraceptives and breast cancer. Review and meta-analysis. Cancer 66:2253, 1990.
98. Rosano, GM and Panina, G: Cardiovascular pharmacology of hormone replacement therapy. Drugs Aging 15:219, 1999.
99. Rossouw, JE: Hormone replacement therapy and cardiovascular disease. Curr Opin Lipidol 10:429, 1999.
100. Roy, S: Effects of smoking on prostacyclin formation and platelet aggregation in users of oral contraceptives. Am J Obstet Gynecol 180(Part 2):S364, 1999.
101. Rozenberg, S, et al: Osteoporosis management. Int J Fertil Womens Med 44:241, 1999.
102. Schein, AB: Pregnancy prevention using emergency contraception: Efficacy, attitudes, and limitations to use. J Pediatr Adolesc Gynecol 12:3, 1999.
103. Seed, M: Hormone replacement therapy and cardiovascular disease. Curr Opin Lipidol 10:581, 1999.
104. Sharpe, RM: Regulation of spermatogenesis. In Knobil, E and Neill, JD (eds): The Physiology of Reproduction, Vol 1, ed 2. Raven Press, New York, 1994.
105. Sherif, K: Benefits and risks of oral contraceptives. Am J Obstet Gynecol 180(Part 2):S343, 1999.
106. Sherman, MR and Stevens, J: Structure of mammalian steroid receptors. Annu Rev Physiol 46:83, 1984.
107. Simoni, M, et al: Role of FSH in male gonadal function. Ann Endocrinol (Paris) 60:102, 1999.
108. Skoog, I and Gustafson, D: HRT and dementia. J Epidemiol Biostat 4:227, 1999.
109. Strobl, JS: Estrogens, progestins, and antiestrogens. In Craig, CR and Stitzel, RE (eds): Modern Pharmacology with Clinical Applications, ed 5. Little Brown, Boston, 1997.
110. Sturdee, DW: Current hormone replacement therapy: What are the shortcomings? Advances in delivery. Int J Clin Pract 53:468, 1999.
111. Sullivan, ML, Martinez, CM, and Gallagher, EJ: Atrial fibrillation and anabolic steroids. J Emerg Med 17:851, 1999.
112. Sullivan, ML, et al: The cardiac toxicity of anabolic steroids. Prog Cardiovasc Dis 41:1, 1998.

113. Tavani, A and La Vecchia, C: The adverse effects of hormone replacement therapy. Drugs Aging 14:347, 1999.
114. Tenover, JL: Testosterone replacement therapy in older adult men. Int J Androl 22:300, 1999.
115. Thein, LA, Thein, JM, and Landry, GL: Ergogenic aids. Phys Ther 75:426, 1995.
116. Vermeulen, A, Goemaere, S, and Kaufman, JM: Testosterone, body composition and aging. J Endocrinol Invest 22(Suppl):110, 1999.
117. Walsh, BW, et al: Effects of postmenopausal estrogen replacement on the concentrations and metabolism of plasma lipoproteins. N Engl J Med 325:1196, 1991.
118. Warren, MP and Shantha, S: Uses of progesterone in clinical practice. Int J Fertil Womens Med 44:96, 1999.
119. Watts, NB: Postmenopausal osteoporosis. Obstet Gynecol Surv 54:532, 1999.
120. Webb, OL, Laskarzewski, PM, and Clueck, CJ: Severe depression of high density lipoprotein cholesterol levels in weight-lifters and bodybuilders by self-administered exogenous testosterone and anabolic-androgenic steroids. Metabolism 33:971, 1984.
121. Wells, G and Herrington, DM: The heart and estrogen/progestin replacement study: What have we learned and what questions remain? Drugs Aging 15:419, 1999.
122. Weryha, G, et al: Selective estrogen receptor modulators. Curr Opin Rheumatol 11:301, 1999.
123. Williams, CL and Stancel, GM: Estrogens and progestins. In Hardman, JG, et al (eds): The Pharmacological Basis of Therapeutics, ed 9. McGraw-Hill, New York, 1996.
124. Wilson, JD: Androgens. In Hardman, JG, et al (eds): The Pharmacological Basis of Therapeutics, ed 9. McGraw-Hill, New York, 1996.
125. Winters, SJ: Current status of testosterone replacement therapy in men. Arch Fam Med 8:257, 1999.
126. Wu, FC: Endocrine aspects of anabolic steroids. Clin Chem 43:1289, 1997.
127. Wuttke, W, et al: Regulation of steroid production and its function within the corpus luteum. Steroids 63:299, 1998.
128. Yesalis, CE and Bahrke, MS: Anabolic-androgenic steroids. Current issues. Sports Med 19:326, 1995.
129. Zeitoun, K and Carr, BR: Is there increased risk of stroke associated with oral contraceptives? Drug Saf 20:467, 1999.

CHAPTER 31

Thyroid and Parathyroid Drugs: Agents Affecting Bone Mineralization

This chapter discusses the function and pharmacologic aspects of two important endocrine structures: the thyroid and parathyroid glands. Hormones secreted from the thyroid gland are involved in controlling metabolism and also work synergistically with other hormones to promote normal growth and development. The parathyroid glands are essential in regulating calcium homeostasis and are important in maintaining proper bone mineralization.

Problems in the function of the thyroid or parathyroid glands are often treated by pharmacologic methods. Pharmacologic management of thyroid and parathyroid function should be of interest to rehabilitation specialists because physical therapists and occupational therapists often treat patients with disorders in bone healing and other endocrine problems related to these glands. This chapter first discusses normal physiologic function of the thyroid gland, followed by the types of drugs used to treat hyperthyroidism and hypothyroidism. Then the function of the parathyroid glands is covered, discussing the role of the parathyroid glands and other hormones in maintaining bone mineral homeostasis. Finally, drugs used to regulate bone calcification are presented.

FUNCTION OF THE THYROID GLAND

The thyroid gland lies on either side of the trachea in the anterior neck region and consists of bilateral lobes that are connected by a central isthmus. The entire gland weighs approximately 15 to 20 g and receives a rich vascular supply, as well as extensive innervation from the sympathetic nervous system.[19]

The thyroid gland synthesizes two primary hormones: thyroxine and triiodothyronine. Discussion of the synthesis and function of these hormones follows.

Synthesis of Thyroid Hormones

The chemical structures of thyroxine and triiodothyronine are shown in Figure 31–1. As shown in this figure, thyroid hormones are synthesized by first adding iodine to residues of the amino acid *tyrosine*. Addition of one iodine atom creates monoiodotyrosine, and the addition of a second iodine creates diiodotyrosine. Two of these iodinated tyrosines are then combined to complete the thyroid hormone. The combination of a monoiodotyrosine and a diiodotyrosine yields triiodothyronine, and the combination of two diiodotyrosines yields thyroxine.[43]

Because thyroxine contains four iodine residues, this compound is also referred to by the abbreviation T_4. Triiodothyronine contains three iodine residues, hence the abbreviation T_3. There has been considerable discussion about which hormone exerts the primary physiologic effects. Plasma levels of T_4 are much higher than T_3 levels, but T_3 may exert most of the physiologic effects on various tissues, suggesting that T_4 is primarily a precursor to T_3 and that conversion of T_4 to T_3 occurs in peripheral tissues.[19] Regardless of which hormone ultimately affects cellular metabolism, both T_4 and T_3 are needed for normal thyroid function.

The primary steps in thyroid hormone biosynthesis are shown schematically in Figure 31–2. Thyroid follicle cells take up and concentrate iodide from the bloodstream, which is significant because there must be a sufficient amount of iodine in the diet to provide the iodide needed for thyroid hormone production.[3] The thyroid cells also manufacture a protein known as thyroglobulin (TGB), which contains tyrosine residues. The TGB molecule is manufactured within the follicle cell and stored in the central lumen of the thyroid follicle (see Fig. 31–2). During hormone synthesis, iodide is oxidized and covalently bonded to the tyrosine residues of the TGB molecule.[14] Two iodinated tyrosine residues combine within the TGB molecule to form T_4 (primarily), with smaller amounts of T_3 also produced. At this point, the hormones are still incorporated within the large

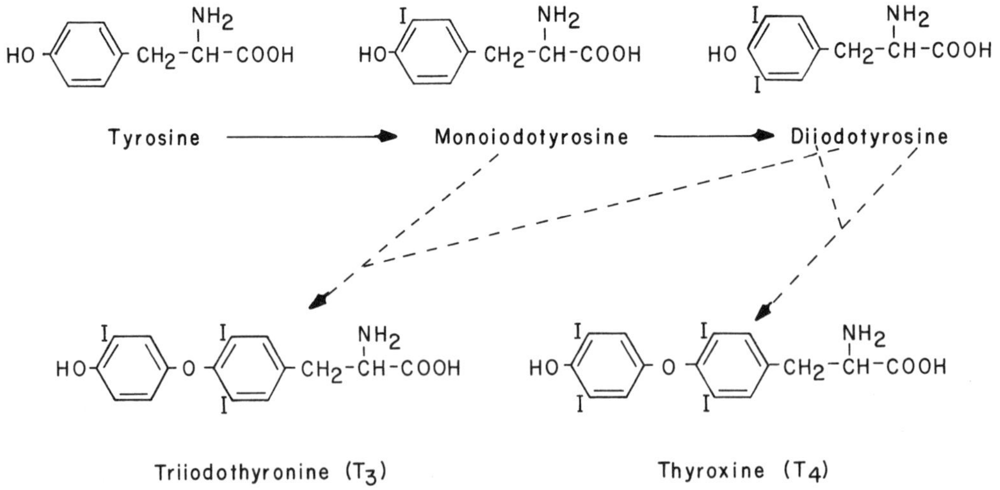

FIGURE 31–1. Structure of the thyroid hormones triiodothyronine (T_3) and thyroxine (T_4). Addition of one iodine atom (I) to tyrosine produces monoiodotyrosine; addition of a second iodine atom produces diiodotyrosine. A monoiodotyrosine and diiodotyrosine combine to form triiodothyronine (T_3). Coupling of two diiodotyrosines forms thyroxine (T_4).

TGB molecule. Hence, the iodinated TGB molecule (TGB containing the iodinated tyrosines) is absorbed back into the follicle cell, where the large molecule is lysed to yield the thyroid hormones. The hormones are then secreted into the systemic circulation, where they can reach various target tissues.

Regulation of Thyroid Hormone Release

Production of the thyroid hormones is controlled by the hypothalamic-pituitary system (see Chap. 28). Thyrotropin-releasing hormone (TRH) from the hypothalamus stimulates the release of thyroid-stimulating hormone (TSH) from the anterior pituitary.[38] TSH then travels via the systemic circulation to the thyroid gland to stimulate the production of thyroxine and triiodothyronine.

Thyroid hormone release is subject to the negative feedback strategy that is typical of endocrine systems controlled by the hypothalamic-pituitary axis. Increased circulating levels of the thyroid hormones (T_4, T_3) serve to limit their own production by inhibiting TSH release from the anterior pituitary.[28,38] The thyroid hormones do not directly inhibit TRH release from the hypothalamus; rather, the primary negative feedback control is at the level of the pituitary gland.[28] This negative feedback control prevents peripheral levels of thyroid hormones from becoming excessively high.

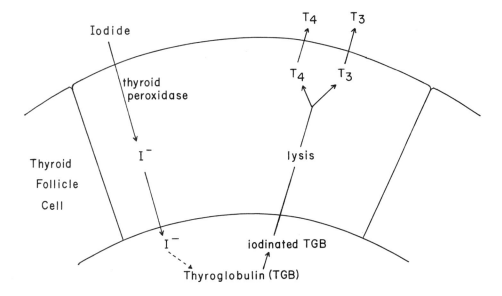

FIGURE 31–2. Thyroid hormone biosynthesis. Iodide is taken into the follicle cell, where it is converted by thyroid peroxidase to an oxidized form of iodine (I^-). I^- is transported to the follicle lumen, where it is bonded to tyrosine residues of the thyroglobulin (TGB) molecule. Iodinated TGB is incorporated back into the cell, where it undergoes lysis to yield the thyroid hormones T_3 and T_4. See text for further discussion.

Physiologic Effects of Thyroid Hormones

Thyroid hormones affect a wide variety of peripheral tissues throughout the entire life of the individual.[19,28] In some situations, these hormones exert a direct effect on cellular function (e.g., T_4 and T_3 appear to increase cellular metabolism by directly increasing oxidative enzyme activity). In other instances, thyroid hormones appear to play a permissive role in facilitating the function of other hormones. For instance, thyroid hormones must be present for growth hormone to function properly. The principal effects of the thyroid hormones are listed here.

Thermogenesis. T_4 and T_3 increase the basal metabolic rate and subsequent heat production from the body, which are important in maintaining adequate body temperature during exposure to cold environments. Increased thermogenesis is achieved by thyroid hormone stimulation of cellular metabolism in various tissues, such as skeletal muscle, cardiac muscle, and liver and kidney cells.

Growth and Development. Thyroid hormones facilitate normal growth and development by stimulating the release of growth hormone and by enhancing the effects of growth hormone on peripheral tissues. Thyroid hormones also directly enhance the development of many physiologic systems, especially the skeletal system and CNS. If thyroid hormones are not present, severe growth restriction and mental retardation (**cretinism**) ensue.

Cardiovascular Effects. Thyroid hormones appear to increase heart rate and myocardial contractility, thus leading to an increase in cardiac output. It is unclear, however, if this occurrence is a direct effect of these hormones or if the thyroid hormones increase myocardial sensitivity to other hormones (norepinephrine and epinephrine).

Metabolic Effects. Thyroid hormones affect energy substrate utilization in a number of ways. For instance, these hormones increase intestinal glucose absorption and increase the activity of several enzymes involved in carbohydrate metabolism. Thyroid hormones enhance lipolysis by increasing the response of fat cells to other lipolytic hormones. In general, these and other metabolic effects help increase the availability of glucose and lipids for increased cellular activity.

Mechanism of Action of Thyroid Hormones

The preponderance of evidence indicates that the thyroid hormones enter the cell and bind to specific receptors located within the cell's nucleus.[63,64] These thyroid hormone receptors act as DNA transcription factors that bind to specific DNA sequences that regulate gene expression. When activated by thyroid hormone, the thyroid receptors induce transcription of specific DNA gene segments, which ultimately results in altered protein synthesis within the cell.[63,64] Most, if not all, of the physiologic effects of the thyroid hormones are related to this alteration in cellular protein production. For instance, thyroid hormones may act through nuclear DNA transcription to stimulate the synthesis of a particular enzymatic protein. Such a protein may increase the transport of specific substances (e.g., amino acids, glucose, sodium) across the cell membrane, or the newly synthesized protein may be directly involved in a metabolic pathway (e.g., glycolysis or lipid oxidation).

TREATMENT OF THYROID DISORDERS

Thyroid disorders can basically be divided into two primary categories: conditions that increase thyroid function (hyperthyroidism) and conditions that decrease thyroid

TABLE 31–1 Primary Types of Hyperthyroidism and Hypothyroidism

Hyperthyroidism (Thyrotoxicosis)	Hypothyroidism (Hypothyroxinemia)

Primary hyperthyroidism
    Graves disease
    Thyroid adenoma/carcinoma
Secondary hyperthyroidism
    Hyperthyroidism induced by
    excessive hypothalamic or
    pituitary stimulation
	Primary hypothyroidism
	    Genetic deficiency of enzymes that synthesize thyroid
	    hormones
	Secondary hypothyroidism
	    Hypothyroidism induced by hypothalamic or pituitary
	    deficiencies
	    Cretinism (childhood hypothyroidism)
	    Myxedema (adult hypothyroidism)
	Other forms of hypothyroidism
	    Hypothyroidism induced by peripheral insensitivity to
	    thyroid hormones, inadequate hormone transport,
	    other causes

function (hypothyroidism).[62] There are several different types of hyperthyroidism and hypothyroidism, depending on the apparent etiology, symptoms, and age of onset of each type. Types of hyperthyroidism and hypothyroidism are listed in Table 31–1. Although we cannot review the causes and effects of all the various forms of thyroid dysfunction at this time, this topic is dealt with extensively elsewhere.[25,28,43,62]

The clinical manifestations of hyperthyroidism and hypothyroidism are listed in Table 31–2. From a pharmacotherapeutic standpoint, hyperthyroidism is treated with drugs that attenuate the synthesis and effects of the thyroid hormones. Hypothyroidism is usually treated by thyroid hormone administration (replacement therapy). The general aspects and more common forms of hyperthyroidism and hypothyroidism are discussed here, along with the drugs used to resolve these primary forms of thyroid dysfunction.

Hyperthyroidism

Hyperthyroidism (**thyrotoxicosis**) results in the increased secretion of thyroid hormones. This condition may occur secondary to a number of reasons, including thyroid tumors and problems in the endocrine regulation of thyroid secretion—for example, ex-

TABLE 31–2 Primary Symptoms of Hyperthyroidism and Hypothyroidism

Hyperthyroidism	Hypothyroidism
Nervousness	Lethargy/slow cerebration
Weight loss	Weight gain (in adult hypothyroidism)
Diarrhea	Constipation
Tachycardia	Bradycardia
Insomnia	Sleepiness
Increased appetite	Anorexia
Heat intolerance	Cold intolerance
Oligomenorrhea	Menorrhagia
Muscle wasting	Weakness
Goiter	Dry, coarse skin
Exophthalmos	Facial edema

Source: Adapted from Kuhn, MA: Thyroid and parathyroid agents. In Kuhn, MA (ed): Pharmacotherapeutics: A Nursing Process Approach, ed 3. FA Davis, Philadelphia, 1994, p 981.

cess TSH secretion (see Table 31–1).[32] Hyperthyroidism is usually associated with en-largement of the thyroid gland, or goiter. One of the more common causes of hyper-thyroidism is diffuse toxic goiter (Graves disease). Graves disease is thought to be caused by a problem in the immune system. Because of a genetic defect, antibodies are synthesized that directly stimulate the thyroid gland, resulting in exaggerated thyroid hormone production.[28,60] There are several other types of hyperthyroidism based on dif-ferent causes and clinical features (see Table 31–1).[28,43]

The principal manifestations of hyperthyroidism are listed in Table 31–2. The treat-ment of this condition often consists of ablation of the thyroid gland, accomplished by direct surgical removal of the thyroid or by administering radioactive iodine. Several pharmacologic agents may also be used in the management of hyperthyroidism in var-ious situations.[17,43] These drugs and their clinical applications are discussed in the fol-lowing sections.

Antithyroid Agents. Antithyroid drugs directly inhibit thyroid hormone synthesis. The antithyroid agents currently in use are propylthiouracil (Propyl-Thyracil) and me-thimazole (Tapazole).[13,17] These drugs inhibit the thyroid peroxidase enzyme necessary for preparing iodide for addition to tyrosine residues (see Fig. 31–2).[43] These agents also prevent coupling of tyrosine residues within the thyroglobulin molecule.[11,17] Propyl-thiouracil also inhibits the effects of the thyroid hormones by blocking the conversion of T_4 to T_3 in peripheral tissues.[11,17] The most common adverse effect of antithyroid drugs is skin rash and itching, although this effect is usually mild and transient. More serious problems involving formed blood elements (agranulocytosis and aplastic anemia) may occur, but the incidence of such problems is relatively small. Finally, excessive inhibi-tion of thyroid hormone synthesis brought about by drug overdosage may cause symp-toms resembling hypothyroidism, such as coldness and lethargy.

Iodide. Relatively large doses of iodide (exceeding 6 mg/day) cause a rapid and dramatic decrease in thyroid function. In sufficient amounts, iodide inhibits virtually all the steps involved in thyroid hormone biosynthesis. For instance, high iodide levels limit the uptake of iodide into thyroid follicle cells, inhibit the formation of T_4 and T_3, and decrease the secretion of the completed hormones from the thyroid cell.

Although iodide is effective in treating hyperthyroidism for short periods, the effects of this drug begin to diminish after about 2 weeks of administration.[17] Con-sequently, iodide is used in limited situations, such as temporary control of hyper-thyroidism prior to thyroidectomy. Also, iodide may cause a severe hypersensitive reaction in susceptible individuals. Therefore, the use of iodide has been replaced some-what by other agents such as the antithyroid drugs and beta blockers.

Radioactive Iodine. A radioactive isotope of iodine (^{131}I) is often used to selectively destroy thyroid tissues in certain forms of hyperthyroidism, such as Graves disease.[17,21] A specific dose of radioactive iodine is administered orally and rapidly sequestered within the thyroid gland. The isotope then begins to emit beta radiation, which selec-tively destroys the thyroid follicle cells. Essentially no damage occurs to surrounding tis-sues because the radioactivity is contained within the thyroid gland. Thus, administra-tion of radioactive iodine is a simple, relatively safe method of permanently ablating the thyroid gland and reducing excess thyroid hormone function.[21] Of course, patients who undergo radioactive destruction of the thyroid gland (or surgical thyroidectomy) must typically be given thyroid hormones as replacement therapy.[17]

Beta-Adrenergic Blockers. Beta-adrenergic blockers are usually associated with the treatment of cardiovascular problems such as hypertension and angina pectoris. Beta blockers may also be helpful as an adjunct in thyrotoxicosis.[15,17] Although these drugs do not directly lower plasma levels of thyroid hormones, they may help suppress symptoms such as tachycardia, palpitations, fever, and restlessness. Consequently, beta blockers are usually not the only drugs used in the long-term control of hyperthyroidism but serve as adjuncts to other medications such as the antithyroid drugs. Beta blockers may be especially helpful in severe, acute exacerbations of thyrotoxicosis (thyroid storm). These drugs are also administered preoperatively to control symptoms until a more permanent means of treating thyrotoxicosis (thyroidectomy) can be implemented.[15] Some beta blockers that have been used effectively in thyrotoxicosis are acebutolol, atenolol, metoprolol, nadolol, oxprenolol, propranolol, and timolol. The pharmacology and adverse effects of these compounds are described in Chapter 20.

Hypothyroidism

There are many forms of hypothyroidism, differing in their cause and age of onset (see Table 31–1). Severe adult hypothyroidism (**myxedema**) may occur idiopathically or may be caused by specific factors such as autoimmune lymphocytic destruction (Hashimoto disease). In the child, thyroid function may be congenitally impaired, and cretinism will result if this condition is untreated. Hypothyroidism may result at any age if the dietary intake of iodine is extremely low. Several other forms of hypothyroidism that have a genetic or familial basis also exist.[25,28,43]

The primary physiologic effects of decreased thyroid function are listed in Table 31–2. Although enlargement of the thyroid gland (*goiter*) is usually associated with hyperthyroidism, goiter may also be present in some forms of hypothyroidism, although for different reasons. For instance, thyroid enlargement occurs during hypothyroidism when there is a lack of dietary iodine (endemic goiter). Under the influence of TSH, the thyroid manufactures large quantities of thyroglobulin. Thyroid hormone synthesis is incomplete, however, because no iodine is available to add to the tyrosine residues. If no thyroid hormones are produced, there is no negative feedback to limit the secretion of TSH. Consequently, the thyroid gland increases in size because of the unabated production of thyroglobulin.

The primary method of treating hypothyroidism is to administer thyroid hormones as replacement therapy. Long-term administration of thyroid hormones is usually a safe, effective means of maintaining optimal patient health in hypothyroidism. Replacement therapy using thyroid hormone preparations is described here.

Thyroid Hormones. Replacement of deficient thyroid hormones with natural and synthetic analogs is necessary in most forms of hypothyroidism.[13,55] Preparations containing T_3, T_4, or both hormones are administered to mimic normal thyroid function whenever the endogenous production of these hormones is impaired. Administration of thyroid hormones is especially important in infants and children with hypothyroidism because adequate amounts of these hormones are needed for normal physical and mental development.[26] Thyroid hormone replacement is likewise necessary following thyroidectomy or pharmacologic ablation of the thyroid gland with radioactive iodine. Thyroid hormones may also be used to prevent and treat cancer of the thyroid gland and to prevent enlargement of the thyroid gland (goiter) caused by other drugs such as lithium. Thyroid hormone maintenance may be beneficial in patients who are in the preliminary or subclinical phase of hypothyroidism. Some clinicians feel that administering these hormones in the early stages may prevent the disease from developing to its full extent.[12,54]

Thyroid hormone preparations used clinically are listed in Table 31–3. The primary problems associated with these agents occur during overdosage. Symptoms of excess

TABLE 31–3 Thyroid Hormones Used to Treat Hypothyroidism

Generic Name	Trade Name(s)	Thyroid Hormone Content	Source
Levothyroxine	Levothroid, Synthroid, others	T_4	Synthetic
Liothyronine	Cytomel	T_3	Synthetic
Liotrix	Thyrolar	T_3 and T_4	Synthetic
Thyroid	Armour Thyroid, others	T_3 and T_4	Natural

T_3 = triiodothyronine; T_4 = thyroxine.

drug levels are similar to the symptoms of hyperthyroidism (see Table 31–2). Presence of these symptoms is resolved by decreasing the dosage or changing the medication.

FUNCTION OF THE PARATHYROID GLANDS

In humans, there are usually four parathyroid glands, which are embedded on the posterior surface of the thyroid gland. Each parathyroid gland is a pea-sized structure weighing about 50 mg. Despite their diminutive size, the parathyroids serve a vital role in controlling calcium homeostasis.[6,18] Because calcium is crucial in many physiologic processes, including synaptic transmission, muscle contraction, and bone mineralization, the importance of parathyroid function is obvious. In fact, removal of the parathyroid glands soon results in convulsions and death because of inadequate plasma calcium levels. The parathyroids control calcium homeostasis through the synthesis and secretion of parathyroid hormone (PTH), and the regulation and function of PTH is discussed here.

Parathyroid Hormone

PTH is a polypeptide hormone that is synthesized within the cells of the parathyroid glands. The primary factor controlling the release of PTH is the amount of calcium in the bloodstream.[18] A calcium-sensing receptor is located on the outer surface of the parathyroid cell membrane, and this receptor monitors plasma calcium levels.[10] A decrease in plasma calcium activates this receptor and causes increased release of PTH. As blood calcium levels increase, the receptor is inhibited, and PTH release is reduced.

The primary effect of PTH is to increase blood calcium levels by altering calcium metabolism in three primary tissues: bone, kidneys, and the gastrointestinal tract.[34,35] PTH directly affects skeletal tissues by increasing bone resorption, thus liberating calcium from skeletal stores.[6] High levels of PTH appear to enhance the development and action of cells (osteoclasts) that break down skeletal tissues.[6,18] Increased osteoclast activity degrades the collagen matrix within the bone, thus releasing calcium into the bloodstream. PTH also increases plasma calcium levels by increasing renal reabsorption of calcium. As renal calcium reabsorption is increased, PTH produces a simultaneous increase in phosphate excretion. Thus, PTH produces a rise in plasma calcium that is accompanied by a decrease in plasma phosphate levels.[18]

Finally, PTH helps increase the absorption of calcium from the gastrointestinal tract. This effect appears to be caused by the interaction between PTH and vitamin D metabolism. PTH increases the conversion of vitamin D to 1,25-dihydroxycholecalciferol (calcitriol).[18] Calcitriol directly stimulates calcium absorption from the intestine.

Consequently, PTH is crucial to maintaining adequate levels of calcium in the body. In addition, PTH works with two other primary hormones—calcitonin and vitamin D—

in regulating calcium homeostasis. These three hormones, as well as several other endocrine factors, are involved in controlling calcium levels for various physiologic needs. Of particular interest to rehabilitation professionals is how these hormones interact in controlling normal bone formation and resorption. Regulation of bone mineral homeostasis and the principal hormones involved in this process are presented in the following section.

REGULATION OF BONE MINERAL HOMEOSTASIS

Bone serves two primary functions: to provide a rigid framework for the body and to provide a readily available and easily interchangeable calcium pool.[41] To serve both functions simultaneously, an appropriate balance must exist between bone formation and bone resorption.[47] As already discussed, bone resorption (breakdown) can supply calcium for various physiologic processes. Mineral resorption, however, occurs at the expense of bone formation. The primary minerals that enable bone to maintain its rigidity are calcium and phosphate. Excessive resorption of these minerals will result in bone demineralization, and the skeletal system will undergo failure (fracture). Also, bone is continually undergoing specific changes in its internal architecture. This process of remodeling allows bone to adapt to changing stresses and optimally resist applied loads.[41]

Consequently, bone is a rather dynamic tissue that is constantly undergoing changes in mineral content and internal structure. The balance between bone resorption and formation is controlled by the complex interaction of local and systemic factors. In particular, there are several hormones that regulate bone formation and help maintain adequate plasma calcium levels. The primary hormones involved in regulating bone mineral homeostasis are described here.

Parathyroid Hormone. The role of the parathyroid gland and PTH in controlling calcium metabolism was discussed previously. Increased secretion of PTH increases blood calcium levels by several methods, including increased resorption of calcium from bone. High levels of PTH accelerate bone breakdown (catabolic effect) to mobilize calcium for other physiologic needs. Low or normal PTH levels, however, may actually enhance bone formation.[42] Moderate amounts of PTH can stimulate osteoblast activity and promote bone formation (anabolic effect). The anabolic effects of low or normal PTH levels seem limited to trabecular or cancellous bone; PTH may still cause breakdown of solid or cortical bone.[18,24] Nonetheless, the possibility that small intermittent doses of PTH may increase certain types of bone formation has sparked interest in using this hormone to prevent or reverse bone demineralization in certain conditions, including osteoporosis.[59] Although it is not currently approved for treating bone mineral loss, additional research should help clarify the therapeutic potential of PTH in treating osteoporosis. PTH therefore plays an important and complex role in regulating bone metabolism. Increased PTH secretion favors bone breakdown, whereas decreased or normal PTH release encourages bone synthesis and remodeling.

Vitamin D. Vitamin D is a steroidlike hormone that can be either obtained from dietary sources or synthesized in the skin from cholesterol derivatives in the presence of ultraviolet light. Vitamin D produces several metabolites that are important in bone mineral homeostasis.[18,35] In general, vitamin D derivatives such as 1,25 dihydroxyvitamin D_3 increase serum calcium and phosphate levels by increasing intestinal calcium and phosphate absorption and by decreasing renal calcium and phosphate excretion.[18] The effects of vitamin D metabolites on bone itself are somewhat unclear. Some metabolites seem to promote bone resorption, and others favor bone formation.[6] The overall influence of vitamin D, however, is to enhance bone formation by increasing the supply of the two primary minerals needed for bone formation (calcium and phosphate). Vitamin D also directly suppresses the synthesis and release of PTH from the parathyroid glands, an effect that tends to promote bone mineralization by limiting the catabolic effects of PTH.[4,7]

Calcitonin. Calcitonin is a hormone secreted by cells located in the thyroid gland. These calcitonin-secreting cells (also known as *parafollicular* or *C cells*) are interspersed between the follicles that produce the thyroid hormones. Basically, calcitonin can be considered the physiologic antagonist of PTH.[18] Calcitonin lowers blood calcium by stimulating bone formation and increasing the incorporation of calcium into skeletal storage. Incorporation of phosphate into bone is also enhanced by the action of calcitonin. Renal excretion of calcium and phosphate is increased by a direct effect of calcitonin on the kidneys, thus further reducing the levels of these minerals in the bloodstream. The effects of calcitonin on bone mineral metabolism, however, are relatively minor compared with PTH, and endogenous production of calcitonin is not essential for normal bone mineral homeostasis.[18] In contrast, PTH is a much more dominant hormone, and the absence of PTH produces acute disturbances in calcium metabolism that result in death. Calcitonin does have an important therapeutic function, and pharmacologic doses of calcitonin may be helpful in preventing bone loss in certain conditions (see "Pharmacologic Control of Bone Mineral Homeostasis").

Other Hormones. A number of other hormones influence bone mineral content.[42] Glucocorticoids produce a general catabolic effect on bone and other supporting tissues (see Chap. 29). Certain prostaglandins are also potent stimulators of bone resorption. Bone formation is generally enhanced by a number of hormones, such as estrogens, androgens, growth hormone, insulin, and the thyroid hormones. In general, the effects of these other hormones are secondary to the more direct effects of PTH, vitamin D, and calcitonin. Nonetheless, all the hormones that influence bone metabolism interact to some extent in the regulation of bone formation and breakdown. Also, disturbances in any of these secondary endocrine systems may produce problems that are manifested in abnormal bone formation, including excess glucocorticoid activity and growth hormone deficiency.

PHARMACOLOGIC CONTROL OF BONE MINERAL HOMEOSTASIS

Satisfactory control of the primary bone minerals is important in both acute and long-term situations. Blood calcium levels must be maintained within a fairly limited range to ensure an adequate supply of free calcium for various physiologic purposes. The normal range of total calcium in the plasma is 8.6 to 10.6 mg/100 mL.[18] If plasma calcium levels fall to below 6 mg/100 mL, tetanic muscle convulsions quickly ensue. Excess plasma calcium (blood levels greater than 12 mg/100 mL) depresses nervous function, leading to sluggishness, lethargy, and possibly coma.

Chronic disturbances in calcium homeostasis can also produce problems in bone calcification. Likewise, various metabolic bone diseases can alter blood calcium levels, leading to hypocalcemia or **hypercalcemia**. Some of the more common metabolic diseases affecting bone mineralization are listed in Table 31–4. Various problems in bone metabolism may produce abnormal plasma calcium levels, thus leading to the aforementioned problems.

Consequently, pharmacologic methods must often be used to help control bone mineral levels in the bloodstream and maintain adequate bone mineralization. Specific

TABLE 31–4 Examples of Metabolic Bone Disease

Disease	Pathophysiology	Primary Drug Treatment
Hypoparathyroidism	Decreased parathyroid hormone secretion; leads to impaired bone resorption and hypocalcemia	Calcium supplements, vitamin D
Hyperparathyroidism	Increased parathyroid hormone secretion, usually caused by parathyroid tumors; leads to excessive bone resorption and hypercalcemia	Usually treated surgically by partial or complete resection of the parathyroid gland
Osteoporosis	Generalized bone demineralization; often associated with effects of aging and hormonal changes in postmenopausal women	Calcium supplements, vitamin D, calcitonin, bisphosphonates, estrogen or SERMs (raloxifene) (see Chap. 30)
Rickets	Impaired bone mineralization in children; caused by a deficiency of vitamin D	Calcium supplements, vitamin D
Osteomalacia	Adult form of rickets	Calcium supplements, vitamin D
Paget disease	Excessive bone formation and resorption (turnover); leads to ineffective remodeling and structural abnormalities within the bone	Calcitonin, bisphosphonates
Renal osteodystrophy	Chronic renal failure; induces complex metabolic changes resulting in excessive bone resorption	Vitamin D, calcium supplements
Gaucher disease	Excessive lipid storage in bone; leads to impaired remodeling and excessive bone loss	No drugs are effective
Hypercalcemia of malignancy	Many forms of cancer accelerate bone resorption, leading to hypercalcemia	Calcitonin, bisphosphonates

drugs used to control bone mineralization and the clinical conditions in which they are used are discussed next.

Calcium Supplements

Calcium preparations are often administered to ensure that adequate calcium levels are available in the body for various physiologic needs, including bone formation. Specifically, calcium supplements can be used to help prevent bone loss in conditions such as osteoporosis, osteomalacia, rickets, and hypoparathyroidism. For instance, calcium supplements alone cannot prevent osteoporosis in postmenopausal women,[9] but these supplements are certainly helpful when combined with other treatments such as estrogen replacement.[44] The use of oral calcium supplements appears to be especially important in individuals who do not receive sufficient amounts of calcium in their diet.[48]

Types of calcium supplements used clinically are listed in Table 31–5. The dose of a calcium supplement should make up the difference between dietary calcium intake and established daily guidelines for each person. The exact dose for a given person therefore depends on factors such as the amount of dietary calcium, age, gender, and hormonal and reproductive status (e.g., women who are pregnant, premenopausal, or postmenopausal).[8] A woman, for example, who is postmenopausal and ingests 500 to 600 mg of dietary calcium per day would need a supplemental dosage of approximately 800 mg/day because the RDA guideline for women after menopause is 1200 to 1500 mg/day.[8]

Clearly, the dosage of a calcium supplement must be determined by the specific needs of each individual. Excessive doses must also be avoided because they may produce symptoms of hypercalcemia, including constipation, drowsiness, fatigue, and headache. As hypercalcemia becomes more pronounced, confusion, irritability, cardiac arrhythmias, hypertension, nausea and vomiting, skin rashes, and pain in bones and muscle may occur. Hypercalcemia is a cause for concern because severe cardiac irregularities may prove fatal.

Vitamin D

Vitamin D is a precursor for a number of compounds that increase intestinal absorption and decrease renal excretion of calcium and phosphate. Metabolites of vitamin

TABLE 31–5 Drugs Used to Control Bone Mineral Homeostasis

General Category	Examples*	Treatment Rationale and Principal Indications
Calcium supplements	Calicum carbonate (BioCal, Os-Cal 500, Tums, others) Calcium citrate (Citracal) Calcium glubionate (Calcionate, Neo-Calglucon) Calcium gluconate Calcium lactate Dibasic calcium phosphate Tribasic calcium phosphate (Posture)	Provide an additional source of calcium to prevent calcium depletion and encourage bone formation in conditions such as osteoporosis, osteomalacia, rickets, and hypoparathyroidism
Vitamin D analogs	Calcifediol (Calderol) Calcitriol (Rocaltrol) Dihydrotachysterol (DHT, Hytakerol) Ergocalciferol (Calciferol, Drisdol)	Generally enhance bone formation by increasing the absorption and retention of calcium and phosphate in the body; useful in treating disorders caused by vitamin D deficiency, including hypocalcemia, hypophosphatemia, rickets, and osteomalacia
Bisphosphonates	Etidronate (Didronel) Pamidronate (Aredia)	Appear to block excessive bone resorption and formation; are used to normalize bone turnover in conditions such as Paget disease and to prevent hypercalcemia resulting from excessive bone resorption in certain forms of cancer
Calcitonin	Human calcitonin (Cibacalcin) Salmon calcitonin (Calcimar, Miacalcin)	Mimics the effects of endogenous calcitonin and increases bone formation in conditions such as Paget disease and osteoporosis; also are used to lower plasma calcium levels in hypercalcemic emergencies

*Common trade names are shown in parentheses.

D and their pharmacologic analogs are typically used to increase blood calcium and phosphate levels and to enhance bone mineralization in conditions such as osteodystrophy, rickets, or other situations when people lack adequate amounts of vitamin D. Vitamin D analogs such as calcitriol have also been combined with calcium supplements to help treat postmenopausal osteoporosis[40,48] and to treat bone loss caused by antiinflammatory steroids (glucocorticoids; see Chap. 29).[2] Specific vitamin D–related compounds and their clinical applications are listed in Table 31–5.

Vitamin D is a fat-soluble vitamin, and excessive doses can accumulate in the body, leading to toxicity. Some early signs of vitamin D toxicity include headache, increased thirst, decreased appetite, metallic taste, fatigue, and gastrointestinal disturbances (nausea, vomiting, constipation, or diarrhea). Increased vitamin D toxicity is associated with hypercalcemia, high blood pressure, cardiac arrhythmias, renal failure, mood changes, and seizures. Vitamin D toxicity is a serious problem that can cause death because of cardiac and renal failure.

Bisphosphonates

The bisphosphonates (also called *diphosphonates*) are a group of inorganic compounds that include etidronate (Didronel), pamidronate (Aredia), and several similar agents. Although their exact mechanism is unclear, these compounds appear to adsorb directly to calcium crystals in the bone and to reduce bone resorption by inhibiting osteoclast activity.[37] Thus, bisphosphonates are often used in Paget disease to help prevent exaggerated bone turnover and promote adequate mineralization.[16] These agents can also be used to inhibit abnormal bone formation in conditions such as heterotopic ossification and to prevent hypercalcemia resulting from increased bone resorption in neoplastic disease.[22,52] Bisphosphonates have also emerged as the treatment of choice for the prevention and treatment of bone loss during prolonged administration of antiinflammatory steroids (glucocorticoids).[1] Bisphosphonates have likewise been used to reduce bone loss in osteoporosis, including osteoporosis associated with estrogen loss in women after menopause.[27,37] These drugs are not typically the first choice for treating postmenopausal osteoporosis, but they may be combined with other agents or used as an alternative in women who cannot take estrogen or other more traditional osteoporosis medications.[36,61]

The primary adverse effect associated with etidronate is tenderness and pain over the sites of bony lesions in Paget disease, leading to fractures if excessive doses are taken for prolonged periods. Pamidronate may cause fever and localized pain and redness at the injection site, but these effects usually last for only a day or two. Bisphosphonates may produce other relatively minor side effects, including gastrointestinal disturbances such as nausea and diarrhea.

Calcitonin

Calcitonin derived from synthetic sources can be administered to mimic the effects of the endogenous hormone. As described previously, endogenous calcitonin decreases blood calcium levels and promotes bone mineralization. Consequently, synthetically derived calcitonin is used to treat hypercalcemia and to decrease bone resorption in Paget disease.[50] Calcitonin has also been used to help prevent bone loss in a variety of other conditions, including rheumatoid arthritis,[51] postmenopausal osteoporosis,[39] and glucocorticoid-induced osteoporosis.[49] Administration of calcitonin can also reduce the risk of vertebral fractures and other fractures,[23] and this hormone may also decrease pain and promote mobility in people who have already sustained a vertebral fracture.[31]

In the past, calcitonin was administered by injection (intramuscular or subcutaneous), but aerosolized versions of calcitonin are now available that allow delivery in the form of nasal sprays.[51,53] Oral delivery of calcitonin is difficult because this hormone is absorbed poorly from the GI tract and because calcitonin is degraded by proteolytic enzymes in the stomach.[29] Nonetheless, efforts are being made to overcome these limitations, and an oral form of calcitonin may be available someday.[29,56]

Hence, calcitonin has emerged as an effective and easy way to treat a variety of conditions that are characterized by increased bone resorption.[45,50] Calcitonin preparations used clinically are either identical to the human form of this hormone (Cibacalcin) or chemically identical to salmon calcitonin (Calcimar, Miacalcin). Redness and swelling may occur locally when these agents are administered by injection. Other side effects include gastrointestinal disturbances (stomach pain, nausea, vomiting, and diarrhea), loss of appetite, and flushing or redness in the head, hands, and feet.

Estrogen Therapy

Estrogen replacement is the primary method used to prevent and treat bone loss in women who lack endogenous estrogen production—that is, following menopause or ovariectomy.[9,44,46,48,57] Estrogen is critical in maintaining adequate bone mineralization in women, and low doses of estrogen alone or estrogen combined with a progestin are often administered whenever endogenous estrogen production is lost. Replacement of estrogen following menopause has been shown to be especially effective, and this treatment can return the rate of bone formation and bone resorption to premenopausal levels.[9] Hence, estrogen replacement, combined with other adjunct treatments (calcium supplements, calcitonin, calcitriol, bisphosphonates), provides some excellent pharmacologic strategies for preventing the rather devastating effects of osteoporosis in postmenopausal women.[61]

The pharmacology and adverse effects of estrogen are discussed in Chapter 30. One of the primary concerns about using estrogen to prevent osteoporosis is that this hormone may increase the risk of certain forms of cancer, especially breast and uterine cancers.[5] This concern led to the development of estrogen-like compounds that activate estrogen receptors on certain tissues such as bone while blocking the effects of estrogen on breast and uterine tissues. These agents are known as selective estrogen receptor modulators (SERMs) because of their ability to preferentially activate certain estrogen receptors on certain types of tissue.[33,58]

The primary SERM used to prevent osteoporosis is raloxifene (Evista).[20,30] This drug binds to and activates estrogen receptors in bone, thus preventing bone loss and demineralization. At the same time, raloxifene blocks estrogen receptors on breast and uterine tissues, thereby preventing excessive stimulation of these receptors that might lead to the development of cancer. Hence, SERMs such as raloxifene provide an alternative to traditional estrogen therapy, and SERMs may be especially useful to women who have a history of breast or uterine cancer. Efforts continue to develop other SERMs that will be effective in preventing osteoporosis while minimizing the risks associated with traditional estrogen replacement therapy.

SPECIAL CONCERNS IN REHABILITATION PATIENTS

Physical therapists and occupational therapists should generally be concerned about potential side effects of the drugs discussed in this chapter. With regard to the treatment of thyroid disorders, excessive doses of drugs used to treat either hyperthyroidism or hypothyroidism tend to produce symptoms of the opposite disorder; that is, overdose of antithyroid drugs can produce signs of hypothyroidism, and vice versa. Therapists should be aware of the signs of thyroid dysfunction (see Table 31–2) and should be able to help detect signs of inappropriate drug dosage. Therapists should also avoid using rehabilitation techniques that may exacerbate any symptoms of thyroid dysfunction. For instance, care should be taken not to overstress the cardiovascular system of a patient with decreased cardiac output and hypotension caused by hypothyroidism (see Table 31–2).

Likewise, physical therapists and occupational therapists should be aware of the potential adverse effects of the drugs that regulate calcium homeostasis. For instance, excessive doses of calcium supplements may alter cardiovascular function, resulting in cardiac arrhythmias. Therapists may help detect these arrhythmias while monitoring pulses or ECG recordings. Finally, therapists may enhance the effects of bone-mineralizing drugs by employing exercise and weight-bearing activities to stimulate bone formation. Also, certain modalities may enhance the effects of bone-mineralizing agents. In particular, ultraviolet light increases endogenous vitamin D biosynthesis, thus facilitating calcium absorption and bone formation (see the Case Study in this chapter).

CASE STUDY

AGENTS AFFECTING BONE MINERAL METABOLISM

Brief History. R.D. is a 74-year-old woman with a history of generalized bone demineralization caused by osteomalacia brought on primarily by poor diet; that is, her total caloric intake and dietary levels of calcium and vitamin D have been very low. The patient is also rather reclusive, spending most of her time indoors. Consequently, she virtually lacks any exposure to natural sunlight. To treat her osteomalacia, she was placed on a regimen of oral calcium supplements and vitamin D. However, she has been reluctant to take these supplements because when she did, she occasionally experienced problems with diarrhea. Recently, she sustained a fracture of the femoral neck during a fall. She was admitted to the hospital, and the fracture was stabilized by open reduction and internal fixation. The patient was referred to physical therapy for strengthening and pre–weight-bearing activities.

Problem/Influence of Medication. During the postoperative period, calcium and vitamin D supplements were reinstituted to facilitate bone formation. The patient, however, soon began to experience bouts of diarrhea, apparently as a side effect of the vitamin D supplements. Consequently, the vitamin D supplements were withdrawn, and only the calcium supplement was continued. Because metabolic by-products of vitamin D accelerate the absorption of calcium from the gastrointestinal tract, both agents should be administered together. This patient, however, was apparently unable to tolerate vitamin D (or its analogs), possibly because of hypersensitivity to these compounds.

Decision/Solution. The physical therapist working with this patient realized that ultraviolet radiation stimulates the production of endogenous vitamin D. Ultraviolet light catalyzes the conversion of a cholesterol-like precursor (7-dehydrocholesterol) to vitamin D_3 within the skin. Vitamin D_3 then undergoes conversions in the liver and kidneys to form specific vitamin D metabolites (i.e., 1,25-dihydroxyvitamin D), which enhance intestinal calcium absorption. After conferring with the physician, the therapist incorporated a program of therapeutic ultraviolet radiation into the treatment regimen. The appropriate dose of ultraviolet exposure was first determined, followed by daily application of whole-body irradiation. Ultraviolet therapy was continued throughout the remainder of the patient's hospitalization, and callus formation at the fracture site was progressing well at the time of discharge.

SUMMARY

The thyroid and parathyroid glands serve a number of vital endocrine functions. The thyroid gland synthesizes and secretes the thyroid hormones T_4 and T_3. These hormones are important regulators of cellular metabolism and metabolic rate. Thyroid hormones also interact with other hormones to facilitate normal growth and development. The parathyroid glands control calcium homeostasis through the release of PTH. This hormone is crucial in maintaining normal blood calcium levels and in regulating bone formation and resorption. PTH also interacts with other hormones such as vitamin D and calcitonin in the control of bone mineral metabolism. Acute and chronic problems in thyroid and parathyroid function are often treated quite successfully with various pharmacologic agents. Rehabilitation specialists should be aware of the general strategies for treating thyroid and parathyroid disorders and of the basic pharmacotherapeutic approach to these problems.

REFERENCES

 1. Adachi, JD, et al: Management of corticosteroid-induced osteoporosis. Semin Arthritis Rheum 29:228, 2000.
 2. Amin, S, et al: The role of vitamin D in corticosteroid-induced osteoporosis: a meta-analytic approach. Arthritis Rheum 42:1740, 1999.
 3. Arthur, JR and Beckett, GJ: Thyroid function. Br Med Bull 55:658, 1999.
 4. Beckerman, P and Silver, J: Vitamin D and the parathyroid. Am J Med Sci 317:363, 1999.
 5. Beral, V, et al: Use of HRT and the subsequent risk of cancer. J Epidemiol Biostat 4:191, 1999.
 6. Bringhurst, FB, Demay, MB, and Kronenberg, HM: Hormones and disorders of mineral metabolism. In Wilson, JD, et al (eds): Williams Textbook of Endocrinology, ed 9. WB Saunders, Philadelphia, 1998.
 7. Brown, AJ and Slatopolsky, E: Vitamin D analogs: Perspectives for treatment. Miner Electrolyte Metab 25:337, 1999.
 8. Celotti, F and Bignamini, A: Dietary calcium and mineral/vitamin supplementation: A controversial problem. J Int Med Res 27:1, 1999.
 9. Christiansen, C: Prevention and treatment of osteoporosis: A review of current modalities. Bone 13:S35, 1992.
10. Coburn, JW, et al: Calcium-sensing receptor and calcimimetic agents. Kidney Int Suppl 73:S52, 1999.
11. Cooper, DS: Antithyroid drugs. N Engl J Med 311:1353, 1984.
12. Cooper, DS, et al: L-thyroxine therapy in subclinical hypothyroidism: A double-blind, placebo-controlled study. Ann Intern Med 101:18, 1984.
13. Corsello, SM, Migneco, MG, and Lovicu, RM: Medical therapy of benign thyroid diseases. Rays 24:315, 1999.
14. Dunn, JT and Dunn, AD: The importance of thyroglobulin structure for thyroid hormone biosynthesis. Biochimie 81:505, 1999.

15. Felz, MW and Stein, PP: The many "faces" of Graves' disease. Part 2. Practical diagnostic testing and management options. Postgrad Med 106:45, 1999.
16. Fleisch, H: Bisphosphonates: Pharmacology. Semin Arthritis Rheum 23:261, 1994.
17. Franklyn, JA: Drug therapy: The management of hyperthyroidism. N Engl J Med 330:1731, 1994.
18. Genuth, SM: Endocrine regulation of the metabolism of calcium and phosphate. In Berne, RM and Levy, MN (eds): Physiology, ed 3. Mosby Year Book, St Louis, 2000.
19. Genuth, SM: Thyroid gland. In Berne, RM and Levy, MN (eds): Physiology, ed 3. Mosby Year Book, St Louis, 2000.
20. Goldfrank, D, et al: Raloxifene, a new selective estrogen receptor modulator. J Clin Pharmacol 39:767, 1999.
21. Gross, MD, Shapiro, B, and Sisson, JC: Radioiodine therapy of thyrotoxicosis. Rays 24:334, 1999.
22. Hasling, C, Charles, P, and Mosekilde, L: Etidronate disodium in the management of malignancy-related hypercalcemia. Am J Med 82(Suppl 2A):51, 1987.
23. Kanis, JA and McClosky, EV: Effect of calcitonin on vertebral and other fractures. QJM 92:143, 1999.
24. Khan, A and Bilezikian, J: Primary hyperparathyroidism: Pathophysiology and impact on bone. CMAJ 163:184, 2000.
25. Lack, EA, Farber, JL, and Rubin, E: The endocrine system. In Rubin, E and Farber, JL (eds): Pathology, ed. 3. Lippincott-Raven, Philadelphia, 1999.
26. LaFranchi, S: Congenital hypothyroidism: Etiologies, diagnosis, and management. Thyroid 9:735, 1999.
27. Lane, JM, Russell, L and Khan, SN: Osteoporosis. Clin Orthop 372:139, 2000.
28. Larsen, PR, Davies, TF, and Hay, ID: The thyroid gland. In Wilson, JD, et al (eds): Williams Textbook of Endocrinology, ed 9. WB Saunders, Philadelphia, 1998.
29. Lee, YH and Sinko, PJ: Oral delivery of salmon calcitonin. Adv Drug Deliv Rev 42:225, 2000.
30. Licata, AA, et al: Raloxifene: A new choice for treating and preventing osteoporosis. Cleve Clin J Med 67:273, 2000.
31. Makysmowych, WP: Managing acute osteoporotic vertebral fractures with calcitonin. Can Fam Physician. 44:2160, 1998.
32. Maussier, ML, et al: Thyrotoxicosis: Clinical and laboratory assessment. Rays 24:263, 1999.
33. McDonnell, DP: Selective estrogen replacement modulators (SERMs): A first step in the development of perfect hormone replacement therapy regimen. J Soc Gynecol Investig 7(Suppl):S10, 2000.
34. Morley, P, Whitfield, JF, and Willick, GE: Design and applications of parathyroid hormone analogues. Curr Med Chem 6:1095, 1999.
35. Mundy, GR and Guise, TA: Hormonal control of calcium homeostasis. Clin Chem 45(Part 2):1347, 1999.
36. Netelenbos, C: Osteoporosis: Intervention options. Maturitas 30:235, 1998.
37. Papapoulos, SE, et al: The use of bisphonates in the treatment of osteoporosis. Bone 13:S41, 1992.
38. Persani, L: Hypothalamic thyrotropin-releasing hormone and thyrotropin biological activity. Thyroid 8:941, 1998.
39. Prelevic, GM and Adashi, EY: Postmenopausal osteoporosis: Prevention and treatment with calcitonin. Gynecol Endocrinol 6:141, 1992.
40. Raisz, LG: Osteoporosis: Current approaches and future prospects in diagnosis, pathogenesis, and management. J Bone Miner Metab 17:79, 1999.
41. Raisz, LG: Physiology and pathophysiology of bone remodeling. Clin Chem 45(Part 2):1353, 1999.
42. Raisz, LG, Kream, BE, and Lorenzo, JA: Metabolic bone disease. In Wilson, JD, et al (eds): Williams Textbook of Endocrinology, ed 9. WB Saunders, Philadelphia, 1998.
43. Reasner, CA and Talbert, RL: Thyroid disorders. In DiPiro, JT, et al (eds): Pharmacotherapy: A Pathophysiologic Approach. Appleton & Lange, Stamford, CT, 1999.
44. Recker, RR: Current therapy for osteoporosis. J Clin Endocrinol Metab 76:14, 1993.
45. Reginster, J-Y: Management of high-turnover osteoporosis with calcitonin. Bone 13:S37, 1992.
46. Reid, IR: Pharmacological management of osteoporosis in postmenopausal women: A comparative review. Drugs Aging 15:349, 1999.
47. Rodan, GA and Martin, TJ: Therapeutic approaches to bone disease. Science 289:1508, 2000.
48. Rozenberg, S, et al: Osteoporosis management. Int J Fertil Womens Med 44:241, 1999.
49. Sambrook, P, et al: Prevention of corticosteroid osteoporosis: A comparison of calcium, calcitriol, and calcitonin. N Engl J Med 328:1747, 1993.
50. Sexton, PM, Findlay, DM, and Martin, TJ: Calcitonin. Curr Med Chem 6:1067, 1999.
51. Sileghem, A, Geusens, P, and Dequeker, J: Intranasal calcitonin for the prevention of bone erosion and bone loss in rheumatoid arthritis. Ann Rheum Dis 51:761, 1992.
52. Singer, FR and Fernandez, M: Therapy of hypercalcemia of malignancy. Am J Med 82(Suppl 2A):34, 1987.
53. Thamsborg, G: Effect of nasal salmon calcitonin on calcium and bone metabolism. Dan Med Bull 46:118, 1999.
54. Tibaldi, J and Barzel, US: Thyroxine supplementations: Method for the prevention of clinical hypothyroidism. Am J Med 79:241, 1985.
55. Toft, AD: Drug therapy: Thyroxine therapy. N Engl J Med 331:174, 1994.
56. Torres-Lugo, M and Peppas, NA: Transmucosal delivery systems for calcitonin: A review. Biomaterials 21:1191, 2000.
57. Watts, NB: Postmenopausal osteoporosis. Obstet Gynecol Surv 54:532, 1999.
58. Weryha, G, et al: Selective estrogen receptor modulators. Curr Opin Rheumatol 11:301, 1999.

59. Whitfield, JF, Morley, P, and Willick, GE: The bone-building action of the parathyroid hormone: Implications for the treatment of osteoporosis. Drugs Aging 15:117, 1999.
60. Wilkin, TJ: Mechanisms of disease: Receptor autoimmunity in endocrine disorders. N Engl J Med 323:1318, 1990.
61. Wimalawansa, SJ: Prevention and treatment of osteoporosis: Efficacy of combination of hormone replacement with other antiresorptive agents. J Clin Densitom 3:187, 2000.
62. Woeber, KA: Update on the management of hyperthyroidism and hypothyroidism. Arch Intern Med 160:1067, 2000.
63. Wu, Y and Koenig, RJ: Gene regulation by thyroid hormone. Trends Endocrinol Metab 11:207, 2000.
64. Zhang, J and Lazar, MA: The mechanism of action of thyroid hormones. Annu Rev Physiol 62:439, 2000.

CHAPTER 32

Pancreatic Hormones and the Treatment of Diabetes Mellitus

The pancreas functions uniquely as both an endocrine and an exocrine gland. The exocrine role of this gland consists of excretion of digestive enzymes into the duodenum via the pancreatic duct. Pancreatic endocrine function consists of the secretion of two principal hormones—insulin and glucagon—into the bloodstream. Insulin and glucagon are involved primarily with the regulation of blood glucose. Insulin also plays a role in protein and lipid metabolism and is important in several aspects of growth and development. Problems with the production and function of insulin cause a fairly common and clinically significant disease known as **diabetes mellitus**.

The purpose of this chapter is to review the normal physiologic roles of the pancreatic hormones and to describe the pathogenesis and treatment of diabetes mellitus. As will be indicated, diabetes mellitus has many sequelae that influence patients' neuromuscular and cardiovascular functioning. Patients with diabetes mellitus often undergo physical rehabilitation for problems related to the condition. Consequently, the nature of diabetes mellitus and the pharmacotherapeutic treatment of this disease are important to physical therapists and occupational therapists.

STRUCTURE AND FUNCTION OF THE ENDOCRINE PANCREAS

The cellular composition of the pancreas has been described in great detail.[18,19,32,94] The bulk of the gland consists of acinar cells that synthesize and release the pancreatic digestive enzymes (thereby providing the exocrine function). Interspersed within the acinar tissues are smaller clumps of tissue known as the *islets of Langerhans*. These islets contain cells that synthesize and secrete the pancreatic hormones, thus constituting the endocrine portion of the gland.

The pancreatic islets consist of three primary cell types: alpha (A) cells, which produce glucagon; beta (B) cells, which produce insulin; and delta (D) cells, which produce somatostatin. As previously mentioned, this chapter focuses on the functions of insulin and glucagon. *Somatostatin* is a polypeptide hormone that appears to affect several physiologic systems, including regulation of gastrointestinal absorption and motility. Although the exact role of pancreatic somatostatin is still somewhat unclear, this hormone may inhibit the release of glucagon and insulin.[5,32]

INSULIN

Insulin is a large polypeptide of 51 amino acids arranged in a specific sequence and configuration. The primary effect of insulin is to lower blood glucose levels by facilitating the entry of glucose into peripheral tissues. The effects of insulin on energy metabolism, specific aspects of insulin release, and insulin's mechanism of action are discussed here.

Effects of Insulin on Carbohydrate Metabolism. Following a meal, blood glucose increases sharply. Insulin is responsible for facilitating the movement of glucose out of the bloodstream and into the liver and other tissues, where it can be stored for future needs.[87] Most tissues in the body (including skeletal muscle cells) are relatively impermeable to glucose and require the presence of some sort of transport system or carrier to help convey the glucose molecule across the cell membrane.[50,87,94] The carrier-mediated transport of glucose into muscle cells is believed to be a form of facilitated diffusion (see Chap. 2). Insulin appears to directly stimulate this facilitated diffusion, resulting in a 10-fold or greater increase in the rate of glucose influx.[37] Possible ways in which insulin affects glucose transport on the cellular level are discussed later in "Cellular Mechanisms of Insulin Action."

Insulin affects uptake and use of glucose in the liver somewhat differently than in skeletal muscle and other tissues. Hepatic cells are relatively permeable to glucose, and glucose enters these cells quite easily, even when insulin is not present. Glucose, however, is also free to leave liver cells just as easily, unless it is trapped in the cells in some manner. Insulin stimulates the activity of the glucokinase enzyme, which phosphorylates glucose and subsequently traps the glucose molecule in the hepatic cell. Insulin also increases the activity of enzymes that promote glycogen synthesis and inhibits enzymes that promote glycogen breakdown. Thus, the primary effect of insulin on the liver is to promote sequestration of the glucose molecule and to increase storage of glucose in the form of hepatic glycogen.

Effects of Insulin on Protein and Lipid Metabolism. Although insulin is normally associated with regulating blood glucose, this hormone also exerts significant effects on proteins and lipids. In general, insulin promotes storage of protein and lipid in muscle and adipose tissue, respectively.[32,94,100] Insulin encourages protein synthesis in muscle cells by stimulating amino acid uptake, increasing DNA/RNA activity related to protein synthesis, and inhibiting protein breakdown. In fat cells, insulin stimulates the synthesis of triglycerides (the primary form of lipid storage in the body), as well as inhibiting the enzyme that breaks down stored lipids (hormone-sensitive lipase). Consequently, insulin is involved in carbohydrate, protein, and lipid metabolism, and disturbances in insulin function (diabetes mellitus) will affect storage and use of all the primary energy substrates.

Cellular Mechanism of Insulin Action

Insulin exerts its effects by first binding to a receptor located on the surface membrane of target cells.[16,94] This receptor is a glycoprotein that is highly specific for insulin.

The complete insulin receptor consists of two matching or paired units, with each unit consisting of an alpha and a beta subunit (Fig. 32–1). The alpha subunit is the binding site for insulin. The beta subunit appears to be an enzyme that functions as a tyrosine kinase, which means that the beta subunit catalyzes the addition of phosphate groups to tyrosine residues within the beta subunit.[16] Thus, binding insulin to the alpha subunit causes the beta subunit to undergo *autophosphorylation;* that is, the receptor adds phosphate groups to itself. This autophosphorylation of the insulin receptor then initiates a series of biochemical changes within the cell.

The way that the insulin-receptor interaction triggers subsequent changes in cellular activity has been the subject of extensive research. When activated, the insulin receptor begins to add phosphate molecules to other large intracellular proteins known as insulin receptor substrates (IRSs).[16,32] Although the exact details need to be elucidated,

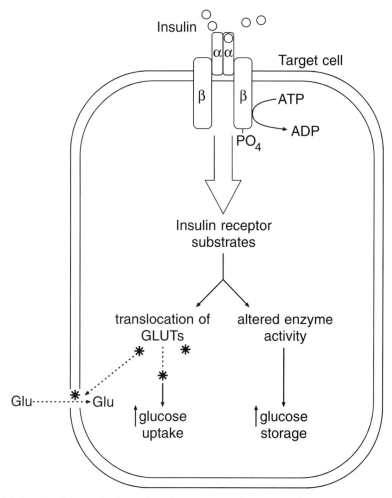

FIGURE 32–1. Possible mechanism of insulin action on glucose metabolism in skeletal muscle cells. An insulin receptor located on the cell's surface consists of 2 alpha (α) and 2 beta (β) subunits. Binding of insulin to the α subunits causes addition of phosphate groups (PO_4) to the β subunits. This receptor autophosphorylation causes activation of 1 or more insulin receptor substrates (IRSs) that promote translocation of glucose carriers (GLUTs) to the cell membrane, where they increase facilitated diffusion of glucose (Glu) into the cell. Activated IRSs also increase the activity of enzymes that promote glucose storage.

IRSs initiate changes in various metabolic pathways that ultimately result in increased glucose uptake, increased protein synthesis, and other changes in cell metabolism.[87] In particular, certain IRSs initiate movement *(translocation)* of glucose transporters from intracellular storage sites to the cell membrane of skeletal muscle cells and other peripheral tissues (see Fig. 32–1). These glucose transporters are proteins that are synthesized and stored within the Golgi system of the cell. Glucose transporters are likewise often referred to as GLUT proteins or simply GLUTs, and several different forms of GLUTs exist, depending on the specific cell affected by insulin. Perhaps the most important GLUT protein is the GLUT4 subtype, which is the glucose transporter in muscle and fat cells.[50] By binding to the insulin receptor on the cell membrane, insulin ultimately causes GLUT4 proteins to travel to the cell membrane, where they can then promote the facilitated diffusion of glucose into the cell (see Fig. 32–1).

Consequently, we now have a fairly clear idea of how insulin binds to a specific receptor and exerts its effects on target cells. Knowledge of exactly how insulin interacts with target tissues is important because defects in receptor binding and problems in the subsequent postreceptor events may be responsible for some of the changes seen in certain forms of diabetes mellitus. The possible role of these receptor-mediated problems in diabetes is discussed later in "Type 2 Diabetes."

GLUCAGON

Glucagon is considered to be the hormonal antagonist of insulin.[32,37] The primary effect of glucagon is to increase blood glucose to maintain normal blood glucose levels and prevent hypoglycemia.[32,37] Glucagon produces a rapid increase in glycogen breakdown *(glycogenolysis)* in the liver, thus liberating glucose into the bloodstream from hepatic glycogen stores. Glucagon then stimulates a more prolonged increase in hepatic glucose production *(gluconeogenesis)*. This gluconeogenesis sustains blood glucose levels even after hepatic glycogen has been depleted.[37]

Glucagon appears to exert its effects on liver cells by a classic adenyl cyclase–cyclic adenosine monophosphate (cAMP) second messenger system (see Chap. 4).[66] Glucagon binds to a specific receptor located on the hepatic cell membrane. This stimulates the activity of the adenyl cyclase enzyme that transforms adenosine triphosphate (ATP) into cAMP. Then, cAMP acts as an intracellular second messenger that activates specific enzymes to increase glycogen breakdown and stimulate gluconeogenesis.

CONTROL OF INSULIN AND GLUCAGON RELEASE

An adequate level of glucose in the bloodstream is necessary to provide a steady supply of energy for certain tissues, especially the brain. Normally, blood glucose is maintained between 80 and 90 mg of glucose per 100 mL of blood.[37] A severe drop in blood glucose *(hypoglycemia)* is a potentially serious problem that can result in coma and death. Chronic elevations in blood glucose (**hyperglycemia**) have been implicated in producing pathologic changes in neural and vascular structures. Consequently, insulin and glucagon play vital roles in controlling glucose levels, and release of these hormones must be closely regulated.

The level of glucose in the bloodstream is the primary factor affecting release of the pancreatic hormones.[32] As blood glucose rises (following a meal), insulin secretion from pancreatic beta cells is increased. Insulin then promotes movement of glucose out of the bloodstream and into various tissues, thus reducing plasma glucose back to normal levels. As blood glucose levels fall (during a sustained fast), glucagon is released from the alpha cells in the pancreas. Glucagon resolves this hypoglycemia by stimulating the synthesis and release of glucose from the liver.

Release of insulin and glucagon may also be governed to some extent by other energy substrates (lipids and amino acids), other hormones (thyroxine, cortisol), and autonomic neural control.[32] Nonetheless, the major factor influencing pancreatic hormone release is blood glucose. Cells located in the pancreatic islets are bathed directly by the blood supply reaching the pancreas. These cells act as glucose sensors, which directly monitor plasma glucose levels. In particular, the beta or insulin-secreting cells act as the primary glucose sensors, and adequate control of insulin release seems to be a somewhat higher priority than control of glucagon function.[78]

An important interaction between insulin and glucagon may also take place directly within the pancreas, and insulin appears to be the dominant hormone controlling this interaction.[78] When the beta cells sense an increase in blood glucose, they release insulin, which in turn inhibits glucagon release from the alpha cells. When insulin release diminishes, the inhibition of glucagon production is removed, and glucagon secretion is free to increase. This intraislet regulation between insulin and glucagon is important during normal physiologic function as well as in pathologic conditions, such as diabetes mellitus.[78] A deficiency of insulin production permits an increase in glucagon release, and the effects of increased glucagon may contribute to some of the metabolic changes in diabetes mellitus (although the exact role of increased glucagon in diabetes remains controversial).[66]

Consequently, insulin and glucagon serve to maintain blood glucose within a fairly finite range. If the endocrine portion of the pancreas is functioning normally, blood glucose levels remain remarkably constant, even in situations such as exercise and prolonged fasting. However, any abnormalities in pancreatic endocrine function can alter the regulation of blood glucose. In particular, problems associated with the production and effects of insulin can produce serious disturbances in glucose metabolism, as well as a number of other metabolic problems. Such problems in insulin production and function are characteristic of a disease known as diabetes mellitus. The pathogenesis and treatment of this disease is presented in the following section.

DIABETES MELLITUS

Diabetes mellitus is a disease caused by insufficient insulin secretion or a decrease in the peripheral effects of insulin. This disease is characterized by a primary defect in the metabolism of carbohydrates and other energy substrates. These metabolic defects can lead to serious acute and chronic pathologic changes. The term *diabetes mellitus* differentiates this disease from an unrelated disorder known as diabetes insipidus. **Diabetes insipidus** is caused by a lack of antidiuretic hormone (ADH) production or insensitivity to ADH. Consequently, the full terminology of "diabetes mellitus" should be used when referring to the insulin-related disease. Most clinicians, however, refer to diabetes mellitus as simply "diabetes."

Diabetes mellitus is a fairly common disease affecting approximately 6 percent of the people in the United States.[86] This disease is a serious problem in terms of the increased morbidity and mortality associated with it. Diabetes mellitus is the leading cause of blindness in adults and is the primary factor responsible for 30 percent of the cases of end-stage renal failure.[86] It is also estimated that 67,000 lower-extremity amputations are performed annually because of complications related to diabetes mellitus.[86] Consequently, this disease is a serious problem affecting the lives of many individuals.

Diabetes mellitus is apparently not a single, homogeneous disease but rather a disease existing in at least two primary forms.[18,19,86] Patients with diabetes mellitus are usually classified as having either type 1 or type 2 diabetes, depending on the pathogenesis of their disease. The primary characteristics of type 1 and type 2 diabetes mellitus are summarized in Table 32–1. Specific aspects of these two primary forms of diabetes mellitus are discussed in more detail here.

Type 1 Diabetes

Type 1 diabetes accounts for approximately 10 percent of the individuals with diabetes mellitus.[86] Patients with type 1 diabetes are unable to synthesize any appreciable amounts of insulin. There appears to be an almost total destruction of pancreatic beta cells in these individuals. Because these patients are unable to produce insulin, type 1 diabetes is also referred to as *insulin-dependent diabetes mellitus* (IDDM); that is, administration of exogenous insulin is necessary for survival. The onset of type 1 diabetes is usually during childhood, so this form of diabetes is sometimes referred to as *juvenile diabetes*. Classic type 1 diabetes, however, can develop in people of all ages.[93] The term *juvenile diabetes* has therefore largely been replaced by the other terms mentioned (i.e., type 1 or IDDM). Patients with type 1 diabetes are typically close to normal body weight or slightly underweight.

The exact cause of type 1 diabetes remains unknown. There is considerable evidence, however, that the beta cell destruction characteristic of this disease may be caused by an autoimmune reaction.[15,18,102] Specifically, a virus or some other antigen may trigger an autoimmune reaction that selectively destroys the insulin-secreting beta cells in susceptible individuals.[35,54,102] The susceptibility of certain patients to such viral-initiated immunodestruction may be because of genetic predisposition, environmental factors, or other factors that remain to be determined.[17,18,52,93,94] The idea that type 1 diabetes may have an autoimmune basis has led to the use of immunosuppressant agents in the early stages of this disease (see "Immunosuppressants" later in this chapter).

Type 2 Diabetes

Type 2 or *non–insulin-dependent diabetes mellitus* (NIDDM) accounts for the other 90 percent of people with diabetes mellitus.[86] This form of diabetes usually occurs in adults, especially in older individuals.[18,19] Type 2 diabetes, however, can also occur in younger people, and there is concern that the incidence of this disease is actually increasing in

TABLE 32–1 Comparison of Type 1 and Type 2 Diabetes Mellitus

Characteristic	Type 1	Type 2
Age at onset	Usually before 20	Usually after 30
Type of onset	Abrupt; often severe	Gradual; usually subtle
Usual body weight	Normal	Overweight
Blood insulin	Markedly reduced	Elevated or normal
Peripheral response to insulin	Normal	Decreased
Clinical management	Insulin and diet	Diet; insulin or oral antidiabetics if diet control alone is ineffective

Source: Adapted from Craighead,[18] p 1208.

certain populations, such as Native American children and other young minority groups.[75] Although the specific factors responsible for this disease are not known, a genetic predisposition combined with poor diet, obesity, and lack of exercise all seem to contribute to the onset of type 2 diabetes.[18,56] Increased body weight is fairly common in people with type 2 diabetes.

Whereas type 1 diabetics simply do not produce any insulin, the problem in type 2 diabetes is somewhat more complex.[67] In most patients with type 2 diabetes, pancreatic beta cells remain intact and are capable of producing insulin. The primary problem in type 2 diabetes is therefore a decreased sensitivity of peripheral tissues to circulating insulin; this is referred to as *insulin resistance*.[19,56,57] For instance, tissues such as the liver and skeletal muscle fail to respond adequately to insulin in the bloodstream.[60,95] Thus, peripheral uptake and use of glucose are blunted, even when insulin is present.

The exact cellular mechanisms responsible for insulin resistance are unknown. This resistance may be caused by a primary (intrinsic) defect at the target cell that results in decreased function of the insulin receptor. For example, insulin resistance could be caused by decreased binding of insulin to the receptor or by a decrease in the total number of functioning insulin receptors on the cell's surface.[19,60] It is even more likely that insulin resistance occurs because of changes in the way the cell responds *after* insulin binds to the surface receptor. Problems in postreceptor signaling, such as decreased protein phosphorylation, impaired production of chemical mediators, and a lack of glucose transporters, have all been suggested as intracellular events that could help explain insulin resistance.[19,57,60] Therefore, even when insulin does bind to the receptor, the cellular response is inadequate. Thus, insulin resistance appears to be a complex phenomenon that may involve a number of changes at the cellular level. The exact changes in receptor or postreceptor function that cause this problem remain to be determined.

A defect in pancreatic beta cell function may also contribute to the manifestations of type 2 diabetes. As indicated, type 2 diabetes is often associated with plasma insulin levels that are normal or even slightly elevated. Insulin release, however, does not follow a normal pattern in people with type 2 diabetes. Normally, insulin is released from the beta cells following a meal, and insulin release decreases substantially during fasting. In most people with type 2 diabetes, insulin is released continuously, even during fasting.[19] Following a meal, beta cells also fail to adequately increase insulin release in proportion to the increased glucose levels in the bloodstream. This abnormal pattern of insulin release suggests beta cell function has been impaired in people with type 2 diabetes. Hence, the combination of peripheral tissue resistance and inappropriate beta cell response creates the fundamental metabolic abnormalities that underlie type 2 diabetes.

Finally, insulin resistance is present in several disease states other than type 2 diabetes mellitus. Patients with conditions such as hypertension, obesity, and certain hyperlipidemias are also found to have decreased tissue sensitivity to circulating insulin.[12,60,88] Although the causes of insulin resistance in nondiabetic conditions are not completely understood, they probably involve a complex series of changes at the systemic, cellular, and subcellular levels.[60] There is consensus, however, that therapeutic strategies for resolving insulin resistance should be considered an important part of the management of various conditions that exhibit this phenomenon.[12,88]

Effects and Complications of Diabetes Mellitus

The most common symptom associated with diabetes mellitus is a chronic elevation of blood glucose (hyperglycemia). Hyperglycemia results from a relative lack of insulin-mediated glucose uptake and use by peripheral tissues. Hyperglycemia then initiates a number of complex and potentially serious acute metabolic changes. For example, hyperglycemia is usually accompanied by increased glucose excretion by the kidneys (**glycosuria**). Glycosuria is caused by an inability of the kidneys to adequately reabsorb the excess amount of glucose reaching the nephron. Increased glucose excretion causes an osmotic force that promotes fluid and electrolyte excretion, thus leading to dehydration and electrolyte imbalance.[83] Also, the loss of glucose in the urine causes a metabolic shift toward the mobilization of fat and protein as an energy source. Increased use of fats and protein leads to the formation of acidic ketone bodies in the bloodstream. Excessive accumulation of ketones lowers plasma pH, producing acidosis (*ketoacidosis*), which can lead to coma and death.[83]

Diabetes mellitus is associated with several other long-term complications involving vascular and neural structures. Perhaps the most devastating complications associated with this disease result from the development of abnormalities in small blood vessels (*microangiopathy*).[19] Small vessels may undergo a thickening of the basement membrane, which can progress to the point of vessel occlusion.[18] The progressive ischemia caused by small-vessel disease is particularly damaging to certain structures such as the retina (leading to blindness) and the kidneys (leading to nephropathy and renal failure).[21,61,77] Problems with large blood vessels (*macroangiopathy*) can also occur in diabetes because of defects in lipid metabolism that lead to atherosclerosis.[7,18] Macroangiopathy is a principal contributing factor in hypertension, myocardial infarction, and cerebral vascular accident in diabetic patients. Finally, peripheral neuropathies are quite common among patients with long-standing diabetes mellitus.[34,104]

The neurovascular complications described previously are directly related to the severity and duration of hyperglycemia in diabetic patients.[19] Although the details are somewhat unclear, prolonged elevations in blood glucose may promote structural and functional changes in vascular endothelial cells and peripheral neurons. These cellular changes are ultimately responsible for the gross pathologic abnormalities characteristic of poorly controlled diabetes mellitus.

Consequently, the primary goal in the treatment of both type 1 and type 2 diabetes mellitus is to control blood glucose levels. Maintenance of blood glucose at or close to normal levels will prevent acute metabolic derangements and greatly reduce the risk of the chronic neurovascular complications associated with this disease.[4,40,62] The pharmacologic agents used to treat diabetes mellitus are described in the next sections.

USE OF INSULIN IN DIABETES MELLITUS

Therapeutic Effects and Rationale for Use

Exogenous insulin is administered to replace normal pancreatic hormone production in type 1 diabetes (insulin-dependent diabetes mellitus). Because beta cell function is essentially absent in type 1 patients, exogenous insulin is crucial in maintaining normal glucose levels and proper metabolic function. Without exogenous insulin, the general health of type 1 patients is severely compromised, and these patients often succumb to the metabolic and neurovascular derangements associated with this disease.

Insulin may also be administered in some cases of type 2 diabetes to complement other drugs (oral antidiabetic agents) and to supplement endogenous insulin release.[13,41,101] In type 2 diabetes (non–insulin-dependent diabetes mellitus), exogenous insulin basically makes up the difference between the patients' endogenous hormone production and their specific insulin requirement. In addition, many patients with advanced cases of type 2 diabetes ultimately require supplemental insulin because other interventions (diet, exercise, other drugs) are not able to adequately control this disease.[25]

Insulin Preparations

There are many different forms of insulin, depending on the source of the hormones and the length of pharmacologic effects. Insulin used in the treatment of diabetes mellitus is derived from three sources: beef insulin, pork insulin, and biosynthetic human insulin. Beef and pork insulin are obtained by extracting the hormone from the pancreas of the respective host animal. These animal forms of insulin are effective in controlling glucose metabolism in humans, even though they have some chemical differences from their human counterpart; that is, the amino acid sequence of beef insulin has three amino acids that differ from human insulin, and pork insulin has one amino acid that is different from the human insulin sequence.[42]

Insulin that is identical to the human form of this hormone has also been produced through the use of cell cultures and recombinant DNA techniques.[44] Biosynthetically produced insulin appears to have some advantages over the animal forms, including more rapid absorption after subcutaneous injection.[36,42] Human insulin is also associated with a lower risk of immunologic reactions than insulin derived from animals.[28] Apparently, beef and pork insulin are sufficiently dissimilar from the human form to evoke antibody production, which can lead to allergic reactions in some individuals. Because insulin obtained from recombinant DNA biosynthesis is identical to the endogenous human hormone, the risk of antibody production is minimal.

More recently, biosynthetic techniques have been used to produce insulin analogs that are slightly different from human insulin. For example, insulin lispro (Humalog; see Table 32–2) is a synthetic insulin in which the sequence of two amino acids has been reversed.[53] This subtle change in the insulin structure allows more rapid absorption than regular human insulin.[64] Insulin lispro can therefore be administered immediately before a meal to more closely mimic the normal release of endogenous insulin.[91,97] Other insulin analogs are currently being developed, and these preparations may provide additional benefits compared with regular human insulin or animal forms of this hormone.[96,98]

TABLE 32–2 Insulin Preparations

Type of Insulin	Effects (hr)			Common Examples*	
	Onset	Peak	Duration	Animal	Human
Rapid-acting					
Insulin lispro	<0.5	0.5–1.5	<5		Humalog
Regular insulin	0.5–1	2–4	5–7	Regular Iletin II	Humulin R
					Novolin R
Intermediate-acting					
Isophane insulin	3–4	6–12	18–28	NPH Insulin	Humulin N
				NPH Purified Insulin	Novolin N
				NPH Iletin II	
Insulin zinc	1–3	8–12	18–28	Lente Insulin	Humulin L
				Lente Insulin III	Novolin L
Long-acting					
Extended insulin zinc	4–6	18–24	36	—	Humulin U

*Examples are trade names of preparations derived from animal sources (beef, pork, or mixed beef and pork) and synthetic human insulin derived from recombinant DNA techniques.

Insulin preparations used in the treatment of diabetes mellitus are listed in Table 32–2, which shows preparations classified according to their length of action. In general, rapid-acting preparations must be administered frequently and are used when control of diabetes is difficult and must be managed closely. Intermediate-acting and long-acting preparations are created by adding acetate buffers and zinc (Lente insulins) or protamine and zinc (NPH insulins) to the insulin molecule. These additions delay the absorption of the insulin molecule, thereby prolonging the effects and decreasing the need for frequent administration. Intermediate- and long-acting preparations are usually reserved for individuals who require less stringent control of blood glucose levels—for example, those who are helping to manage their condition through dietary and weight control. Also, combinations of different preparations may be used to manage diabetes in specific situations. For instance, a long-acting preparation may be supplemented by occasional administration of a rapid-acting agent to provide optimal glycemic control.

Administration of Insulin

Insulin, a large polypeptide, is not suitable for oral administration. Even if the insulin molecule survived digestion by proteases in the stomach and small intestine, this compound is much too large to be absorbed through the gastrointestinal wall. Consequently, insulin is usually administered through subcutaneous injection. In emergency situations (e.g., diabetic coma), insulin may be administered by the intravenous route.

Patients on long-term insulin therapy are usually trained to administer their own medication. Important factors in safe insulin use include adequate (refrigerated) storage of the preparation, maintenance of sterile syringes, accurate dose measurement and filling of the syringe, and proper injection technique. Patients should rotate the sites of administration (abdomen, upper thighs, upper arms, back, and buttocks) to avoid local damage caused by repeated injection.

The optimal dosage of insulin varies greatly from patient to patient, as well as within each patient. Factors such as exercise and dietary modification can change the insulin requirements for each individual. Consequently, the dose of insulin is often adjusted periodically by monitoring the patient's blood glucose level. Adjustment of insulin dosage in poorly controlled diabetes mellitus is usually done under the close supervision of a physician. Advancements in glucose-monitoring devices that can be used in the home, however, now permit patients to routinely check their own blood glucose levels. Many patients can make their own insulin adjustments based on periodic blood glucose measurement. This process of glucose self-monitoring and insulin dose adjustment permits optimal management of blood glucose levels on a day-to-day basis.

To avoid some of the problems of repeated subcutaneous injection, several alternative ways to administer insulin have been explored. Insulin pumps, for example, can be used to deliver a continuous (background) infusion of insulin that can also be supplemented at mealtime by manually activating the pump. These pumps can be worn outside the body, with insulin administered subcutaneously through a small catheter and needle that is held in place by skin tape.[46] Alternatively, small implantable pumps are available that can be placed surgically under the skin and programmed to release insulin as needed.[48,81] Insulin pumps are obviously much more convenient than a hypodermic syringe to make multiple injections each day. These pumps may also provide better control over blood glucose levels while reducing the risk of side effects such as severe hypoglycemia.[8,24] The major drawback at the present time is that insulin pumps can malfunction, primarily because the catheter delivering insulin becomes occluded or obstructed.[24,81] Patients using insulin pumps must also monitor their glucose levels several times each day, and they must understand how to correctly use the pump to deliver the appropriate amount of insulin. Nonetheless, insulin pumps currently offer a convenient way to administer insulin, and technologic improvements in these devices may result in more extensive use in the future.[48]

Alternative routes for administering insulin are also being considered.[14] In particular, a form of insulin may ultimately be available that can be administered by inhalation or nasal spray, thus precluding the need for subcutaneous injection.[38,58,92] Other modifications of the insulin molecule or use of chemical enhancers may eventually increase the permeability of this hormone so that insulin can be administered through the skin (transcutaneously) or even via oral or buccal routes.[38,92] Technologic and practical advancements in insulin delivery continue to be explored, and methods for administering insulin may be much safer and more convenient in the future.

Intensive Insulin Therapy

As indicated previously, the ultimate goal in the treatment of diabetes mellitus is to maintain blood glucose in the normal physiologic range as much as possible. To achieve this goal, an administration strategy known as intensive insulin therapy has been developed for people who require exogenous insulin.[40,65] The idea of intensive insulin therapy is that the patient frequently monitors his or her blood glucose level and self-administers several (three or more) doses of insulin per day, with each dose adjusted carefully to meet the patient's needs throughout the day.[40,90] Basically, several relatively small doses of insulin are able to maintain blood glucose in the appropriate range much better than one or two relatively large doses. Likewise, different types of insulin can be combined to provide optimal results. For example, daily regimens can be designed that provide several doses of short-acting insulin (including the newer insulin analogs like insulin lispro), along with one or more doses of intermediate-acting insulin.[40] The short-acting doses can be administered at mealtimes or whenever immediate control of glucose levels is needed, and the intermediate-acting form can be administered once or twice a day to provide lower, background levels of insulin throughout the day or night.[43]

Of course, intensive insulin therapy requires more motivation and compliance on the part of the patient. Intensive therapy may also be associated with a somewhat greater risk of severe hypoglycemia if the insulin dosage does not carefully match the patient's needs throughout the day.[9] There is, nonetheless, considerable evidence that this strategy reduces the long-term complications associated with diabetes, including a lower incidence of neuropathies, renal disease, and other complications related to microangiopathy.[72,90,103] Hence, intensive insulin therapy may be worth the extra effort because this strategy can help prevent the devastating complications that are typically associated with poorly controlled diabetes mellitus.

Adverse Effects of Insulin Therapy

The primary problem associated with insulin administration is *hypoglycemia*.[9,89] Because insulin lowers blood glucose, exogenous insulin may produce a dramatic fall in blood glucose levels. Hypoglycemia may occur during insulin therapy if the dose of insulin is too high for the patient's particular needs. Missing a meal or receiving a delayed meal may also precipitate hypoglycemia. During insulin treatment, insulin is not released exclusively after a meal, as it would be during normal function. Insulin administered from an exogenous source may be present in the bloodstream even if the patient fails to provide glucose by eating. Hence, insulin may reduce blood glucose below normal levels because of the lack of a periodic replenishment of blood glucose from dietary sources.

Strenuous physical activity may promote hypoglycemia during insulin therapy. Exercise generally produces an insulin-like effect, meaning that exercise accelerates the movement of glucose out of the bloodstream and into peripheral tissues (skeletal muscle) where it is needed. The combined effects of exercise and insulin may produce an exaggerated decrease in blood glucose, thus leading to hypoglycemia. To avoid exercise-induced hypoglycemia, the insulin dose should be decreased by 30 to 35 percent.[10] Careful measurement of blood glucose before and after exercise can help predict how much the insulin dose should be adjusted in each patient.

Initial symptoms of hypoglycemia include headache, fatigue, hunger, tachycardia, sweating, anxiety, and confusion. Symptoms progressively worsen as blood glucose continues to decrease, and severe hypoglycemia may lead to loss of consciousness, convulsions, and death. Consequently, early detection and resolution of hypoglycemia are imperative. In the early stages, hypoglycemia can usually be reversed if the patient ingests foods containing glucose (soft drinks, fruit juice, glucose tablets, etc.). Typically, administration of the equivalent of 15 to 20 g of D-glucose is recommended to restore blood glucose in the early stages of hypoglycemia.[86]

Other problems that may be encountered are related to the immunologic effects of insulin use. Certain forms of insulin may evoke an immune reaction and stimulate antibody production. These anti-insulin antibodies may cause an allergic reaction in some individuals, as well as resistance to the exogenous insulin molecule. As discussed previously, the incidence of these immunologic reactions seems to be greater when animal (beef and pork) forms of insulin are used. Consequently, these problems are often resolved by switching the patient to another type of preparation, preferably biosynthetic human insulin.

ORAL ANTIDIABETIC DRUGS

Several agents are now available that can be administered by mouth to help control blood glucose levels in people with type 2 (NIDDM) diabetes mellitus. These drugs tend to be most effective if some endogenous insulin production is present but insulin secretion is relatively inadequate and the peripheral tissues are resistant to the effects of the endogenous insulin. These agents are therefore not effective for treating type 1 diabetes, but they can be used along with diet and exercise for the long-term management of type 2 diabetes.

Oral antidiabetic drugs do not offer a cure for type 2 diabetes, and their effectiveness varies considerably from patient to patient. Still, it appears that early and aggressive use of one or more of these agents can substantially reduce the complications associated with this disease. What follows is a brief description of currently available oral antidiabetic agents. Agents categorized as sulfonylureas will be addressed first, followed by a fairly diverse group of newer orally acting agents.

Sulfonylureas

The oldest and largest group of oral agents are classified chemically as *sulfonylureas*. These drugs act directly on pancreatic beta cells and stimulate the release of insulin. This insulin is released directly into the hepatic portal vein and subsequently travels to the liver and inhibits hepatic glucose production.[23] Increased plasma levels of insulin also help facilitate glucose entry into muscle and other peripheral tissues. The combined effect of decreased hepatic glucose production and increased glucose uptake by muscle helps lower blood sugar in many people with type 2 diabetes. These drugs seem to be most effective in people who are in the early stages of type 2 diabetes and still have reasonable functioning of their beta cells.[23,39]

Specific sulfonylureas used clinically are listed in Table 32–3. These agents are all fairly similar in their pharmacologic efficacy and are distinguished primarily by individual potencies and pharmacokinetic properties (rate of absorption, duration of action, etc.).[23] The principal adverse effect of these drugs is hypoglycemia.[39] As with insulin therapy, hypoglycemia may be precipitated by sulfonylureas if the dose is excessive, if a meal is skipped, or if the patient increases his or her level of activity. Consequently, patients should be observed for any indications of low blood glucose, such as anxiety, confusion, headache, and sweating.[86] Other side effects that may occur include heartburn, gastrointestinal distress (nausea, vomiting, stomach pain, and diarrhea), headache, dizziness, skin rashes, and hematologic abnormalities (e.g., leukopenia, agranulocytosis). These side effects are usually fairly mild and transient but may require attention if they are severe or prolonged.

TABLE 32–3 Oral Antidiabetic Agents

Classification and Examples*	Mechanism of Action and Effects	Primary Adverse Effects
Sulfonylureas		
Acetohexamide (Dymelor) Chlorpropamide (Diabinese) Glimepiride (Amaryl) Glipizide (Glucotrol) Glyburide (DiaBeta, Micronase) Tolazamide (Tolinase) Tolbutamide (Orinase)	Increase insulin secretion from pancreatic beta cells; increased insulin release helps reduce blood glucose by increasing glucose storage in muscle and by inhibiting hepatic glucose production	Hypoglycemia (the most common and potentially serious side effect of the sulfonylureas); other bothersome effects (GI disturbances, headache, etc.) may also occur, depending on the specific agent
Biguanides		
Metformin (Glucophage)	Act directly on the liver to decrease hepatic glucose production; also increase sensitivity of peripheral tissues (muscle) to insulin	Gastrointestinal disturbances; lactic acidosis may also occur in rare cases, which could be severe or fatal
Alpha-glucosidase inhibitors Acarbose (Precose) Miglitol (Glyset)	Inhibit sugar breakdown in the intestines and delay glucose absorption from the GI tract	Gastrointestinal disturbances
Thiazolidinediones Rosiglitazone (Avandia) Troglitazone (Rezulin)	Similar to the biguanides (metformin)	Headache, dizziness, fatigue or weakness, back pain; rare but potentially severe cases of hepatic toxicity may also occur
Benzoic acid derivatives Repaglinide (Prandin)	Similar to the sulfonylureas	Hypoglycemia, bronchitis, upper respiratory tract infections, joint pain and back pain, GI disturbances, headache

*Examples include generic names with trade names listed in parentheses.

Other Orally Active Drugs

In addition to the sulfonylureas, several other agents are currently available that can also be administered orally to manage type 2 diabetes (Table 32–3).[11,23] These drugs differ in their chemical classification and mechanism of action, but they all attempt to normalize blood glucose levels in type 2 patients. Metformin (Glucophage), for example, is classified chemically as a biguanide agent that acts primarily on the liver to inhibit glucose production.[99] Metformin also increases the sensitivity of peripheral tissues to insulin, an effect that helps treat the fundamental problem in type 2 diabetes (i.e., decreased tissue sensitivity to insulin).[99] Acarbose (Precose) and miglitol (Glyset) are characterized as alpha-glucosidase inhibitors because they inhibit enzymes that break down sugars in the GI tract.[23,80] This effect helps delay glucose absorption from the intestines, thereby slowing the entry of glucose into the bloodstream and allowing time for the beta cells to respond to hyperglycemia after a meal.[23]

Troglitazone (Rezulin) and rosiglitazone (Avandia) are members of a drug group called the thiazolidones.[3,71,79] These agents work like metformin; that is, they decrease hepatic glucose production and increase tissue sensitivity to insulin.[22,45] Repaglinide (Prandin) is classified as a benzoic acid derivative, and this drug acts like the sulfonylureas because it directly increases the release of insulin from pancreatic beta cells.[68] Efforts continue to develop other thiazolidones and benzoic acid derivatives, and we may ultimately see additional drugs become available in the future.[26]

The adverse side effects of these orally acting drugs are summarized in Table 32–3. These drugs provide alternative treatments for patients who do not respond to sulfonylureas. These drugs can also be combined with one another or with a sulfonylurea to provide optimal glucose control in certain patients.[29,55,73] Treatment of type 2 diabetes will undoubtedly continue to improve as more is learned about the best way to use existing oral drugs, and as other new oral antidiabetic agents become available.[2]

OTHER DRUGS USED IN THE MANAGEMENT OF DIABETES MELLITUS

Glucagon

Glucagon is sometimes used to treat acute hypoglycemia induced by insulin or oral hypoglycemic agents.[86] As discussed previously, the initial effect of glucagon is to mobilize the release of glucose from hepatic glycogen stores. Consequently, the patient must have sufficient liver glycogen present for glucagon to be effective.

When used to treat hypoglycemia, glucagon is administered by injection (intravenous, intramuscular, or subcutaneous). Glucagon should reverse symptoms of hypoglycemia (including coma) within 5 to 20 minutes after administration.[86] The primary adverse effects associated with glucagon are nausea and vomiting (although these effects may result directly from hypoglycemia). Glucagon may also cause an allergic reaction (skin rash, difficulty in breathing) in some individuals.

Immunosuppressants

As indicated earlier, type 1 diabetes is caused by an autoimmune response that selectively attacks and destroys pancreatic beta cells in susceptible individuals. Drugs that suppress this autoimmune response may therefore be helpful in limiting beta cell destruction and thereby decreasing the severity of this disease.[6] Several immunosuppressant agents have been investigated as a way to potentially minimize beta cell loss from the autoimmune reactions that underlie type 1 diabetes. In particular, cyclosporine (Sandimmune) is a powerful immunosuppressant drug that is often used to prevent tissue rejection following organ transplants (see Chap. 37). There is also some indication that this drug may help attenuate the autoimmune response that appears to be responsible for beta cell destruction in type 1 diabetes mellitus.[49] Other immunosuppressants that may be helpful in this situation include azathioprine, cyclophosphamide, methotrexate, and glucocorticoids.[6,82] The pharmacology of these immunosuppressants is discussed in more detail in Chapter 37.

Clinical trials therefore continue to assess whether immunosuppressant drugs can prevent beta cell destruction in people who are at risk for developing type 1 diabetes. There is some evidence that certain immunosuppressants may blunt the severity of this disease in certain individuals.[6] Response to immunosuppressants, however, may vary greatly from person to person, and certain patients may relapse when immunosuppressant therapy is discontinued.[6] Immunosuppressant drugs are likewise notorious for producing severe side effects, especially when used at high doses for prolonged periods (see Chap. 37). Nonetheless, efforts continue to clarify the role of immunosuppressants and immune system modulators in preventing type 1 diabetes. We may someday be able to administer effective immunosuppressants that negate the autoimmune destruction of beta cells, thereby preventing type 1 diabetes.[82]

Aldose Reductase Inhibitors

Drugs that selectively inhibit the aldose reductase enzyme represent a method for reducing peripheral neuropathies associated with poorly controlled type 1 or type 2 diabetes.[70] This enzyme, which is located in neurons and other cells, is responsible for converting glucose to another sugar known as sorbitol. The excessive accumulation of sorbitol within the cell may lead to structural and functional changes that are ultimately responsible for the complications associated with diabetes mellitus, especially peripheral neuropathies.[33,51,70] Consequently, aldose reductase inhibitors (ARIs) such as tolrestat, zenarestat, and epalrestat may be useful in preventing these complications by inhibiting the formation and accumulation of sorbitol within peripheral neurons.

Clinical trials using ARIs have been somewhat disappointing, however.[27] Although treatment with these drugs may slow the progression of diabetic neuropathy, ARIs do not appear to reverse any pre-existing nerve damage.[70] Likewise, ARIs must be administered in a dose that is sufficient to inhibit more than 80 percent of the sorbitol production in the nerve cell.[33] That is, even relatively small amounts of sorbitol produced in the nerve can have a harmful effect. ARIs may therefore provide some benefit for people who show early signs of diabetic neuropathy, but the extensive use of these drugs in people with diabetes remains questionable.[69]

NONPHARMACOLOGIC INTERVENTION IN DIABETES MELLITUS

Dietary Management and Weight Reduction

Despite advancements in the pharmacologic treatment of diabetes mellitus, the most important and effective factor in controlling this disease is still proper nutrition.[59]

In both type 1 and type 2 diabetes, total caloric intake, as well as the percentage of calories from specific sources (carbohydrates, fats, or proteins), is important in controlling blood glucose. Also, weight loss is a significant factor in decreasing the patient's need for drugs such as insulin and the oral hypoglycemic agents.[30] By losing weight, the patient may reduce the amount of tissue that requires insulin, thereby reducing the need for exogenous drugs. Because obesity is quite prevalent in type 2 diabetics, weight loss seems to be especially effective in reducing drug requirements in these individuals.[76]

Exercise

Exercise appears to be beneficial in diabetes mellitus for several reasons. Physical training may help facilitate weight loss, thus helping to decrease body mass and drug requirements.[30] Regular exercise also appears to increase the sensitivity of peripheral tissues to insulin; that is, training helps overcome insulin resistance.[1] The exact reason for this training effect is not clear. Finally, a program of physical training will improve the general health and well-being in diabetic patients, making them less susceptible to various problems such as cardiovascular disease.[1] Of course, patients beginning a program of regular exercise should first undergo a complete physical examination, and the frequency and intensity of the exercise should be closely monitored.

Tissue Transplants and Gene Therapy

A relatively new approach in treating diabetes mellitus is the transplantation of tissues containing pancreatic beta cells into patients with this disease.[20,74] For example, islet tissues containing functioning beta cells can be harvested from adult, neonatal, or fetal pancreatic tissues and surgically transplanted into the pancreas of patients who lack adequate insulin production (type 1 diabetics). Likewise, the entire pancreas can be transplanted from organ donors into people with type 1 diabetes, and this procedure may be done simultaneously with a kidney transplant in people with diabetic nephropathy.[47,85] If successful, these tissue transplants can provide the patient with an endogenous source of insulin that will decrease or eliminate the need for insulin therapy. The success rates of these transplants is likewise improving steadily, primarily because newer immunosuppressant agents are available to prevent tissue rejection.[47,84]

New molecular strategies are also being investigated that could re-establish insulin production and insulin sensitivity by transplanting insulin-related genes into the cells of patients with diabetes mellitus.[31,63] These techniques basically attempt to either deliver insulin genes directly into cells of people with type 1 or type 2 diabetes or focus on transplanting genetically altered cells that will produce or respond to insulin in these patients.[31] Although techniques such as tissue transplants and gene therapy are still relatively experimental, these techniques may eventually be developed to provide a more permanent means of treating diabetes mellitus.

SIGNIFICANCE OF DIABETES MELLITUS IN REHABILITATION

Patients often undergo rehabilitation for complications arising from diabetes mellitus. For instance, peripheral neuropathies may produce functional deficits that require physical therapy and occupational therapy. Small-vessel angiopathy may cause decreased peripheral blood flow, resulting in tissue ischemia and ulceration. This ischemia can lead to tissue necrosis and subsequent amputation, especially in the lower extremities. In advanced stages of diabetes, general debilitation combined with specific conditions (e.g., end-stage renal failure) creates multiple problems that challenge the health of the individual. Consequently, rehabilitation specialists will be involved in the treatment of various sequelae of diabetes mellitus throughout the course of this disease.

Physical therapists and occupational therapists must be aware of the possibility that acute metabolic derangements exist in their patients who have diabetes mellitus. Therapists should realize that patients on insulin and oral hypoglycemic medications may experience episodes of hypoglycemia because of an exaggerated lowering of blood glucose by these drugs. Hypoglycemia may be precipitated if the patient has not eaten or is engaging in relatively strenuous physical activity. Therapists must ensure that patients are maintaining a regular dietary schedule and have not skipped a meal prior to the therapy session. Likewise, therapists should be especially alert for any signs of hypoglycemia during and after exercise in diabetic patients.

Therapists should note any changes (confusion, fatigue, sweating, nausea) in the patient that may signal the onset of hypoglycemia. If these symptoms are observed, administration of a high-glucose snack is typically recommended. Therapists working with diabetic patients should have sources of glucose on hand to reverse these hypoglycemic symptoms. Some sources of glucose include soft drinks, fruit juices, and tablets containing D-glucose.[86]

Finally, physical therapists and occupational therapists may help reinforce the importance of patient compliance during pharmacologic management of diabetes mellitus. Therapists can question whether patients have been taking their medications on a routine basis. Regular administration of insulin is essential in preventing a metabolic shift toward ketone body production and subsequent ketoacidosis, especially in the type 1 patient. Also, therapists can help explain that adequate control of blood glucose not only prevents acute metabolic problems but also seems to decrease the incidence of the neurovascular complications associated with this disease. Likewise, rehabilitation specialists can encourage patient compliance in the nonpharmacologic management of their disease. Therapists can emphasize the importance of an appropriate diet and adequate physical activity in both type 1 and type 2 diabetes. Therapists may also play an important role in preventing the onset of diabetic foot ulcers and infection by educating the patient in proper skin care and footwear.

CASE STUDY

DIABETES MELLITUS

Brief History. W.S. is an 18-year-old woman who began experiencing problems with glucose metabolism following a viral infection when she was 12. She was subsequently diagnosed as having type 1 diabetes mellitus. Since that time, her condition has been successfully managed by insulin administration combined with dietary control. Once-daily administration of intermediate-acting insulin combined with periodic administration of a short-acting insulin usually provides optimal therapeutic effects. She is also very active athletically and was a member of her high school soccer team. Currently, she is entering her first year of college and is beginning preseason practice with the college's soccer team. The physical therapist who serves as the team's athletic trainer was apprised of her condition.

Problem/Influence of Medication. Exercise produces an insulin-like effect; that is, it lowers blood glucose by facilitating the movement of glucose out of the bloodstream and into peripheral tissues. Because insulin also lowers blood glucose, the additive effects of insulin and exercise may produce profound hypoglycemia. As a result, a lower dose of insulin is usually required on days that involve strenuous activity. The physical therapist was aware of this and other potential problems in the diabetic athlete.

Decision/Solution. The therapist reminded the athlete to monitor her blood glucose levels before and after each practice session and to adjust her insulin dosage accordingly. During some of the initial practice sessions, blood glucose was also monitored during practice to ensure that insulin doses were adequate. On practice days, insulin was injected into abdominal sites rather than around exercising muscles (thighs), in order to prevent the insulin from being absorbed too rapidly from the injection site. The therapist also reminded the athlete to eat a light meal before each practice and to be sure to eat again afterward. The therapist maintained a supply of glucose tablets and fruit juice on the practice field. The athlete was questioned periodically to look for early signs of hypoglycemia (confusion, nausea, etc.), and ingestion of carbohydrates was encouraged whenever appropriate. Finally, the therapist assigned a teammate to check on the athlete within an hour after practice ended to ensure that no delayed effects of hypoglycemia were apparent. With these precautions, the athlete successfully completed preseason training as well as the entire soccer season without any serious incident.

SUMMARY

The islet cells of the pancreas synthesize and secrete insulin and glucagon. These hormones are important in regulating glucose uptake and use, as well as other aspects of energy metabolism. Problems in the production and effects of insulin are typical of a disease known as diabetes mellitus. Diabetes mellitus can be categorized into two primary forms: type 1 diabetes, which is caused by an absolute deficiency of insulin, and type 2 diabetes, which is caused by decreased peripheral insulin effects, combined with abnormal insulin release. Administration of exogenous insulin is required in the treatment of type 1 diabetes mellitus. Patients with type 2 diabetes may be treated with insulin or with oral antidiabetic drugs, depending on the severity of their disease. In both forms of diabetes mellitus, dietary control and adequate physical activity may help reduce the need for drug treatment, as well as improve the general health and well-being of the patient. Physical therapists and occupational therapists play an important role in helping treat the complications of diabetes mellitus and in promoting good patient compliance in the management of this disease. Therapists must be cognizant of the potential problems that may occur when working with diabetic patients (hypoglycemia) and should be able to recognize and deal with these problems before a medical emergency arises.

REFERENCES

1. Arakawa, K: Exercise, a measure to lower blood pressure and reduce other risks. Clin Exp Hypertens 21:797, 1999.
2. Bailey, CJ: Potential new treatments for type 2 diabetes. Trends Pharmacol Sci 21:259, 2000.

3. Balfour, JA and Plosker, GL: Rosiglitazone. Drugs 57:921, 1999.
4. Barranco, JG: Glucose control guidelines: Current concepts. Clin Nutr 17(Suppl 2):7, 1998.
5. Benali, N, et al: Somatostatin receptors. Digestion 62(Suppl 1):27, 2000.
6. Bertera, S, et al: Immunology of type 1 diabetes. Intervention and prevention strategies. Endocrinol Metab Clin North Am 28:841, 1999.
7. Best, JD and O'Neal, DN: Diabetic dyslipidaemia: Current treatment recommendations. Drugs 59:1101, 2000.
8. Boland, EA, et al: Continuous subcutaneous insulin infusion. A new way to lower risk of severe hypoglycemia, improve metabolic control, and enhance coping in adolescents with type 1 diabetes. Diabetes Care 22:1779, 1999.
9. Bolli, GB: How to ameliorate the problem of hypoglycemia in intensive as well as nonintensive treatment of type 1 diabetes. Diabetes Care 22(Suppl 2):B43, 1999.
10. Brannon, FJ, et al: Cardiac Rehabilitation: Basic Theory and Application, ed 3. FA Davis, Philadelphia, 1998.
11. Brown, DL and Brillon, D: New directions in type 2 diabetes mellitus: An update on current oral antidiabetic therapy. J Natl Med Assoc 91:389, 1999.
12. Buhler, FR, Julius, S, and Reaven, GM: A new dimension in hypertension: Role of insulin resistance. J Cardiovasc Pharmacol 15(Suppl 5):S1, 1990.
13. Buse, J: Combining insulin and oral agents. Am J Med 108(Suppl 6a):23S, 2000.
14. Chetty, DJ and Chien, YW: Novel methods of insulin delivery: An update. Crit Rev Ther Drug Carrier Syst 15:629, 1998.
15. Choudhuri, K and Vergani, D: MHC restriction to T-cell autoaggression: An emerging understanding of IDDM pathogenesis. Diabetes Metab Rev 14:285, 1998.
16. Combettes-Souverain, M and Issad, T: Molecular basis of insulin action. Diabetes Metab 24:477, 1998.
17. Cooper, GS, Miller, FW, and Pandey, JP: The role of genetic factors in autoimmune disease: Implications for environmental research. Environ Health Perspect 107(Suppl 5):693, 1999.
18. Craighead, JE: Diabetes. In Rubin, E and Farber, JL (eds): Pathology, ed 3. Lippincott-Raven, Philadelphia, 1999.
19. Crawford, JM and Cotran, RS: The pancreas. In Cotran, RS, Kumar, V, and Collins, T (eds): The Pathologic Basis of Disease, ed 6. WB Saunders, Philadelphia, 1999.
20. Cretin, N, et al: Human islet allotransplantation: World experience and current status. Dig Surg 15:656, 1998.
21. Dalla Vestra, M, et al: Structural involvement in type 1 and type 2 diabetic nephropathy. Diabetes Metab 26(Suppl 4):8, 2000.
22. Day, C: Thiazolidinediones: A new class of antidiabetic drugs. Diabet Med 16:179, 1999.
23. DeFronzo, RA: Pharmacologic therapy for type 2 diabetes mellitus. Ann Intern Med 131:281, 1999.
24. Dunn, FL, et al: Long-term therapy of IDDM with an implantable insulin pump. The Implantable Insulin Pump Trial Study Group. Diabetes Care 20:59, 1997.
25. Evans, AJ and Krentz, AJ: Benefits and risks of transfer from oral agents to insulin in type 2 diabetes mellitus. Drug Saf 21:7, 1999.
26. Evans, AJ and Krentz, AJ: Recent developments and emerging therapies for type 2 diabetes mellitus. Drugs R D 2:75, 1999.
27. Fedele, D and Giugliano, D: Peripheral diabetic neuropathy. Current recommendations and future prospects for its prevention and management. Drugs 54:414, 1997.
28. Fineberg, SE, et al: Immunologic improvement resulting from the transfer of animal insulin treated diabetic subjects to human insulin (recombinant-DNA). Diabetes Care 5(Suppl 2):107, 1982.
29. Florence, JA and Yeager, BF: Treatment of type 2 diabetes mellitus. Am Fam Physician 59:2835, 1999.
30. Foreyt, JP and Poston, WS: The challenge of diet, exercise, and lifestyle modification in the management of the obese diabetic patient. Int J Obes Relat Metab Disord 23(Suppl 7):S5, 1999.
31. Freeman, DJ, Leclerc, I, and Rutter, GA: Present and potential future use of gene therapy for the treatment of non-insulin dependent diabetes mellitus. Int J Mol Med 4:585, 1999.
32. Genuth, SM: Hormones of the pancreatic islets. In Berne, RM and Levy, MN (eds): Physiology, ed 3. Mosby Year Book, St. Louis, 2000.
33. Greene, DA, Arezzo, JC, and Brown, MB: Effect of aldose reductase inhibition on nerve conduction and morphometry in diabetic neuropathy. Zenarestat Study Group. Neurology 53:580, 1999.
34. Greene, DA, et al: Glucose-induced oxidative stress and programmed cell death in diabetic neuropathy. Eur J Pharmacol 375:217, 1999.
35. Greene, EA and Flavell, RA: The initiation of autoimmune diabetes. Curr Opin Immunol 11:663, 1999.
36. Gulan, M, Gottesman, IS, and Zinman, B: Biosynthetic human insulin improves postprandial glucose excursions in type 1 diabetes. Ann Intern Med 107:506, 1987.
37. Guyton, AC and Hall, JE: Textbook of Medical Physiology, ed 9. WB Saunders, Philadelphia, 1996.
38. Haak, T: New developments in the treatment of type 1 diabetes mellitus. Exp Clin Endocrinol Diabetes 107(Suppl 3):S108, 1999.
39. Harrower, AD: Comparative tolerability of sulphonylureas in diabetes mellitus. Drug Saf 22:313, 2000.
40. Havas, S: Educational guidelines for achieving tight control and minimizing complications of type 1 diabetes. Am Fam Physician 60:1985, 1999.

41. Heine, RJ: Current therapeutic options in type 2 diabetes. Eur J Clin Invest 29(Suppl 2):17, 1999.
42. Heinemann, L and Richter, B: Clinical pharmacology of human insulin. Diabetes Care 16:90, 1993.
43. Hirsch, IB: Type 1 diabetes mellitus and the use of flexible insulin regimens. Am Fam Physician 60:2343, 1999.
44. Home, PH and Alberti, KGMM: The new insulins: Their characteristics and clinical implications. Drugs 24:401, 1982.
45. Horikoshi, H, Hashimoto, T, and Fujiwara, T: Troglitazone and emerging glitazones: New avenues for potential therapeutic benefits beyond glycemic control. Prog Drug Res 54:191, 2000.
46. Hotta, SS and Adams, D: Reassessment of external insulin infusion pumps. J Pharm Technol 8:252, 1992.
47. Hricik, DE: Kidney-pancreas transplantation for diabetic nephropathy. Semin Nephrol 20:188, 2000.
48. Jaremko, J and Rorstad, O: Advances toward the implantable artificial pancreas for treatment of diabetes. Diabetes Care 21:444, 1998.
49. Jaworski, MA, et al: Immunosuppression in autoimmune disease: The double-edged sword. Clin Invest Med 10(Suppl):488, 1987.
50. Jung, CY and Lee, W: Glucose transporters and insulin action: Some insights into diabetes management. Arch Pharm Res 22:329, 1999.
51. Kador, PF and Kinoshita, JH: Role of aldose reductase in the development of diabetes-associated complications. Am J Med 79(Suppl 5A):8, 1985.
52. Knip, M and Akerblom, HK: Environmental factors in the pathogenesis of type 1 diabetes mellitus. Exp Clin Endocrinol Diabetes 107(Suppl 3):S93, 1999.
53. Koivisto, VA: The human insulin analogue insulin lispro. Ann Med 30:260, 1998.
54. Kukreja, A and Maclaren, NK: Autoimmunity and diabetes. J Clin Endocrinol Metab 84:4371, 1999.
55. Lebovitz, HE: Effects of oral antihyperglycemic agents in modifying macrovascular risk factors in type 2 diabetes. Diabetes Care 22(Suppl 3):C41, 1999.
56. Lebovitz, HE: Type 2 diabetes: An overview. Clin Chem 45:1339, 1999
57. Le Marchand-Brustel, Y: Molecular mechanisms of insulin action in normal and insulin-resistant states. Exp Clin Endocrinol Diabetes 107:126, 1999.
58. Leslie, CA: New insulin replacement technologies: Overcoming barriers to tight glycemic control. Cleve Clin J Med 66:293, 1999.
59. Lipkin, E: New strategies for the treatment of type 2 diabetes. J Am Diet Assoc 99:329, 1999.
60. Moller, DE and Flier, JS: Mechanisms of disease: Insulin resistance—mechanisms, syndromes, and implications. N Engl J Med 325:938, 1991.
61. Nathan, DM: Medical progress: Long-term complications of diabetes mellitus. N Engl J Med 328:1676, 1993.
62. Nathan, DM: The rationale for glucose control in diabetes mellitus. Endocrinol Metab Clin 21:221, 1992.
63. Newgard, CB: Cellular engineering and gene therapy strategies for insulin replacement in diabetes. Diabetes 43:341, 1994.
64. Noble, SK, Johnston, E, and Walton, B: Insulin lispro: A fast-acting insulin analog. Am Fam Physician 57:279, 1998.
65. Nolte, MS: Insulin therapy in insulin-dependent (type 1) diabetes mellitus. Endocrinol Metab Clin 21:281, 1992.
66. Norman, AW and Litwack, G: Pancreatic hormones: Insulin and glucagon. In Hormones, ed 2. Academic Press, San Diego, 1997.
67. Olefsky, JM: Pathogenesis of insulin resistance and hyperglycemia in non–insulin-dependent diabetes mellitus. Am J Med 79(Suppl 3B):1, 1985.
68. Owens, DR: Repaglinide—prandial glucose regulator: A new class of oral antidiabetic drugs. Diabet Med 15(Suppl 4):S28, 1998.
69. Parry, GJ: Management of diabetic neuropathy. Am J Med 107(Suppl 2b):27S, 1999.
70. Pfeifer, MA, Schumer, MP, and Gelber, DA: Aldose reductase inhibitors: The end of an era or the need for different trial designs? Diabetes 46(Suppl 2):S82, 1997.
71. Plosker, GL and Faulds, D: Troglitazone: A review of its use in the management of type 2 diabetes mellitus. Drugs 57:409, 1999.
72. Reichard, P, Nilsson, B-Y, and Rosenquist, U: The effect of long-term intensified insulin treatment on the development of microvascular complications of diabetes mellitus. N Engl J Med 329:304, 1993.
73. Riddle, M: Combining sulfonylureas and other oral agents. Am J Med 108(Suppl 6a):15S, 2000.
74. Rosenberg, L: Clinical islet cell transplantation. Are we there yet? Int J Pancreatol 24:145, 1998.
75. Rosenbloom, AL, et al: Emerging epidemic of type 2 diabetes in youth. Diabetes Care 22:345, 1999.
76. Ross, R, Janssen, I, and Tremblay, A: Obesity reduction through lifestyle modification. Can J Appl Physiol 25:1, 2000.
77. Rossert, J, Terraz-Durasnel, C, and Brideau, G: Growth factors, cytokines, and renal fibrosis during the course of diabetic nephropathy. Diabetes Metab 26(Suppl 4):16, 2000.
78. Samols, E and Stagner, JI: Intra-islet regulation. Am J Med 85(Suppl 5A):31, 1988.
79. Scheen, AJ and Lefebvre, PJ: Troglitazone: Antihyperglycemic activity and potential role in the treatment of type 2 diabetes. Diabetes Care 22:1568, 1999.
80. Scott, LJ and Spencer, CM: Miglitol: A review of its therapeutic potential in type 2 diabetes mellitus. Drugs 59:521, 2000.

81. Selam, JL, et al: Clinical trial of programmable implantable insulin pump for type 1 diabetes. Diabetes Care 15:877, 1992.
82. Simone, EA, Wegmann, DR, and Eisenbarth, GS: Immunologic "vaccination" for the prevention of autoimmune diabetes (type 1A). Diabetes Care 22(Suppl 2):B7, 1999.
83. Siperstein, MD: Diabetic ketoacidosis and hyperosmolar coma. Endocrinol Metab Clin 21:415, 1992.
84. Steen, DC: The current state of pancreas transplantation. AACN Clin Issues 10:164, 1999.
85. Stegall, MD, et al: Pancreas transplantation for the prevention of diabetic nephropathy. Mayo Clin Proc 75:49, 2000.
86. Steil, CF: Diabetes mellitus. In DiPiro, JT, et al (eds): Pharmacotherapy: A Pathophysiologic Approach, ed 4. Appleton & Lange, Stamford, CT, 1999.
87. Summers, SA, et al: Signaling pathways mediating insulin-stimulated glucose transport. Ann NY Acad Sci 892:169, 1999.
88. Symposium (various authors): Insulin sensitivity: Cardioprotection versus metabolic disorders. J Cardiovasc Pharmacol 20(Suppl 11):S1, 1992.
89. Tamborlane, WV and Amiel, SA: Hypoglycemia in the treated diabetic patient: A risk of intensive insulin therapy. Endocrinol Metab Clin 21:313, 1992.
90. The Diabetes Control and Complications Trial Research Group: The effect of intensive treatment of diabetes on the development and progression of long-term complications in insulin-dependent diabetes mellitus. N Engl J Med 329:977, 1993.
91. Toth, EL and Lee, KC: Guidelines for using insulin lispro. Can Fam Physician. 44:2444, 1998.
92. Trehan, A and Ali, A: Recent approaches in insulin delivery. Drug Dev Ind Pharm 24:589, 1998.
93. Trevisan, R, Vedovato, M, and Tiengo, A: The epidemiology of diabetes mellitus. Nephrol Dial Transplant 13(Suppl 8):2, 1998.
94. Unger, RH and Foster, DW: Diabetes mellitus. In Wilson, JD, et al (eds): Textbook of Endocrinology, ed 9. WB Saunders, Philadelphia, 1998.
95. Vaag, A: On the pathophysiology of late onset non-insulin dependent diabetes mellitus. Current controversies and new insights. Dan Med Bull 46:197, 1999.
96. Vaidyanathan, B and Menon, PS: Insulin analogues and management of diabetes mellitus. Indian J Pediatr 67:435, 2000.
97. Vajo, Z and Duckworth, WC: Genetically engineered insulin analogs: Diabetes in the new millenium. Pharmacol Rev 52:1, 2000.
98. White, JR, Campbell, RK, Hirsch, I: Insulin analogues: new agents for improving glycemic control. Postgrad Med 101:58, 1997.
99. Wiernsperger, NF and Bailey, CJ: The antihyperglycaemic effect of metformin: Therapeutic and cellular mechanisms. Drugs 58(Suppl 1):31, 1999.
100. Wolfe, RR: Effects of insulin on muscle tissue. Curr Opin Clin Nutr Metab Care 3:67, 2000.
101. Yki-Jarvinen, H, et al: Comparison of insulin regimens in patients with non–insulin-dependent diabetes mellitus. N Engl J Med 327:1426, 1992.
102. Yoon, JW and Jun, HS: Cellular and molecular roles of beta cell autoantigens, macrophages and T cells in the pathogenesis of autoimmune disease. Arch Pharm Res 22:437, 1999.
103. Zinman, B: Glucose control in type 1 diabetes: From conventional to intensive therapy. Clin Cornerstone 1:29, 1998.
104. Zochodne, DW: Diabetic neuropathies: Features and mechanisms. Brain Pathol 9:369, 1999.

Chemotherapy of Infectious and Neoplastic Diseases

CHAPTER 33

Treatment of Infections I: Antibacterial Drugs

This chapter and the next two chapters in this text address drugs used to treat infections caused by pathogenic microorganisms and parasites. Microorganisms such as bacteria, viruses, and protozoa, as well as larger multicellular parasites, frequently invade human tissues and are responsible for various afflictions, ranging from mild, annoying symptoms to life-threatening disease. Often, the body's natural defense mechanisms are unable to deal with these pathogenic invaders, and pharmacologic treatment is essential in resolving infections and promoting recovery. Drugs used to treat infection represent one of the most significant advances in medical history, and these agents are among the most important and widely used pharmacologic agents throughout the world.

Drugs used to treat infectious diseases share a common goal of **selective toxicity,** meaning they must selectively kill or attenuate the growth of the pathogenic organism without causing excessive damage to the host (human) cells. In some cases, the pathogenic organism may have some distinctive structural or biochemical feature that allows the drug to selectively attack the invading cell. For instance, drugs that capitalize on certain differences in membrane structure, protein synthesis, or other unique aspects of cellular metabolism in the pathogenic organism will be effective and safe anti-infectious agents. Of course, selective toxicity is a relative term, because all of the drugs discussed in the following chapters exert some adverse effects on human tissues. However, drugs used to treat various infections generally impair function much more in the pathogenic organism than in human tissues.

Several other general terms are also used to describe the drugs used to treat infectious disease. Agents used specifically against small, unicellular organisms (e.g., bacteria, viruses) are often referred to as *antimicrobial drugs*. Antimicrobial agents are also commonly referred to as *antibiotics,* indicating that these substances are used to kill other living organisms (i.e., anti-"bios," or life). To avoid confusion, various drugs in this text are classified and identified according to the primary type of infectious organism they are used to treat—that is, whether they are antibacterial, antiviral, antifungal, and so on.

This chapter discusses the drugs used to treat bacterial infections. Drugs used to treat and prevent viral infections are presented in Chapter 34, followed by the pharmacologic management of other parasitic infections (antifungal, antiprotozoal, and anthelmintic drugs) in Chapter 35. Because infectious disease represents one of the most common forms of illness, many patients undergoing physical rehabilitation take one or more of these drugs. Physical therapists and occupational therapists will undoubtedly deal with patients undergoing chemotherapy for infectious disease on a routine basis. The pharmacotherapeutic management of infectious disease presented in Chapters 33 through 35 should be of interest to all rehabilitation specialists.

BACTERIA: BASIC CONCEPTS

Bacterial Structure and Function

Bacteria are unicellular microorganisms, ranging in size from 0.8 to 15.0 μm in diameter.[37] Bacteria are distinguished from other microorganisms by several features, including a rigid cell wall that surrounds the bacterial cell and the lack of a true nuclear membrane (i.e., the genetic material within the bacterial cell is not confined by a distinct membrane).[38] Bacteria usually contain the basic subcellular organelles needed to synthesize proteins and maintain cellular metabolism, including ribosomes, enzymes, and cytoplasmic storage granules. Bacteria, however, must depend on some kind of nourishing medium to provide metabolic substrates to maintain function. Hence, these microorganisms often invade human tissues to gain access to a supply of amino acids, sugars, and other substances.

Pathogenic Effects of Bacteria

Bacterial infections can be harmful to host organisms in several ways.[12,37] Bacteria multiply, competing with host (human) cells for essential nutrients. Bacteria also may directly harm human cells by releasing toxic substances. Plus, bacteria may cause an immune response that ultimately damages human tissues and the invading bacteria. Of course, not all bacteria in the human body are harmful. For example, certain bacteria in the gastrointestinal system inhibit the growth of other microorganisms and assist in the digestion of food and synthesis of certain nutrients. Also, many bacteria that enter the body are adequately dealt with by normal immunologic responses. However, invasion of pathogenic bacteria can lead to severe infections and death, especially if the patient is debilitated or the body's endogenous defense mechanisms are unable to combat the infection. In some cases, bacteria may establish areas of growth or colonies that remain fairly innocuous for extended periods. This colonization may, however, begin to proliferate and become a health threat when the patient succumbs to some other disorder or illness. Consequently, the chance of severe, life-threatening infections is especially high in individuals who are debilitated or have some immune system defect.

Bacterial Nomenclature and Classification

Bacteria are usually named according to their genus and species, with these names identified in italic typeset.[38] For instance, *Escherichia coli* refers to bacteria from the *Escherichia* genus, *coli* species. According to this nomenclature, the genus is capitalized and refers to bacteria with common genetic, morphologic, and biochemical characteristics. The species name is not capitalized and often refers to some physical, pathogenic, or

TABLE 33–1 Types of Bacteria

Type	Principal Features	Common Examples
Gram-positive bacilli	Generally rod-shaped; retain color when treated by Gram's method of staining	*Bacillus anthracis, Clostridium tetani*
Gram-negative bacilli	Rod-shaped; do not retain color of Gram's method	*Escherichia coli, Klebsiella pneumoniae, Pseudomonas aeruginosa*
Gram-positive cocci	Generally spherical or ovoid in shape; retain color of Gram's method	*Staphylococcus aureus, Streptococcus pneumoniae*
Gram-negative cocci	Spherical or ovoid; do not retain color of Gram's method	*Neisseria gonorrhoeae* (gonococcus), *N. meningitidis* (meningococcus)
Acid-fast bacilli	Rod-shaped; retain color of certain stains even when treated with acid	*Mycobacterium leprae, M. tuberculosis*
Spirochetes	Slender, spiral shape; able to move about without flagella (intrinsic locomotor ability)	Lyme disease agent; *Treponema pallidum* (syphilis)
Actinomycetes	Thin filaments that stain positively by Gram's method	*Actinomyces israelii; Nocardia*
Others		
Mycoplasmas	Spherical; lack the rigid, highly structured cell wall found in most bacteria	*Mycoplasma pneumoniae*
Rickettsiae	Small, gram-negative bacteria	*Rickettsia typhi, R. rickettsii*

other characteristic of the species. For example, *Streptococcus pyogenes* refers to bacteria from the *Streptococcus* genus that are commonly associated with pyogenic or pus-producing characteristics.

Because of the diverse bacterial genera, bacteria are often categorized according to common characteristics, such as the shape and histologic staining of the bacterial cell.[38] For example, *gram-positive cocci* refers to spherical bacteria (cocci) that retain the discoloration of a particular staining technique (Gram's method of staining). However, development of a comprehensive taxonomy that neatly categorizes all bacteria is difficult because of the diverse morphologic and biochemical characteristics of the various bacterial families and genera.

For the purpose of this chapter, bacteria are categorized according to the criteria outlined in Table 33–1. This classification scheme does not fully identify all of the various characteristics of the many bacterial families. The classifications listed in Table 33–1 are used here only to categorize bacteria according to the use of antibacterial agents, which are discussed later in this chapter under "Specific Antibacterial Agents."

TREATMENT OF BACTERIAL INFECTIONS: BASIC PRINCIPLES

Spectrum of Antibacterial Activity

Some drugs are effective against a variety of bacteria; these are usually referred to as *broad-spectrum agents*. For example, a drug such as tetracycline is considered to have a broad spectrum of activity because this drug is effective against many gram-negative, gram-positive, and other types of bacteria. In contrast, a drug such as isoniazid is fairly specific for the bacillus that causes tuberculosis (i.e., *Mycobacterium tuberculosis*), and its spectrum of activity is relatively narrow. Hence, antibacterial spectrum is one property of an antibacterial drug that determines the clinical applications of that agent. Other factors, including patient tolerance, bacterial resistance, and physician preference, also influence the selection of a particular drug for a particular condition. The clinical use of antibacterial drugs relative to specific bacterial pathogens is discussed in "Clinical Use of Antibacterial Drugs: Relationship to Specific Bacterial Infections."

Bactericidal versus Bacteriostatic Activity

The term **bactericidal** refers to drugs that typically kill or destroy bacteria. In contrast, drugs that do not actually kill bacteria but limit the growth and proliferation of bacterial invaders are referred to as **bacteriostatic**. Antibacterial drugs are usually classified as either bactericidal or bacteriostatic, depending on their mechanism of action. Also, the classification of whether a drug is bactericidal or bacteriostatic may depend on the dosage of the drug. For instance, drugs such as erythromycin exhibit bacteriostatic activity at lower doses but are bactericidal at higher doses.

BASIC MECHANISMS OF ANTIBACTERIAL DRUGS

As mentioned previously, antibacterial and other antimicrobial drugs must be selectively toxic to the infectious microorganism, without causing excessive damage to human cells. Drugs that exert selective toxicity against bacteria generally employ one of the mechanisms shown in Figure 33–1. These mechanisms include (1) inhibition of bacterial cell wall synthesis and function, (2) inhibition of bacterial protein synthesis, and (3) inhibition of bacterial DNA/RNA function. The details of these mechanisms, along with the reasons why each mechanism is specific for bacterial (versus human) cells, are discussed next.

Inhibition of Bacterial Cell Wall Synthesis and Function

Penicillin, cephalosporins, and several other commonly used drugs exert their antibacterial effects by inhibiting the synthesis of bacterial cell walls.[38] These drugs are selectively toxic because the bacterial cell walls differ considerably from those of their mammalian counterparts. The membrane surrounding most bacterial cells (with the exception of the *Mycoplasma* genus) is a relatively rigid, firm structure.[20] This rigidity appears to be essential in constraining the high osmotic pressure within the bacterial cell.[20] This behavior contrasts with the relatively supple, flexible membrane encompassing the mammalian cell.

The increased rigidity of bacterial cell walls is caused by the presence of protein-polysaccharide structures known as *peptidoglycans*.[38] Peptidoglycan units (known also as mureins) within the cell wall are cross-linked to one another in such a way as to provide a remarkable amount of rigidity and firmness to the cell. If these peptidoglycans are not present, the bacterial membrane will lack integrity and cause altered function and impaired homeostasis within the bacterial cell. Also, the lack of adequate membrane cytoarchitecture appears to initiate a suicidal autolysis, whereby bacterial hydrolases released from lysosomes begin to break down the cell wall, thus further contributing to destruction of the microorganism.[38]

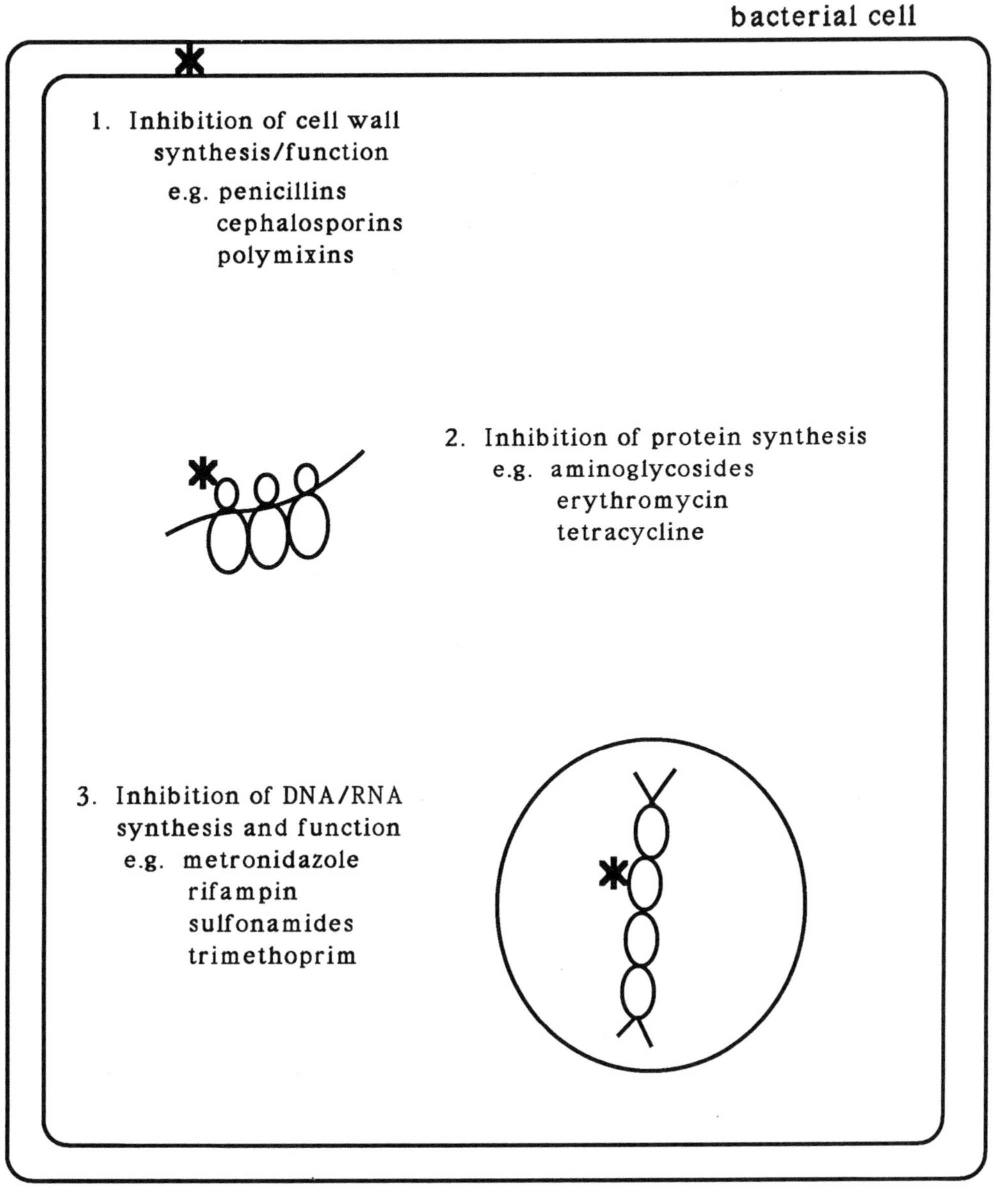

bacterial cell

1. Inhibition of cell wall
   synthesis/function
   e.g. penicillins
        cephalosporins
        polymixins

2. Inhibition of protein synthesis
   e.g. aminoglycosides
        erythromycin
        tetracycline

3. Inhibition of DNA/RNA
   synthesis and function
   e.g. metronidazole
        rifampin
        sulfonamides
        trimethoprim

FIGURE 33–1. Primary sites of antibacterial drug action on bacterial cells. See text for discussion.

Consequently, drugs that cause inadequate production of peptidoglycans or other structural components within the cell wall may produce a selective bactericidal effect. Also, a limited number of antibacterial agents directly punch holes in the bacterial cell membrane, destroying the selective permeability and separation of internal from external environment, which is crucial for the life of the microorganism.[9] These agents include the polymyxin antibiotics (polymyxin B, colistin). These drugs are cationic compounds that are attracted to negatively charged phospholipids in the bacterial cell membrane. The selectivity of these agents for bacterial cell membranes may be due to a greater attraction to certain bacterial phospholipids, as opposed to human cell membrane phospholipids. In any event, these drugs penetrate and disrupt the architecture and integrity of the surface membrane. In essence, these drugs act as detergents that break apart the phospholipid bilayer, creating gaps and leaks in the bacterial cell membrane.[9] The loss of cell membrane integrity leads to rapid death of the bacteria.

Inhibition of Bacterial Protein Synthesis

Bacteria, like most living organisms, must continually synthesize specific proteins to carry out various cellular functions, including enzymatic reactions and membrane transport. A fairly large and well-known group of antibacterial agents work by inhibiting or impairing the synthesis of these bacterial proteins. Drugs that exert their antibacterial effects in this manner include the aminoglycosides (e.g., gentamicin, streptomycin), erythromycin, the tetracyclines, and several other agents.[12,38,44]

Generally, drugs that inhibit bacterial protein synthesis enter the bacterial cell and bind to specific ribosomal subunits.[38] Antibacterial drugs that work by this mechanism have a much greater affinity for bacterial ribosomes than for human ribosomes, hence their relative specificity in treating bacterial infections. Binding of the drug to the ribosome either blocks protein synthesis or causes the ribosome to misread the messenger RNA (mRNA) code, resulting in the production of meaningless or nonsense proteins.[12,38] The lack of appropriate protein production impairs bacterial cell membrane transport and metabolic function, resulting in retarded growth or death of the bacteria.

Inhibition of Bacterial DNA/RNA Synthesis and Function

As in any cell, bacteria must be able to replicate their genetic material to reproduce and function normally. An inability to produce normal DNA and RNA will prohibit the bacteria from mediating continued growth and reproduction. Drugs that exert their antibacterial activity by directly or indirectly interfering with the structure, synthesis, and function of DNA and RNA in susceptible bacteria include the fluoroquinolones, sulfonamides, and several other agents.[25,38] Apparently, these drugs are able to selectively impair bacterial DNA/RNA function because they have a greater affinity for bacterial genetic material and enzymes related to bacterial DNA/RNA synthesis.

Several antibacterial drugs inhibit bacterial nucleic acid synthesis by inhibiting the production of folic acid.[25] Folic acid serves as an enzymatic cofactor in a number of reactions, including synthesis of bacterial nucleic acids and certain essential amino acids. The pathway for synthesis of these folic acid cofactors is illustrated in Figure 33–2. Certain antibacterial drugs block specific steps in the folate pathway, thus impairing the production of this enzymatic cofactor and ultimately impairing the production of nucleic acids and other essential metabolites. Examples of drugs that exert antibacterial effects by this mechanism are trimethoprim and the sulfonamide drugs (e.g., sulfadiazine, sulfamethoxazole).[25]

SPECIFIC ANTIBACTERIAL AGENTS

Considering the vast number of antibacterial drugs, we cannot explore the pharmacokinetic and pharmacologic details of each individual agent. For the purposes of this chapter, the major groups of antibacterial drugs are categorized according to the basic

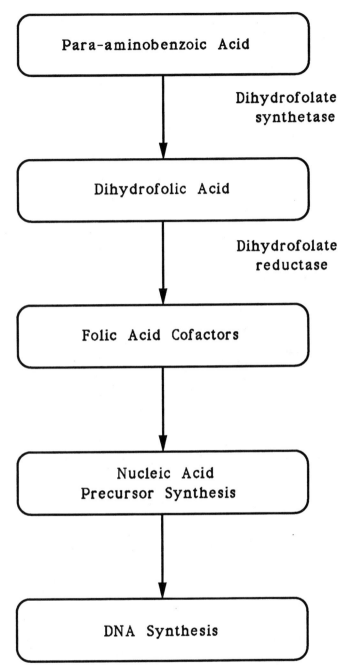

FIGURE 33–2. Folic acid metabolism in bacterial cells. Certain antibacterial drugs (e.g., sulfonamides and trimethoprim) inhibit the dihydrofolate synthetase and reductase enzymes, thus interfering with DNA biosynthesis.

modes of antibacterial action that were just discussed (inhibition of cell wall synthesis, etc.). Pertinent aspects of each group's actions, uses, and potential side effects are briefly discussed. For a more detailed description of any specific agent, the reader is referred to one of the current drug indexes, such as the *Physician's Desk Reference (PDR).*

ANTIBACTERIAL DRUGS THAT INHIBIT BACTERIAL CELL WALL SYNTHESIS AND FUNCTION

Table 33–2 lists drugs that exert their primary antibacterial effects by impairing bacterial cell membrane synthesis and function. Clinical use and specific aspects of these drugs are presented here.

Penicillins

Penicillin, the first antibiotic, was originally derived from mold colonies of the *Penicillium* fungus during the early 1940s. Currently, there are several forms of natural and semisynthetic penicillins (see Table 33–2). These agents have a chemical structure and mode of action similar to the cephalosporin drugs and several other agents. Collectively, the penicillins and these other drugs are known as *beta-lactam antibiotics* because they share a common structure known as a *beta-lactam ring*.[15]

Penicillin and other beta-lactam agents exert their effects by binding to specific enzymatic proteins within the bacterial cell wall. These enzymatic proteins, known as penicillin-binding proteins (PBPs), are responsible for the normal synthesis and organization of the bacterial cell wall. In particular, PBPs help manufacture the peptidoglycans, which are essential for normal membrane structure and function. Penicillins and other beta-lactam drugs attach to the PBPs and inhibit their function.[21] Thus, construction of the bacterial cell wall is impaired, and the cell dies from an inability of the membrane to serve as a selective barrier and contain the high internal osmotic pressure of the bacterial cell.

CLASSIFICATION AND USE OF PENICILLINS

As indicated in Table 33–2, penicillins can be classified according to their chemical background, spectrum of antibacterial activity, or pharmacokinetic features.[54] The naturally occurring penicillins (penicillin G and V) can be administered orally but have a relatively narrow antibacterial spectrum. Some semisynthetic penicillins (amoxicillin, ampicillin) have a broader antibacterial spectrum and may be administered either orally or parenterally, depending on the specific agent. Penicillinase-resistant forms of penicillin were developed to overcome strains of bacteria that contain an enzyme known as a penicillinase or beta-lactamase. This enzyme destroys natural and some semisynthetic penicillins, rendering these drugs ineffective in bacteria containing this enzyme. For penicillinase-containing bacteria, semisynthetic forms of penicillin that are resistant to destruction by the penicillinase must be used (see Table 33–2).

Discussing all the clinical applications of the penicillins goes well beyond the scope of this chapter. These agents are a mainstay in the treatment of infection and remain the drugs of choice in a diverse array of clinical disorders. Tables 33–3a to 33–3d give some indication of the clinical uses of the penicillins. Clearly, these agents continue to be one of the most important and effective antibacterial regimens currently available.

ADVERSE EFFECTS

One of the primary problems with penicillin drugs is the potential for allergic reactions. **Hypersensitivity** to penicillin is exhibited by skin rashes, hives, itching, and difficulty in breathing. In some individuals, these reactions may be fairly minor and can

TABLE 33–2 Drugs That Inhibit Bacterial Cell Membrane Synthesis

Penicillins	Cephalosporins	Other Agents	Penicillin and Beta-Lactamase Combinations
Natural penicillins	First-generation cephalosporins	Aztreonam (Azactam)	Ampicillin and clavulanate (Augmentin)
Penicillin G (Bicillin, Wycillin, many others)	Cefadroxil (Duricef)	Bacitracin (Bacitracin ointment)	Ampicillin and sulbactam (Unasyn)
Penicillin V (Beepen-VK, V-Cillin K, others)	Cefazolin (Ancef, Kefzol)	Colistin (Coly-Mycin S)	Piperacillin and tazobactam (Zosyn)
Penicillinase-resistant penicillins	Cephalexin (Keflex, Keftab)	Cycloserine (Seromycin)	Ticarcillin and clavulanate (Timentin)
Cloxacillin (Cloxapen, Tegopen)	Cephalothin (Keflin)	Imipenem/cilastatin (Primaxin)	
Dicloxacillin (Dycill, Dynapen, Pathocil)	Cephapirin (Cefadyl)	Meropenem (Merrem I.V.)	
Methicillin (Staphcillin)	Cephradine (Velosef)	Polymyxin B (generic)	
Nafcillin (Unipen)	Second-generation cephalosporins	Vancomycin (Vancocin)	
Oxacillin (Bactocill, Prostaphilin)	Cefaclor (Ceclor)		
Aminopenicillins	Cefamandole (Mandol)		
Amoxicillin (Amoxil, Polymox, others)	Cefonicid (Monocid)		
Ampicillin (Omnipen, Polycillin, others)	Cefotetan (Cefotan)		
Bacampicillin (Spectrobid)	Cefoxitin (Mefoxin)		
Extended-spectrum penicillins	Cefprozil (Cefzil)		
Carbenicillin (Geocillin, Geopen, Pyopen)	Cefuroxime (Ceftin, Kefurox, Zinacef)		
Mezlocillin (Mezlin)	Third-generation cephalosporins		
Piperacillin (Pipracil)	Cefixime (Suprax)		
Ticarcillin (Ticar)	Cefoperazone (Cefobid)		
	Cefotaxime (Claforan)		
	Cefpodoxime (Vantin)		
	Ceftazidime (Fortaz, Tazicef, others)		
	Ceftibuten (Cedax)		
	Ceftizoxime (Cefizox)		
	Ceftriaxone (Rocephin)		
	Moxalactam (Moxam)		
	Fourth-generation cephalosporins		
	Cefepime (Maxipime)		

often be resolved by changing the type of penicillin or the method of administration. In others, however, penicillin hypersensitivity may be severe and lead to an *anaphylactic reaction* (severe bronchoconstriction and cardiovascular collapse).

During prolonged administration, penicillin drugs may also cause central nervous system (CNS) problems (e.g., confusion, hallucinations), as well as certain blood disorders, such as hemolytic anemia and thrombocytopenia. Other relatively minor side effects of penicillin drugs include gastrointestinal problems such as nausea, vomiting, and diarrhea.

Cephalosporins

The cephalosporin drugs, which are also classified as beta-lactam antibiotics, exert their bactericidal effects in a manner similar to that of the penicillins (inhibition of PBPs, resulting in inadequate peptidoglycan production).[27] Generally, the cephalosporins serve as alternative agents to penicillins if penicillin drugs are ineffective or poorly tolerated by the patient. Cephalosporins may also be the drugs of choice in certain types of urinary tract infections (see Tables 33–3a to 33–3d).

Cephalosporins can be subdivided into first-, second-, third-, and fourth-generation groups according to their spectrum of antibacterial activity (see Table 33–2). First-generation cephalosporins, which are generally effective against gram-positive cocci, may also be used against some gram-negative bacteria. Second-generation cephalo-

TABLE 33–3a Treatment of Common Infections Caused by Gram-Positive Bacilli

Bacillus	Disease	Primary Agent(s)	Alternative Agent(s)
Bacillus anthracis	Anthrax; pneumonia	Penicillin G	Doxycycline; erythromycin; a cephalosporin; chloramphenicol
Clostridium difficile	Antibiotic-associated colitis	Metronidazole	Vancomycin
Clostridium perfringens	Gas gangrene	Penicillin G	A cephalosporin; clindamycin; doxycycline; imipenem; chloramphenicol
Clostridium tetani	Tetanus	Penicillin G; vancomycin	Clindamycin; doxycycline
Corynebacterium diphtheriae	Pharyngitis; laryngo-tracheitis; pneumonia; other local lesions	Erythromycin	A cephalosporin; clindamycin; rifampin
Corynebacterium species	Endocarditis; infections in various other tissues	Penicillin G ± an aminoglycoside; vancomycin	Rifampin + penicillin G; ampicillin-sulbactam
Erysipelothrix rhusiopathiae	Erysipeloid	Penicillin G	Chloramphenicol; doxycycline; erythromycin
Listeria mono-cytogenes	Bacteremia; meningitis	Ampicillin or penicillin G ± gentamicin	Chloramphenicol; erythromycin; trimethoprim-sulfamethoxazole

Source: Adapted from Chambers, HF and Sande, MA: Antimicrobial agents. In Hardman, JG, et al (eds): The Pharmacological Basis of Therapeutics, ed 9. McGraw-Hill, New York, 1996, with permission of McGraw-Hill, Inc.

TABLE 33–3b Treatment of Common Infections Caused by Gram-Negative Bacilli

Bacillus	Disease	Primary Agent(s)	Alternative Agent(s)
Acinetobacter	Infections in various tissues; hospital-acquired infections	An aminoglycoside; imipenem	A cephalosporin; trimethoprim-sulfamethoxazole
Brucella	Brucellosis	Doxycycline + gentamicin; doxycycline + rifampin; trimethoprim + rifampin	Chloramphenicol; trimethoprim-sulfamethoxazole ± gentamicin
Calymmatobacterium granulomatis	Granuloma inguinale	Doxycycline	Trimethoprim-sulfamethoxazole
Campylobacter fetus	Bacteremia; endocarditis; meningitis	Ampicillin; gentamicin	Ceftriaxone; chloramphenicol; ciprofloxacin or ofloxacin; imipenem
Campylobacter jejuni	Enteritis	Ciprofloxacin or ofloxacin	Azithromycin or clarithromycin; clindamycin; erythromycin
Enterobacter species	Urinary tract and other infections	An aminoglycoside; imipenem	Ciprofloxacin or ofloxacin; a broad-spectrum penicillin; trimethoprim-sulfamethoxazole
Escherichia coli	Bacteremia; urinary tract infections; infections in other tissues	Ampicillin ± an aminoglycoside; a cephalosporin; ciprofloxacin or ofloxacin; trimethoprim-sulfamethoxazole	An aminoglycoside; aztreonam; doxycycline; nitrofurantoin; a penicillin + a penicillinase inhibitor
Flavobacterium meningosepticum	Meningitis	Vancomycin	Rifampin; trimethoprim-sulfamethoxazole
Franciscella tularensis	Tularemia	Gentamicin or streptomycin	Chloramphenicol; ciprofloxacin; doxycycline
Fusobacterium nucleatum	Empyema; genital infections; gingivitis; lung abscesses; ulcerative pharyngitis	Clindamycin; penicillin G	Cefoxitin; a cephalosporin; chloramphenicol; doxycycline; erythromycin; metronidazole
Haemophilus ducreyi	Chancroid	Ceftriaxone; erythromycin; trimethoprim-sulfamethoxazole	Ciprofloxacin; doxycycline; a sulfonamide
Haemophilus influenzae	Epiglottitis, meningitis	Ceftriaxone or cefotaxime; chloramphenicol	Ampicillin-sulbactam; trimethoprim-sulfamethoxazole
Haemophilus influenzae	Otitis media; pneumonia, sinusitis	Amoxicillin-clavulanate; trimethoprim-sulfamethoxazole	Amoxicillin or ampicillin; azithromycin; cefuroxime; ciprofloxacin
Klebsiella pneumoniae	Pneumonia; urinary tract infection	A cephalosporin ± an aminoglycoside	Aztreonam; ciprofloxacin or ofloxacin; mezlocillin or piperacillin; a penicillin + a penicillinase inhibitor imipenem; trimethoprim-sulfamethoxazole

(continued)

TABLE 33–3b Treatment of Common Infections Caused by
Gram-Negative Bacilli *(Continued)*

Bacillus	Disease	Primary Agent(s)	Alternative Agent(s)
Legionella pneumophila	Legionnaires' disease	Erythromycin ± rifampin	Azithromycin or clarithromycin; ciprofloxacin; trimethoprim-sulfamethoxazole
Pasteurella multocida	Abscesses; bacteremia; meningitis; wound infections (animal bites)	Amoxicillin-clavulanate; penicillin G	A cephalosporin; doxycycline
Proteus mirabilis	Urinary tract and other infections	Ampicillin or amoxicillin	An aminoglycoside; a cephalosporin; ciprofloxacin or ofloxacin
Proteus, other species	Urinary tract and other infections	An aminoglycoside; a cephalosporin	Aztreonam; imipenem; penicillin + a beta-lactamase inhibitor
Pseudomonas aeruginosa	Bacteremia, pneumonia	A broad-spectrum penicillin + an aminoglycoside	Aztreonam + an aminoglycoside; ceftazidime + an aminoglycoside; ciprofloxacin + a broad-spectrum penicillin or an aminoglycoside; imipenem + an aminoglycoside
Pseudomonas aeruginosa	Urinary tract infection	Ceftazidime; ciprofloxacin or ofloxacin; a broad-spectrum penicillin	An aminoglycoside; aztreonam; imipenem or meropenem
Pseudomonas mallei	Glanders	Streptomycin + tetracycline	Streptomycin + chloramphenicol
Pseudomonas pseudomallei	Melioidosis	Ceftazidime or ceftriaxone; trimethoprim-sulfamethoxazole	Chloramphenicol; imipenem
Salmonella	Acute gastroenteritis	Ciprofloxacin or norfloxacin	Ampicillin; trimethoprim-sulfamethoxazole
Salmonella	Bacteremia; paratyphoid fever; typhoid fever	Ceftriaxone; ciprofloxacin or ofloxacin; trimethoprim-sulfamethoxazole	Ampicillin; chloramphenicol
Serratia	Various opportunistic and hospital-acquired infections	Cefoxitin, cefotetan, or a third-generation cephalosporin; imipenem; a broad-spectrum penicillin + an aminoglycoside	Aztreonam; piperacillin-tazobactam or ticarcillin-clavulanate
Shigella	Acute gastroenteritis	Ciprofloxacin or norfloxacin	Ampicillin; trimethoprim-sulfamethoxazole
Streptobacillus moniliformis	Abscesses; arthritis; bacteremia; endocarditis	Penicillin G	Chloramphenicol; doxycycline; erythromycin; streptomycin
Vibrio cholerae	Cholera	Ciprofloxacin or ofloxacin; doxycycline	Chloramphenicol; trimethoprim-sulfamethoxazole

TABLE 33–3b Treatment of Common Infections Caused by
Gram-Negative Bacilli *(Continued)*

Bacillus	Disease	Primary Agent(s)	Alternative Agent(s)
Yersinia entero-colitica	Sepsis, yersiniosis	An aminoglycoside; chloramphenicol; trimethoprim-sulfamethoxazole	A cephalosporin; ciprofloxacin or ofloxacin
Yersinia pestis	Plague	Streptomycin ± a tetracycline	Chloramphenicol; ciprofloxacin; doxycycline

Source: Adapted from Chambers, HF and Sande, MA: Antimicrobial agents. In Hardman, JG, et al (eds): The Pharmacological Basis of Therapeutics, ed 9. McGraw-Hill, New York, 1996, with permission of McGraw-Hill, Inc.

sporins are also effective against gram-positive cocci, but they are somewhat more effective than first-generation agents against gram-negative bacteria. Third-generation cephalosporins have the broadest spectrum of activity against gram-negative bacteria, but they have limited effectiveness against gram-positive cocci. Fourth-generation agents have the broadest antibacterial spectrum of the cephalosporins, and they are effective against gram-positive and gram-negative organisms. Specific indications for cephalosporins are listed in Tables 33–3a to 33–3d.

ADVERSE EFFECTS

In some patients, cephalosporins may cause an allergic reaction similar to the penicillin hypersensitivity just described. Often a cross-sensitivity exists: a patient who is allergic to penicillin drugs will also display hypersensitivity to cephalosporin agents. Other principal adverse effects of cephalosporins include gastrointestinal problems such as stomach cramps, diarrhea, nausea, and vomiting.

Other Agents That Inhibit Bacterial Cell Wall Synthesis

Aztreonam. Aztreonam (Azactam) is another type of beta-lactam antibiotic, but this drug is classified as a carbapenam agent rather than a penicillin or cephalosporin.[2] Nonetheless, aztreonam acts like the other beta-lactam agents and inhibits the synthesis and structure of the cell membrane in susceptible bacteria. Aztreonam has a fairly limited spectrum, but it may be useful against serious infections caused by certain gram-negative bacilli *(Enterobacter aerogenes* and *Pseudomonas aeruginosa).* The principal problems associated with aztreonam include skin rashes, redness, and itching because of hypersensitivity in susceptible individuals.

Bacitracin. Bacitracin refers to a group of polypeptide antibiotics that have similar chemical and pharmacologic properties. These compounds inhibit bacterial cell wall synthesis by inhibiting the incorporation of amino acids and nucleic acid precursors into the bacterial cell wall. Bacitracin compounds, which have a fairly broad range of antibacterial activity, are effective against many gram-positive bacilli and gram-positive cocci, as well as several other microorganisms. Bacitracin is usually applied topically to prevent and treat infection in superficial skin wounds and certain ophthalmic infections. Commercial preparations containing bacitracin may also contain other antibiotics, such as neomycin and polymyxin B. The primary problem associated with bacitracin is local hypersensitivity, as indicated by skin rashes and itching.

Coccus	Disease	Primary Agent(s)	Alternative Agent(s)
Enterococcus	Endocarditis or other serious infections (bacteremia)	Gentamicin + penicillin G or ampicillin	Vancomycin + gentamicin
Enterococcus	Urinary tract infection	Ampicillin or penicillin	Ciprofloxacin; vancomycin
Staphylococcus aureus	Abscesses; bacteremia; cellulitis; endocarditis; osteomyelitis; pneumonia; others	If methicillin-sensitive: nafcillin or oxacillin; if methicillin-resistant: vancomycin	A cephalosporin; clindamycin; erythromycin; other combinations
Streptococcus agalactiae (group B)	Bacteremia; endo-carditis; meningitis	Ampicillin or penicillin G ± an aminoglycoside	A cephalosporin; chloramphenicol; vancomycin
Streptococcus bovis	Bacteremia; endo-carditis	Penicillin G ± gentamicin	Ceftriaxone; vancomycin
Streptococcus pneumoniae	Arthritis; otitis; pneumonia; sinusitis	If penicillin sensitive: amoxicillin; penicillin. If penicillin resistant: ceftriaxone or cefotaxime; penicillin (large doses); vancomycin.	A cephalosporin; chloramphenicol; clindamycin; a macrolide; trimethoprim-sulfamethoxazole
Streptococcus pyogenes (group A)	Bacteremia; cellulitis; pharyngitis; pneumonia; scarlet fever; other local and systemic infections	Amoxicillin; penicillin	A cephalosporin; clindamycin; erythromycin; vancomycin
Streptococcus (anaerobic species)	Bacteremia; brain and other abscesses; endocarditis; sinusitis	Penicillin G	A cephalosporin; clindamycin; chloramphenicol; erythromycin
Streptococcus (*viridans* group)	Bacteremia; endocarditis	Penicillin G ± gentamicin	Ceftriaxone; vancomycin
Moraxella catarrhalis	Otitis; pneumonia; sinusitis	Amoxicillin + clavulanate; ampicillin + sulbactam; trimethoprim-sulfamethoxazole	A cephalosporin; ciprofloxacin; erythromycin; tetracycline
Neisseria gonorrhoeae (gonococcus)	Arthritis-dermatitis syndrome; genital infections	If penicillin sensitive: ampicillin or amoxicillin + probenecid; penicillin G. If penicillinase-producing: cefixime or ceftriaxone	Cefixime, cefoxitin, or ceftriaxone; ciprofloxacin or ofloxacin; doxycycline; erythromycin; spectinomycin
Neisseria meningitidis (meningococcus)	Meningitis	Penicillin G	Cefotaxime or ceftriaxone; chloramphenicol

Source: Adapted from Chambers, HF and Sande, MA: Antimicrobial agents. In Hardman, JG, et al (eds): The Pharmacological Basis of Therapeutics, ed 9. McGraw-Hill, New York, 1996, with permission of McGraw-Hill, Inc.

TABLE 33–3d Treatment of Infections Caused by Acid-Fast Bacilli,
Spirochetes, Actinomycetes, and Other Microorganisms

Microorganism	Disease	Primary Agent(s)	Alternative Agent(s)
Acid-fast bacillus			
Mycobacterium avium intra-cellulare	Disseminated diseases in AIDS	Clarithromycin + ethambutol ± clofazimine ± ciprofloxacin	Amikacin; rifabutin; rifampin
Mycobacterium leprae	Leprosy	Dapsone + rifampin	Clofazimine, ofloxacin
Mycobacterium tuberculosis	Pulmonary, renal, meningeal, and other tuberculosis infections	Isoniazid + rifampin + pyrazinamide + ethambutol	Various combinations of the primary drugs ± streptomycin
Spirochetes			
Borrelia burgdorferi	Lyme disease	Stage 1: doxycycline Stage 2: ceftriaxone	Stage 1: amoxicillin; azithromycin or clarithromycin; ceftriaxone Stage 2: penicillin G; tetracycline
Borrelia recurrentis	Relapsing fever	Doxycycline	Erythromycin; penicillin G
Leptospira	Meningitis, Weil's disease	Penicillin G	Doxycycline
Treponema pallidum	Syphilis	Penicillin G	Ceftriaxone; doxycycline
Treponema pertenue	Yaws	Penicillin G; streptomycin	Doxycycline
Actinomycetes			
Actinomyces israelii	Cervicofacial, abdominal, thoracic, and other lesions	Penicillin G or ampicillin	Doxycycline; erythromycin
Nocardia asteroides	Brain abscesses; pulmonary and other lesions	A sulfonamide; trimethoprim-sulfamethoxazole	Amikacin; amoxicillin-clavulanate; ceftriaxone; minocycline ± a sulfonamide
Other microorganisms			
Chlamydia psittaci	Ornithosis	Doxycycline	Chloramphenicol
Chlamydia pneumoniae	Pneumonia	Doxycycline	Azithromycin or clarithromycin; erythromycin
Chlamydia trachomatis	Blennorrhea; lymphogranuloma venereum; non-specific urethritis; trachoma	Doxycycline	Azithromycin; erythromycin; a sulfonamide
Mycoplasma pneumoniae	"Atypical" pneumonia	Doxycycline; erythromycin	Azithromycin or clarithromycin
Pneumocystis carinii	Pneumonia (in impaired host)	Trimethoprim-sulfamethoxazole	Mild-moderate disease: atovaquone; clindamycin-primaquine; trimethoprim-dapsone. Moderately severe-severe disease: Clindamycin-primaquine; pentamidine; trimetrexate

(*continued*)

TABLE 33–3d Treatment of Infections Caused by Acid-Fast Bacilli, Spirochetes, Actinomycetes, and Other Microorganisms *(Continued)*

Microorganism	Disease	Primary Agent(s)	Alternative Agent(s)
Rickettsia	Q fever; rickettsial-pox; Rocky Mountain spotted fever; typhus fever, other diseases	Doxycycline	Chloramphenicol
Ureaplasma urealyticum	Nonspecific urethritis	Doxycycline	Erythromycin

Source: Adapted from Chambers, HF and Sande, MA: Antimicrobial agents. In Hardman, JG, et al (eds): The Pharmacological Basis of Therapeutics, ed 9. McGraw-Hill, New York, 1996, with permission of McGraw-Hill, Inc.

Colistin. Colistin (also known as *colistimethate* or *polymyxin E*) is similar to poly-myxin B in terms of pharmacologic mechanism and antibacterial effects.[9] Colistin is used primarily in combination with other agents (neomycin and hydrocortisone) to treat lo-cal infections of the external auditory canal. Adverse effects are relatively rare during lo-cal, topical use of this drug.

Cycloserine. Cycloserine inhibits bacterial wall synthesis by interfering with the fi-nal stage of peptidoglycan synthesis. Synthesis of peptidoglycans is completed by adding two units of the amino acid D-alanine. Cycloserine, which is similar in structure to D-alanine, competitively inhibits the enzyme that adds the final D-alanine units onto the peptidoglycan structures. Cycloserine is considered to be a broad-spectrum antibi-otic but is used primarily as an adjunct in the treatment of tuberculosis. The primary adverse effect of this drug is CNS toxicity, which may occur during prolonged use at relatively high dosages.

Imipenem and Cilastatin. Imipenem is a beta-lactam drug that is classified as a car-bapenam antibiotic. Imipenem exerts bactericidal effects similar to the other beta-lactam agents (penicillins and cephalosporins); that is, imipenem inhibits PBP function and peptidoglycan synthesis. This drug is typically administered along with a second agent, cilastatin. Cilastatin itself does not have any antibacterial activity, but it enhances the bactericidal effects of imipenem by inhibiting metabolic inactivation of imipenem within the kidneys.[31] Imipenem has one of the broadest antibacterial spectrums of the beta-lactam drugs and may be useful against a variety of aerobic gram-positive bacteria, gram-negative bacteria, and some anaerobic bacterial strains.[31] Adverse side effects as-sociated with imipenem include nausea, hypotension, and hypersensitivity (skin rashes, redness, itching). CNS abnormalities such as confusion, tremors, and even seizures have also been reported in certain patients. The risk of imipenem-induced seizures is in-creased in patients who have a pre-existing seizure disorder or if the dose is too high, based on the patients body weight.

Meropenem. Meropenem is a carbapenam antibacterial with effects and spectrum similar to imipenem.[31] Meropenem, however, does not need to be administered with cilastatin. This agent may likewise be effective against certain forms of gram-positive and gram-negative bacteria that are resistant to other beta-lactam drugs. Meropenem may cause CNS problems including seizures, but the risk of seizures is relatively low when compared with the risk of seizures with imipenem.[31]

Polymyxin B. Polymyxin antibiotics are cationic compounds that are attracted to negatively charged phospholipids in the bacterial cell membrane. These drugs penetrate and disrupt the architecture and integrity of the surface membrane. Essentially, poly-myxins act as detergents that break apart the phospholipid bilayer, creating gaps in the bacterial cell wall, which lead to the subsequent destruction of the bacteria.[9]

Polymyxin B is effective against many gram-negative bacteria, including *E. coli*, *Klebsiella*, and *Salmonella*. Systemic administration of this drug, however, is often associated with extreme nephrotoxicity. Hence, this agent is used primarily for the treatment of local, superficial infections of the skin, eyes, and mucous membranes. When applied topically for these conditions, adverse reactions are relatively rare. Polymyxin B is often combined with other antibiotics such as bacitracin and neomycin in commercial topical preparations.

Vancomycin. Vancomycin appears to bind directly to bacterial cell wall precursors such as D-alanine and to impair the incorporation of these precursors into the cell wall. Vancomycin is effective against gram-positive bacilli and cocci and serves primarily as an alternative to the penicillins in a variety of infections (see Tables 33–3a to 33–3d).[34] The emergence of bacteria that are resistant to vancomycin, however, has generated concern about the continued use of this drug (see "Resistance to Antibacterial Drugs" later in this chapter). The primary adverse effects associated with vancomycin include hypersensitivity (e.g., skin rashes), a bitter or unpleasant taste in the mouth, and gastrointestinal disturbances (nausea and vomiting). Vancomycin also has the potential to cause nephrotoxicity and **ototoxicity**.

Use of Beta-Lactamase Inhibitors

A primary problem in using penicillins, cephalosporins, and other beta-lactam antibiotics is that certain bacteria produce enzymes known as beta-lactamases.[39] These beta-lactamase enzymes bind to the beta-lactam drug and destroy the drug before it can exert an antibacterial effect. Bacteria that produce these beta-lactamase enzymes are therefore resistant to penicillin and other beta-lactam antibacterial drugs[21] (problems related to antibacterial drug resistance are discussed later in this chapter; see "Resistance to Antibacterial Drugs"). Fortunately, several drugs are available that inhibit these beta-lactamase enzymes.[47] These drugs include clavulanate, sulbactam, and tazobactam. These beta-lactamase inhibitors are typically combined with a specific type of penicillin to treat infections caused by bacteria that produce beta-lactamase enzymes.[54] The beta-lactamase inhibitor prevents the beta-lactamase enzyme from destroying the penicillin, thus allowing the penicillin to remain intact and effective against the bacterial infection.

Some common combinations of penicillins and specific beta-lactamase inhibitors are listed in Table 33–2. Administration of these drug combinations may produce side effects that are caused primarily by the penicillin component; that is, penicillin-related side effects such as headache, gastrointestinal problems, and allergic reactions may occur. Nonetheless, combining a beta-lactamase inhibitor with a penicillin can be an effective way of treating bacterial infections that might otherwise be resistant to traditional antibacterial therapy.

DRUGS THAT INHIBIT BACTERIAL PROTEIN SYNTHESIS

Drugs that exert their primary antibacterial effects by inhibiting protein synthesis are listed in Table 33–4 and discussed here.

TABLE 33–4 Drugs That Inhibit Bacterial Protein Synthesis

Aminoglycosides	Erythromycins	Tetracyclines	Other Agents
Amikacin (Amikin)	Erythromycin (ERYC, E-Mycin, others)	Demeclocycline (Declomycin)	Chloramphenicol (Chloromycetin)
Gentamicin (Garamycin)	Erythromycin estolate (Ilosone)	Doxycycline (Monodox, Vibramycin, others)	Clindamycin (Cleocin)
Kanamycin (Kantrex)	Erythromycin ethylsuccinate (E.E.S., EryPed)	Minocycline (Minocin)	Ethionamide (Trecator-SC)
Neomycin (generic)	Erythromycin gluceptate (Ilotycin)	Oxytetracycline (Terramycin)	Lincomycin (Lincocin, Lincorex)
Netilmicin (Netromycin)	Erythromycin lactobionate (Erythrocin)	Tetracycline (Achromycin V, others)	
Streptomycin (generic)	Erythromycin stearate (Erythrocin, Erythrocot, others)		
Tobramycin (Nebcin)			

Aminoglycosides

The aminoglycosides are a group of antibacterial agents that include streptomycin, gentamicin, neomycin, and similar agents (see Table 33–4). These agents bind irreversibly to certain parts of bacterial ribosomes and cause several changes in protein synthesis, including alterations in the ability of the ribosome to read the mRNA genetic code.[6,7] This misreading results in improper synthesis of proteins that control specific aspects of cell function, such as membrane structure and permeability.[6] The lack of normal cell proteins leads to the death of the bacterial cell.

ANTIBACTERIAL SPECTRUM AND GENERAL INDICATIONS

Aminoglycosides have a very broad spectrum of antibacterial activity and are effective against many aerobic gram-negative bacteria, including *E. coli, Pseudomonas,* and *Salmonella.*[6] Aminoglycosides are also active against some aerobic gram-positive bacteria, such as certain species of *Staphylococcus,* and many anaerobic bacteria. Consequently, aminoglycosides are used to treat a variety of tissue and wound infections (see Tables 33–3a to 33–3d).

ADVERSE EFFECTS

Aminoglycoside use is limited somewhat by problems with toxicity.[6] Nephrotoxicity, as indicated by bloody urine, acute renal tubular necrosis, and so on, is one of the more common and serious adverse effects.[51] Ototoxicity, as indicated by dizziness and ringing or fullness in the ears, may also occur. This effect can be irreversible in severe cases.[10,11] Toxicity may occur more frequently in certain individuals, such as patients with liver or kidney failure, or elderly patients. To reduce the risk of toxicity, drug levels in the bloodstream must be periodically monitored so dosages can be adjusted for individual patients. Other adverse effects include hypersensitivity (e.g., skin rashes, itching) in susceptible individuals.

Erythromycin and Other Macrolides

Erythromycin and its chemical derivatives (azithromycin, clarithromycin, dirithromycin) comprise a group of agents known as macrolide antibiotics.[1] These drugs inhibit bacterial protein synthesis by binding to specific parts of the ribosomes in susceptible bacteria. This binding impairs protein synthesis primarily by inhibiting the formation of peptide bonds between adjacent amino acids. In particular, erythromycin seems to encourage the dissociation of transfer RNA (tRNA) units from their binding site on the ribosome.[4,29] Normally, the tRNAs bring amino acids to the ribosome, where the amino acids are linked together to form proteins. By stimulating the detachment of tRNA, peptide bond formation is averted.

ANTIBACTERIAL SPECTRUM AND GENERAL INDICATIONS

Erythromycin and the other macrolides exhibit a very broad spectrum of antibacterial activity and are active against many gram-positive bacteria, as well as some gram-negative bacteria. These agents are often used as the primary or alternative drug in a variety of clinical conditions (see Tables 33–3a to 33–3d). Macrolides may be especially useful in patients who are allergic to penicillin.

ADVERSE EFFECTS

When given in high (bactericidal) doses, gastrointestinal distress is a common problem with erythromycin administration. Stomach cramps, nausea, vomiting, and diarrhea may occur. Hence, erythromycin is usually given in doses that only impair the growth of bacteria (bacteriostatic doses). Some of the newer macrolides (clarithromycin, dirithromycin) may be somewhat safer and produce fewer side effects than erythromycin.[28] However, various degrees of allergic reactions, ranging from mild skin rashes to acute anaphylaxis, may occur when these drugs are used in susceptible individuals.

Tetracyclines

Tetracycline and tetracycline derivatives (see Table 33–4) inhibit protein synthesis by binding to several components of the ribosomal apparatus in susceptible bacteria. Hence, these drugs may cause misreading of the mRNA code, as well as impair the formation of peptide bonds at the bacterial ribosome. Thus, tetracyclines are very effective in preventing bacterial protein synthesis.

ANTIBACTERIAL SPECTRUM AND GENERAL INDICATIONS

Tetracyclines are active against a variety of bacteria, including many gram-positive and gram-negative bacteria, as well as other bacterial microorganisms (*Rickettsia*, spirochetes).[41] Their use as a broad-spectrum antibiotic has diminished somewhat, however, because of the development of tetracycline-resistant bacterial strains. (The problem of drug-resistant bacteria is discussed in more detail in "Resistance to Antibacterial Drugs.") Some of the newer tetracycline derivatives, however, may be used to overcome bacterial strains that are resistant to the traditional drugs.[44] Currently, tetracyclines are used to treat specific infections relating to such bacilli as *Chlamydia*, *Rickettsia*, and certain spirochetes (see Tables 33–3a to 33–3d). Tetracyclines may also be used as alternative agents in treating bacterial strains that are resistant to other drugs, such as chloramphenicol, streptomycin, and various penicillins.

ADVERSE EFFECTS

Gastrointestinal distress (nausea, vomiting, diarrhea) may be a problem with tetracycline use. Hypersensitivity reactions (such as rashes) may also occur, as well as increased sensitivity of the skin to ultraviolet light (photosensitivity).[17] Tetracyclines form chemical complexes with calcium that may impair the growth and development of calcified tissues such as bone and teeth, especially in children.[41] Tetracyclines also cause discoloration of teeth in children and pregnant women, apparently because of this tetracycline-calcium interaction.[41] As mentioned previously, development of tetracycline-resistant strains and resulting superinfections may be a serious problem during tetracycline therapy.

Other Agents That Inhibit Bacterial Protein Synthesis

Chloramphenicol. Chloramphenicol (Chloromycetin) is a synthetically produced agent that exerts antibacterial effects similar to those of erythromycin; that is, it binds to the 50S subunit of bacterial ribosomes and inhibits peptide bond formation. Chloramphenicol is a broad-spectrum antibiotic that is active against many gram-negative and gram-positive bacteria. This drug is administered systemically to treat serious infections such as typhoid fever, *Haemophilus* infections such as osteomyelitis, rickettsial infections such as Rocky Mountain spotted fever, and certain forms of meningitis. Chloramphenicol may also be administered topically to treat various skin, eye, and ear infections.

The most serious problem associated with chloramphenicol is the potential for bone marrow aplasia, which can lead to aplastic anemia and possibly death.[18] There is some suggestion that chloramphenicol may lead to chromosomal changes in certain tissues and that the possibility for genotoxicity with prolonged chloramphenicol use should be considered.[18]

Clindamycin. Clindamycin (Cleocin) is derived from lincomycin. Both drugs are similar in structure and function to erythromycin and inhibit protein synthesis by binding to the 50S ribosomal subunit of susceptible bacteria. These agents are effective against most gram-positive bacteria and some gram-negative microorganisms.[18] Typically, clindamycin and lincomycin are reserved as alternative drugs (rather than primary agents) in the treatment of local and systemic infections and may be especially useful if patients are unable to tolerate either penicillin or erythromycin. The principal adverse effects associated with these drugs include gastrointestinal distress (nausea, diarrhea, colitis) and various allergic reactions, ranging from mild skin rashes to anaphylactic shock.

Ethionamide. Ethionamide (Trecator-SC) appears to inhibit bacterial protein synthesis, but the exact mechanism of action is unknown. This drug may act in a manner similar to that of some of the other drugs discussed previously in this section (binding to bacterial ribosomes), or it may mediate its effect by some other means. Ethionamide is effective against *M. tuberculosis* and is used primarily in the treatment of tuberculosis. This drug is usually used as a secondary agent when the primary antituberculosis drugs are ineffective. Gastrointestinal distress (nausea, vomiting) is the most frequent problem encountered with ethionamide use. CNS disorders (drowsiness, mental depression, etc.), as well as severe postural hypotension, may also occur.

Lincomycin. Lincomycin (Lincocin, Lincorex) is similar in mechanism of action, clinical indications, and adverse side effects to clindamycin (see previously in this section).

DRUGS THAT INHIBIT BACTERIAL DNA/RNA SYNTHESIS AND FUNCTION

Table 33–5 lists drugs that exert their primary antibacterial effects by impairing the synthesis and replication of bacterial DNA and RNA. These agents are presented here.

Aminosalicylic Acid

Aminosalicylic acid (Paser, PAS) exerts its effects in a manner similar to the sulfonamide drugs; that is, aminosalicylic acid is structurally similar to para-aminobenzoic acid (PABA) and inhibits folic acid synthesis by competing with PABA in tuberculosis bacteria. This drug is used as an adjunct to the primary antitubercular agents isoniazid and rifampin. Adverse effects are fairly common with aminosalicylic acid use and include gastrointestinal problems, hypersensitivity reactions, and blood dyscrasias (e.g., agranulocytosis, thrombocytopenia).

TABLE 33–5 Drugs That Inhibit Bacterial DNA/RNA Synthesis and Function

Fluoroquinolones	Sulfonamides	Others
Ciprofloxacin (Cipro)	Sulfacytine (Renoquid)	Aminosalicylic acid (Tubasal)
Enoxacin (Penetrex)	Sulfadiazine (Silvadene)	Clofazimine (Lamprene)
Grepafloxacin (Raxar)	Sulfamethizole (Thiosulfil Forte)	Dapsone (Avlosulfon)
Lomefloxacin (Maxaquin)	Sulfamethoxazole (Gantanol, Urobak)	Ethambutol (Myambutol)
Levofloxacin (Levaquin)	Sulfisoxazole (Gantrisin)	Metronidazole (Flagyl,
Norfloxacin (Noroxin)		Protostat, others)
Ofloxacin (Floxin)		Rifampin (Rifadin, Rimactane)
Sparfloxacin (Zagam)		Trimethoprim (Proloprim,
		Trimpex)

Clofazimine

Although the exact mechanism of clofazimine (Lamprene) is unclear, this drug appears to bind directly to bacterial DNA in susceptible microorganisms. Binding of the drug may prevent the double-stranded DNA helix from unraveling to allow replication of the DNA genetic code. An inability to replicate its genetic material will prevent the bacteria from undergoing mitosis.

Clofazimine, which is effective against *Mycobacterium leprae,* is used primarily as an adjunct in the treatment of leprosy. During clofazimine therapy, many patients experience problems with red to brownish-black discoloration of the skin. Although this discoloration is reversible, it may take several months to years before skin color returns to normal after the drug is discontinued. Other adverse effects include abdominal pain, nausea, vomiting, and rough, scaly skin.

Dapsone

Dapsone (Avlosulfon) is a member of a class of chemical agents known as the sulfones. Dapsone is especially effective against *M. leprae* and is used with rifampin as the primary method of treating leprosy. Dapsone appears to exert its antibacterial effects in a manner similar to that of the sulfonamide drugs; that is, dapsone impairs folic acid synthesis by competing with PABA in bacterial cells. Primary adverse effects associated with dapsone include peripheral motor weakness, hypersensitivity reactions (skin rashes, itching), fever, and blood dyscrasias, such as hemolytic anemia.

Ethambutol

The mechanism of ethambutol (Myambutol) is not fully understood. This drug apparently suppresses RNA synthesis in susceptible bacteria, but the exact manner by which this occurs is unknown. Ethambutol is primarily effective against *M. tuberculosis* infections and is a secondary agent in the treatment of tuberculosis.[49] Adverse effects associated with this drug include joint pain, nausea, skin rash and itching, and CNS abnormalities (dizziness, confusion, hallucinations).

Fluoroquinolones

The fluoroquinolone antibiotics include ciprofloxacin (Cipro), enoxacin (Penetrex), grepafloxacin (Raxar), levofloxacin (Levaquin), lomefloxacin (Maxaquin), norfloxacin (Noroxin), ofloxacin (Floxin), and sparfloxacin (Zagam). These drugs inhibit the twisting or supercoiling of DNA necessary for bacterial nucleic acid replication. Evidently, a specific enzyme known as DNA-gyrase is responsible for promoting the DNA supercoiling in bacterial cells. Fluoroquinolone antibiotics inhibit this DNA-gyrase enzyme, thus impairing normal DNA structure and function.[16,52]

Fluoroquinolones are effective against a wide range of gram-positive and gram-negative aerobic bacteria and are especially useful in urinary tract infections caused by *E. coli, Klebsiella, Proteus,* and *Enterobacter aerogenes.*[35,40,52] Other indications include treatment of gastrointestinal infections, respiratory infections, osteomyelitis, and certain sexually transmitted diseases (gonorrhea).[32] Primary adverse effects include CNS toxicity, manifested by visual disturbances, headache, and dizziness. Gastrointestinal distress (nausea, vomiting, diarrhea) and allergic reactions (skin rashes, itching) may also occur.[43] These drugs produce photosensitivity and increase the skin's sensitivity to ultraviolet light.[3,43] Rare but potentially serious cases of nephrotoxicity may occur in certain patients.[22,24]

Finally, these drugs may cause tendon pain and inflammation (tendinopathy) that can be severe and ultimately lead to tendon rupture in some patients. Tendinopathy seems to occur most commonly in the Achilles tendon, but other tendons such as the patellar tendon and supraspinatus tendon may also be affected.[5,14] Although the overall incidence of tendinopathy is fairly low, patients may be more susceptible if they are older, have renal failure, are taking glucocorticoids, or have a history of fluoroquinolone-induced tendinopathy.[14] Although all of the fluoroquinolones can potentially cause tendinopathy, the risk of tendon damage seems highest with ofloxacin.[48] Hence, complaints of pain in any tendon should be carefully evaluated in patients taking fluoroquinolones, and the affected tendon(s) should not be exercised until the cause of tendinopathy can be determined. If it seems that fluoroquinolones are causing tendinopathy, these drugs should be discontinued, and efforts should be made to protect the tendon from excessive stress until the tendinopathy is resolved.

Metronidazole

The exact mechanism of metronidazole (Flagyl, Protostat, others) is not fully understood. This drug appears to be incorporated into bacterial cells, where it undergoes chemical reduction. Apparently, the reduced metabolite of metronidazole interacts with bacterial DNA and causes the DNA to lose its characteristic double-helix structure. This leads to the disintegration of DNA molecules and loss of the ability to replicate and carry out normal genetic functions. Further details of this bactericidal effect remain to be determined, however.

Metronidazole, effective against most anaerobic bacteria, is useful in treating serious infections caused by *Bacteroides, Fusobacterium,* and other anaerobic bacteria. Metronidazole, which is also effective against certain protozoa, is discussed in Chapter 35 with regard to its antiprotozoal effects. Common side effects associated with metronidazole include gastrointestinal distress (nausea, diarrhea), allergic reactions (such as rashes), and CNS symptoms (confusion, dizziness, mood changes). This drug may also cause peripheral neuropathies as indicated by numbness and tingling in the hands and feet.

Rifampin

Rifampin (Rifadin, Rimactane) directly impairs DNA replication by binding to and inhibiting the DNA-dependent RNA polymerase enzyme in susceptible bacteria. This enzyme initiates the replication of genetic material by generating the formation of RNA strands from the DNA template. By inhibiting this enzyme, rifampin blocks RNA chain synthesis and subsequent replication of the nucleic acid code in bacterial cells.

Rifampin is effective against many gram-negative and gram-positive bacteria and is also one of the principal agents used to treat tuberculosis and leprosy. Typically, this drug is combined with another agent—for example, rifampin plus dapsone for leprosy, or rifampin plus isoniazid for tuberculosis—to increase effectiveness and prevent the development of resistance to rifampin. Rifampin is also used in combination with erythromycin to treat Legionnaires' disease and certain forms of meningitis (see Tables 33–3a to 33–3d).

Common adverse effects with rifampin include gastrointestinal distress (nausea, vomiting, stomach cramps) and various hypersensitivity reactions (rashes and fever). Disturbances in liver function have also been noted, and serious hepatic abnormalities may occur in patients with pre-existing liver disease.

Sulfonamides

The sulfonamides include sulfadiazine, sulfamethizole, and similar agents (see Table 33–5). Sulfonamides interfere with bacterial nucleic acid production by disrupting folic acid synthesis in susceptible bacteria. Sulfonamide drugs are structurally similar to PABA, which is the substance used in the first step of folic acid synthesis in certain types of bacteria (see Fig. 33–2). Sulfonamides either directly inhibit the enzyme responsible for PABA utilization or become a substitute for PABA and result in the abnormal synthesis of folic acid. In either case, folic acid synthesis is reduced, and bacterial nucleic acid synthesis is impaired.

Sulfonamides have the potential to be used against a wide variety of bacteria, including gram-negative and gram-positive bacilli and cocci. The development of resistance in various bacteria, however, has limited the use of these drugs somewhat. Currently, sulfonamides are used systemically to treat certain urinary tract infections and infections caused by Nocardia bacteria (see Tables 33–3a to 33–3d). Sulfonamides may also be applied topically to treat vaginal infections, ophthalmic conditions, and other local infections. A specific agent, sulfadiazine, can also be combined with silver nitrate to form silver sulfadiazine, which is often applied topically to control bacterial infection in burns.[19]

The problems encountered most frequently with sulfonamide drugs include gastrointestinal distress, increased sensitivity of the skin to ultraviolet light, and allergic reactions. Fairly serious disturbances in the formed blood elements, including blood dyscrasias such as agranulocytosis and hemolytic anemia, may also occur during systemic sulfonamide therapy.

Trimethoprim

Trimethoprim (Proloprim, Trimpex) interferes with the bacterial folic acid pathway by inhibiting the dihydrofolate reductase enzyme in susceptible bacteria (see Fig. 33–2). This enzyme converts dihydrofolic acid to tetrahydrofolic acid during the biosynthesis of folic acid cofactors. By inhibiting this enzyme, trimethoprim directly interferes with the production of folic acid cofactors, and subsequent production of vital bacterial nucleic acids is impaired.

Trimethoprim is effective against several gram-negative bacilli, including *E. coli*, *Enterobacter*, *Proteus mirabilis*, and *Klebsiella*. Trimethoprim is used primarily in the treatment of urinary tract infections caused by these and other susceptible bacteria (see Tables 33–3a to 33–3d). Trimethoprim is frequently used in combination with the sulfonamide drug sulfamethoxazole.[42] Primary adverse effects associated with trimethoprim include headache, skin rashes and itching, decreased appetite, an unusual taste in the mouth, and gastrointestinal problems (nausea, vomiting, diarrhea). Trimethoprim may also cause excessively high levels of potassium in the blood (hyperkalemia), especially in older adults.[26,33]

OTHER ANTIBACTERIAL DRUGS

Several other antibacterial drugs work by mechanisms that are either unknown or are different from the classical antibacterial mechanisms described previously. These drugs are discussed individually here.

Capreomycin

Capreomycin (Capastat) is used as an adjunct or alternative drug for the treatment of tuberculosis. The mechanism of action of this drug is unknown. The primary problems associated with this drug include ototoxicity and nephrotoxicity.

Isoniazid

Isoniazid (INH, Nydrazid, other names) is one of the primary drugs used to treat tuberculosis.[49] Although the exact mechanism of action is unknown, this drug appears to interfere with several enzymatic pathways involving protein, lipid, carbohydrate, and nucleic acid metabolism in susceptible bacteria. Adverse reactions to isoniazid are fairly common, and patients may develop disorders such as hepatitis and peripheral neuropathies.

Methenamine

Methenamine (Hiprex, Mandelamine, Urex) exerts antibacterial properties in a unique fashion. In an acidic environment, this drug decomposes into formaldehyde and ammonia. Formaldehyde is bactericidal to almost all bacteria, and bacteria do not develop resistance to this toxin. This mechanism enables methenamine to be especially useful in treating urinary tract infections, because the presence of this drug in acidic urine facilitates the release of formaldehyde at the site of infection (i.e., within the urinary tract). Use of methenamine is fairly safe, although high doses are associated with gastrointestinal upset and problems with urination (bloody urine, pain while urinating).

Pyrazinamide

Pyrazinamide (generic) is used primarily as an adjunct to other drugs in treating tuberculosis. The mechanism of action of this drug against *M. tuberculosis* is unknown. Problems associated with pyrazinamide include hepatotoxicity and lower-extremity joint pain.

Nitrofurantoin

Nitrofurantoin (Macrobid, Macrodantin, others) is reduced by bacterial enzymes to a metabolite that is toxic to the bacterial cell. This toxic metabolite inhibits bacterial metabolic function by interfering with ribosomal function and other molecules involved in energy production and utilization in the bacterial cell. Nitrofurantoin is primarily used to treat urinary tract infections caused by a number of gram-negative and some gram-positive bacteria. Adverse effects associated with this drug include gastrointestinal distress (nausea, vomiting, diarrhea) and neurotoxicity (as indicated by headache, numbness, and excessive fatigue). Acute pneumonitis (as indicated by coughing, chills, fever, and difficulty in breathing) may also occur soon after nitrofurantoin is initiated. This pneumonitis appears to be a direct chemical effect of the drug and usually disappears within hours after the drug is withdrawn.

CLINICAL USE OF ANTIBACTERIAL DRUGS: RELATIONSHIP TO SPECIFIC BACTERIAL INFECTIONS

An incredible array of antibacterial agents are currently being used clinically. As mentioned previously, selection of a particular agent is based on the effectiveness of the drug against a range or spectrum of different bacteria. The clinical application of antibacterial drugs according to their effectiveness against specific bacteria is summarized in Tables 33–3a to 33–3d. As this table indicates, various antibacterial drugs can serve as either the primary or alternative agents against specific bacterial infections. The actual selection of an antibacterial agent is often highly variable, depending on the particular patient, the type and location of the infection, the experience of the physician, and many other factors.

RESISTANCE TO ANTIBACTERIAL DRUGS

One of the most serious problems of antibacterial therapy is the potential for development of strains of bacteria that are resistant to one or more antibacterial agents.[50,53] Certain bacterial strains have a natural or acquired defense mechanism against specific antibacterial drugs. This enables the strain to survive the effects of the drug and continue to grow and reproduce similar resistant strains, thus representing a genetic selection process in which only the resistant strains survive the drug. As a result, bacteria that are invulnerable to the drug can breed. If other drugs are not effective against the resistant strain, or if cross-resistance to several antibacterial drugs occurs, the resistant bacteria become especially dangerous because of their immunity from antibacterial chemotherapy.[8,34,36]

Bacterial resistance can occur as a result of several mechanisms.[53] Certain bacterial strains may be able to enzymatically destroy the antibacterial drug. The best example is the beta-lactamase enzyme that is found in bacteria that are resistant to beta-lactam drugs (penicillins and cephalosporins).[47] As previously discussed, bacteria containing this enzyme can destroy certain penicillin and cephalosporin drugs, thus rendering the drug ineffective against these resistant strains. Resistance may also occur because the bacterial cell modifies or masks the site where the antibacterial drug typically binds on or within the cell. For instance, penicillins, aminoglycosides, vancomycin, and other drugs must bind to membrane proteins, intracellular proteins, ribosomes, and the like to exert their effect. Differences in the affinity of these binding sites may be acquired by bacterial mutation, thus decreasing the effectiveness of the drug.[13] Bacteria may also develop resistance through mutations that change the enzymes targeted by certain drugs. For example, fluoroquinolones, rifampin, and other drugs that normally inhibit enzymes responsible for bacterial DNA/RNA function will be ineffective if these enzymes are modified within resistant bacteria.[39]

Resistance can likewise occur if the drug's ability to penetrate the bacterial cell is reduced. Most drugs must first penetrate the cell membrane and enter the bacterial cell to exert their bactericidal effects. Specific bacteria that have a natural or acquired opposition to drug penetration render the drug useless, thus leading to the development of strains that are resistant to aminoglycosides and other agents.[39] Certain bacteria also develop drug efflux pumps that expel the drug from the bacterial cell, thus rendering the drug ineffective.[27] These pumps may be the reason that bacteria develop resistance to tetracyclines and a number of other antimicrobial agents.[30]

Consequently, a number of factors may be responsible for mediating the formation of bacterial resistance to penicillins, cephalosporins, aminoglycosides, tetracyclines, and other antibacterial agents. Antibacterial resistance is typically categorized according to the name of the drug and the associated resistant bacterial strain. For example, some of the best known and most important types of resistance include vancomycin-resistant *Staphylococcus aureus* (VRSA), methicillin-resistant *S. aureus* (MRSA), vancomycin-resistant *Enterococcus* (VRE), and penicillin-resistant *Streptococcus pneumoniae* (PRSP).[13] Even though a resistant organism may be linked by name to a specific drug, the organism is typically resistant to other drugs as well (multidrug resistance).[13]

Development of resistant bacteria is understandably a very serious problem in contemporary drug therapy.[8] In addition, the number of resistant bacterial strains continues to progressively increase in certain institutions.[8,45] To limit the development of resistant strains, antibacterial drugs should be used judiciously and not overused.[13,23] For instance, the effort to perform culture and sensitivity tests on sputum, blood, and other body fluids is worthwhile because the pathogenic bacteria can be identified, leading to the use of highly selective agents. Administering selective agents as opposed to broad-spectrum antibiotics may help attenuate and kill resistant strains more effectively.[23] The selective use of current antibacterial drugs and the development of new bactericidal agents are needed to help control the problem of bacterial resistance.[46]

SPECIAL CONCERNS IN REHABILITATION PATIENTS

Patients undergoing physical therapy and occupational therapy will be taking antibacterial drugs for any number of reasons. Antibacterial drugs may be administered to prevent or treat infection in conditions relating directly to the rehabilitation program. For instance, therapists are often involved with administering topical antibacterial agents (e.g., sulfadiazine) to patients with burns. Infection in other conditions that relate to rehabilitation, such as bone infections (osteomyelitis), infections sustained from trauma and various wounds, and infections following joint replacement and other types of surgery, will also require antibacterial therapy. Other types of infection not directly related to rehabilitation (e.g., urinary tract infection, pneumonia) are also very common, frequently occurring in hospitalized patients as well as those receiving outpatient physical therapy and occupational therapy. Consequently, therapists will routinely be working with patients who are receiving antibacterial treatment.

Therapists should generally be aware of the possible adverse effects of antibacterial drugs. Many of these agents have the potential to cause hypersensitivity reactions including skin rashes, itching, and respiratory difficulty (such as wheezing). Therapists may recognize the onset of such reactions when working with these patients. Other common side effects including gastrointestinal problems (nausea, vomiting, diarrhea) are usually not serious but may be bothersome if they continually interrupt physical therapy and occupational therapy. Therapists may have to alter the time of the rehabilitation session to work around these effects, especially if gastrointestinal and similar annoying side effects tend to occur at a specific time of the day (e.g., early morning, late afternoon).

Certain agents may have adverse effects that directly interact with specific rehabilitation treatments. In particular, tetracyclines, sulfonamides, and fluoroquinolones (ciprofloxacin, norfloxacin, etc.) cause increased sensitivity of the skin to ultraviolet light. This problem is obvious if the therapist is administering ultraviolet treatments. Therapists must be especially careful to establish an accurate minimal erythemal dosage to ultraviolet light. Therapists should also be prepared to adjust the ultraviolet light treatments in accordance with changes in dosage of the antibacterial drug.

Finally, therapists play a vital role in preventing the spread of bacterial and other infections. Therapists must maintain appropriate sterile technique when dealing with open wounds. Adequate sterilization of whirlpools with strong disinfectants is also critical in preventing the spread of infection from patient to patient in a rehabilitation setting. Therapists must also recognize the importance of hand washing in preventing the spread of infection and must not neglect to wash their own hands between patients.

CASE STUDY

ANTIBACTERIAL DRUGS

Brief History. J.B. is a 40-year-old former truck driver who was injured in a traffic accident 5 years ago, sustaining a spinal cord transection that resulted in complete paraplegia at the L1–2 level. He underwent extensive physical rehabilitation, including vocational retraining, and had recently been working as a computer programmer when he began to develop a pressure area in the region of the right ischial tuberosity. Despite conservative management, a pressure ulcer developed. Because the patient was in relatively good health otherwise, the ulcer was treated with local debridement and reconstructive surgery, using skin flaps. The patient was admitted to the hospital, and a routine preoperative culture of the ulcer revealed the presence of *E. coli*. The patient had a history of sensitivity to penicillin drugs and was therefore given a tetracycline antibiotic (Achromycin V, 250 mg orally every 6 hours) to resolve the infection prior to surgery. Physical therapy and occupational therapy were also requested to help maintain the patient's upper body strength and functional activity while awaiting surgery. The physical therapist also suggested that ultraviolet radiation might be helpful in resolving the infection.

Problem/Influence of Medication. Tetracyclines and several other antibacterial agents increase the sensitivity of the skin to ultraviolet light.

Decision/Solution. The therapist carefully determined the minimal erythemal dosage for the patient prior to initiating ultraviolet treatments. Also, using careful draping techniques, the therapist confined the treatment to the ulcer site, so that a minimum of the surrounding skin was exposed to the ultraviolet light. This approach ensured that the surrounding tissues would not be endangered if the patient's response to the ultraviolet treatment changed during the course of tetracycline treatment. The combination of drug therapy and ultraviolet radiation quickly resolved the infection, allowing the surgery to proceed as planned.

SUMMARY

Antibacterial drugs are used to prevent and treat infection in a variety of clinical situations. Some drugs are effective against a fairly limited number of bacteria (narrow-spectrum), whereas other agents may be used against a relatively wide variety of bacterial pathogens (broad-spectrum). Specific agents may exert their antibacterial effects by preventing bacterial cell wall synthesis and function, or by inhibiting either bacterial protein synthesis or bacterial DNA/RNA synthesis and function. Although most bacterial infections can be effectively treated with one or more agents, the development of bacterial strains that are resistant to drug therapy continues to be a serious problem. Rehabilitation specialists will routinely treat patients receiving antibacterial drugs for conditions that are directly or indirectly related to the need for physical therapy and occupational therapy. Therapists should be cognizant of the potential side effects of these drugs and how these drugs may interfere with specific physical therapy and occupational therapy procedures.

REFERENCES

1. Alvarez-Elcoro, S and Enzler, MJ: The macrolides: Erythromycin, clarithromycin, and azithromycin. Mayo Clin Proc 74:613, 1999.
2. Asbel, LE and Levison, ME: Cephalosporins, carbapenems, and monobactams. Infect Dis Clin North Am 14:435, 2000.
3. Blondeau, JM: Expanded activity and utility of the new fluoroquinolones: A review. Clin Ther 21:3, 1999.
4. Brisson-Noel, A, Trieu-Cuot, P, and Courvalin, P: Mechanism of action of spiramycin and other macrolides. J Antimicrob Chemother 22(Suppl B):13, 1988.
5. Casparian, JM, et al: Quinolones and tendon ruptures. South Med J 93:488, 2000.
6. Chambers, HF and Sande, MA: The aminoglycosides. In Hardman JG, et al (eds): The Pharmacological Basis of Therapeutics, ed 9. McGraw-Hill, New York, 1996.
7. Davies, BD: The lethal action of aminoglycosides. J Antimicrob Chemother 22:1, 1988.
8. Elliott, TS and Lambert, PA: Antibacterial resistance in the intensive care unit: Mechanisms and management. Br Med Bull 55:259, 1999.
9. Evans, ME, Feola, DJ, and Rapp, RP: Polymixin B sulfate and colistin: Old antibiotics for emerging multiresistant gram-negative bacteria. Ann Pharmacother 33:960, 1999.
10. Fischel-Ghodsian, N: Genetic factors in aminoglycoside toxicity. Ann N Y Acad Sci 884:99, 1999.
11. Forge, A and Schacht, J: Aminoglycoside antibiotics. Audiol Neurootol 5:3, 2000.
12. Genta, RM and Connor, DH: Infectious and parasitic diseases. In Rubin, E and Farber, JL (eds): Pathology, ed 3. JB Lippincott, Philadelphia, 1998.
13. Hand, WL: Current challenges in antibiotic resistance. Adolesc Med 11:427, 2000.
14. Harrell, RM: Fluoroquinolone-induced tendinopathy: What do we know? South Med J 92:622, 1999.
15. Holten, KB and Onusko, EM: Appropriate prescribing of oral beta-lactam antibiotics. Am Fam Physician 62:611, 2000.
16. Hooper, DC and Wolfson, JS: Drug therapy: Fluoroquinolone antimicrobial agents. N Engl J Med 324:384, 1991.

17. Kapusnik-Uner, JE, Sande, MA, and Chambers, HF: Tetracyclines, chloramphenicol, erythromycin, and miscellaneous antibacterial agents. In Hardman, JG, et al (eds): The Pharmacological Basis of Therapeutics, ed 9. McGraw-Hill, New York, 1996.
18. Kasten, MJ: Clindamycin, metronidazole, and chloramphenicol. Mayo Clin Proc 74:825, 1999.
19. Klasen, HJ: A historical review of the use of silver in the treatment of burns. II. Renewed interest for silver. Burns 26:131, 2000.
20. Koch, AL: The exoskeleton of bacterial cells (sacculus): Still a highly attractive target for antibacterial agents that will last for a long time. Crit Rev Microbiol 26:1, 2000.
21. Kotra, LP and Mobashery, S: Mechanistic and clinical aspects of beta-lactam antibiotics and beta-lactamases. Arch Immunol Ther Exp (Warsz) 47:211, 1999.
22. Lipsky, BA and Baker, CA: Fluoroquinolone toxicity profiles: A review focusing on newer agents. Clin Infect Dis 28:352, 1999.
23. Livermore, DM: Epidemiology of antibiotic resistance. Intensive Care Med 26(Suppl 1):S14, 2000.
24. Lomaestro, BM: Fluoroquinolone-induced renal failure. Drug Saf 22:479, 2000.
25. Mandell, GL and Petri, WA: Sulfonamides, trimethoprim-sulfamethoxazole, quinolones, and agents for urinary tract infection. In Hardman, JG, et al (eds): The Pharmacological Basis of Therapeutics, ed 9. McGraw-Hill, New York, 1996.
26. Marinella, MA: Trimethoprim-induced hyperkalemia: An analysis of reported cases. Gerontology 45:209, 1999.
27. Marshall, WF and Blair, JE: The cephalosporins. Mayo Clin Proc 74:187, 1999.
28. McConnell, SA and Amsden, GW: Review and comparison of advanced-generation macrolides clarithromycin and dirithromycin. Pharmacotherapy 19:404, 1999.
29. Menninger, JR: Functional consequences of binding macrolides to ribosomes. J Antimicrob Chemother 16(Suppl A):23, 1985.
30. Nikaido, H: Multiple antibiotic resistance and efflux. Curr Opin Microbiol 1:516, 1998.
31. Norrby, SR: Carbapenems in serious infections: A risk-benefit assessment. Drug Saf 22:191, 2000.
32. O'Donnell, JA and Gelone, SP: Fluoroquinolones. Infect Dis Clin North Am 14:489, 2000.
33. Perazella, MA: Trimethoprim-induced hyperkalemia: Clinical data, mechanism, prevention and management. Drug Saf 22:227, 2000.
34. Perl, TM: The threat of vancomycin resistance. Am J Med 106(Suppl 5a):26S, 1999.
35. Ronald, A: The quinolones and renal infection. Drugs 58(Suppl 2):96, 1999.
36. Rubinstein, E: Antimicrobial resistance: Pharmacological solutions. Infection 27(Suppl 2):S32, 1999.
37. Samuelson, J: Infectious diseases. In Cotran, RS, Kumar, V, and Collins, T (eds): Pathologic Basis of Disease, ed 6. WB Saunders, Philadelphia, 1999.
38. Schaechter, M: Biology of infectious agents. In Schaechter, M, et al (eds): Mechanisms of Microbial Disease, ed 3. Lippincott Williams & Wilkins, Philadelphia, 1999.
39. Schlessinger, D and Eisenstein, BI: Biological basis for antibacterial action. In Schaechter, M, et al (eds): Mechanisms of Microbial Disease, ed 3. Lippincott Williams & Wilkins, Philadelphia, 1999.
40. Scully, BE: Pharmacology of the fluoroquinolones. Urology 35(Suppl 1):8, 1990.
41. Smilack, JD: The tetracyclines. Mayo Clin Proc 74:727, 1999.
42. Smilack, JD: Trimethoprim-sulfamethoxazole. Mayo Clin Proc 74:730, 1999.
43. Stahlmann, R and Lode, H: Toxicity of quinolones. Drugs 58(Suppl 2):37, 1999.
44. Sum, PE, Sum, FW, and Projan, SJ: Recent developments in tetracycline antibiotics. Curr Pharm Des 4:119, 1998.
45. Talon, D: The role of the hospital environment in the epidemiology of multi-resistant bacteria. J Hosp Infect 43:13, 1999.
46. Tan, YT, Tillett, DJ, and McKay, IA: Molecular strategies for overcoming antibiotic resistance in bacteria. Mol Med Today 6:309, 2000.
47. Therrien, C and Levesque, RC: Molecular basis of antibiotic resistance and beta-lactamase inhibition by mechanism-based inactivators: Perspectives and future directions. FEMS Microbiol Rev 24:251, 2000.
48. Van der Linden, PD, et al: Achilles tendinitis associated with fluoroquinolones. Br J Clin Pharmacol 48:433, 1999.
49. Van Scoy, RE and Wilkowske, CJ: Antimycobacterial therapy. Mayo Clin Proc 74:1038, 1999.
50. Virk, A and Steckelberg, JM: Clinical aspects of antimicrobial resistance. Mayo Clin Proc 75:200, 2000.
51. Walker, PD, Barri, Y, and Shah, SV: Oxidant mechanisms in gentamicin nephrotoxicity. Ren Fail 21:433, 1999.
52. Walker, RC: The fluoroquinolones. Mayo Clin Proc 74:1030, 1999.
53. Walsh, C: Molecular mechanisms that confer antibacterial drug resistance. Nature 406:775, 2000.
54. Wright, AJ: The penicillins. Mayo Clin Proc 74:290, 1999.

CHAPTER 34

Treatment of Infections II: Antiviral Drugs

A virus is one of the smallest microorganisms, consisting of only a nucleic acid core surrounded by a protein shell.[32] Several types of viruses commonly infect human cells and are responsible for a diverse range of pathologies. Viral infections extend from relatively mild disorders such as the common cold to serious, life-threatening conditions such as AIDS. Viruses are somewhat unique in that they must rely totally on the metabolic processes of the host (human) cell to function.[77] Hence, the pharmacologic treatment of viral infections is complex, because selective destruction of the virus without destroying human cells is often difficult.

This chapter describes the basic characteristics of viruses and the relatively limited number of drugs that can act selectively as antiviral agents. Methods of preventing viral infections (antiviral vaccines) are also briefly discussed. Finally, the current methods of treating a specific viral-induced disease, AIDS, are presented. Rehabilitation specialists often treat patients who are in the active stages of viral infection, as well as those suffering from the sequelae of viral disorders, such as gastroenteritis, encephalitis, and influenza. Hence, the pharmacotherapeutic treatment and prophylaxis of viral infections should concern physical therapists and occupational therapists.

VIRAL STRUCTURE AND FUNCTION

Classification of Viruses

Viruses are classified according to several criteria, including physical, biochemical, and pathogenic characteristics.[64,77] The classifications of some of the more common viruses affecting humans and their associated diseases are listed in Table 34–1. This table shows that viruses can be divided into basically two categories, depending on the type of genetic material contained in the virus (DNA or RNA viruses). Families within each major subdivision are classified according to physical characteristics (configuration of the genetic material, shape of the virus capsule) and other functional criteria.

567

TABLE 34–1 Common Viruses Affecting Humans

Family	Virus	Related Infections
DNA viruses		
Adenoviridae	Adenovirus, types 1–33	Respiratory tract and eye infections
Hepatitis B	Hepatitis B virus	Hepatitis B
Herpesviridae	Cytomegalovirus	Cytomegalic inclusion disease (i.e., widespread involvement of virtually any organ, especially the brain, liver, lung, kidney, and intestine)
	Epstein-Barr virus	Infectious mononucleosis
	Herpes simplex, types 1 and 2	Local infections of oral, genital, and other mucocutaneous areas; systemic infections
	Varicella-zoster virus	Chickenpox; herpes zoster (shingles); other systemic infections
Poxviridae	Smallpox virus	Smallpox
RNA viruses		
Coronaviridae	*Coronavirus*	Upper respiratory tract infection
Flaviviridae	Hepatitis C virus	Hepatitis C
Orthomyxoviridae	*Influenzavirus,* types A and B	Influenza
Paramyxoviridae	Measles virus	Measles
	Mumps virus	Mumps
	Respiratory syncytial virus	Respiratory tract infection in children
Picornaviridae	Hepatitis A virus	Hepatitis A
	Polioviruses	Poliomyelitis
	Rhinovirus, types 1–89	Common cold
Retroviridae	Human immunodeficiency virus (HIV)	AIDS
Rhabdoviridae	Rabies virus	Rabies
Togaviridae	*Alphavirus*	Encephalitis
	Rubella virus	Rubella

Characteristics of Viruses

Viruses are somewhat unique in structure and function as compared with other microorganisms. The basic components of viral microorganisms are illustrated in Figure 34–1. A virus essentially consists of a core of viral DNA or RNA.[32,41] The genetic core is surrounded by a protein shell, or *capsid*. This structure—the capsid enclosing the nucleic acid core—is referred to as the *nucleocapsid*. In some viruses, the nucleocapsid is also surrounded by a viral membrane, or envelope, which is composed of glycoproteins extending outward from a lipid bilayer.

The virus, however, does not contain any of the cellular components necessary to replicate itself or synthesize proteins and other macromolecules; that is, the virus lacks ribosomes, endoplasmic reticulum, and so on.[32,41] The virus contains only the genetic code (viral genome) that will produce additional viruses. To replicate itself, the virus must rely on the biochemical machinery of the host cell.[77] In essence, the virus invades the host cell, takes control of the cell's metabolic function, and uses the macromolecular-synthesizing apparatus of the host cell to crank out new viruses. Specific steps in the viral replication process are described in the next section.

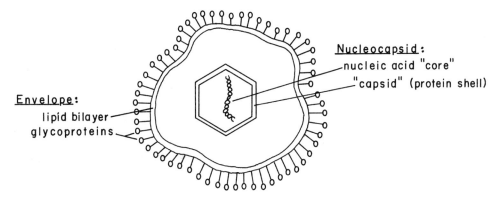

FIGURE 34–1. Basic components of a virus. Note the relative lack of most cellular organelles (ribosomes, endoplasmic reticulum, etc.).

Viral Replication

Self-replication of a virus occurs in several distinct steps.[32] These steps are (1) adsorption, (2) penetration and uncoating, (3) biosynthesis, and (4) maturation and release. These four basic steps are illustrated in Figure 34–2. Each step is also briefly discussed here.

Adsorption. Initially, the virus attaches or adsorbs to the surface of the host cell. Most viruses are attracted to the host cell because of the interaction between proteins on the outer surface of the virus and receptor-like proteins on the host-cell membrane. The interaction of the virus with these surface proteins causes the virus to adhere to the outer surface of the host-cell membrane.

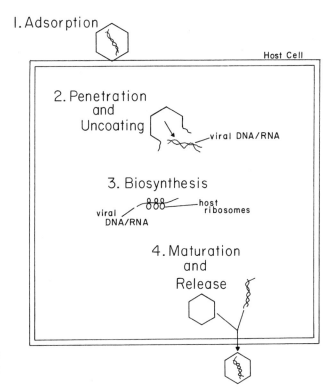

FIGURE 34–2. Basic sequence of viral replication. See text for details.

Penetration and Uncoating. The virus enters the host cell either by passing directly through the cell membrane or by fusing with the host-cell membrane and releasing the viral genetic material into the host cell. Once inside the host cell, any coating that remains on the virus is removed, usually by proteolytic enzymes of the host cell.

Biosynthesis. When the viral genetic material is released within the host cell, the virus takes control of the cell's molecular synthesizing machinery to initiate the biosynthesis of new viral enzymes and proteins. Different viruses exert their effects on the host cell in different ways, but many viruses control the host cell through a direct effect on the cell's nucleus. Some viruses, including the virus that causes AIDS, actually insert their genetic material directly into the host cell's DNA, thereby becoming integrated within the genetic control of the infected cell.

Regardless of the exact mechanism of infection, the virus essentially commands the cell to synthesize enzymes that produce more copies of the viral DNA or RNA and to synthesize structural proteins that will ultimately be used to form new viral shells or capsids. Thus, the virus uses the biosynthetic machinery as well as the structural components and nutrients of the cell (amino acids, nucleic acids, etc.) to replicate itself. Likewise, the virus often incapacitates the cell so that the infected cell cannot carry out its normal physiologic activities.

Maturation and Release. The component parts of the virus (the genetic core and surrounding shell) are assembled into mature viruses and released from the host cell. In some cases, the virus may be released by a process of exocytosis, leaving the host cell relatively intact (although still infected with the original virus). Alternatively, the host cell may simply be destroyed (undergo lysis), thus releasing the viral offspring. Lysis of the host cell not only results in release of the virus and death of the cell but also may stimulate the production of inflammatory mediators (prostaglandins, kinins, etc.), which create a hypersensitivity response.

The steps involved in viral replication are important pharmacologically because antiviral drugs may interrupt this process at one or more of the steps. Specific agents that are currently used as antiviral drugs and their pharmacodynamic aspects are discussed next.

SPECIFIC ANTIVIRAL DRUGS

The primary agents that are approved for use as antiviral drugs are listed in Tables 34–2 and 34–3. Each agent is also briefly discussed below.

Acyclovir and Valacyclovir

Antiviral Efficacy and Clinical Use. Acyclovir (Zovirax) is effective against herpesvirus infections, especially those involving herpes simplex types I and II.[26,51,96] Acyclovir is the principal drug used to treat genital herpes and herpes simplex–related infections in other mucosal and cutaneous areas (lips and face).[28,100] Acyclovir is also effective against other members of the herpesvirus family, including varicella-zoster and Epstein-Barr virus.[28,68] This agent may be used to treat varicella-zoster–related infections such as herpes zoster and chickenpox. Epstein-Barr virus infections, including infectious mononucleosis, may also respond to acyclovir.

Acyclovir can be applied topically as a cream to treat cutaneous and mucosal infections. This drug can also be administered systemically by the oral route or by intravenous administration in severe, acute infections.

TABLE 34–2 Antiviral Drugs*

Generic Name	Trade Name(s)	Principal Indication(s)
Acyclovir	Zovirax	Treatment of initial and recurrent herpesvirus infections, including herpes simplex, herpes zoster, and varicella (chicken-pox) infections
Amantadine	Symmetrel	Prevention and treatment of influenza A infections (also used as an antiparkinson drug; see Chap. 10)
Cidofovir	Vistide	Treatment of cytomegalovirus (CMV) retinitis in immunocompromised patients
Famciclovir	Famvir	Treatment and suppression of herpesvirus infections, including herpes simplex (genital herpes) and herpes zoster (shingles)
Foscarnet	Foscavir	Treatment of cytomegalovirus (CMV) retinitis and other CMV and herpes virus infections in immunocompromised patients
Ganciclovir	Cytovene	Treatment of CMV infections in immunocompromised patients
Penciclovir	Denavir	Topical application for treatment of recurrent herpes simplex infections (cold sores)
Ribavirin	Virazole	Treatment of severe viral pneumonia caused by respiratory syncytial virus in infants and young children
Rimantadine	Flumadine	Prevention and treatment of influenza A infections
Valacyclovir	Valtrex	Treatment of initial and recurrent herpesvirus infections, including herpes simplex (genital herpes) and herpes zoster (shingles)
Vidarabine	Vira-A	Local (ophthalmic) administration for treatment of herpes simplex keratoconjunctivitis

*Drugs listed here are used to treat infections caused by viruses other than human immunodeficiency virus (HIV). Specific anti-HIV drugs are listed in Table 34–3.

TABLE 34–3 Agents Used to Inhibit Human Immunodeficiency Virus (HIV) Replication

Generic Name	Trade Name(s)
Nucleoside reverse transcriptase inhibitors (NRTIs)	
Abacavir	Ziagen
Didanosine	Videx
Lamivudine	Epivir
Stavudine	Zerit
Zalcitabine	HIVID
Zidovudine	Retrovir
Nonnucleoside reverse transcriptase inhibitors (NNRTIs)	
Delavirdine	Rescriptor
Efavirenz	Sustiva
Nevirapine	Viramune
Protease inhibitors	
Amprenavir	Agenerase
Indinavir	Crixivan
Nelfinavir	Viracept
Ritonavir	Norvir
Saquinavir	Fortovase, Invirase

Valacyclovir (Valtrex) is the precursor or "prodrug" of acyclovir.[68,69] When administered orally, valacyclovir is converted to acyclovir in the intestinal tract and liver. This conversion typically results in higher levels of acyclovir eventually appearing in the bloodstream, because valacyclovir is absorbed more readily from the gastrointestinal tract than acyclovir.[26] Thus, administration of valacyclovir is a more effective way to achieve the therapeutic effects of acyclovir when these drugs are administered orally.[69]

Mechanism of Action. Acyclovir inhibits viral DNA replication by inhibiting the function of the DNA polymerase enzyme.[20,43] This drug is taken into virus-infected cells and converted to acyclovir triphosphate by an enzyme known as viral thymidine kinase.[43] The phosphorylated drug directly inhibits the function of the viral DNA polymerase, thus impairing the replication of viral genetic material. The virus also incorporates the drug into viral DNA strands, thus halting further production of DNA because of the presence of a false nucleic acid.[20]

The antiviral specificity of acyclovir is due to the much higher affinity of this drug for viral DNA polymerase rather than the analogous enzyme in human cells.[43] Also, the first step in the phosphorylation of acyclovir is greatly accelerated in virus-infected cells versus healthy cells. Hence, the amount of the activated (phosphorylated) form of acyclovir is much greater in the cells that really need it—that is, cells infected with the virus.

Adverse Effects. Topical application of acyclovir may produce local irritation of cutaneous and mucosal tissues. Prolonged systemic administration of acyclovir or valacyclovir may cause headaches, dizziness, skin rashes, and gastrointestinal problems (nausea, vomiting, and diarrhea).

Amantadine and Rimantadine

Antiviral Efficacy and Clinical Use. Amantadine (Symmetrel) and rimantadine (Flumadine) are used in the prevention and treatment of infections caused by the influenza A virus.[42,54] When administered prophylactically, these drugs appear to be approximately 70 to 90 percent effective in preventing influenza A infections.[43] Also, these drugs usually decrease the severity and duration of flu symptoms in people infected with influenza A if drug therapy is initiated when symptoms first appear.[43] As discussed in Chapter 10, amantadine is also effective in alleviating some of the motor abnormalities of Parkinson disease. It is not exactly clear, however, why this antiviral agent is effective in treating parkinsonism.

Amantadine and rimantadine are administered to individuals already infected with influenza A to lessen the extent of the illness associated with this virus. These drugs are also given prophylactically to individuals who may have been exposed to influenza A and to high-risk patients such as the elderly or those with cardiopulmonary and other diseases. These drugs are typically administered orally, either in capsule form or in a syrup preparation.

Mechanism of Action. Amantadine and rimantadine appear to inhibit one of the early steps in influenza A replication by blocking the uncoating of the virus and preventing release of viral nucleic acid within the host cell.[43] These drugs may also interfere with assembly of viral components, thus inhibiting one of the final steps in the replication process.[43] This dual inhibitory effect on the early and late steps of viral replication accounts for the antiviral effectiveness of these drugs.

Adverse Effects. These drugs may produce CNS symptoms such as confusion, loss of concentration, mood changes, nervousness, dizziness, and light-headedness. These

symptoms may be especially problematic in elderly patients. Excessive doses of amantadine and rimantadine may increase the severity of these CNS symptoms, and overdose
may cause seizures.

Cidofovir

Antiviral Efficacy and Clinical Use. Cidofovir (Vistide) is used primarily to treat
CMV retinitis in people with AIDS.[45,72] When used clinically, this drug is often combined
with probenecid, an agent that inhibits renal excretion of cidofovir, thereby providing
higher plasma levels of this antiviral agent.

Mechanism of Action. Cidofovir works like acyclovir and ganciclovir; these drugs
inhibit viral DNA replication by inhibiting DNA polymerase activity and by halting
elongation of viral DNA chains.[19]

Adverse Effects. Cidofovir may cause nephrotoxicity, especially at higher doses.
This drug may also decrease the number of neutrophilic leukocytes, resulting in neutropenia and related symptoms such as fever, chills, and sore throat. Other bothersome
side effects include headache and gastrointestinal disturbances (anorexia, nausea, diarrhea).

Famciclovir and Penciclovir

Antiviral Efficacy and Clinical Use. Penciclovir (Denavir) is similar to acyclovir in
terms of antiviral effects and clinical indications. Penciclovir, however, is absorbed
poorly from the gastrointestinal tract. This drug is primarily administered topically to
treat recurrent herpes simplex infections of the lips and face (cold sores). Famciclovir
(Famvir) is the precursor (prodrug) to penciclovir, and famciclovir is converted to penciclovir following oral administration.[100] This situation is analogous to the relationship
between acyclovir and valacyclovir, where it is advantageous to administer the prodrug
because it will be absorbed much more completely and ultimately result in higher
plasma levels of the active form of the drug. Hence, famciclovir is administered orally
to treat infections related to herpes simplex (e.g., genital herpes) and varicella zoster
(e.g., herpes zoster).[28,90,100] However, the actual antiviral effects of famciclovir occur because this drug is converted to penciclovir within the body.

Mechanism of Action. Penciclovir acts like acyclovir (see earlier); that is, penciclovir is activated (phosphorylated) within virus-infected cells, where it subsequently
inhibits viral DNA synthesis and viral replication. As indicated, famciclovir exerts its antiviral effects after being converted to penciclovir in vivo.

Adverse Effects. Topical application of penciclovir may cause some skin reactions
(rashes, irritation) at the application site, but the incidence of these reactions is fairly low.
Systemic (oral) administration of famciclovir is generally tolerated well, with only minor side effects such as headache, dizziness, and gastrointestinal disturbances.

Foscarnet

Antiviral Efficacy and Clinical Use. Foscarnet (Foscavir) is primarily given to treat
cytomegalovirus (CMV) retinitis in patients with AIDS.[27,45] This agent may also help
control other infections in patients with a compromised immune system, including se-

rious cytomegaloviral infections (pneumonia, gastrointestinal infections) and some herpesvirus infections (herpes simplex, varicella-zoster).

Mechanism of Action. Foscarnet works somewhat like acyclovir and ganciclovir; that is, foscarnet inhibits the DNA polymerase enzyme necessary for viral DNA replication. Foscarnet differs from these other antiviral drugs, however, in that it does not require phosphorylation (activation) by enzymes such as viral thymidine kinase. Certain strains of viruses are thymidine-kinase deficient, meaning that these viruses lack the enzyme needed to activate antiviral agents such as acyclovir and ganciclovir. Hence, foscarnet is often used in patients who exhibit these thymidine-kinase–resistant viruses and do not respond to acyclovir or ganciclovir.

Adverse Effects. The primary problem associated with foscarnet is impaired renal function, including acute tubular necrosis. Hematologic disorders (anemia, granulocytopenia, leukopenia), gastrointestinal disturbances (cramps, nausea, vomiting), and CNS toxicity (confusion, dizziness) may also occur during foscarnet treatment.

Ganciclovir

Antiviral Efficacy and Clinical Use. Ganciclovir (Cytovene) is given primarily to patients with AIDS to treat problems related to CMV infection, including CMV retinitis, polyradiculopathy, and other systemic CMV infections.[45,51]

Mechanism of Action. Ganciclovir, like acyclovir, inhibits viral DNA replication by inhibiting DNA polymerase activity and by halting elongation of viral DNA chains.

Adverse Effects. The most serious problems associated with ganciclovir include anemia, granulocytopenia, thrombocytopenia, and related hematologic disorders. Ganciclovir may also cause gastrointestinal disturbances (anorexia, nausea) and CNS disturbances (mood changes, nervousness, tremor).

Protease Inhibitors

Antiviral Efficacy and Clinical Use. These drugs inhibit an enzyme known as HIV protease. This enzyme is needed for the manufacture of specific HIV proteins, including enzymes such as the HIV reverse transcriptase enzyme and structural proteins that comprise the HIV molecule.[75,84] By inhibiting this enzyme, protease inhibitors prevent the synthesis and maturation of HIV, thus helping to prevent HIV replication and progression of HIV-related disease.[35,87] The protease inhibitors currently available include amprenavir (Agenerase), indinavir (Crixivan), nelfinavir (Viracept), ritonavir (Norvir), and saquinavir (Fortovase, Invirase) (see Table 34–3). Use of these drugs in combination with other anti-HIV agents is discussed in more detail later in this chapter (see "HIV and the Treatment of AIDS").

Mechanism of Action. Protease inhibitors bind to the HIV protease and prevent this enzyme from acting on HIV substrates.[35,53] This effect negates the ability of the protease enzyme to cleave polypeptide precursors from larger, polypeptide chains.[75,84] If these precursors are not available for the manufacture of HIV proteins, the virus cannot fully develop.[87] Treatment with protease inhibitors therefore results in the manufacture of incomplete and noninfectious fragments of HIV rather than the mature virus.[75]

Adverse Effects. Protease inhibitors may cause alterations in fat deposition in the body (lipodystrophy); fat deposits atrophy in the limbs, but excess fat is deposited in the abdomen.[11,29] Blood lipids may also be adversely affected, resulting in increased plasma cholesterol, increased triglycerides, and decreased high-density lipoproteins.[70] These drugs may also cause other metabolic disturbances, including insulin resistance.[11,29] Other bothersome side effects include diarrhea, headache, and fatigue.[72,74,79]

Reverse Transcriptase Inhibitors

Antiviral Efficacy and Clinical Use. Reverse transcriptase inhibitors (RTIs) are used to inhibit the replication and proliferation of type I human immunodeficiency virus (HIV-1). These agents act on a specific enzyme (HIV reverse transcriptase; see the next section) and inhibit a key step in HIV replication. Although these drugs do not eliminate the virus from infected cells, they are often effective in reducing HIV proliferation and the spread of HIV to noninfected cells. These drugs are therefore beneficial in preventing or delaying the progression of HIV and AIDS. The use of RTIs in treating HIV infection is discussed in more detail later in this chapter.

Zidovudine (Retrovir), also known generically as azidothymidine or AZT, was the first RTI approved for treating people who are infected with HIV.[82] Other zidovudine-like drugs have also been developed, and currently available agents include abacavir (Ziagen), didanosine (Videx), lamivudine (Epivir), stavudine (Zerit), and zalcitabine (HIVID).[86] These RTIs can also be subclassified as nucleoside reverse transcriptase inhibitors (NRTIs) because they share a common chemical background (see Table 34–3).

More recently, RTIs that are chemically distinct from zidovudine and other NRTIs have also been developed (see Table 34–3). These agents are known as nonnucleoside reverse transcriptase inhibitors (NNRTIs), and this group includes drugs such as delavirdine (Rescriptor), efavirenz (Sustiva), and nevirapine (Viramune).[40,50] These drugs also inhibit the reverse transcriptase enzyme, but act at a different site on the enzyme than their NRTI counterparts.

Several types of RTIs are therefore available that can help prevent HIV replication and inhibit the proliferation and spread of this virus to noninfected cells. Although these drugs do not kill HIV, RTIs are the cornerstone of treatment for preventing the progression of HIV disease. Use of the various RTIs in combination with each other and with other anti-HIV drugs is discussed in more detail in "HIV and the Treatment of AIDS" later in this chapter.

Mechanism of Action. RTIs impair HIV replication by inhibiting the reverse transcriptase enzyme that is needed to convert viral RNA to viral DNA (Fig. 34–3). With regard to zidovudine and the other NRTIs, these agents enter viral-infected cells, where they are progressively phosphorylated (activated) by various intracellular enzymes.[43] The phosphorylated version of the drug then acts as a false nucleic acid that competes with the real nucleic acid (thymidine) for incorporation into growing viral DNA strands. This competition slows down the reverse transcriptase enzyme because the enzyme cannot handle the false nucleic acid (the drug) as easily as the real nucleic acid (thymidine). Even if the reverse transcriptase is successful in incorporating the drug into viral DNA strands, this action prematurely terminates DNA strand synthesis because a false nucleic acid has been added to the viral DNA instead of the real nucleic acid.

The newer agents (NNRTIs) such as delavirdine, efavirenz, and nevirapine directly inhibit the reverse trancriptase enzyme by binding to the active (catalytic) site on the enzyme and preventing this enzyme from converting viral RNA to viral DNA. Thus, these agents offer an alternative way to impair reverse transcriptase function and prevent viral replication.

Adverse Effects. RTIs are associated with a number of bothersome side effects, and certain agents can also cause potentially serious problems. The most common problems

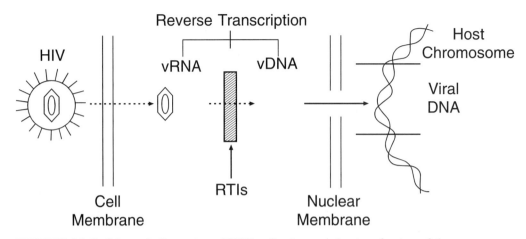

FIGURE 34–3. Schematic illustration of HIV replication and the site of action of the reverse transcriptase inhibitors (RTIs). These drugs interfere with the process of reverse transcription by inhibiting the enzyme that converts viral RNA (vRNA) to viral DNA (vDNA). See text for further discussion.

associated with zidovudine are blood dyscrasias, such as anemia and granulocytopenia. Other symptoms that may occur during zidovudine administration include fever, chills, nausea, diarrhea, dizziness, headache, and excessive fatigue. This drug may also cause myopathy, as indicated by skeletal muscle tenderness, weakness, and atrophy. Considering, however, that this drug is often used in severely immunocompromised patients (such as patients with AIDS), some adverse effects may be caused by other sequelae of AIDS rather than directly by the effects of this drug.

Peripheral neuropathies are fairly common with didanosine, lamivudine, stavudine, and zalcitabine, especially when higher doses are administered.[62,63] Blood dyscrasias such as anemia, leukopenia, and thrombocytopenia can also occur with these drugs, especially if hematologic function has already been impaired by HIV infection. Other effects associated with these NRTIs include pancreatitis, CNS toxicity (headache, irritability, insomnia), and gastrointestinal disturbances (nausea, diarrhea).

Abacavir can cause an allergic (hypersensitivity) reaction that produces symptoms such as fever, joint and muscle pain, skin rashes, abdominal pain, nausea, diarrhea, and vomiting.[83] In severe cases, this reaction can progress to anaphylactic shock and possibly death.

Skin rashes are the most common side effect of the NNRTIs, and efavirenz may also cause nervous system symptoms such as headache, dizziness, and insomnia.[2,40]

Ribavirin

Antiviral Efficacy and Clinical Use. Ribavirin (Virazole) is active against several RNA and DNA viruses, including respiratory syncytial virus (RSV).[43] Clinically, this drug is used to treat severe RSV pneumonia in infants and young children[6,76] and RSV in certain adult populations, including the elderly, people with cardiopulmonary problems, and people with a compromised immune system.[31] Ribavirin may also be useful as a secondary agent in the treatment of influenza A and B in young adults. The combination of ribavirin and interferons (see later) is often the treatment of choice in treating chronic hepatitis C infection.[7,21,59]

Ribavirin is administered through oral inhalation. This drug is suspended in an aerosol form and administered to the patient by a mechanical aerosol generator and a ventilation mask, mouthpiece, or hood.

Mechanism of Action. The mechanism of action of this drug is not fully understood. Ribavirin appears to impair viral messenger RNA synthesis, probably by selectively inhibiting enzymes responsible for RNA replication.[43] Inadequate viral mRNA production leads to impaired viral protein synthesis, which ultimately curtails viral replication.

Adverse Effects. Ribavirin produces relatively few adverse effects when administered by inhalation. Most of the drug's action is confined to local pulmonary tissues, and severe systemic effects are rare. One adverse effect that may occur is local irritation of the eyes (conjunctivitis) because of direct contact of the aerosol with the eyes. This occurrence may be a problem if the drug is administered via some sort of hood or tent that encloses the patient's entire head.

Vidarabine

Antiviral Efficacy and Clinical Use. Vidarabine (Vira-A) is effective against several members of the herpesvirus family, including CMV, herpes simplex virus, and varicella-zoster virus.[43] Clinically, this drug can be administered by continuous intravenous infusion to treat severe systemic infections caused by these viruses, but systemic use of vidarabine has been replaced somewhat by safer and more effective drugs, such as foscarnet. Vidarabine is currently used primarily to treat local viral infections of the eye (e.g., herpes simplex keratoconjunctivitis); it is applied topically by ophthalmic ointment to treat these infections.

Mechanism of Action. Vidarabine appears to exert its antiviral effects in a manner similar to acyclovir (see "Acyclovir"). Both drugs selectively inhibit viral enzymes that are responsible for viral DNA replication.[43]

Adverse Effects. The primary problems associated with systemic administration of vidarabine include gastrointestinal distress (nausea, vomiting, diarrhea) and CNS disturbances (dizziness, hallucinations, mood changes). Ophthalmic application may produce local irritation (itching, redness, swelling) in some individuals.

INTERFERONS

Interferons are a group of proteins that produce a number of beneficial pharmacologic and physiologic effects.[9,43] These agents were first recognized as endogenous substances that exert nonspecific antiviral activity; that is, interferons enable healthy cells to resist infection from a variety of viruses.[22] Interferons produce other beneficial effects, including controlling cell differentiation, limiting excessive cell proliferation, and modifying certain immune processes.[43]

There are three primary classes of human interferons: alpha, beta, and gamma (Table 34–4). Each primary interferon class is produced by certain cells and tissues. Of these three types, alpha and beta interferons are often grouped together as type I interferons, and these type I interferons seem more important in terms of antiviral activity.[88] Type II (gamma) interferons appear to be more important in regulating other aspects of the immune response and are responsible for promoting the growth of T lymphocytes.[43]

The possibility that interferons can be used as pharmacologic agents has aroused a great deal of interest. Recombinant DNA techniques and cell tissue cultures have been used

TABLE 34–4 Types of Interferons

Type and Subtype	Specific Agents*	Primary Indications
Type I		
Alpha	Alfacon-1 (Infergen)	Chronic hepatitis C
	Alfa-2a (Roferon-A)	Hairy cell leukemia; Kaposi sarcoma (AIDS related)
	Alfa-2b (Intron A)	Hairy cell leukemia; Kaposi sarcoma (AIDS related); chronic hepatitis B; condyloma acuminatum
	Alfa-n3 (Alferon N)	Condyloma acuminatum
Beta	Beta-1A (Avonex)	Multiple sclerosis
	Beta-1B (Betaseron)	Multiple sclerosis
Type II		
Gamma	Gamma-1b (Actimmune)	Chronic granulomatous disease

*Specific agents are synthesized using recombinant DNA techniques to mimic the effects of naturally occurring type I or type II interferons.

to produce sufficient quantities of interferons for clinical drug trials. The rationale is that exogenously administered interferons will produce antiviral and other beneficial effects in healthy cells in a manner similar to their endogenously produced counterparts. Some of the pertinent aspects of interferon action and clinical applications are presented here.

Synthesis and Cellular Effects of Interferons

The basic sequence of events in the cellular production and antiviral action of interferons is illustrated in Figure 34–4. Virtually all cells in the body are capable of producing interferons, and these substances serve as an early step in preventing the virus from infecting healthy cells.[22] As illustrated in Figure 34–4, cells that have been infected by a virus produce interferons that are subsequently released from the infected cell. These interferons then travel to noninfected cells, where they bind to specific receptors located on the surface of the healthy cells. Binding of the interferon induces the healthy cell to synthesize its own antiviral proteins. Interferons apparently direct the healthy cell to synthesize enzymes that inhibit viral messenger RNA and protein synthesis.[43] Thus, even if the virus does penetrate into the healthy cell, the virus cannot replicate because of an inability to synthesize viral proteins.

The manner in which interferons control cell growth and proliferation is not fully understood. Interferons may limit excessive cell division by controlling specific gene segments in normal and cancerous cells.[91] In particular, interferons may inhibit specific gene-regulatory segments of tumor cells known as *oncogenes*. Inhibition of the oncogenes would attenuate the excessive proliferation and lack of cell differentiation that typify neoplastic disease.[91] Interferons may also limit cancer growth by activating certain aspects of the immune system, including increased activity of natural killer cells and other cytotoxic cells that attack cancerous tissues.[91] Hence, interferons have proved effective in controlling several forms of cancer (see Table 34–4), and the use of these agents as anticancer drugs is discussed in more detail in Chapter 36.

Pharmacologic Applications of Interferons

When interferons were first discovered, there was a great deal of optimism about their use as antiviral agents. Although early clinical trials with interferons were some-

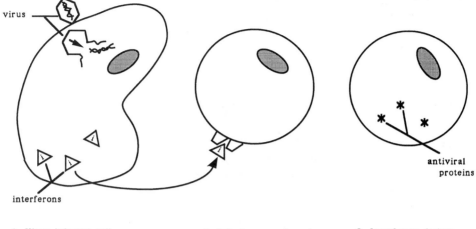

1. Virus infected cell produces interferons

2. Interferons released, bind to non-infected cells.

3. Interferons induce synthesis of new antiviral proteins in non-infected cell.

FIGURE 34–4. Antiviral effects of interferons.

what disappointing, their use as antiviral agents gained acceptance as more was learned about the three primary classes and subclasses of the interferons. We now realize that interferons cannot be used interchangeably as antiviral drugs, but that certain types of interferons can be administered to treat specific viruses (see Table 34–4). Currently, type I interferons (interferons alpha and beta) seem especially beneficial in treating hepatitis B and C infections.[10,89,101] These interferons can also be injected locally to treat certain forms of viral-induced warts such as condyloma acuminatum (see Table 34–4). The clinical use of interferons as antiviral drugs should continue to increase as more is learned about various interferon subclasses and other factors influencing their effectiveness.[43]

As mentioned, interferons also help control abnormal cell proliferation, and these drugs have been approved for use in certain cancers. Interferons are often used as part of the treatment for certain leukemias, lymphomas, and several other forms of cancer (see Table 34–4). Interferon use in cancer chemotherapy is discussed in more detail in Chapter 36.

Finally, certain interferons may decrease exacerbations of multiple sclerosis (MS).[15,38] Specifically, interferon beta-1a (Avonex) and interferon beta-1b (Betaseron) may help reduce the incidence and severity of relapses in exacerbating-remitting MS.[3,94] This effect seems to occur because these beta interferons prevent gamma interferons from participating in the autoimmune response that initiates the pathological changes associated with MS.[38]

Adverse Effects of Interferons

Interferons may cause flulike symptoms including fever, sweating, chills, muscle aches, and general malaise. Other side effects such as loss of appetite, nausea and vomiting, diarrhea, and unusual tiredness can also occur, depending on the type of interferon and the dosage. Interferons may also cause behavioral side effects such as depression, presumably because these drugs inhibit serotonin activity in the brain.[24,61] When interferons are administered by intramuscular or subcutaneous injection, some irritation may develop around the injection site. Finally, anti-interferon antibodies may be produced by the immune system, especially when interferons are administered for prolonged periods.[38] These antibodies can neutralize the interferons, thus decreasing their effectiveness in controlling viral infections and other conditions, such as cancer and MS.

CONTROL OF VIRAL INFECTION WITH VACCINES

Vaccines prevent viral infection by stimulating the endogenous production of immune factors that will selectively destroy the invading virus. Hence, the vaccine can be administered to healthy individuals to provide them with immunity from certain viral infections. Basically, a vaccine acts as an antigen that induces the immune system to generate virus-specific antibodies. The vaccine, however, does not cause any appreciable viral infection because the vaccine contains a virus that has been modified in some way so that it retains its antigenic properties but lacks the ability to produce infection. Vaccines, for example, typically consist of a whole virus or part of the virus (viral particle or fragment) that has been completely inactivated (killed vaccines) or partially inactivated (live attenuated vaccines).[8] Thus, most antiviral vaccinations are accomplished by administering small amounts of the modified virus.

In general, it is somewhat easier to develop vaccines that prevent viral infection than to develop drugs that destroy the virus once it has infected human cells. This notion is reasonable when one considers that the virus is essentially coexisting with the host cell. As indicated previously, there are currently only a limited number of drugs that are able to selectively inhibit the virus without harming the host cell. A more practical strategy is to use vaccines to enable the body to destroy the virus before an infection is established.

At present, vaccines are available for several serious viral infections including polio, smallpox, rabies, measles, mumps, rubella, hepatitis A and B, and influenza. In some situations, vaccination against certain viral infections is routine. For instance, school children must periodically show evidence of polio, measles, and other vaccinations according to state and local laws. In other cases, vaccines are administered prior to potential exposure to the virus or in high-risk groups. For example, influenza vaccinations are often administered to elderly and debilitated patients during seasonal influenza outbreaks.[8]

Although vaccines exist for many serious viral infections, some drawbacks still exist. Some vaccines are only partially effective, and viral infection still occurs in a significant percentage of vaccinated individuals. Other vaccines, especially killed vaccines, often require periodic readministration (boosters) to help maintain antiviral immunity. Also, certain types of viruses still lack an effective vaccination. For example, no vaccine is currently approved for the HIV that causes AIDS.[30,65] Hence, the improvement of existing vaccines and the development of new vaccines remain two of the more important aspects of antiviral chemotherapy.[85]

HIV AND THE TREATMENT OF AIDS

HIV is a member of the retrovirus family (see Table 34–1).[17,60] HIV selectively attacks certain cells in the immune system such as CD4[1] (T-helper) lymphocytes.[34,47] Destruction of immune system components often leads to the severe immunocompromised state known as AIDS. This virus exists in at least two forms: HIV-1 and HIV-2. Both forms of the virus are capable of causing AIDS, but HIV-1 is the more prevalent form of the virus.[34] Hence, HIV-1 is also referred to informally as the "AIDS virus." Because there is currently no effective way to kill the AIDS virus in humans, there is no cure for AIDS.

AIDS is a life-threatening disorder because of the susceptibility of the immuno-compromised patient to severe infections and certain forms of cancer.[4,14,16,44,55,93] In particular, patients with AIDS often suffer from severe viral infections (CMV, various herpesvirus infections), bacterial infections (*Mycobacterium tuberculosis*), protozoal infections (*Pneumocystis carinii* pneumonia), and infections caused by various other microbes and parasites. Patients with AIDS also develop relatively unusual neoplastic diseases, such as Kaposi sarcoma.

Considerable neuromuscular involvement also occurs in patients with AIDS.[99] Peripheral neuropathies, myopathies, and various CNS manifestations (dementia, other psychological manifestations) can occur directly from HIV infection or secondary to some other opportunistic infection.[58,80,98,99] Likewise, peripheral neuropathies are a common side effect of certain anti-HIV drugs (didanosine, zalcitabine), and myopathies are a side effect of zidovudine therapy. Patients with HIV disease often have painful symptoms such as joint pain, back pain, and pain related to neuropathies and myopathies.[67,81] Hence, HIV disease can often be regarded as a degenerative neuromuscular disorder from the standpoint of a rehabilitation professional. Therapists can help improve function and decrease pain in patients with HIV infection and AIDS.[1,37,97]

Individuals who are infected with HIV may remain totally asymptomatic for several years before developing the full-blown clinical picture of AIDS. Even people exposed to HIV who do not initially develop AIDS carry the virus for the rest of their lives and are thus capable of transmitting the virus to others. Transmission of HIV from one individual to another occurs primarily through intimate sexual contact and through sharing intravenous needles. Transfusions of blood from HIV-infected donors are also a potential source of HIV transmission. Hence, practices such as safe sex, not sharing needles, and improved blood-screening techniques are crucial in preventing the transmission of HIV and the subsequent risk of developing AIDS.

The treatment of patients with AIDS and individuals infected by HIV is continually being modified as new drugs become available and more information is gained about the nature of the AIDS virus. Currently, the pharmacologic management of HIV-infected patients consists of two principal strategies: (1) controlling the proliferation and effects of HIV in individuals infected with this virus and (2) treatment and prevention of various opportunistic infections that attempt to take advantage of the compromised immune system in patients with AIDS. The pharmacologic methods used to accomplish these principal strategies are presented here.

Inhibition of HIV Proliferation in Infected Individuals

No drugs currently are available that selectively kill HIV in humans, hence the lack of a cure for this viral infection. Nonetheless, several antiviral drugs are given to inhibit the replication of this virus, thus decreasing the morbidity and mortality of HIV infection. These drugs are usually specific for the HIV-1 form of this virus, because HIV-1 is the more prevalent type of virus found in people infected by HIV. Several pharmacologic strategies for treating HIV infection are currently available, and these strategies are discussed briefly here.

Zidovudine (Retrovir, AZT) was the first drug approved as an anti-HIV agent.[82] Other agents that act like zidovudine were subsequently approved to prevent HIV replication. These drugs include abacavir (Ziagen), didanosine (Videx, ddI), lamivudine (Epivir), stavudine (Zerit), and zalcitabine (HIVID, ddC) (see Table 34–3). As discussed in "Specific Antiviral Drugs," zidovudine and similar drugs are classified as nucleoside reverse transcriptase inhibitors (NRTIs) because they share a common mechanism of action that is illustrated in Figure 34–3; that is, these drugs inhibit the reverse transcriptase enzyme that HIV uses to synthesize viral DNA from viral RNA. This action impairs one of the early steps in viral replication, thus slowing the progression of HIV infection and the development of AIDS.

Protease inhibitors were the second major breakthrough in the pharmacologic treatment of HIV infection. Protease inhibitors are typically identified by generic names that contain an "-avir" suffix. Currently available protease inhibitors include amprenavir (Agenerase), indinavir (Crixivan), nelfinavir (Viracept), ritonavir (Norvir), and saquinavir (Fortovase, Invirase). As indicated earlier, these drugs impair the HIV protease enzyme that is responsible for several steps in HIV replication. Like the NRTIs, these drugs do not kill the virus but can slow its replication and prevent the spread of HIV to noninfected cells.

The third strategy developed to inhibit HIV replication is the nonnucleoside reverse transcriptase inhibitors (NNRTIs). These drugs include delavirdine (Rescriptor), efavirenz (Sustiva), and nevirapine (Viramune). Like their nucleoside counterparts, the NNRTIs also inhibit the ability of the reverse transcriptase enzyme to perform one of the initial steps in HIV replication. The NNRTIs, however, directly inhibit the active (catalytic) site on this enzyme, whereas zidovudine and other NRTIs serve as false substrates that take the place of the substance (thymidine) normally acted on by this enzyme (see "Reverse Transcriptase Inhibitors: Mechanism of Action"). Hence, the NNRTIs provide another way to impair one of the key steps in HIV replication, and these drugs can be used along with other agents (NRTIs, protease inhibitors) to provide optimal benefits in preventing HIV replication and proliferation (see the next section).

The arsenal of anti-HIV agents has grown steadily since the development of the first anti-HIV drug (zidovudine). In addition, other drugs and strategies that inhibit HIV infection continue to be explored.[43] As more is learned about the structure and function of this virus, drugs can be developed that impair specific steps in the absorption and replication of HIV in human cells. If clinical trials using these other drugs are favorable, they may also be approved for future use in individuals infected with HIV.

Anti-HIV Drug Combinations: Use of Highly Active Antiretroviral Therapy

Several anti-HIV drugs are often administered simultaneously to provide optimal inhibition of HIV replication and proliferation. This idea of combining several agents is referred to as highly active antiretroviral therapy, or HAART.[78] HAART often involves the simultaneous use of at least three anti-HIV agents.[49,56] A typical HAART strategy, for example, involves the use of two RTIs and one protease inhibitor.[73] There are, however, many variations of the specific drug combinations used during HAART. Other HAART regimens may, for instance, combine two protease inhibitors with two RTIs, or they may combine a nonnucleoside RTI with two nucleoside RTIs.[33] The exact number and type of drugs used during HAART are selected based on the specific needs of each patient.

Regardless of the exact drugs used, there is ample evidence that HAART can successfully delay the progression of HIV disease in people infected with this virus. In many cases, strict adherence to HAART regimens can reduce the viral load (that is, the amount of viral RNA present in the bloodstream) to levels that are undetectable with current testing procedures.[33] This fact does not mean that HAART has successfully eliminated the virus from the infected host or that the person infected with HIV has been cured. Even if HAART successfully reduces evidence of the virus in the plasma, the virus can be sequestered into T cells and other tissue "reservoirs" so that viral components cannot be detected in the bloodstream.[46,92] Still, HAART regimens can prevent the progression of HIV infection and help sustain immune function by allowing increases in the number of functioning CD4 lymphocytes.[18] The use of HAART is therefore associated with a substantial reduction in the incidence of AIDS and with improved clinical outcomes (fewer infections, decreased cancers, prolonged survival) in people who are infected with HIV.[4,18,23,49]

HAART regimens are, however, associated with several problems and limitations. A certain percentage of people with HIV do not respond adequately to HAART; that is, HAART may not be totally successful in producing a sustained and complete reduction in viral load in anywhere from 20 to 50 percent of individuals receiving these regimens.[73] Adherence to HAART can also be a problem because of the potential for side effects with these drugs and because of difficulties in remembering the complicated dosage regimens associated with taking three or more agents.[5,13,57] Resistance to anti-HIV drugs may develop,[66,71] especially if there is poor adherence to HAART regimens.[5,12,78] As mentioned earlier, HAART does not completely eliminate the virus from the infected host, because some of the viral components remain sequestered within tissues, where they remain hidden from the HAART drugs.[73]

Nonetheless, HAART can suppress HIV disease in many people who are infected with this virus. Drug combinations can be used successfully for the long-term management of HIV disease, and they offer hope that people with HIV do not have to progress inexorably toward AIDS and death. Research continues to find the best way to combine existing agents and to incorporate new agents into a comprehensive and successful regimen for people infected with HIV.

HIV Vaccines

An HIV vaccine has not yet been successfully developed and approved for use in the United States. As indicated earlier, vaccines are typically an altered form of the original virus that is administered to stimulate the immune system, so that the immune system can recognize and destroy the virus if a person is exposed to that virus. Creation of an HIV vaccine is understandably a complicated endeavor, given the complexity of this virus and the tendency for this virus to evolve and mutate into different types of HIV.[95] Nonetheless, the development of a safe, effective vaccine remains the best pharmacologic method for dealing with the spread of this virus, especially in underdeveloped nations that continue to experience a rise in the incidence of HIV and AIDS.[25,52]

Hence, efforts continue to develop an HIV vaccine that will produce adequate immunity from HIV infection without severe untoward side effects.[30,36] There is concern, however, than a successful vaccine may be very difficult to produce.[48,65] For example, development of an HIV vaccine that is not 100 percent effective might give recipients a false sense of security; that is, a vaccine that confers only partial immunity (e.g., a 50 to 75 percent reduction in the risk of contracting HIV) might encourage the recipient to forgo other precautions, such as safe sex, not sharing intravenous needles, and so forth. Likewise, the question arises about whether a single vaccine will be successful in providing immunity from all the various HIV strains and subtypes.[39,65] An HIV vaccine is urgently needed and would undoubtedly be received as one of the most important pharmacologic advancements of our time. The development of such a vaccine may be delayed, however, until we have a better understanding of HIV and how to best modify this virus into a successful vaccine.

We must therefore remember that zidovudine and other drugs currently available for treating HIV are not curative and may be helpful only in delaying or reducing AIDS-related deaths. A cure for AIDS, if at all possible, will take several years or even several decades before becoming a reality. As with many viruses, developing a vaccine against the AIDS virus is somewhat easier than making a drug that selectively destroys HIV. The development of an HIV vaccine, however, is probably still years away. Until a vaccine is developed, preventing transmission of HIV remains the best method of controlling the spread of AIDS.

Management of Opportunistic Infections

Because of a virtual lack of immunologic defenses, AIDS patients usually succumb to a variety of opportunistic infections.[34,47] Essentially, these patients simply do not have the ability to fight off various viral, bacterial, and other microbial invaders.[34] Consequently, much of the pharmacologic approach to the treatment of AIDS is associated with trying to curtail various infections by using the respective antimicrobial drugs that are currently available.

It is beyond the scope of this chapter to give a detailed description of the pharmacologic treatment of all the possible opportunistic infections that occur in patients with AIDS. Nonetheless, some of the more common types of opportunistic infections and the drugs commonly used to treat them are listed in Table 34–5. Because the patient essentially lacks an endogenous defense system, drug therapy must often be continued indefinitely, or the infection will recur. Also, early recognition of infectious symptoms is crucial in helping initiate drug therapy before the infection becomes uncontrollable.[34] Strategies for dealing with various infections are constantly changing, however, and drug therapy for these opportunistic infections will surely be modified as new antimicrobial agents are developed and new evidence is provided about how these agents can be used in various infections.

RELEVANCE OF ANTIVIRAL CHEMOTHERAPY IN REHABILITATION PATIENTS

The major significance of antiviral drugs to rehabilitation specialists and other health-care professionals is the potential for controlling or eliminating infectious disease at present and in the future. As indicated in this chapter, only a few drugs can really effectively resolve viral infections in humans at the present time. Nonetheless, the development of new antiviral agents and the improved use of existing compounds such as the interferons are exciting and important areas of pharmacology. Also, viral prophylaxis through vaccination has virtually eliminated some types of serious infections, and the possibility of new and improved antiviral vaccines may enhance the health and welfare of patients throughout the world.

TABLE 34–5 Treatment of Common Opportunistic Infections in Patients with AIDS

Organism	Type of Infection	Drug Treatment*
Viral infections		
Cytomegalovirus	Pneumonia; hepatitis; chorioretinitis; involvement of many other organs	Foscarnet or ganciclovir
Herpes simplex	Unusually severe vesicular and necrotizing lesions of mucocutaneous areas (mouth, pharynx) and GI tract	Acyclovir, famciclovir, or valacyclovir
Varicella-zoster	Painful, vesicular eruption of skin according to dermatomal boundaries (shingles)	Acyclovir, famciclovir, or valacyclovir
Bacterial infections		
Mycobacterium avium complex	Involvement of bone marrow, reticuloendothelial tissues	Clarithromycin plus ethambutol; rifabutin
Mycobacterium tuberculosis	Tuberculosis	Isoniazid plus pyridoxine; rifampin (if isoniazid resistant)
Salmonella	Enterocolitis and bacteremia	Ciprofloxacin or trimethoprim
Fungal infections		
Candida	Inflammatory lesions in oropharyngeal region and esophagus	Oral infections: clotrimazole, fluconazole, or nystatin; Esophageal infections: fluconazole or ketoconazole
Coccidioides	Primarily affects lungs but may disseminate to other tissues	Amphotericin B
Cryptococcus	Meningoencephalitis	Amphotericin B ± flucytosine, followed by fluconazole
Histoplasma capsulatum	Affects various tissues including lungs, lymphatics, and mucocutaneous tissues; also causes blood dyscrasias (anemias, leukopenia)	Amphotericin B or itraconazole
Protozoal infections		
Pneumocystis carinii	Pneumonia	Trimethoprim-sulfamethoxazole, pentamidine, or atovaquone
Toxoplasma	CNS infections (cerebral degeneration, meningoencephalitis)	Pyrimethamine plus sulfadiazine

*Choice of specific drugs varies according to disease status, presence of other infections, and so forth. Pharmacotherapeutic rationale is also changing constantly as new agents are developed and tested.

Consequently, physical therapists and occupational therapists should keep abreast of advances in treating and preventing viral infections. This notion is especially true for the AIDS crisis, which promises to be a major health issue for some time. By keeping informed of current developments in antiviral pharmacology, health-care professionals will enrich their own knowledge while serving as a reliable source of information for their patients.

CASE STUDY

ANTIVIRAL DRUGS

Brief History. R.K. is a 28-year-old man who was infected with HIV after sharing hypodermic syringes with a fellow drug abuser. He began a pharmacologic regimen of highly active antiretroviral therapy, consisting of two reverse transcriptase inhibitors (zidovudine [Retrovir], 600 mg/d and didanosine [Videx], 400 mg/d) and one protease inhibitor (indinavir [Crixivan], 2400 mg/d). This regimen was initially successful in controlling HIV replication and proliferation, but the patient began to lapse into periods of noncompliance and frequently failed to take his medications according to the proper dosing schedule. Hence, HIV proliferated and suppressed immune function to the point where he was considered to have developed AIDs. Recently, he developed a fever and respiratory infection due to *Pneumocystis carinii* pneumonia. He was admitted to the hospital and treated with a combination of pentamidine and trimethoprim-sulfamethoxazole. The patient also exhibited muscular weakness and began to develop burning pain in both lower extremities. The weakness and pain were attributed to radiculopathy caused by infection of peripheral nerves by HIV or by some other opportunistic infection. The physical therapy department was consulted to determine what could be done to alleviate the neuropathic pain and dysfunction.

Decision/Solution. The therapist initiated a program of transcutaneous electrical nerve stimulation (TENS) along the affected nerve pathways. The patient was instructed in the use of the TENS unit, and intensity and other stimulation parameters were adjusted to tolerance by the patient. The therapist also found that cold neon laser treatment helped decrease pain and increase function along the more severely affected nerves, and daily laser treatments were instituted. The combined use of TENS and laser helped decrease pain in this viral-related disorder, thus improving the patient's well-being without the use of additional pharmacologic agents (pain medications). Progressive involvement of other peripheral neurons occurred over the course of the next few weeks, however, and the patient eventually died of respiratory failure.

SUMMARY

Viruses present a unique problem in terms of the pharmacologic treatment of infectious disease. These microorganisms rely totally on the metabolic function of host (human) cells to function and replicate more viruses. Hence, there are currently only a limited number of effective antiviral agents that selectively kill or attenuate the virus without seriously harming the human cells. Developing and administering antiviral vaccines that stimulate the immunity of the host to specific viral infections is often more practical. In the future, the development of new antiviral agents and vaccines may help treat and eliminate viral infections that currently pose a serious health threat.

REFERENCES

1. Abbaticola, MM: A team approach to the treatment of AIDS wasting. J Assoc Nurses AIDS Care 11:45, 2000.
2. Adkins, JC and Noble, S: Efavirenz. Drugs 56:1055, 1998.
3. Arnason, BG: Treatment of multiple sclerosis with interferon beta. Biomed Pharmacother 53:344, 1999.
4. Ashley, EA, Johnson, MA, and Lipman, MC: Human immunodeficiency virus and respiratory infection. Curr Opin Pulm Med 6:240, 2000.
5. Back, DJ: Pharmacological issues relating to viral resistance. Infection 27(Suppl 2):S42, 1999.
6. Baker, KA and Ryan, ME: RSV infection in infants and young children. What's new in diagnosis, treatment, and prevention? Postgrad Med 106:97, 1999.
7. Battaglia, AM and Hagmeyer, KO: Combination therapy with interferon and ribavirin in the treatment of chronic hepatitis C infection. Ann Pharmacother 34:487, 2000.

8. Bertino, JS and Casto, DT: Vaccines, toxoids, and other immunobiologics. In DiPiro, JT, et al (eds): Pharmacotherapy: A Pathophysiologic Approach, ed 4. Appleton & Lange, Stamford, CT, 1999.
9. Bogdan, C: The function of type I interferons in antimicrobial immunity. Curr Opin Immunol 12:419, 2000.
10. Bonkovsky, HL and Woolley, JM: Outcomes research in chronic viral hepatitis C: effects of interferon therapy. Can J Gastroenterol 14(Suppl B):21B, 2000.
11. Carr, A: HIV protease inhibitor-related lipodystrophy syndrome. Clin Infect Dis 30(Suppl 2):S135, 2000.
12. Chesney, MA, et al: Adherence: A necessity for successful HIV combination therapy. AIDS 13(Suppl A):S271, 1999.
13. Chesney, MA, Morin, M, and Sherr, L: Adherence to HIV combination therapy. Soc Sci Med 50:1599, 2000.
14. Cheung, TW and Teich, SA: Cytomegalovirus infection in patients with HIV infection. Mt Sinai J Med 66:113, 1999.
15. Chofflon, M: Recombinant human interferon beta in relapsing-remitting multiple sclerosis: A review of the major clinical trials. Eur J Neurol 7:369, 2000.
16. Clifford, DB: Opportunistic viral infections in the setting of human immunodeficiency virus. Semin Neurol 19:185, 1999.
17. Coffin, KM: Retroviridae: The viruses and their replication. In Fields, BN, Knipe, DM, and Howley, PM (eds): Fundamental Virology, ed 3. Lippincott-Raven, Philadelphia, 1996.
18. Cooper, DA: Immunological effects of antiretroviral therapy. Antivir Ther 3(Suppl 4):19, 1998.
19. Cundy, KC: Clinical pharmacokinetics of the antiviral nucleotide analogues cidofovir and adefovir. Clin Pharmacokinet 36:127, 1999.
20. Darby, G: The acyclovir legacy: Its contribution to antiviral drug discovery. J Med Virol 1(Suppl):134, 1993.
21. Davis, GL: Current therapy for chronic hepatitis C. Gastroenterology 118(Suppl 1):S104, 2000.
22. De Maeyer, E and De Maeyer-Guignard, J: Type I interferons. Int Rev Immunol 17:53, 1998.
23. Dezube, BJ: Acquired immunodeficiency syndrome-related Kaposi's sarcoma: Clinical features, staging, and treatment. Semin Oncol 27:424, 2000.
24. Dierperink, E, Willenbring, M, and Ho, SB: Neuropsychiatric symptoms associated with hepatitis C and interferon alpha: A review. Am J Psychiatry 157:867, 2000.
25. D'Souza, MP, Cairns, JS, and Plaeger, SF: Current evidence and future directions for targeting HIV entry: Therapeutic and prophylactic strategies. JAMA 284:215, 2000.
26. Emmert, DH: Treatment of common cutaneous herpes simplex virus infections. Am Fam Physician 61:1697, 2000.
27. Eong, KG, Beatty, S, and Charles, SJ: Cytomegalovirus retinitis in patients with acquired immune deficiency syndrome. Postgrad Med J 75:585, 1999.
28. Erlich, KS: Management of herpes simplex and varicella-zoster virus infections. West J Med 166:211, 1997.
29. Eron, JJ: HIV-1 protease inhibitors. Clin Infect Dis 30(Suppl 2):S160, 2000.
30. Esparza, J and Bhamarapravati, N: Accelerating the development and future availability of HIV-1 vaccines: Why, when, where, and how? Lancet 355:2061, 2000.
31. Falsey, AR and Walsh, EE: Respiratory syncytial virus infection in adults. Clin Microbiol Rev 13:371, 2000.
32. Fields, BN: Biology of viruses. In Schaechter, M, et al (eds): Mechanisms of Microbial Disease, ed 3. Lippincott Williams & Wilkins, Philadelphia, 1999.
33. Fischl, MA: Antiretroviral therapy in 1999 for antiretroviral-naive individuals with HIV infection. AIDS 13(Suppl 1):S49, 1999.
34. Fletcher, CV: Human immunodeficiency virus infection. In DiPiro, JT, et al (eds): Pharmacotherapy: A Pathophysiologic Approach, ed 4. Appleton & Lange, Stamford, CT, 1999.
35. Flexner, C: Dual protease inhibitor therapy in HIV-infected patients: Pharmacologic rationale and clinical benefits. Annu Rev Pharmacol Toxicol 40:649, 2000.
36. Frey, SE: HIV vaccines. Infect Dis Clin North Am 13:95, 1999.
37. Galantino, ML, et al: Physical therapy management for the patient with HIV. Lower extremity challenges. Clin Podiatr Med Surg 15:329, 1998.
38. Gidal, BE, Fleming, JO, and Dalmady-Israel, C: Multiple sclerosis. In DiPiro, JT, et al (eds): Pharmacotherapy: A Pathophysiologic Approach, ed 4. Appleton & Lange, Stamford, CT, 1999.
39. Girard, M, Habel, A, and Chanel, C: New prospects for the development of a vaccine against human immunodeficiency virus type 1. An overview. C R Acad Sci III 322:959, 1999.
40. Harris, M and Montaner, JS: Clinical uses of non-nucleoside reverse transcriptase inhibitors. Rev Med Virol 10:217, 2000.
41. Harrison, S, Skehel, JJ, and Wiley, DC: Principles of viral structure. In Fields, BN, Knipe, DM, and Howley, PM (eds): Fundamental Virology, ed 3. Lippincott-Raven, Philadelphia, 1996.
42. Hayden, FG: Prevention and treatment of influenza in immunocompromised patients. Am J Med 102(Suppl 3A):55, 1997.
43. Hayden, FG: Antiviral agents. In Hardman, JB, et al (eds): The Pharmacological Basis of Therapeutics, ed 9. McGraw-Hill, New York, 1996.
44. Hermans, P: Opportunistic AIDS-associated malignancies in HIV-infected patients. Biomed Pharmacother 54:32, 2000.
45. Holland, GN: New strategies for the management of AIDS-related CMV retinitis in the era of potent antiretroviral therapy. Ocul Immunol Inflamm 7:179, 1999.
46. Isada, CM and Calabrese, LH: AIDS update 1999: Viral reservoirs and immune-based therapies. Cleve Clin J Med 66:267, 1999.

47. Johnson, KJ, Chensue, SW, and Ward, PA: Immunopathology. In Rubin, E and Farber, JL (eds): Pathology, ed 3. Lippincott-Raven, Philadelphia, 1999.
48. Joy, AK, Dale, CJ, and Kent, SJ: Can HIV be prevented with a vaccine? Drugs RD 1:431, 1999.
49. Kak, V, MacArthur, RD, and Crane, LR: Treatment of HIV disease in the new millenium. Semin Thorac Cardiovasc Surg 12:140, 2000.
50. Katlama, C: Review of NNRTIs: Today and tomorrow. Int J Clin Pract Suppl 103:16, 1999.
51. Keating, MR: Antiviral agents for non-human immunodeficiency virus infections. Mayo Clin Proc 74:1266, 1999.
52. Klein, M: AIDS and HIV vaccines. Vaccine 17(Suppl 2):S65, 1999.
53. Lebon, F and Ledecq, M: Approaches to the design of effective HIV-1 protease inhibitors. Curr Med Chem 7:455, 2000.
54. Long, JK, Mossad, SB, and Goldman, MP: Antiviral agents for treating influenza. Cleve Clin J Med 67:92, 2000.
55. Marra, CM: Bacterial and fungal brain infections in AIDS. Semin Neurol 19:177, 1999.
56. Matsushita, S: Current status and future issues in the treatment of HIV-1 infection. Int J Hematol 72:20, 2000.
57. Max, B and Sherer, R: Management of the adverse effects of antiretroviral therapy and medication adherence. Clin Infect Dis 30(Suppl 2):S96, 2000.
58. McArthur, JC, Sacktor, N, and Selnes, O: Human immunodeficiency virus-associated dementia. Semin Neurol 19:129, 1999.
59. McHutchison, JG and Younossi, Z: Treatment strategies for hepatitis C: Making the best of limited options. Cleve Clin J Med 67:476, 2000.
60. Meissner, C and Coffin, JM: The human retroviruses: AIDS and other diseases. In Schaechter, M, et al (eds): Microbial Disease, ed 3. Lippincott Williams & Wilkins, Philadelphia, 1999.
61. Menkes, DB and MacDonald, JA: Interferons, serotonin, and neurotoxicity. Psychol Med 30:259, 2000.
62. Moyle, GJ and Gazzard, BG: Finding a role for zalcitabine in the HAART era. Antivir Ther 3:125, 1998.
63. Moyle, GJ and Sadler, M: Peripheral neuropathy with nucleoside antiretrovirals: Risk factors, incidence, and management. Drug Saf 19:481, 1998.
64. Murphy, FA: Virus taxonomy. In Fields, BN, Knipe, DM, and Howley, PM (eds): Fundamental Virology, ed 3. Lippincott-Raven, Philadelphia, 1996.
65. Nathanson, N and Mathieson, BJ: Biological considerations in the development of a human immunodeficiency virus vaccine. J Infect Dis 182:579, 2000.
66. O'Brien, WA: Resistance against reverse transcriptase inhibitors. Clin Infect Dis 30(Suppl 2):S185, 2000.
67. O'Neill, WM and Sherrard, JS: Pain in human immunodeficiency disease: A review. Pain 54:3, 1993.
68. Ormod, D and Goa, K: Valaciclovir: A review of its use in the management of herpes zoster. Drugs 59:1317, 2000.
69. Ormod, D, Scott, LJ, and Perry, CM: Valaciclovir: A review of its long term utility in the management of genital herpes simplex virus and cytomegalovirus infections. Drugs 59:839, 2000.
70. Penzak, SR and Chuck, SK: Hyperlipidemia associated with HIV protease inhibitor use: Pathophysiology, prevalence, risk factors, and treatment. Scan J Infect Dis 32:111, 2000.
71. Pillay, D, Taylor, S, and Richman, DD: Incidence and impact of resistance against approved antiviral drugs. Rev Med Virol 10:231, 2000.
72. Plosker, GL and Noble, S: Cidofovir: A review of its use in cytomegalovirus retinitis in patients with AIDS. Drugs 58:325, 1999.
73. Powderly, WG: Current approaches to treatment for HIV-1 infection. J Neurovirol 6(Suppl 1):S8, 2000.
74. Powderly, WG and Tebas, P: Nelfinavir, a new protease inhibitor: Early clinical results. AIDS 13(Suppl 1):S41, 1999.
75. Rana, KZ and Dudley, MN: Human immunodeficiency virus protease inhibitors. Pharmacotherapy 19:35, 1999.
76. Rodriguez, WJ: Management strategies for respiratory syncytial virus infections in infants. J Pediatr 135(Part 2):45, 1999.
77. Samuelson, J: Infectious diseases. In Cotran, RS, Kumar, V, and Collins, T (eds): The Pathologic Basis of Disease, ed 6. WB Saunders, Philadelphia, 1999.
78. Shafer, RW and Vuitton, DA: Highly active antiretroviral therapy (HAART) for the treatment of infections with human immunodeficiency virus type 1. Biomed Pharmacother 53:73, 1999.
79. Sherman, DS and Fish, DN: Management of protease inhibitor-associated diarrhea. Clin Infect Dis 30:908, 2000.
80. Simpson, DM: Human immunodeficiency virus-associated dementia: Review of pathogenesis, prophylaxis, and treatment studies of zidovudine therapy. Clin Infect Dis 29:19, 1999.
81. Singer, EJ, et al: Painful symptoms reported by ambulatory HIV-infected men in a longitudinal study. Pain 54:15, 1993.
82. Sperling, R: Zidovudine. Infect Dis Obstet Gynecol 6:197, 1998.
83. Staszewski, S: Coming therapies: Abacavir. Int J Clin Pract Suppl 103:35, 1999.
84. Swanstrom, R and Erona, J: Human immunodeficiency virus type-1 protease inhibitors: Therapeutic successes and failures, suppression and resistance. Pharmacol Ther 86:145, 2000.
85. Talwar, GP, et al: The impact of new technologies on vaccines. Natl Med J India 12:274, 1999.

86. Temesgen, Z and Wright, AJ: Antiretrovirals. Mayo Clin Proc 74:1284, 1999.
87. Tomasselli, AG and Heinrikson, RL: Targeting the HIV-protease in AIDS therapy: A current clinical perspective. Biochem Biophys Acta 1477:189, 2000.
88. Tompkins, WA: Immunomodulation and therapeutic effects of the oral use of interferon-alpha: Mechanism of action. J Interferon Cytokine Res 19:817, 1999.
89. Torresi, J and Locarnini, S: Antiviral chemotherapy for the treatment of hepatitis B virus infection. Gastroenterology 118(Suppl 1):S83, 2000.
90. Tyring, SK: Advances in the treatment of herpesvirus infection: The role of famciclovir. Clin Ther 20:661, 1998.
91. Valley, AW and Balmer, CM: Cancer treatment and chemotherapy. In DiPiro, JT, et al (eds): Pharmacotherapy: A Pathophysiologic Approach, ed 4. Appleton & Lange, Stamford, CT, 1999.
92. Volberding, PA: Advances in the medical management of patients with HIV-1 infection: An overview. AIDS 13(Suppl 1):S1, 1999.
93. Wakefield, AE, et al: Genetics, metabolism and host specificity of *Pneumocystis carinii*. Med Mycol 36(Suppl 1):183, 1998.
94. Weinstock-Guttman, B and Jacobs, LD: What is new in the treatment of multiple sclerosis? Drugs 59:401, 2000.
95. Weiss, RA: Getting to know HIV. Trop Med Int Health 5:A10, 2000.
96. Whitley, RJ and Gnann, JW: Drug therapy: Acyclovir—A decade later. N Engl J Med 327:782, 1992.
97. Williams, B, Waters, D, and Parker, K: Evaluation and treatment of weight loss in adults with HIV disease. Am Fam Physician 60:843, 1999.
98. Wulff, EA and Simpson, DM: Neuromuscular complications of the human immunodeficiency virus type 1 infection. Semin Neurol 19:157, 1999.
99. Wulff, EA, Wang, AK, and Simpson, DM: HIV-associated peripheral neuropathy: Epidemiology, pathophysiology, and treatment. Drugs 59:1251, 2000.
100. Wutzler, P: Antiviral therapy for herpes simplex and varicella-zoster virus infections. Intervirology 40:343, 1997.
101. Zein, NN: Interferons in the management of viral hepatitis. Cytokines Cell Mol Ther 4:229, 1998.

CHAPTER 35

Treatment of Infections III: Antifungal and Antiparasitic Drugs

In additional to bacteria and viruses, several parasitic microorganisms may produce infections in humans. In particular, certain species of fungi, protozoa, and helminths (worms) frequently cause infections in humans. Although some types of parasitic infections are limited or unknown in developed nations such as the United States, parasitic infections generally represent the most common form of disease worldwide. These infections are especially prevalent in tropical and subtropical environments and in impoverished areas of the world where sanitation and hygiene are inadequate. Also, the incidence of serious fungal and other parasitic infections has been increasing even in industrialized nations because of the increased susceptibility of immunocompromised patients, such as patients with AIDS, to these infections.[1,15,26] Hence, effective pharmacologic treatment of these infections remains one of the most important topics in the global management of disease.

The pharmacologic treatment of parasitic infections is a fairly complex and extensive topic. In a limited space, it is difficult to describe the many species of each parasite, all the diseases caused by these parasites, and the chemical methods currently available to selectively destroy various fungi, protozoa, and helminths in humans. Consequently, the general aspects of each type of parasitic infection are reviewed briefly, followed by the primary drugs used to treat specific fungal, protozoal, and helminthic infections. This discussion will acquaint physical therapists and occupational therapists with the nature of these types of infections and the basic chemotherapeutic techniques and agents that are used to treat these problems.

ANTIFUNGAL AGENTS

Fungi are plantlike microorganisms that exist ubiquitously throughout the soil and air and in plants and animals. Although abundant in nature (about 100,000 species exist), only a few species produce infections in humans.[9,18,32] A disease caused by fungal

590

infection is also referred to as a *mycosis*. Some fungal infections are relatively local or superficial, affecting cutaneous and mucocutaneous tissue. Examples of common superficial fungal infections include the tinea (ringworm) infections that cause problems such as athlete's foot. Common mucocutaneous fungal infections include candidiasis and yeast infections of vaginal tissues. Other fungal infections are deeper or more systemic. For instance, fungal infections may affect the lungs, CNS, or other tissues and organs throughout the body.[9]

Often, fungal infections are relatively innocuous because they can be destroyed by the body's normal immune defense mechanisms. Some infections require pharmacologic treatment, especially if the patient's endogenous defense mechanisms are compromised in some way. For instance, individuals undergoing immunosuppressive drug treatment with glucocorticoids or certain antibiotics may develop systemic fungal infections. Also, diseases that attack the immune system, such as AIDS, leave the patient vulnerable to severe fungal infections (see Chap. 34). Fungal infections that are relatively easy to treat in the immunocompetent person may become invasive and life-threatening in those who lack adequate immune function. Hence, there is currently a significant need for effective systemic antifungal agents in certain high-risk patients.

Agents used to treat common fungal infections are listed in Tables 35–1 and 35–2. As indicated in Table 35–1, certain drugs can be administered systemically to treat infections in various tissues. Other agents are more toxic, and their use is limited to local or topical application for fungal infections in the skin and mucous membranes (Table 35–2). The use of systemic and topical antifungal agents is addressed in more detail below.

Systemic Antifungal Agents

Listed here are the antifungal agents that can be administered systemically by oral or intravenous routes. These agents are often used to treat invasive (deep) fungal infec-

TABLE 35–1 Use of Systemic Antifungal Agents in Invasive and Disseminated Mycoses*

Type of Infection	Principal Sites of Infection	Principal Agent(s)	Alternative/ Secondary Agent(s)
Aspergillosis	Lungs, other organs, body orifices	Amphotericin B	Itraconazole
Blastomycosis	Lungs, skin; may disseminate to other tissues	Amphotericin B	Itraconazole, ketoconazole
Candidiasis	Intestinal tract, skin, mucous membranes (mouth, pharynx, vagina)	Amphotericin B, fluconazole	Flucytosine, itraconazole, ketoconazole
Coccidioidomycosis	Lungs, skin, subcutaneous tissues; may form disseminated lesions throughout the body	Amphotericin B	Flucytosine, itraconazole, ketoconazole
Cryptococcosis	Lungs, meninges, other tissues	Amphotericin B, fluconazole	Flucytosine, itraconazole
Histoplasmosis	Lungs, spleen	Amphotericin B, itraconazole	Ketoconazole
Tinea (ringworm) infections	Skin, subcutaneous tissues	Griseofulvin	Itraconazole, terbinafine

*Drugs indicated here are administered systemically (orally, intravenously) to treat widespread or invasive fungal infections. Some of these agents are also available in topical preparations, especially in the treatment of candidiasis and tinea infections in the skin and mucocutaneous tissues (see text).

TABLE 35–2 Topical Antifungals

Generic Name	Trade Name	Type of Preparation	Primary Indication(s)
Azoles			
Butoconazole	Femstat 3	Vaginal cream; vaginal suppositories	Vulvovaginal candidiasis
Clotrimazole	Gyne-Lotrimin, Fem Care, others	Vaginal cream; vaginal tablets	Vulvovaginal candidiasis
	Mycelex Troches	Lozenges	Oropharyngeal candidiasis
	Mycelex Creme, Lotrimin, others	Cream; lotion; solution	Cutaneous candidiasis, tinea (ringworm) infections
Econazole	Spectazole	Cream	Cutaneous candidiasis, tinea (ringworm) infections
Miconazole	Femizol-M, Monistat, others	Vaginal cream; vaginal suppositories; vaginal tampons	Vulvovaginal candidiasis
Oxiconazole	Oxistat	Cream; lotion	Tinea (ringworm) infections
Sulconazole	Exelderm	Cream; solution	Tinea (ringworm) infections
Terconazole	Terazol	Vaginal cream; vaginal suppositories	Vulvovaginal candidiasis
Tioconazole	Monistat 1, Vagistat-1	Vaginal ointment; vaginal suppositories	Vulvovaginal candidiasis
Other Topical Agents			
Naftifine	Naftin	Cream; gel	Tinea (ringworm) infections
Nystatin	Mycostatin, Nilstat, others	Lozenges; oral suspension; tablets	Oropharyngeal candidiasis
	Mycostatin; Nilstat; Nystex	Cream; ointment; powder	Cutaneous and mucocutaneous candidiasis
	Generic	Vaginal cream; vaginal tablets	Vulvovaginal candidiasis
Tolnaftate	Aftate, Tinactin, many others	Aerosol powder; aerosol solution; powder; solution	Tinea (ringworm) infections

*Drugs listed here are available only in topical or local preparations. Certain systemic agents listed in Table 35–1 can also be applied locally to treat various superficial fungal infections.

tions in the body, or they can be administered systemically to treat more superficial infections that are disseminated over a fairly large area of the skin or subcutaneous tissues. The clinical use, mechanism of action, and potential adverse effects of these drugs are addressed here.

AMPHOTERICIN B

Clinical Use. Amphotericin B (Amphocin, Fungizone Intravenous) is one of the primary drugs used to treat severe systemic fungal infections.[22,35] This drug is often chosen to treat systemic infections and meningitis caused by *Candida, Cryptococcus*, and several other species of pathogenic fungi (see Table 35–1). Typically, this drug is administered by slow intravenous infusion. Local and topical administration may also be used to treat more limited infections caused by susceptible fungi.

Several newer forms of amphotericin B (Abelcet, AmBisome, Amphotec) have also been developed. Here the drug is encapsulated in small lipid spheres (liposomes) and then injected slowly by intravenous infusion.[30,35] These lipid-based preparations appear to deliver higher doses of amphotericin B more directly to the site of fungal infections, thereby reducing the risk of adverse effects such as renal toxicity.[5,13,30] Further research should help clarify the optimal way that these lipid forms can be used to treat serious fungal infections while reducing the risk of nephrotoxicity and other side effects.[11]

Mechanism of Action. Amphotericin B appears to work by binding to specific steroidlike lipids (sterols) located in the cell membrane of susceptible fungi.[10] This binding causes increased permeability in the cell membrane, leading to a leaky membrane and loss of cellular components.

Adverse Effects. The effectiveness of amphotericin B against serious systemic fungal infections is tempered somewhat by a high incidence of side effects.[35] Most patients experience problems such as headache, fever, muscle and joint pain, muscle weakness, and gastrointestinal distress (nausea, vomiting, and stomach pain or cramping). As indicated, nephrotoxicity may also occur in some patients, but use of the lipid-based formulations of this drug may reduce the risk of this adverse effect. Considering the life-threatening nature of some fungal infections such as meningitis, certain side effects of amphotericin B must often be tolerated while the drug exerts its antifungal actions.

FLUCONAZOLE

Clinical Use. Fluconazole (Diflucan) can be administered orally to treat serious systemic fungal infections.[17] This drug is often the primary treatment for urinary tract infections, pneumonia, and infections of the mouth and esophagus caused by the *Candida* species of fungus.[5] This agent may also be used to treat cryptococcal meningitis and may help prevent recurrence of cryptococcal infections in patients with AIDS. Because this drug is somewhat less toxic than more traditional agents such as amphotericin B, fluconazole has emerged as the drug of choice in treating many fungal infections that were previously treated with other drugs.[6,11,34] Fluconazole can be administered orally, which is also an advantage over amphotericin B.

Mechanism of Action. Fluconazole and similar drugs (itraconazole, ketoconazole) inhibit certain enzymes in fungal cells that are responsible for the synthesis of important steroidlike compounds (sterols).[10] A deficiency of these sterols results in impaired membrane function and other metabolic abnormalities within the fungal cell. Fluconazole also directly damages the fungal membrane by destroying certain membrane components such as triglycerides and phospholipids. Loss of normal membrane structure and function results in the destruction of the fungus.

Adverse Effects. Hepatotoxicity is the most serious adverse effect of fluconazole, and this drug should be used cautiously in patients with impaired liver function. Other common side effects include headache and gastrointestinal disturbances (abdominal pain, nausea, vomiting).

FLUCYTOSINE

Clinical Use. The antifungal spectrum of flucytosine (Ancobon) is limited primarily to the *Candida* and *Cryptococcus* species.[39] This drug is used systemically to treat endocarditis, urinary tract infections, and presence of fungi in the bloodstream (*fungemia*) during candidiasis. Flucytosine is also used to treat meningitis and severe pulmonary infections caused by cryptococcosis. This drug is often combined with amphotericin B to provide optimal effects and decrease the chance of fungal resistance.[38,39]

Mechanism of Action. Flucytosine is incorporated into susceptible fungi, where it then undergoes enzymatic conversion to fluorouracil.[10] Fluorouracil then acts as an antimetabolite during RNA synthesis in the fungus. Fluorouracil is incorporated into RNA chains but acts as a false nucleic acid. This event ultimately impairs protein synthesis, thus disrupting the normal function of the fungus.

Adverse Effects. Flucytosine may cause hepatotoxicity and may also impair bone marrow function, resulting in anemia, leukopenia, and several other blood dyscrasias.[39] This drug may also produce severe gastrointestinal disturbances, including nausea, vomiting, diarrhea, and loss of appetite.

GRISEOFULVIN

Clinical Use. Griseofulvin (Fulvicin, Grisactin, other names) is used primarily in the treatment of common fungal infections of the skin known as tinea or ringworm infections.[3,4] For example, this drug is administered to treat fungal infections of the feet (tinea pedis, or "athlete's foot"), infections in the groin area (tinea cruris, or "jock rash"), and similar infections of the skin, nails, and scalp. Griseofulvin is administered orally to treat these infections.

Mechanism of Action. Griseofulvin enters susceptible fungal cells and binds to the mitotic spindle during cell division. This binding impairs the mitotic process, thus directly inhibiting the ability of the cell to replicate itself.

Adverse Effects. Common side effects of griseofulvin administration include headache, which may be severe, and gastrointestinal disturbances (nausea, vomiting, diarrhea). Some individuals may exhibit hypersensitivity to this drug as evidenced by skin rashes. Skin photosensitivity (increased reaction to ultraviolet light) may also occur.

ITRACONAZOLE

Clinical Use. Itraconazole (Sporanox) is an azole antifungal agent that is effective against many systemic fungal infections.[7,34] This drug is, for example, used to treat blastomycosis and histoplasmosis infections in the lungs and other tissues, especially in patients with a compromised immune system.[22] Itraconazole may also be used as the primary or alternative treatment for other fungal infections such as aspergillosis, chromomycosis, coccidioidomycosis, and various infections caused by *Candida* species. Like fluconazole, itraconazole offers the advantage of oral administration in treating these systemic infections.[34]

Mechanism of Action. Itraconazole works like fluconazole and similar azoles. These drugs disrupt membrane function of the fungal cell by inhibiting the synthesis of key membrane components such as sterols and by directly damaging other membrane components such as phospholipids. Impaired membrane function leads to metabolic abnormalities and subsequent death of the fungal cell.

Adverse Effects. Side effects associated with itraconazole include headache, gastrointestinal disturbances (nausea, vomiting), and skin rash.

KETOCONAZOLE

Clinical Use. Ketoconazole (Nizoral) is used to treat a variety of superficial and deep fungal infections.[22] This drug can be administered orally to treat pulmonary and systemic infections in candidiasis, coccidioidomycosis, histoplasmosis, and several other types of deep fungal infections. Oral administration is also used to treat tinea infections of the skin, scalp, and other body areas. Ketoconazole is also available in topical preparations for the treatment of tinea infections and other relatively localized infections, including certain vaginal infections.

Mechanism of Action. Ketoconazole selectively inhibits certain enzymes that are responsible for the synthesis of important steroidlike compounds (sterols) in fungal cells.[10] A deficiency of these sterols results in impaired membrane function and other metabolic abnormalities within the fungal cell. At higher concentrations, ketoconazole may also directly disrupt the cell membrane, resulting in the destruction of the fungus.

Adverse Effects. Gastrointestinal disturbances (e.g., nausea, vomiting, stomach pain) are the most common adverse effects when ketoconazole is administered systemically. Some degree of hepatotoxicity may occur, and severe or even fatal hepatitis has been reported on rare occasions. In large, prolonged doses, this drug may also impair testosterone and adrenocorticosteroid synthesis, resulting in breast tenderness and enlargement (gynecomastia) and decreased sex drive in some men.

TERBINAFINE

Clinical Use. Terbinafine (Lamisil), effective against a broad spectrum of fungi, can be administered systemically to treat infections in the toenails and fingernails (onchomycosis) caused by various fungi.[12,21] Oral administration of this drug may also be useful in treating ringworm infections such as tinea corporis (ringworm of the body), tinea capitis (ringworm of the scalp), and tinea cruris (ringworm of the groin, jock rash), especially if these infections do not respond to topical treatment. Terbinafine is likewise available in creams and solutions for topical treatment of various tinea infections, including tinea pedis (athlete's foot) and tinea versicolor.

Mechanism of Action. Terbinafine inhibits a specific enzyme (squalene epoxidase) that is responsible for sterol synthesis in the fungal cell membrane. This action impairs cell wall synthesis, with subsequent loss of cell membrane function and integrity. Inhibition of this enzyme likewise causes squalene to accumulate in the fungal cell, which can also impair cell function and lead to death of the fungus.

Adverse Effects. Systemic administration of terbinafine may cause a hypersensitivity reaction (skin rashes, itching) and gastrointestinal problems such as nausea, vomiting, and diarrhea. This drug may also cause a change or loss of taste, an effect that may last several weeks after the drug is discontinued. Topical administration is generally well tolerated, although signs of local irritation (itching, redness, peeling skin) may indicate a need to discontinue this drug.

Topical Antifungal Agents

As mentioned earlier, certain antifungals are too toxic to be administered systemically, but these drugs can be applied topically to treat fungal infections in the skin and mucous membranes. These drugs are therefore commonly used to treat various fungal infections in the skin (dermatophytosis), including tinea (ringworm) infections such as tinea pedis (athlete's foot), and tinea cruris (jock rash). These drugs can also be applied locally to treat *Candida* infections in the mucous membranes of the mouth, pharynx, and vagina. The primary topical antifungals are listed in Table 35–2, and they are addressed briefly here.

TOPICAL AZOLE ANTIFUNGALS

Clinical Use. Azole antifungals that are administered topically include clotrimazole, miconazole, and other topical agents listed in Table 35–2. These drugs are related to the systemic azoles (fluconazole, itraconazole, ketoconazole; see earlier), sharing a common chemical background, mechanism of action, and antifungal spectrum. The topical azoles, however, are too toxic for systemic use and are therefore restricted to local application. Nonetheless, these drugs are valuable in controlling fungal infections in the skin and mucocutaneous tissues (see Table 35–2). For example, azoles such as butoconazole, clotrimazole, miconazole, terconazole, and tioconazole can be applied via creams, ointments, and suppositories to treat vaginal *Candida* infections. Other agents such as econazole, oxiconazole, and sulconazole can be applied via creams, solutions, or powders to treat tinea infections that cause athlete's foot (tinea pedis) and jock rash (tinea cruris). Certain azoles can also be applied locally via lozenges or elixirs (syrups) to treat oral candidiasis infections that occur in patients with a compromised immune system (see Table 35–2). Hence, these agents are used to treat local mycoses that occur in a variety of clinical situations.

Mechanism of Action. Like the systemic azoles, clotrimazole and other topical antifungal azoles work by inhibiting the synthesis of key components of the fungal cell membrane; that is, these drugs impair production of membrane sterols, triglycerides, and phospholipids.[10] Loss of these components results in an inability of the membrane to maintain intracellular homeostasis, leading to death of the fungus.

Adverse Effects. Side effects are relatively few when these drugs are applied locally. Gastrointestinal distress (cramps, diarrhea, vomiting) can occur if azole lozenges are swallowed. Other problems associated with topical use include local burning or irritation of the skin or mucous membranes.

OTHER TOPICAL AGENTS

Clinical Use. Other topical antifungals include nystatin (Mycostatin, Nilstat, others), naftifine (Naftin), and tolnaftate (Aftate, Tinactin, many other names) (see Table 35–2). Nystatin has a wide spectrum of activity against various fungi but is not used to treat systemic infections because it is not absorbed from the gastrointestinal tract. Nystatin is therefore administered via several topical preparations to treat cutaneous, oropharyngeal, or vaginal candidiasis. Topical and local (oropharyngeal) use of nystatin is especially important in treating candidiasis in immunocompromised patients, including people with AIDS.[28] Naftifine and tolnaftate are used primarily to treat local and superficial cases of tinea (ringworm) infection. These agents are found in several popular over-the-counter products that are administered topically to treat tinea infections such as tinea pedis (athlete's foot) and tinea cruris (jock rash).

Mechanism of Action. Nystatin exerts its antifungal effects in a manner similar to that of amphotericin B; that is, this drug binds to sterols in the cell membrane, causing an increase in membrane permeability and loss of cellular homeostasis. The exact mechanism of naftifine is unclear, although this drug probably inhibits the synthesis of membrane sterols, resulting in loss of membrane integrity and death of the fungus. Tolnaftate appears to stunt the growth of fungal cell bodies, but the exact mechanism of this drug is not known.

Adverse Effects. Nystatin is generally well tolerated when applied locally. Systemic absorption through mucous membranes may cause some gastrointestinal disturbances (nausea, vomiting, diarrhea), but these side effects are generally mild and transient. Topical use of naftifine and tolnaftate is likewise fairly safe, although local burning and irritation of the skin may occur in some individuals.

ANTIPROTOZOAL AGENTS

Protozoa are single-celled organisms that represent the lowest division of the animal kingdom. Of the several thousand species of protozoa, approximately 35 represent a threat of parasitic infection in humans.[9] One relatively common disease caused by protozoal infection is malaria. Malaria is caused by several species of a protozoan parasite known as plasmodia. Although this disease has been virtually eliminated in North America and Europe, malaria continues to be the primary health problem throughout many other parts of the world.[9] Individuals who live in these areas, as well as those traveling to parts of the world where malaria is prevalent, must often undergo antimalarial chemotherapy. Hence, drugs that prevent and treat malaria are extremely important.

In addition to malaria, several other serious infections may occur in humans because of parasitic invasion by protozoa.[9] Severe intestinal infections (dysentery) produced by various protozoa occur quite frequently, especially in areas where contaminated food and drinking water are prevalent. Infections in tissues such as the liver, heart, lungs, brain, and other organs may also occur because of protozoal infestation. As mentioned in the introduction to this chapter, individuals with a compromised immune system may be especially susceptible to these intestinal and extraintestinal infections.[26]

The primary agents used to treat protozoal infections are listed in Table 35–3 and Table 35–4, and each agent is described subsequently. Drugs that are used primarily to treat and prevent malaria are grouped together, followed by drugs that are used to treat other types of protozoal infections (intestinal and extraintestinal infections).

Antimalarial Agents

CHLOROQUINE

Clinical Use. Chloroquine (Aralen) is often the drug of choice in preventing and treating most forms of malaria.[29] This agent is administered routinely to individuals who are traveling to areas of the world where they may be exposed to malaria infection.[27] Certain strains of the parasite that causes malaria (the *Plasmodium* ameba) are resistant to chloroquine, however.[14] If these chloroquine-resistant strains are encountered, other antimalarial drugs such as mefloquine must be used (see Table 35–3).

Chloroquine is also used for the treatment of conditions other than malaria. This drug is effective against other types of protozoal infections such as amebiasis and may be used with iodoquinol or emetine to treat infections in the liver and pericardium. As discussed in Chapter 16, chloroquine is effective in rheumatoid disease and is used in

TABLE 35–3 Treatment of Malaria

Type of Malaria	Primary Agent(s)	Alternative/Secondary Agent(s)
Chloroquine-sensitive	Chloroquine	Primaquine
Chloroquine-resistant	Mefloquine, pyrimethamine-sulfadoxine, quinine	Antibacterials (e.g., sulfamethoxazole, tetracycline) may be added to the primary agent(s)

TABLE 35–4 Treatment of Other Protozoal Infections

Type of Infection	Principal Site(s) of Infection	Primary Agent(s)	Alternative/ Secondary Agent(s)
Amebiasis	Intestinal tract; liver; lungs	Metronidazole	Diloxanide furoate, emetine, iodoquinol, antibacterials (paromomycin, tetracycline)
Balantidiasis	Lower gastro-intestinal tract	Iodoquinol (tetracycline antibiotics are also effective)	Metronidazole
Giardiasis	Small intestine	Metronidazole; antimalarial drugs (e.g., quinacrine)	—
Leishmaniasis	Skin; mucocutaneous tissues, viscera	Sodium stibogluconate	Amphotericin B, itraconazole, ketoconazole pentamidine
Pneumocystis carinii	Lungs (pneumonia)	Trimethoprim-sulfamethoxazole (see Chap. 33)	Atovaquone, pentamidine
Trichomoniasis	Vagina, genitourinary tract	Metronidazole	—
Toxoplasmosis	Lymph nodes, many organs and tissues	Pyrimethamine-sulfadiazine (see antimalarial drugs); other antibacterials (clindamycin)	—
Trypanosomiasis (Chagas disease; African sleeping sickness)	Heart, brain, many other organs	Nifurtimox, melarsoprol, suramin	Pentamidine

the treatment of conditions such as rheumatoid arthritis and systemic lupus erythematosus. However, the reasons why this antiprotozoal agent is also effective against rheumatoid disease are unclear. Chloroquine is administered orally.

Mechanism of Action. Although the exact mechanism is unknown, chloroquine may impair metabolic and digestive function in the protozoa by becoming concentrated within subcellular vacuoles and raising the pH of these vacuoles.[29] This effect may inhibit the ability of the parasite to digest hemoglobin from the blood of the host erythrocytes. Impaired hemoglobin digestion leads to the accumulation of toxic heme by-products in the protozoa, which subsequently leads to death of this parasite.[29] Chloroquine may also bind directly to DNA within susceptible parasites and inhibit DNA/RNA function and subsequent protein synthesis. The ability to impair protein synthesis may contribute to the antiprotozoal actions of this drug.

Adverse Effects. The most serious problem associated with chloroquine is the possibility of toxicity to the retina and subsequent visual disturbances. This issue is usually insignificant, however, when this drug is used for short periods of time in relatively low doses (see Chap. 16). Other relatively mild side effects may occur, including gastrointestinal distress (nausea, vomiting, stomach cramps, diarrhea), behavior and mood changes (irritability, confusion, nervousness, depression), and skin disorders (rashes, itching, discoloration).

HYDROXYCHLOROQUINE

Hydroxychloroquine (Plaquenil) is derived chemically from chloroquine and is similar to it in clinical use, mechanism of action, and adverse effects. Hydroxychloroquine does not have any distinct therapeutic advantages over chloroquine, but it may be substituted in certain individuals who do not respond well to chloroquine.

MEFLOQUINE

Clinical Use. Mefloquine (Lariam) has emerged as one of the most important antimalarial agents.[14] This drug is especially important in the prevention and treatment of malaria that is resistant to traditional antimalarial drugs such as chloroquine and quinine.[14,31] Mefloquine is often the drug of choice for antimalarial prophylaxis, especially in areas of the world where chloroquine-resistant strains of malaria are common.[33]

Mechanism of Action. Although the exact mechanism of action of this drug is unknown, mefloquine may exert antimalarial effects similar to chloroquine; that is, these drugs inhibit hemoglobin digestion in malarial parasites, thus causing heme by-products to accumulate within the protozoa and cause toxicity and death of this parasite.[29]

Adverse Effects. Mefloquine is fairly safe and well tolerated when used at moderate doses to prevent malarial infection. At higher doses, such as those used to treat infection, mefloquine may cause dizziness, headache, fever, joint and muscle pain, and gastrointestinal problems (abdominal pain, nausea, vomiting, diarrhea). These side effects, however, may be difficult to distinguish from the symptoms associated with malaria.

PRIMAQUINE

Clinical Use. Primaquine is used in rather extreme circumstances to cure certain forms of malaria[37] and is generally administered in acute, severe exacerbations or when other drugs (chloroquine, mefloquine) are ineffective in suppressing malarial attacks. Primaquine may also be used to prevent the onset of malaria in individuals who are especially at risk because of prolonged exposure to this disease.[14] This drug is administered orally.

Mechanism of Action. Primaquine appears to impair DNA function in susceptible parasites. The exact manner in which this occurs is unknown, however.

Adverse Effects. Gastrointestinal disturbances (nausea, vomiting, abdominal pain), headache, and visual disturbances may occur during primaquine therapy. A more serious side effect, acute hemolytic anemia, may occur in patients who have a deficiency in the enzyme glucose-6-phosphate dehydrogenase. This enzymatic deficiency is more common in certain black, Mediterranean, and Asian individuals; hence there is an increased risk of hemolytic anemia in these groups.[37]

PYRIMETHAMINE

Clinical Use. When used alone, pyrimethamine (Daraprim) is only of minor use in treating and preventing malaria. However, the antimalarial effectiveness of pyrimethamine is increased dramatically by combining it with the antibacterial drug sulfadoxine.[37] The combination of these two drugs (known commercially as Fansidar) is often used to prevent or treat certain forms of chloroquine-resistant malaria (see Table 35–3).[37] Pyrimethamine may also be combined with a sulfonamide drug like dapsone, sulfadiazine, or sulfamethoxazole to treat protozoal infections that cause toxoplasmosis or *Pneumocystis carinii* pneumonia. These agents are administered orally.

Mechanism of Action. Pyrimethamine blocks the production of folic acid in susceptible protozoa by inhibiting the function of the dihydrofolate reductase enzyme. Folic acid helps catalyze the production of nucleic and amino acids in these parasites. Therefore, this drug ultimately impairs nucleic acid and protein synthesis by interfering with folic acid production. The action of sulfadoxine and other sulfonamide antibacterial agents was discussed in Chapter 33. These agents also inhibit folic acid synthesis in certain bacterial and protozoal cells.

Adverse Effects. The incidence and severity of side effects from pyrimethamine-sulfadoxine are related to the dosage and duration of therapy. Toxicity is fairly common when these drugs are given in high doses for prolonged periods, and adverse effects include gastrointestinal disturbances (vomiting, stomach cramps, loss of appetite), blood dyscrasias (agranulocytosis, leukopenia, thrombocytopenia), CNS abnormalities (tremors, ataxia, seizures), and hypersensitivity reactions (skin rashes, anaphylaxis, liver dysfunction). Resistance may also occur during repeated use, and this drug strategy may be ineffective in certain strains of malaria that have already developed resistant mechanisms. Hence, pyrimethamine-sulfadoxine is usually administered on a very limited basis, such as a single dose at the onset of malarial symptoms.

QUININE

Clinical Use. Quinine is one of the oldest forms of antimalarial chemotherapy, having been obtained from the bark of certain South American trees as early as the 1600s.[37] Although quinine was the principal method of preventing and treating malaria for many years, the use of this drug has diminished somewhat because it is relatively toxic and expensive to produce.[37] Hence, the routine use of this drug has largely been replaced by newer, safer agents such as chloroquine and mefloquine. Quinine, however, remains one of the most effective antimalarial drugs and is currently used to treat malaria that is resistant to other drugs. Quinine sulfate is administered orally, and quinine dihydrochloride is administered by slow intravenous infusion.

Mechanism of Action. The exact mechanism of quinine is not known. This drug probably exerts antimalarial effects similar to those of chloroquine—that is, inhibition of hemoglobin digestion and subsequent accumulation of toxic heme by-products that lead to death in susceptible protozoa.[29]

Adverse Effects. Quinine is associated with many adverse effects involving several primary organ systems. This drug may produce disturbances in the CNS (headache, visual disturbances, ringing in the ears), gastrointestinal system (nausea, vomiting, abdominal pain), and cardiovascular system (cardiac arrhythmias). Problems with hypersensitivity, blood disorders, liver dysfunction, and hypoglycemia may also occur in some individuals.

OTHER ANTIMALARIALS: USE OF ARTEMISININ DERIVATIVES

Clinical Use. Artemisinin derivatives are naturally occurring compounds that appear to be effective against many forms of the protozoa that cause malaria.[41] These drugs consist of the parent compound (artemisinin) and several products that can be synthesized from artemisinin such as artesunate, artemether, and arteether.[42] It does not appear that any one derivative is superior to another in treating malaria, hence the term *artemisinin derivative* can be used to collectively describe this group.[24] These agents act rapidly and appear to be effective against all malarial parasites that infect humans.[42] Artemisinin derivatives can likewise be used alone or combined with other antimalarials (quinine, mefloquine) to improve efficacy and reduce the chance of resistance to these drugs.

Mechanism of Action. Artemisinin derivatives appear to work by a two-step process that occurs within the malarial parasite.[25] In the first step, the drug is activated when it is cleaved by the heme-iron component within the protozoa. This cleavage forms a highly reactive free radical that, in the second step, reacts with and destroys essential protozoal proteins.[25] Destruction of these proteins results in loss of cellular function and subsequent death of the protozoa.

Adverse Effects. Because these drugs are fairly new, the potential for side effects remains to be fully determined. Studies on animals suggested that these drugs may be neurotoxic, but this effect has not been proven conclusively in humans.[42] Future research should help determine the relative risks and benefits of these agents, as well as how artemisinin derivatives can complement other drugs in the antimalarial armamentarium.

Drugs Used to Treat Protozoal Infections in the Intestines and Other Tissues

ATOVAQUONE

Clinical Use. Atovaquone (Mepron) is effective against the *Plasmodia* parasite that causes *Pneumocystis carinii* pneumonia (PCP) in immunocompromised patients.[37] This drug is not typically the primary treatment for PCP but is often reserved for patients who cannot tolerate more traditional PCP treatments using sulfamethoxazole and trimethoprim (see Chap. 34) or pentamidine (see later).

Mechanism of Action. Atovaquone appears to selectively inhibit electron transport in the *Plasmodium* protozoa. This inhibition directly decreases production of ATP in the protozoa and may also interfere with nucleic acid synthesis, ultimately resulting in death of this parasite.

Adverse Effects. Atovaquone may cause side effects such as fever, skin rash, cough, headache, and gastrointestinal problems (nausea, vomiting, diarrhea).

EMETINE AND DEHYDROEMETINE

Clinical Use. Emetine and dehydroemetine (Mebadin) are used primarily to treat protozoal infections in the intestinal tract and extraintestinal sites such as the lungs and liver. These drugs are powerful amebicides and are generally reserved for severe, acute cases of intestinal amebiasis (dysentery).[37] Because of potential adverse effects, these drugs are no longer marketed in the United States, and safer agents like metronidazole are often used in their place. Emetine and dehydroemetine are typically administered by deep subcutaneous injection or intramuscular injection.

Mechanism of Action. These drugs exert a direct effect on susceptible protozoa by causing degeneration of subcellular components such as the nucleus and reticular system within the parasite.

Adverse Effects. As indicated earlier, the effectiveness of emetine and dehydroemetine is limited by a number of potentially serious side effects. In particular, problems with cardiotoxicity may occur, as reflected by arrhythmias, palpitations, and other changes in cardiac conduction and excitability. Gastrointestinal disturbances such as diarrhea, nausea, and vomiting are also quite common. Generalized muscular aches and weakness may occur, as well as localized myositis near the site of administration. Hence, these drugs are administered under close medical supervision and are withdrawn as soon as the amebicidal effects are apparent.

IODOQUINOL

Clinical Use. Iodoquinol (Diquinol, Yodoxin, others) is used primarily to treat protozoal infections within the intestinal tract,[37] and it is often combined with a second tissue amebicide, which kills protozoa at extraintestinal sites. For instance, iodoquinol may be combined with metronidazole to ensure destruction of parasites throughout the body. Iodoquinol is usually administered orally. Because iodoquinol is relatively toxic, the routine use of this drug has been replaced somewhat by other agents such as diloxanide furoate, which may be somewhat safer.

Mechanism of Action. The mechanism of action of iodoquinol as an amebicide is unknown.

Adverse Effects. Iodoquinol is neurotoxic and may produce optic and peripheral neuropathies when administered in large doses for prolonged periods. Problems with muscle weakness and ataxia may also occur because of the neurotoxic effects of this drug. Other adverse effects include gastrointestinal distress (e.g., nausea, vomiting, cramps) and various skin reactions (rashes, itching, discoloration), but these effects are relatively mild and transient.

PAROMOMYCIN

Clinical Use. Paromomycin (Humatin) is an aminoglycoside antibacterial (see Chap. 33) that is used primarily to treat mild to moderate intestinal infections (amebiasis). This drug may also be used as an adjunct to other amebicides during the treatment of more severe protozoal infections. Paromomycin is also effective against some bacteria and tapeworms and may be used as a secondary agent in certain bacterial or helminthic infections. This drug is administered orally.

Mechanism of Action. Paromomycin acts selectively on protozoa within the intestinal lumen and destroys these parasites by a direct toxic effect.

Adverse Effects. Paromomycin is not absorbed from the intestine to any great extent, so adverse effects are fairly limited. Nonetheless, problems with gastrointestinal distress (nausea, vomiting, abdominal pain) may occur as this drug exerts amebicidal effects within the intestine.

METRONIDAZOLE

Clinical Use. Metronidazole (Flagyl, Protostat, other names) is effective against a broad spectrum of protozoa and is often the primary agent used against protozoal infections in intestinal as well as extraintestinal tissues.[37] Metronidazole, for example, is often the drug of choice for treating several intestinal infections (amebiasis, giardiasis) and amebic abscesses in other tissues such as the liver. Metronidazole is also the primary drug used to treat trichomoniasis, a sexually transmitted protozoal disease affecting the vagina and male genitourinary tract. As indicated in Chapter 33, metronidazole has bactericidal effects and is used in certain gram-negative bacterial infections. This drug may be administered orally or intravenously.

Mechanism of Action. The exact mechanism of action of this drug is not known. Metronidazole is believed to be reduced chemically within the parasitic cell to a metabolite that impairs nucleic acid and DNA synthesis.[37] The exact nature of this metabolite, however, and other features of the cytotoxic effects of this drug remain to be determined.

Adverse Effects. Gastrointestinal disturbances including nausea, vomiting, diarrhea, stomach pain, and an unpleasant taste in the mouth are relatively common with metronidazole. Other adverse effects such as hypersensitivity reactions, peripheral neuropathy, hematologic abnormalities, and genitourinary problems have been reported, but their incidence is relatively low.

PENTAMIDINE

Clinical Use. Pentamidine (Nebupent, Pentam, others) is effective against several types of extraintestinal protozoal infections, including *P. carinii* pneumonia, certain forms of trypanosomiasis (African sleeping sickness), and visceral infections caused by *Leishmania* protozoa. Typically, pentamidine is reserved as a secondary agent in treating these infections and is used when the principal drug in each case is not available or is poorly tolerated (see Table 35–4). Use of this drug as a primary agent has increased, however, in the treatment of *P. carinii* infections in patients with AIDS.[23,40] This drug is usually administered by parenteral routes such as deep intramuscular injection or slow intravenous infusion. Pentamidine may also be administered by oral inhalation to treat lung infections, and this strategy is now commonly used as prophylaxis and treatment of *P. carinii* pneumonia (PCP) in patients with AIDS.[37]

Mechanism of Action. The exact mechanism of this drug is not clear, and pentamidine may affect different parasites in different ways. Some possible antiprotozoal actions of this drug include inhibition of protein and nucleic acid synthesis, cellular metabolism, and oxidative phosphorylation in susceptible parasites.

Adverse Effects. The primary adverse effect of systemic pentamidine administration is renal toxicity. Renal function may be markedly impaired in some patients, but kidney function usually returns to normal when the drug is withdrawn. Other adverse effects include hypotension, hypoglycemia, gastrointestinal distress, blood dyscrasias (leukopenia, thrombocytopenia), and local pain and tenderness at the site of injection. Adverse effects are reduced substantially when this drug is given by inhalation, and this method of administration is desirable when pentamidine is used to prevent PCP in patients with HIV disease.

Other Antiprotozoal Drugs

Several additional agents have been developed to treat intestinal and extraintestinal infections caused by various protozoa. These agents include diloxanide furoate, eflornithine, melarsoprol, nifurtimox, sodium stibogluconate, and suramin. The use and distribution of these drugs, however, is quite different from the agents described previously. In the United States, these additional drugs are usually available only from the Centers for Disease Control (CDC), in Atlanta, Georgia. At the request of the physician, the CDC dispenses the drug to the physician, who then provides the agent to the patient.

Clinical applications of individual drugs in this category are indicated in Table 35–4. In general, these drugs are reserved for some of the more serious or rare types of protozoal infections. As might be expected, adverse side effects of these drugs are quite common. Yet these drugs may be lifesaving in some of the more severe infections, which is why the CDC controls their distribution. For more information about specific agents in this group, the reader is referred to other sources.[37]

ANTHELMINTICS

Infection from helminths, or parasitic worms, is the most common form of disease in the world.[9,36] There are several types of worms that may invade and subsist from human tissues.[9,19,20] Common examples include tapeworms (cestodes), roundworms (nematodes), and flukes (trematodes).[32] Worms can enter the body by various routes but often are ingested as eggs in contaminated food and water. Once in the body, the eggs hatch, and adult worms ultimately lodge in various tissues, especially the digestive tract. Some types (flukes) may also lodge in blood vessels such as the hepatic portal vein. Depending on the species, adult worms may range from a few millimeters to several meters in length. The adult worms begin to steal nutrients from their human host and may begin to obstruct the intestinal lumen or other ducts if they reproduce in sufficient numbers.

Some of the common **anthelmintics** used to kill the basic types of worms in humans are listed in Table 35–5. These agents are often very effective, a single oral dose being sufficient to selectively destroy the parasite. Brief descriptions of the basic pharmacologic effects and possible adverse effects of the primary anthelmintic agents are presented here. The pharmacologic treatment of helminthic infections has also been reviewed extensively by several authors.[2,8,16,36]

Albendazole

Albendazole (Albenza) is used primarily to treat infections caused by the larval form of certain cestodes (tapeworms). These infections often cause cysts (hydatid disease) in the liver, lungs, and other tissues, and albendazole is used as an adjunct to surgical removal of these cysts or as the primary treatment if these cysts are inoperable. This drug is also effective against many gastrointestinal roundworms and hookworms, and it is typically used as a secondary agent if other anthelmintics are not effective in treating these infections.

Albendazole exerts its anthelmintic effects by acting on the intestinal cells of para-

TABLE 35–5 Treatment of Common Helminthic Infections

Parasite	Primary Agent(s)	Secondary Agent(s)
Roundworms (nematodes)		
Ascariasis (roundworm)	Albendazole, mebendazole, pyrantel pamoate	Piperazine citrate
Filariasis	Diethylcarbamazine, ivermectin	—
Hookworm	Albendazole, mebendazole	Pyrantel pamoate, thiabendazole
Pinworm	Albendazole, mebendazole, pyrantel pamoate	Piperazine citrate
Trichinosis	Thiabendazole	Mebendazole
Tapeworms (cestodes)		
Beef tapeworm	Niclosamide, praziquantel	—
Pork tapeworm	Albendazole, praziquantel	Niclosamide
Fish tapeworm	Niclosamide, praziquantel	—
Flukes (trematodes)		
Blood flukes	Praziquantel	Oxamniquine
Fluke infections in other organs	Praziquantel	—

sitic worms and by inhibiting glucose uptake and glycogen storage by these parasites. This effect ultimately leads to lack of energy production, degeneration of intracellular components, and subsequent death of the parasite. Albendazole is usually well tolerated when used for short-term treatment of infections in gastrointestinal or other tissues. Long-term treatment for conditions such as hydatid disease may result in abnormal liver function tests (e.g., increased serum aminotransferase activity), and liver function should therefore be monitored periodically to prevent hepatotoxicity if this drug is used for extended periods.

Diethylcarbamazine

Diethylcarbamazine (Hetrazan) is used to treat certain roundworm infections of the lymphatics and connective tissues, including loiasis, onchocerciasis, and Bancroft filariasis. This agent immobilizes immature roundworms (microfilariae) and facilitates the destruction of these microfilariae by the body's immune system. Diethylcarbamazine is also effective against the adult forms of certain roundworms, but the mechanism of this anthelmintic action against mature nematodes is not known.

Side effects associated with diethylcarbamazine include headache, malaise, weakness, and loss of appetite. More severe reactions (fever, acute inflammatory response) may also occur following diethylcarbamazine use, but these reactions may be caused by release of antigenic substances from the dying roundworms rather than from the drug itself.

Ivermectin

Ivermectin (Mectizan, Stromectol) is the primary treatment for filarial nematode infections (onchocerciasis) that invade ocular tissues and cause loss of vision (river blindness). Ivermectin may also be used in filarial infections in other tissues (lymphatics, skin). This drug is a secondary agent for treating intestinal nematodes such as strongyloidosis.

Ivermectin binds to chloride ion channels in parasitic nerve and muscle cells, thereby increasing membrane permeability to chloride. Increased intracellular chloride results in hyperpolarization of nerve and muscle tissues, which results in paralysis and death of the parasite. Ivermectin is well tolerated during short-term use in mild to moderate infections. Administration in more severe infection may cause swollen or tender lymph glands, fever, skin rash, itching, and joint and muscle pain, but these reactions may be caused by the death of the infectious parasites rather than by the drug itself.

Mebendazole

Mebendazole (Vermox) is effective against many types of roundworms and a few tapeworms that parasitize humans. Like albendazole, this drug selectively damages intestinal cells in these worms, thus inhibiting the uptake and intracellular transport of glucose and other nutrients into these parasites. This activity leads to destruction of the epithelial lining and subsequent death of the parasite. Mebendazole is a relatively safe drug, although some mild, transient gastrointestinal problems may occur.

Niclosamide

Niclosamide (Niclocide) is effective against several types of tapeworm (see Table 35–5). This drug inhibits certain mitochondrial enzymes in these parasites. This inhibition ultimately results in the breakdown of the protective integument of the worm, thus allowing the digestive enzymes in the host (human) intestine to attack the parasite. Ultimately, the worm is digested and expelled from the gastrointestinal tract. There are relatively few adverse effects of niclosamide treatment, probably because the drug is not absorbed to any great extent from the human intestine. Thus, the drug remains in the intestinal lumen, where it can act directly on the tapeworm.

Oxamniquine

Oxamniquine (Vansil) is effective against a genus of parasitic worms known as blood flukes (schistosomes). These parasites typically adhere to the wall of blood vessels such as the hepatic portal vein. Oxamniquine inhibits muscular contraction of the sucker that holds the fluke to the vessel wall, thus allowing the worm to dislodge and travel to the liver. In the liver, the parasite is engulfed and destroyed by hepatic phagocytes. Common side effects associated with this drug include headache, dizziness, and drowsiness. These adverse effects are generally mild and transient, however.

Piperazine Citrate

Piperazine citrate is typically used as a secondary agent in ascariasis (roundworm) and enterobiasis (pinworm) infections (see Table 35–5). This drug appears to paralyze the worm by blocking the effect of acetylcholine at the parasite's neuromuscular junction. The paralyzed worm can then be dislodged and expelled from the host (human) intestine during normal bowel movements. Side effects such as headache, dizziness, and gastrointestinal disturbance may occur during piperazine citrate administration, but these effects are generally mild and transient.

Praziquantel

Praziquantel (Biltricide), one of the most versatile and important anthelmintic agents, is the drug of choice in treating all major trematode (fluke) infections and several common types of tapeworm infections (see Table 35–5). The exact mechanism of action of this drug is not known. Praziquantel may stimulate muscular contraction of the parasite, resulting in a type of spastic paralysis, which causes the worm to lose its hold on intestinal or vascular tissue. At higher concentrations, this drug may initiate destructive changes in the integument of the worm, allowing the host defense mechanisms (e.g., enzymes, phagocytes) to destroy the parasite. Praziquantel is associated with a number of frequent side effects including gastrointestinal problems (such as abdominal pain, nausea, vomiting), CNS effects (headache, dizziness), and mild hepatotoxicity. These adverse effects can usually be tolerated, however, for the relatively short time that the drug is in effect.

Pyrantel Pamoate

Pyrantel pamoate (Antiminth, several other names) is one of the primary agents used in several types of roundworm and pinworm infections (see Table 35–5). This drug stimulates acetylcholine release and inhibits acetylcholine breakdown at the neuromuscular junction, thus producing a prolonged state of excitation and muscular contraction that causes spastic paralysis of the worm. The worm is unable to retain its hold on the intestinal tissue and can be expelled from the digestive tract by normal bowel movements. This drug is generally well tolerated, with only occasional problems of mild gastrointestinal disturbances.

Thiabendazole

Thiabendazole (Mintezol) is the primary drug used in trichinosis and several other types of roundworm infections (see Table 35–5). The anthelmintic mechanism of this drug is not fully understood, but selective inhibition of certain key metabolic enzymes in susceptible parasites is probable. The most common side effects associated with this drug involve gastrointestinal distress (nausea, vomiting, and loss of appetite). Allergic reactions (e.g., skin rash, itching, chills) may also occur in some individuals.

SIGNIFICANCE OF ANTIFUNGAL AND ANTIPARASITIC DRUGS IN REHABILITATION

The drugs discussed in this chapter are relevant because they relate largely to specific groups of patients seen in a rehabilitation setting. Therapists working in sports physical therapy may deal frequently with topical antifungal agents in the treatment of cutaneous ringworm infections. For instance, physical therapists and athletic trainers may be responsible for recognizing and helping treat tinea pedis, tinea cruris, and similar infections. Therapists and trainers can make sure the drugs are being applied in the proper fashion and as directed by the physician. Therapists may also play a crucial role in preventing the spread of these infections by educating athletes about how to prevent transmission among team members (e.g., not sharing towels and combs).

Physical therapists and occupational therapists working with patients who have AIDS will frequently encounter patients taking systemic antifungal and antiprotozoal drugs. The use of these agents is critical in controlling parasitic infections in patients with AIDS and other individuals with a compromised or deficient immune system.

Finally, the drugs discussed in this chapter will have particular importance to therapists working in or traveling to parts of the world where parasitic infections remain a primary health problem and source of human suffering. Therapists involved in the Peace Corps or similar organizations will routinely treat patients taking these drugs. Also, therapists working in these areas may be taking some of these drugs themselves, such as the prophylactic antimalarial agents chloroquine and mefloquine. Hence, therapists should be aware of the pharmacology and potential side effects of these agents, both in their patients and in themselves. Of course, therapists working in North America should know that individuals who have returned from or immigrated from certain geographic areas may carry various fungal and parasitic infections and that these patients will also require chemotherapy using the drugs discussed in this chapter.

CASE STUDY

ANTIFUNGAL DRUGS

Brief History. A physical therapist working with a college football team was taping a team member's ankle when he noticed redness and inflammation between the athlete's toes. The athlete reported that the redness and itching had developed within the last few days and was becoming progressively worse. The therapist suspected a cutaneous fungal infection (probably tinea pedis) and reported this information to the team physician.

Decision/Solution. The physician prescribed a topical antifungal preparation containing miconazole (Monistat-Derm). The athlete was instructed to apply this preparation twice daily. The physical therapist also instructed the athlete in proper skin hygiene (such as thoroughly washing and drying the feet, wearing clean socks). In addition, the physical therapist had the locker room floors and shower areas thoroughly disinfected to prevent transmission of the fungus to other team members. This isolated case of tinea pedis was resolved without further incident.

SUMMARY

This chapter presented three general groups of drugs that are used to treat infection caused by specific microorganisms in humans. Antifungal drugs are used against local or systemic infections caused by pathogenic fungi. Antiprotozoal agents are used to prevent and treat protozoal infections such as malaria, severe intestinal infection (dysentery), and infections in other tissues and organs. Anthelmintic drugs are used against parasitic worms (tapeworm, roundworm, etc.) that may infect the human intestinal tract and other tissues. Although the use of some of these agents is relatively limited in the United States, these drugs tend to be some of the most important agents in controlling infection and improving health on a worldwide basis. Also, the use of some of these agents has increased lately in treating opportunistic fungal and protozoal infections in patients who have AIDS and other individuals with compromised immune systems. Physical therapists and occupational therapists may be involved with treating specific groups of patients taking these drugs, including patients with AIDS and patients located in geographic areas where these types of infections are prevalent.

REFERENCES

1. Ablordeppey, SY, et al: Systemic antifungal agents against AIDS-related opportunistic infections: Current status and emerging drugs in development. Curr Med Chem 6:1151, 1999.
2. Anandan, JV: Parasitic diseases. In DiPiro, JT, et al (eds): Pharmacotherapy: A Pathophysiologic Approach, ed 4. Appleton & Lange, Stamford, CT, 1999.
3. Bennett, JE: Antimicrobial agents: Antifungal agents. In Hardman, JG, et al (eds): The Pharmacological Basis of Therapeutics, ed 9. McGraw-Hill, New York, 1996.
4. Bennett, ML, et al: Oral griseofulvin remains the treatment of choice for tinea capitis in children. Pediatr Dermatol 17:304, 2000.
5. De Marie, S: New developments in the diagnosis and management of invasive fungal infections. Haematologica 85:88, 2000.
6. De Pauw, BE, Donnelly, JP, and Kullberg, BJ: Treatment of fungal infections in surgical patients using conventional antifungals. J Chemother 11:494, 1999.
7. De Rosso, JQ and Gupta, AK: Oral itraconazole therapy for superficial, subcutaneous, and systemic infections. A panoramic view. Postgrad Med 75:46, 1999.

8. De Silva, N, Guyatt, H, and Bundy, D: Anthelmintics. A comparative review of their clinical pharmacology. Drugs 53:769, 1997.
9. Genta, RM and Connor, DH: Infectious and parasitic diseases. In Rubin, E and Farber, JL (eds): Pathology, ed 3. Lippincott-Raven, Philadelphia, 1999.
10. Ghannoum, MA and Rice, LB: Antifungal agents: Mode of action, mechanisms of resistance, and correlation of these mechanisms with bacterial resistance. Clin Microbiol Rev 12:501, 1999.
11. Graybill, JR: Changing strategies for treatment of systemic mycoses. Braz J Infect Dis 4:47, 2000.
12. Hay, RJ: Therapeutic potential of terbinafine in subcutaneous and systemic mycoses. Br J Dermatol 141(Suppl 56):36, 1999.
13. Jones, E and Goldman, M: Lipid formulations of amphotericin B. Cleve Clin J Med 65:423, 1998.
14. Juckett, G: Malaria prevention in travelers. Am Fam Physician 59:2523, 1999.
15. Kappe, R, et al: Recent advances in cryptococcosis, candidiasis and coccidioidomycosis complicating HIV infection. Med Mycol 36(Suppl 1):207, 1998.
16. Katz, M: Anthelmintics. Current concepts in the treatment of helminthic infections. Drugs 32:358, 1986.
17. Kauffman, CA and Carver, PL: Antifungal agents in the 1990s. Current status and future developments. Drugs 53:539, 1997.
18. Kobayashi, GS and Medoff, G: Introduction to the fungi and mycoses. In Schaechter, M, et al (eds): Microbial Disease, ed 3. Lippincott Williams & Wilkins, Philadelphia, 1999.
19. Krogstad, DJ and Engleberg, NC: Intestinal helminths. In Schaechter, M, et al (eds): Microbial Disease, ed 3. Lippincott Williams & Wilkins, Philadelphia, 1999.
20. Krogstad, DJ and Engleberg, NC: Tissue and blood helminths. In Schaechter, M, et al (eds): Microbial Disease, ed 3. Lippincott Williams & Wilkins, Philadelphia, 1999.
21. Lesher, JL: Oral therapy of common superficial fungal infections of the skin. J Am Acad Dermatol 40(Part 2):S31, 1999.
22. Lortholary, O, Denning, DW, and Dupont, B: Endemic mycoses: A treatment update. J Antimicrob Chemother 43:321, 1999.
23. Masur, H: Drug therapy: Prevention and treatment of Pneumocystis pneumonia. N Engl J Med 327:1853, 1992.
24. McIntosh, HM and Olliaro, P: Treatment of uncomplicated malaria with artemisinin derivatives. A systematic review of randomized controlled trials. Med Trop 58(Suppl):57, 1998.
25. Meshnick, SR: Artemisinin antimalarials: Mechanism of action and resistance. Med Trop 58(Suppl):13, 1998.
26. Miller, RF: Clinical presentation and significance of emerging opportunistic infections. J Eukaryot Microbiol 47:21, 2000.
27. Pellegrini, M and Ruff, TA: Malaria. The latest in advice for travelers. Aust Fam Physician 28:683, 1999.
28. Powderly, WG, Mayer, KH, and Perfect, JR: Diagnosis and treatment of oropharyngeal candidiasis in patients infected with HIV: A critical reassessment. AIDS Res Hum Retroviruses 15:1405, 1999.
29. Raynes, K: Bisquinoline antimalarials: Their role in malaria chemotherapy. Int J Parasitol 29:367, 1999.
30. Robinson, RF and Nahata, MC: A comparative review of conventional and lipid formulations of amphotericin B. J Clin Pharm Ther 24:249, 1999.
31. Rosenblatt, JE: Antiparasitic agents. Mayo Clin Proc 74:1161, 1999.
32. Samuelson, J: Infectious diseases. In Cotran, RS, Kumar, V, and Collins, T: Pathologic Basis of Disease, ed 6. WB Saunders, Philadelphia, 1999.
33. Schlagenhauf, P: Mefloquine for malaria chemoprophylaxis 1992–1998: A review. J Travel Med 6:122, 1999.
34. Sheehan, DJ, Hitchcock, CA, and Sibley, CM: Current and emerging azole antifungal agents. Clin Microbiol Rev 12:40, 1999.
35. Slain, D: Lipid-based amphotericin B for the treatment of fungal infections. Pharmacotherapy 19:306, 1999.
36. Tracy, JW and Webster, LT: Drugs used in the chemotherapy of helminthiasis. In Hardman, JG, et al (eds): The Pharmacological Basis of Therapeutics, ed 9. McGraw-Hill, New York, 1996.
37. Tracy, JW and Webster, LT: Drugs used in the chemotherapy of protozoal infections: Malaria. In Hardman, JG, et al (eds): The Pharmacological Basis of Therapeutics, ed 9. McGraw-Hill, New York, 1996.
38. Verduyn Lunel, FM, Meis, JF, and Voss, A: Nosocomial fungal infections: Candidemia. Diagn Microbiol Infect Dis 34:213, 1999.
39. Vermes, A, Guchelaar, HJ, and Dankert, J: Flucytosine: A review of its pharmacology, clinical indications, pharmacokinetics, toxicity, and drug interactions. J Antimicrob Chemother 46:171, 2000.
40. Vohringer, HF and Arasteh, K: Pharmacokinetic optimisation in the treatment of Pneumocystis carinii pneumonia. Clin Pharmacokinet 24:388, 1993.
41. Vroman, JA, Alvim-Gaston, M, and Avery, MA: Current progress in the chemistry, medicinal chemistry, and drug design of artemisinin based antimalarials. Curr Pharm Des 5:101, 1999.
42. White, NJ and Olliaro, P: Artemisinin and derivatives in the treatment of uncomplicated malaria. Med Trop (Mars) 58(Suppl):54, 1998.

CHAPTER 36

Cancer Chemotherapy

Cancer encompasses a group of diseases that are marked by rapid, uncontrolled cell proliferation and a conversion of normal cells to a more primitive and undifferentiated state.[14,53] Excessive cell proliferation may form large tumors, or *neoplasms*. Although some types of tumors are well contained, or benign, **malignant tumors** continue to proliferate within local tissues and possibly spread (**metastasize**) to other tissues in the body. *Cancer* specifically refers to the malignant forms of neoplastic disease that are often fatal as tumors invade and destroy tissues throughout the body. However, benign tumors can also be life-threatening; for example, a large benign tumor may produce morbidity and mortality by obstructing the intestinal tract or pressing on crucial CNS structures. Cancer cells, however, are unique in their progressive invasion of local tissues and ability to metastasize to other tissues.[53]

Cancer ranks second to cardiovascular disease as the leading cause of death in the United States.[63] There are many different types of cancer, and malignancies are classified by the location and type of tissue from which the cancer originated.[14,53] For instance, cancers arising from epithelial tissues (e.g., skin, gastrointestinal lining) are labeled as *carcinomas;* cancers arising from mesenchymal tissues (e.g., bone, striated muscle) are labeled as *sarcomas*. Also, cancers associated with the formed blood elements are connoted by the "-emia" suffix (e.g., "leukemia," cancerous proliferation of leukocytes). Many other descriptive terms are used to describe various malignancies, and certain forms of cancer are often named after a specific person (e.g., Hodgkin disease, Wilms tumor). We cannot, however, describe all the various types of malignancies. The reader may want to consult a pathology text[14,53] or similar reference for more information about the location and morphology of particular forms of cancer.

The exact cause of many cases of neoplastic disease is unknown. However, a great deal has been learned about possible environmental, viral, genetic, and other possible elements, or **carcinogens,** that may cause or increase susceptibility to various types of cancer. Conversely, certain positive lifestyles, including adequate exercise, a high-fiber diet, and avoidance of tobacco products, may be crucial in preventing certain forms of cancer. Of course, routine checkups and early detection play a crucial role in reducing cancer mortality.

When cancer is diagnosed, three primary treatment modalities are available: surgery, radiation treatment, and cancer chemotherapy. The purpose of this chapter is to describe the basic rationale of cancer **chemotherapy** and to provide an overview of the drugs that are currently available to treat specific forms of cancer. Rehabilitation specialists will routinely be working with patients undergoing cancer chemotherapy. For reasons that will become apparent in this chapter, these drugs tend to produce toxic effects that directly influence physical therapy and occupational therapy procedures. Therefore, this chapter should provide therapists with a better understanding of the pharmacodynamic principles and beneficial effects, as well as the reason for the potential adverse effects of these important drugs.

GENERAL PRINCIPLES

Cytotoxic Strategy

The basic strategy of anticancer drugs is to limit cell proliferation by killing or attenuating the growth of the cancerous cells. However, the pharmacologic treatment of cancer represents a unique and perplexing problem. Although cancer cells have become more primitive and have lost much of their normal appearance, they are still human cells that have simply gone wild. Plus, they cannot be easily destroyed without also causing some harm to the healthy human tissues. The concept of selective toxicity becomes much more difficult to achieve when using anticancer drugs versus drugs that attack foreign invaders and parasites such as antibacterial drugs or antiprotozoal drugs (see Chaps. 33 through 35).

Hence, most anticancer drugs rely on the basic strategy of inhibiting DNA/RNA synthesis and function, or they directly inhibit cell division (mitosis). Cancerous cells are believed to have a much greater need to replicate their genetic material and undergo mitosis than noncancerous cells. Healthy cells will, of course, also suffer to some extent because anticancer drugs typically lack specificity and impair function in noncancerous tissues as well as cancerous cells.[33,38] The cancerous cells, however, will be affected to a greater extent because of their need to undergo mitosis at a much higher rate than most healthy cells.

Cell-Cycle–Specific versus Cell-Cycle–Nonspecific Drugs

Antineoplastic drugs are sometimes classified by whether they act at a specific phase of cell division.[10] Cancer cells and most normal cells typically undergo a life cycle that can be divided into several distinct phases: resting phase (G_0), pre-DNA synthesis phase (also the phase of normal cell metabolism—G_1), period of DNA synthesis (S), post-DNA synthesis phase (G_2), and the period of actual cell division or mitosis (M).[10,63] Certain antineoplastic drugs are referred to as cell-cycle–specific because they exert their effects only when the cancer cell is in a certain phase. For instance, most antimetabolites (cytarabine, methotrexate, others) act when the cell is in the S phase. Other drugs are classified as cell-cycle–nonspecific because they exert antineoplastic effects on the cell regardless of the phase of the cell cycle. Examples of cell-cycle–nonspecific agents include most alkylating agents and antineoplastic antibiotics.

The significance of cell-cycle specificity or nonspecificity is fairly obvious. Cell-cycle–specific drugs will be effective only in cells that are progressing through the cell cycle—that is, cells that are not remaining in the resting (G_0) phase. Cell-cycle–nonspecific agents have a more general effect and should inhibit replication in all the cells reached by the drug.

Concepts of Growth Fraction and Total Cell Kill

Cancer cells are not all uniform in their rate of replication and proliferation. In any given tumor or type of disseminated cancer, certain cells do not proliferate, while other cells reproduce at variable rates. The term *growth fraction* refers to the percentage of proliferating cells relative to total neoplastic cell population.[63] The cells included in the growth fraction are more susceptible to antineoplastic drugs because these are the cells that must synthesize and replicate their genetic material. Fortunately, these are also the cells that must be killed to prevent the cancer from spreading.

The concept of *total cell kill* refers to the fact that virtually every tumor cell capable of replicating must be killed to eliminate the cancer totally.[10,63] Even one single surviving malignant cell could eventually replicate in sufficient numbers to cause death. The difficulty of achieving total cell kill is illustrated by the following example. The number of malignant cells in a patient with acute lymphocytic leukemia could be as high as 10^{12} cells. If an anticancer drug kills 99.99 percent of these cells, one might think that the drug would be successful in resolving the cancer. However, 10^8, or approximately 1 billion, cells would still remain alive and capable of advancing the leukemia. Obviously, total cell kill is always a chemotherapeutic goal but may sometimes be difficult to achieve.

Prevalence and Management of Adverse Effects

Because antineoplastic agents also impair replication of normal tissues, these drugs are generally associated with a number of common and relatively severe adverse effects. Normal human cells must often undergo controlled mitosis to sustain normal function. This fact is especially true for certain tissues such as hair follicles, bone marrow, immune system cells, and epithelial cells in the skin and gastrointestinal tract. Obviously, these tissues will also be affected to some extent by most cancer chemotherapy agents. In fact, the primary reason for most of the common adverse effects (e.g., hair loss, anemia, anorexia) is that normal cells are also experiencing the same toxic changes as the tumor cells. The cancer cells, however, tend to suffer these toxic effects to a greater extent because of their increased rate of replication and cell division. Still, healthy cells often exhibit some toxic effects, even at the minimum effective doses of the chemotherapeutic agents.

Consequently, antineoplastic drugs typically have a very low therapeutic index compared with drugs that are used to treat less serious disorders (see Chap. 1). Considering that cancer is usually life-threatening, these toxic effects must be expected and tolerated during chemotherapeutic treatments. Occasionally, some side effects can be treated with other drugs. In particular, gastrointestinal disturbances (e.g., nausea, vomiting, loss of appetite) may be relieved to some extent by administering traditional antiemetic agents such as glucocorticoids (dexamethasone) or drugs that block dopamine receptors (metoclopramide).[18] In addition, newer antiemetic and antinausea agents such as dolasetron (Anzemet), granisetron (Kytril), and ondansetron (Zofran) have been developed to treat chemotherapy-induced nausea and vomiting. These newer agents, which block a specific type of serotonin receptor known as the 5-hydroxytryptamine type 3 (5-HT_3) receptor have become very helpful in preventing or reducing the severity of gastrointestinal distress commonly associated with cancer chemotherapy agents.[46,49]

Other forms of supportive care can also be helpful in improving the quality of life for people with cancer. Analgesics (see Chaps. 14 and 15) are often needed to help patients cope with cancer pain and make the rigors of chemotherapy treatment more tolerable.[20] A variety of other medications can also be used to treat specific symptoms such as anemia, cough, weight loss, and constipation.[5,44,66] Support from medical, nursing, and other health-care providers (including physical therapists and occupational therapists) can likewise help immeasurably in reassuring the patient that chemotherapy-induced side effects are normal—and even necessary—for the cancer chemotherapy drugs to exert their antineoplastic effects.

SPECIFIC DRUGS

Drugs used against cancer can be classified by their chemical structure, source, or mechanism of action. The primary groups of antineoplastic drugs are the alkylating agents, antimetabolites, antineoplastic antibiotics, plant alkaloids, antineoplastic hormones, and several other miscellaneous drug groups and individual agents. These principal antineoplastic medications are presented here.

Alkylating Agents

Alkylating agents exert cytotoxic effects by inducing binding within DNA strands and by preventing DNA function and replication.[7,60] Essentially, the drug causes cross-links to be formed between the strands of the DNA double helix or within a single DNA strand (Fig. 36–1). In either case, these cross-links effectively tie up the DNA molecule, eliminating the ability of the DNA double helix to untwist. If the DNA double helix cannot unravel, the genetic code of the cell cannot be reproduced, and cell reproduction is arrested. Also, cross-linking within the double helix impairs cellular protein synthesis because the DNA double helix cannot unwind to allow formation of messenger RNA strands. The cell therefore cannot synthesize vital cellular proteins (enzymes, transport proteins, etc.). By disrupting DNA function, alkylating agents likewise initiate a process of cell death (apoptosis), in which several degradative enzymes (nucleases, proteases) are released and begin to destroy the cell.[7,16]

Alkylating agents are so named because they typically generate a chemical alkyl group on one of the bases such as guanine in the DNA chain. This alkyl group acts as the bridge that ultimately links two bases in the DNA molecule (see Fig. 36–1). The bonds formed by this cross-linking are strong and resistant to breakage. Thus the DNA double helix remains tied up for the life of the cell. Anticancer drugs that work primarily as alkylating agents are listed in Table 36–1. As indicated, these agents represent the largest category of anticancer drugs and are used to treat a variety of leukemias, carcinomas, and other neoplasms. Common adverse side effects of alkylating agents are also listed in Table 36–1. As previously discussed, most of these adverse effects are caused by the effect of the alkylating agent on DNA replication in normal, healthy tissues.

Antimetabolites

Cells are able to synthesize genetic material (DNA, RNA) from endogenous metabolites known as purine and pyrimidine nucleotides (Fig. 36–2). Certain anticancer drugs are structurally similar to these endogenous metabolites and compete with these compounds during DNA/RNA biosynthesis. These drugs are therefore called **antimetabolites** because they interfere with the normal metabolites during cellular biosynthesis.[3,63]

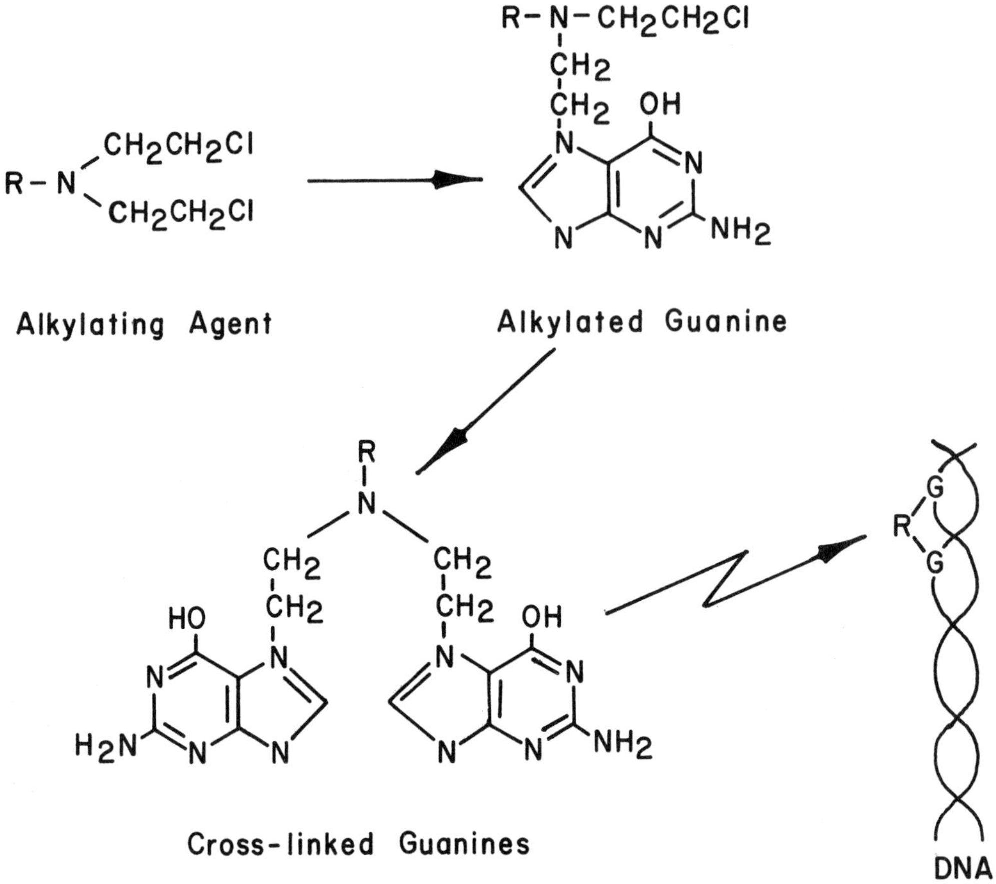

FIGURE 36–1. Mechanism of action of anticancer alkylating agents. The alkylating agent (R) causes alkylation of guanine nucleotides located in the DNA strand. Cross-links are then formed between two alkylated guanines, thus creating strong bonds between or within the DNA strands that inhibit DNA function and replication.

Antimetabolites can impair the biosynthesis of genetic material in two primary ways.[63] First, the drug may be incorporated directly into the genetic material, thus forming a fake and nonfunctional genetic product. This effect would be like baking a cake but substituting an inappropriate ingredient (salt) for a normal ingredient (flour). Obviously, the end product would not work (or taste) very well. A second manner in which antimetabolites may impair DNA/RNA biosynthesis is by occupying the enzymes that synthesize various components of the genetic material. These enzymes do not recognize the difference between the antimetabolite drug and the normal metabolite and waste their time trying to convert the antimetabolite into a normal metabolic product. The enzyme, however, cannot effectively act on the drug, so the normal metabolic products are not formed. In either case, the cell's ability to synthesize normal DNA and RNA is impaired, and the cell cannot replicate its genetic material or carry out normal protein synthesis because of a lack of functional DNA and RNA.

Cancer chemotherapeutic agents that act as antimetabolites and the principal neoplastic diseases for which they are indicated are listed in Table 36–2. As stated previously, these drugs interrupt cellular pathways that synthesize DNA and RNA, and the primary sites where specific antimetabolites interrupt these pathways are indicated in

TABLE 36–1 Alkylating Agents

Generic Name	Trade Name	Primary Antineoplastic Indication(s)*	Common Adverse Effects
Busulfan	Myleran	Chronic myelocytic leukemia	Blood disorders (anemia, leukopenia, thrombocytopenia); metabolic disorders (hyperuricemia, fatigue, weight loss, other symptoms)
Carmustine	BCNU, BiCNU	Primary brain tumors; Hodgkin disease; non-Hodgkin lymphomas; multiple myeloma	Blood disorders (thrombocytopenia, leukopenia); GI distress (nausea, vomiting); hepatotoxicity; pulmonary toxicity
Chlorambucil	Leukeran	Chronic lymphocytic leukemia; Hodgkin disease; non-Hodgkin lymphomas	Blood disorders (leukopenia, thrombocytopenia, anemia); skin rashes and itching; pulmonary toxicity; seizures
Cyclophosphamide	Cytoxan, Neosar	Acute and chronic lymphocytic leukemia; acute and chronic myelocytic leukemia; carcinoma of ovary, breast; Hodgkin disease; non-Hodgkin lymphomas; multiple myeloma	Blood disorders (anemia, leukopenia, thrombocytopenia); GI distress (nausea, vomiting, anorexia); bladder irritation; hair loss; cardiotoxicity; pulmonary toxicity
Dacarbazine	DTIC-Dome	Malignant melanoma; refractory Hodgkin lymphomas	GI distress (nausea, vomiting, anorexia); blood disorders (leukopenia, thrombocytopenia)
Ifosfamide	Ifex	Testicular cancer	Blood disorders (leukopenia, thrombocytopenia); CNS effects (agitation, confusion, dizziness); urotoxicity; GI distress (nausea, vomiting)
Lomustine	CeeNU	Brain tumors; Hodgkin disease	Blood disorders (anemia, leukopenia); GI disorders (nausea, vomiting)
Mechlorethamine	Mustargen, nitrogen mustard	Bronchogenic carcinoma; chronic leukemia; Hodgkin disease; non-Hodgkin lymphomas; blood disorders (leukopenia, thrombocytopenia); skin rashes and itching	Blood disorders (anemia, leukopenia, thrombocytopenia); GI distress (nausea, vomiting); CNS effects (headache, dizziness, convulsions); local irritation at injection site

(continued)

TABLE 36–1 Alkylating Agents *(Continued)*

Generic Name	Trade Name	Primary Antineoplastic Indication(s)*	Common Adverse Effects
Melphalan	Alkeran	Ovarian carcinoma; multiple myeloma	Blood disorders (leukopenia, thrombocytopenia); skin rashes and itching
Procarbazine	Matulane	Hodgkin disease	Blood disorders (leukopenia, thrombocytopenia); GI distress (nausea, vomiting); CNS toxicity (mood changes, incoordination, motor problems)
Streptozocin	Zanosar	Pancreatic carcinoma	Nephrotoxicity; GI distress (nausea, vomiting); blood disorders (anemia, leukopenia, thrombocytopenia); local irritation at injection site
Thiotepa	Thioplex	Carcinoma of breast, ovary, and bladder; Hodgkin disease	Blood disorders (anemia, leukopenia, thrombocytopenia, pancytopenia)
Uracil mustard	—	Chronic lymphocytic leukemia; chronic myelocytic leukemia; non-Hodgkin lymphomas	Blood disorders (anemia, leukopenia, thrombocytopenia); GI distress (nausea, vomiting, diarrhea, anorexia)

*Only the indications listed in the U.S. product labeling are included here. Many anticancer drugs are used for additional types of neoplastic disease.

616

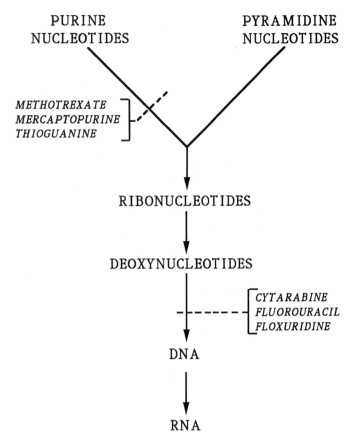

FIGURE 36–2. Sites of action of anticancer antimetabolites. Various drugs interfere with DNA/RNA production by inhibiting nucleic acid biosynthesis at specific sites indicated by the dashed lines.

Figure 36–2. As with most anticancer drugs, these agents are especially toxic to cells that have a large growth fraction and undergo extensive replication. These cells have an especially great need to synthesize nucleic acids—hence the preferential effect of antimetabolites on these cells.

Antibiotics

Several anticancer drugs are chemically classified as antibiotics but are usually reserved for neoplastic diseases because of their relatively high toxicity. The exact mechanism of action for these antibiotics to exert antineoplastic effects is still being investigated. These drugs may act directly on DNA by becoming intercalated (inserted) between base pairs in the DNA strand. This insertion would cause a general disruption or even lysis of the DNA strand, thus preventing DNA replication and RNA synthesis.[21] Alternatively, these antibiotics may act in other ways, including direct effects on the cancerous cell membrane, inhibition of DNA-related enzymes, and formation of highly reactive free radicals that directly damage the DNA molecule.[21,63] Regardless of their exact mechanism, these agents play a role in the treatment of several neoplastic diseases. Antibiotic agents used for cancer chemotherapy are listed in Table 36–3.

TABLE 36-2 Antimetabolites

Generic Name	Trade Name	Primary Antineoplastic Indication(s)*	Common Adverse Effects
Capecitabine	Xeloda	Breast cancer	Blood disorders (anemia, neutropenia, thrombocytopenia); GI distress (abdominal pain, nausea, vomiting); dermatitis; stomatitis; unusual tiredness
Cladribine	Leustatin	Hairy cell leukemia	Blood disorders (anemia, neutropenia, thrombocytopenia); fever; infection; GI distress (anorexia, nausea, vomiting); skin rash; headache; unusual tiredness
Cytarabine	Cytosar-U, DepoCyt	Several forms of acute and chronic leukemia; non-Hodgkin lymphomas	Blood disorders (anemia, megaloblastosis, reticulocytopenia, others); GI distress (nausea, vomiting); skin rashes; hair loss
Floxuridine	FUDR	Carcinoma of the GI tract and liver	GI disorders (nausea, vomiting, anorexia); skin disorders (discoloration, rashes, hair loss)
Fludarabine	Fludara	Chronic lymphocytic leukemia	Blood disorders (anemia, leukopenia, thrombocytopenia); infection; pneumonia; GI distress (nausea, vomiting, diarrhea); skin rash; unusual tiredness; hair loss
Fluorouracil	Adrucil	Carcinoma of colon, rectum, stomach, and pancreas	GI distress (anorexia, nausea); blood disorders (anemia, leukopenia, thrombocytopenia); skin disorders (rashes, hair loss)
Gemcitabine	Gemzar	Carcinoma of the pancreas; non–small-cell lung cancer	Blood disorders (anemia, leukopenia, neutropenia, thrombocytopenia); dyspnea; edema; fever; skin rash; hematuria; GI distress (nausea, vomiting, constipation, diarrhea)
Mercaptopurine	Purinethol	Acute lymphocytic and myelocytic leukemia; chronic myelocytic leukemia	Blood disorders (anemia, leukopenia, thrombocytopenia); GI distress (nausea, anorexia); hepatotoxicity
Methotrexate	Folex, Mexate	Acute lymphocytic leukemia; meningeal leukemia; carcinoma of head and neck region, lung; non-Hodgkin lymphomas	Blood disorders (anemia, leukopenia, thrombocytopenia); GI distress (including ulceration of GI tract); skin disorders (rashes, photosensitivity, hair loss); hepatotoxicity; CNS effects (headaches, drowsiness, fatigue)
Pentostatin	Nipent	Hairy cell leukemia	Blood disorders (anemia, leukopenia, thrombocytopenia); allergic reaction; CNS toxicity (unusual tiredness, anxiety, confusion); headache; muscle pain; GI distress (nausea, vomiting, diarrhea)
Thioguanine	Lanvis	Acute lymphocytic leukemia; acute and chronic myelocytic leukemia	Blood disorders (anemia, leukopenia, thrombocytopenia); GI distress (nausea, vomiting); hepatotoxicity

*Only the indications listed in the U.S. product labeling are included here. Many anticancer drugs are used for additional types of neoplastic disease.

TABLE 36–3 Antineoplastic Antibiotics

Generic Name	Trade Name	Primary Antineoplastic Indication(s)*	Common Adverse Effects
Bleomycin	Blenoxane	Carcinoma of head, neck, cervical region, skin, penis, vulva, and testicle; Hodgkin disease; non-Hodgkin lymphomas	Pulmonary toxicity (interstitial pneumonitis); skin disorders (rashes, discoloration); mucosal lesions; fever; GI distress; general weakness and malaise
Dactinomycin	Cosmegen	Carcinoma of testicle and endometrium; carcinosarcoma of kidney (Wilms tumor); Ewing sarcoma; rhabdomyosarcoma	Blood disorders (leukopenia, thrombocytopenia, others); GI distress (nausea, vomiting, anorexia); mucocutaneous lesions; skin disorders (rashes, hair loss); local irritation at injection site
Daunorubicin	Cerubidine, DaunoXome	Several forms of acute leukemia	Blood disorders (anemia, leukopenia, thrombocytopenia); cardiotoxicity (arrhythmias, congestive heart failure); GI distress (nausea, vomiting, GI tract ulceration); hair loss
Doxorubicin	Adriamycin RDF, Rubex, others	Acute leukemias; carcinoma of bladder, breast, ovary, thyroid, and other tissues; Hodgkin disease; non-Hodgkin lymphomas; several sarcomas	Similar to daunorubicin
Idarubicin	Idamycin	Acute myelocytic leukemia	Similar to daunorubicin
Mitomycin	Mutamycin	Carcinoma of stomach and pancreas; chronic myelocytic leukemia	Blood disorders (leukopenia, thrombocytopenia); GI distress (nausea, vomiting, GI irritation and ulceration); nephrotoxicity; pulmonary toxicity
Mitoxantrone	Novantrone	Carcinoma of the prostate; acute nonlymphocytic leukemia	Cough, shortness of breath; leukopenia or infection; stomatitis and mucositis; GI problems (stomach pain, nausea, vomiting, diarrhea, GI bleeding)
Plicamycin	Mithracin	Testicular carcinoma	Blood disorders (leukopenia, thrombocytopenia); GI distress (nausea, vomiting, diarrhea, GI tract irritation); general weakness and malaise

*Only the indications listed in the U.S. product labeling are included here. Many anticancer drugs are used for additional types of neoplastic disease.

619

Plant Alkaloids

Alkaloids are nitrogen-based compounds frequently found in plants. The plant alkaloids used in treating cancer in humans include traditional agents, such as vincristine and vinblastine, and newer agents, such as vinorelbine, paclitaxel, and docetaxel (Table 36–4). These agents are also known as antimitotic drugs because they directly impair cell division. These drugs exert their antimitotic effects by binding to cellular microtubules and altering the function of these microtubules.[12] In particular, these drugs disrupt the function of microtubules that are involved in the mitotic apparatus of the cell (the mitotic spindle). Certain agents (vincristine, vinblastine, and vinorelbine) inhibit the formation of the mitotic apparatus, whereas others (paclitaxel, docetaxel) inhibit breakdown of these microtubules, thereby creating a stable but nonfunctional mitotic apparatus.[63] In either situation, these drugs disrupt the normal function of the mitotic apparatus and prevent the cell from dividing and proliferating. In fact, when the cell attempts to divide, the nuclear material becomes disrupted and dispersed throughout the cytosol. This effect causes damage directly to the chromosomes, leading to subsequent cell dysfunction and death.

Other drugs classified as plant alkaloids include etoposide, irinotecan, teniposide, and topotecan (see Table 36–4). Rather than directly affecting the mitotic apparatus, these drugs inhibit specific enzymes known as topoisomerase enzymes, necessary for DNA replication. Inhibition of these enzymes causes a break in both strands of the DNA double helix, which leads to DNA destruction and death of the cell. Etoposide and teniposide inhibit the topoisomerase I form of this enzyme, and irinotecan and topotecan inhibit the topoisomerase II form of this enzyme. These drugs are therefore used to limit cell division and cancer growth in various types of neoplastic disease (see Table 36–4).

Hormones

Several forms of cancer are referred to as hormone sensitive because they tend to be exacerbated by certain hormones and attenuated by others. In particular, adrenocorticosteroids (see Chap. 29) and the sex hormones (androgens, estrogens, and progesterone; see Chap. 30) may influence the proliferation of certain tumors. Hence, drugs that either mimic or block (antagonize) the effects of these hormones may be useful in treating certain hormone-sensitive forms of cancer.[17,63] Hormonal anticancer drugs are typically used as adjuvant therapy; that is, they are used in conjunction with surgery, radiation treatments, and other anticancer drugs.

The primary drugs that inhibit neoplasms via hormonal mechanisms are listed in Table 36–5. In some cases, these drugs work by direct inhibitory effects on cancerous cells (e.g., adrenocorticoid suppression of lymphocyte function) or by negative feedback mechanisms that decrease endogenous hormonal stimulation of the tumor (e.g., gonadotropin-releasing hormones). In other cases, drugs can directly block the effects of the endogenous hormone and prevent that hormone from stimulating specific tumors. In particular, androgen receptor blockers (flutamide) can treat prostate cancer by blocking the effects of testosterone on the prostate gland.[4,8,29] Estrogen receptor blockers (tamoxifen) can likewise help prevent and treat breast and uterine cancers that are stimulated by estrogen.[43,48] As indicated in Chapter 30, tamoxifen is actually classified as a selective estrogen receptor modulator (SERM), meaning that this drug blocks estrogen receptors on certain tissues (breast, uterus) while stimulating other estrogen receptors in bone, cardiovascular tissues, skin, and so forth.[43] Refer to Chapter 30 for more details about the effects of androgens, estrogens, and their respective receptor blocking agents.

TABLE 36–4 Plant Alkaloids

Generic Name	Trade Name	Primary Antineoplastic Indication(s)*	Common Adverse Effects
Docetaxel	Taxotere	Breast cancer	Blood disorders (anemia, leukopenia, neutropenia); fever; fluid retention; paresthesias and dysthesias; skin rashes and itching; stomatitis; GI distress (nausea, diarrhea)
Etoposide	Etopophos, VePesid	Carcinoma of lung, testes	Blood disorders (anemia, leukopenia, thrombocytopenia); GI distress (nausea, vomiting); hypotension, allergic reactions; hair loss; neurotoxicity (peripheral neuropathies, CNS effects)
Irinotecan	Camptosar	Colorectal cancer	Blood disorders (anemia, leukopenia, neutropenia); dyspnea; GI distress (nausea, vomiting, diarrhea, constipation, anorexia, abdominal cramps)
Paclitaxel	Taxol	Carcinoma of the breast, ovaries; Kaposi sarcoma; non–small-cell lung cancer	Blood disorders (anemia, leukopenia, neutropenia, thrombocytopenia); hypersensitivity reaction (skin rashes and itching, shortness of breath); joint and muscle pain; peripheral neuropathies; GI distress (nausea, vomiting, diarrhea)
Teniposide	Vumon	Acute lymphocytic leukemia	Blood disorders (anemia, leukopenia, neutropenia, thrombocytopenia); hypersensitivity reaction; mucositis; GI distress (nausea, vomiting, diarrhea)
Topotecan	Hycamtin	Ovarian cancer; small lung cell carcinoma	Blood disorders (anemia, leukopenia, neutropenia, thrombocytopenia); dyspnea; fever; neurological effects (muscle weakness, paresthesias); stomatitis; GI distress (abdominal pain, anorexia, nausea, vomiting, diarrhea, constipation)
Vinblastine	Velban, Velsar	Carcinoma of breast, testes, other tissues; Hodgkin disease; non-Hodgkin lymphomas; Kaposi sarcoma	Blood disorders (primarily leukopenia); GI distress (nausea, vomiting); hair loss; central and peripheral neuropathies; local irritation at injection site
Vincristine	Oncovin, Vincasar	Acute lymphocytic leukemia; neuroblastoma; Wilms tumor; Hodgkin disease; non-Hodgkin lymphomas; Ewing sarcoma	Neurotoxicity (peripheral neuropathies, CNS disorders); hair loss; local irritation at injection site
Vinorelbine	Navelbine	Non–small-cell lung cancer	Blood disorders (anemia, granulocytopenia, leukopenia); unusual weakness or fatigue; GI distress (anorexia, nausea, vomiting, constipation); hair loss

*Only the indications listed in the U.S. product labeling are included here. Many anticancer drugs are used for additional types of neoplastic disease.

621

TABLE 36–5 Antineoplastic Hormones

Types of Hormones	Primary Antineoplastic Indication(s)*	Common Adverse Effects

Adrenocorticosteroids
  Prednisone
  Prednisolone
  Others
	Acute lymphoblastic leukemia; chronic lymphocytic leukemia; Hodgkin disease	Adrenocortical suppression; general catabolic effect on supporting tissues (see Chap. 29)

Androgens
  Fluoxymesterone
  Methyltestosterone
  Testosterone
	Advanced, inoperable breast cancer in postmenopausal women	Masculinization in women (see Chap. 30)

Antiandrogens Flutamide	Inhibits the cellular uptake and effects of androgens in advanced, metastatic prostate cancer	Nausea, vomiting, diarrhea; decreased sex drive

Estrogens
  Diethylstilbestrol
  Estradiol
  Others
	Advanced, inoperable breast cancer in selected men and postmenopausal women; advanced, inoperable prostate cancer in men	Cardiovascular complications (including stroke and heart attack—especially in men); many other adverse effects (see Chap. 30)

Antiestrogens Tamoxifen	Acts as an estrogen antagonist to decrease the recurrence of cancer following mastectomy or to reduce tumor growth in advanced stages of breast cancer	Nausea, vomiting, hot flashes (generally well tolerated relative to other antineoplastic hormones)

Progestins
  Hydroxyprogesterone
  Medroxyprogesterone
  Megestrol
	Carcinoma of the breast and endometrium; advanced prostate cancer; advanced renal cancer	Menstrual irregularities; hyperglycemia; edema; mood changes; unusual tiredness; abdominal pain and cramps

Gonadotropin-releasing
  hormone drugs
  Leuprolide
  Goserelin
	Work by negative feedback mechanisms to inhibit testosterone or estrogen production; used primarily in advanced prostate cancer or breast cancer	Hot flashes; bone pain; CNS effects (e.g., headache, dizziness); GI disturbances (nausea, vomiting)

*Administration of hormonal agents in neoplastic disease is frequently palliative; that is, these drugs may offer some relief of symptoms but are not curative. Also, hormones are usually combined with other antineoplastic drugs or are used as an adjuvant to surgery and radiation treatment.

Biologic Response Modifiers

Agents such as the interferons and interleuklin-2 are classified as biologic response modifiers because they affect the body's ability to deal with neoplasms; that is, these drugs are not necessarily toxic to the cancerous cells, but they affect the mechanisms that regulate cell division or influence specific aspects of immune function that help inhibit or destroy the cancerous tissues.

The chemistry and pharmacology of the interferons were discussed in Chapter 34. Basically, these peptide compounds exert a number of beneficial effects, including antiviral and antineoplastic activity. The exact mechanism of action for interferons to impair cancerous cell growth is not clear, however. It is possible that interferons affect several aspects of tumor growth, including inhibition of cancerous genes (oncogenes), activation of cytotoxic immune cells (natural killer cells), and inhibition of other aspects of cell metabolism and proliferation in cancerous tissues.[63] These agents are currently used to treat certain types of leukemias, lymphomas, Kaposi sarcoma, and cancer in other organs and tissues (Table 36–6).[1,57]

Interleukin-2 (IL-2) is an endogenous cytokine that normally exerts a number of beneficial immunologic responses. In particular, IL-2 stimulates the growth and differentiation of T-cell lymphocytes that are selectively toxic for tumor cells.[12] Hence, recombinant DNA techniques are now used to synthesize IL-2 so that this agent can be used to treat cancers such as renal cancer and malignant melanoma (see Table 36–6). Research continues to identify the antineoplastic role of interleukins, interferons, and other cytokines and to define how these agents can be used alone or in combination to treat various forms of cancer.[9]

Heavy Metal Compounds

Heavy metal compounds used to treat cancer include cisplatin and carboplatin (see Table 36–6). These heavy metal drugs, which contain platinum, are also known as platinum coordination complexes.[12] These drugs act like the alkylating agents; that is, they form strong cross-links between and within DNA strands, thereby preventing DNA translation and replication. The chemical nature of these cross-links, however, involves the platinum component of the drug rather than actual formation of an alkyl side group. These heavy metal compounds are especially important in treating certain epithelial cancers, including testicular cancer, ovarian cancer, bladder cancer, and other cancers[12] (see Table 36–6).

Aspirin and Other NSAIDs

Considerable evidence exists that aspirin and similar nonsteroidal anti-inflammatory drugs (NSAIDs) may help prevent cancer in the colon and rectum.[2,32,39,45] This effect seems to be dose-related, with increased protection occurring in people who use aspirin on a regular basis.[58,61] The exact reason for this anticancer effect is not known.[2,32] As indicated in Chapter 15, aspirin and similar drugs inhibit the cyclooxygenase enzyme that synthesizes prostaglandins in various cells in the body. It is not clear, however, if these drugs reduce the risk of colorectal cancer by inhibiting prostaglandin synthesis or through some other mechanism that remains to be determined. More information will surely be forthcoming about how aspirin and other NSAIDs can help prevent specific types of cancer.

TABLE 36–6 Other Antineoplastic Drugs

Drug(s)	Primary Antineoplastic Indication(s)*	Common Adverse Effects
Biologic response modifiers		
Interferons		
Interferon alfa-2a (Roferon-A)	Hairy-cell leukemia, Kaposi sarcoma, chronic myelocytic leukemia, renal and bladder cancers	Flulike syndrome (mild fever, chills, malaise)
Interferon alfa-2b (Intron-A)		
Interleukin-2 Aldesleukin (Proleukin)	Renal carcinoma	Blood disorders (anemia, eosinophilia, leukopenia, thrombocytopenia); cardiac arrhythmias; hypotension; pulmonary toxicity; renal toxicity; neuropsychiatric effects; hypothyroidism
Heavy metal compounds		
Carboplatin (Paraplatin)	Carcinoma of the ovaries	Blood disorders (anemia, leukopenia, neutropenia, thrombocytopenia); unusual tiredness; GI distress (nausea, vomiting)
Cisplatin (Platinol)	Carcinoma of bladder, ovaries, testicles, and other tissues	Nephrotoxicity; GI distress (nausea, vomiting); neurotoxicity (cranial and peripheral nerves); hypersensitive reactions (e.g., flushing, respiratory problems, tachycardia)
Miscellaneous agents		
Asparaginase (Elspar)	Acute lymphocytic leukemia	Allergic reactions; renal toxicity; hepatic toxicity; delayed hemostasis; CNS toxicity (fatigue, mood changes); GI distress (nausea, vomiting); pancreatitis
Estramustine (Emcyt)	Prostate cancer	Sodium and fluid retention; blood disorders (leukopenia, thrombocytopenia); thrombosis; GI distress (nausea, diarrhea)
Hydroxyurea (Hydrea)	Carcinoma of the ovaries, head and neck region, other tissues; chronic myelocytic leukemia; melanomas	Blood disorders (primarily leukopenia); GI distress (nausea, vomiting, anorexia, GI tract irritation and ulceration); skin rashes
Mitotane (Lysodren)	Suppresses adrenal gland; used primarily to treat adrenocortical carcinoma	GI distress (nausea, vomiting, diarrhea, anorexia); CNS toxicity (lethargy, fatigue, mood changes); skin rashes
Tretinoin (Vesanoid)	Acute promyelocytic leukemia	Cardiac arrhythmias; edema; blood pressure abnormalities (hypotension, hypertension); phlebitis; respiratory tract problems; muscle pain; paresthesias; CNS toxicity (depression, anxiety, confusion); skin rash; GI distress (abdominal distension, nausea, vomiting)

*Only the indications listed in the U.S. product labeling are included here. Many anticancer drugs are used for additional types of neoplastic disease.

Miscellaneous Agents

Asparaginase. Asparaginase (Elspar) is an enzyme that converts the amino acid asparagine into aspartic acid and ammonia. Most normal cells are able to synthesize sufficient amounts of asparagine to function properly. Some tumor cells (especially certain leukemic cells) must rely on extracellular sources for a supply of asparagine, however. By breaking down asparagine in the bloodstream and extracellular fluid, asparaginase deprives tumor cells of their source of asparagine, thus selectively impairing cell metabolism in these cells.[63] Asparaginase is used primarily in the treatment of acute lymphocytic leukemia (see Table 36–6).

Estramustine. Chemically, estramustine (Emcyt) is a combination of mechlorethamine (an alkylating agent) and estrogen. It is not clear, however, how this drug exerts antineoplastic effects. Beneficial effects of this drug are probably not related to any alkylating effects. Rather, they may be the direct result of its estrogenic component or perhaps its inhibitory effect on the microtubules that comprise the mitotic apparatus.[63] This drug is typically used for the palliative treatment of advanced prostate cancer.

Hydroxyurea. Hydroxyurea (Hydrea) is believed to impair DNA synthesis by inhibiting a specific enzyme (ribonucleoside reductase) that is involved in synthesizing nucleic acid precursors.[63] Uses of hydroxyurea are listed in Table 36–6.

Mitotane. Although the exact mechanism of this drug is unknown, mitotane (Lysodren) selectively inhibits adrenocortical function. This agent is used exclusively to treat carcinoma of the adrenal cortex.

Tretinoin. Tretinoin (Vesanoid), known also as all-*trans*-retinoic acid, is derived from vitamin A (retinol).[63] This drug is not cytotoxic, but it may help cells differentiate and replicate at a more normal rate. However, the exact way that this agent affects cell differentiation is not known. Tretinoin is used primarily to treat certain forms of leukemia.

COMBINATION CHEMOTHERAPY

Frequently, several different anticancer drugs are administered simultaneously. This process of combination chemotherapy increases the chance of successfully treating the cancer because of an additive and synergistic effect of each agent. Often, different types of anticancer drugs are combined in the same regimen to provide optimal results.[63] For instance, a particular drug regimen may include an alkylating agent, an antineoplastic antibiotic, a hormonal agent, or some other combination of anticancer drugs.

Some common anticancer drug combinations and the types of cancer in which they are used are listed in Table 36–7. These drug combinations are often indicated by an acronym of the drug names. For instance, "FAC" indicates a regimen of fluorouracil, Adriamycin (doxorubicin), and cyclophosphamide. These abbreviations are used to summarize drug therapy in a patient's medical chart, so therapists should be aware of the more common chemotherapy combinations.

USE OF ANTICANCER DRUGS WITH OTHER TREATMENTS

Cancer chemotherapy is only one method of treating neoplastic disease. The other primary weapons in the anticancer arsenal are surgery and radiation treatment.[40,65] The choice of one or more of these techniques depends primarily on the patient, type of can-

TABLE 36–7 Frequently Used Combination Chemotherapy Regimens

Type of Cancer	Therapy	Components of Therapy Regimen
Breast	FAC	5-Fluorouracil, doxorubicin (Adriamycin), cyclophosphamide (Cytoxan)
	CMF	Cyclophosphamide (Cytoxan), methotrexate, 5-fluorouracil
	Cooper regimen (CVFMP)	5-Fluorouracil, methotrexate, vincristine (Oncovin), cyclophosphamide (Cytoxan), prednisone
Hodgkin disease	MOPP	Mustargen (mechlorethamine), Oncovin (Vincristine), procarbazine, prednisone
	ABVD	Doxorubicin (Adriamycin), bleomycin (Blenoxane), vinblastine (Velban), dacarbazine (DTIC)
Leukemia	OAP	Oncovin, Ara-C (cytarabine), prednisone
	COAP	Cyclophosphamide, Oncovin (vincristine), Ara-C (cytarabine), prednisone
	Ad-OAP	Adriamycin (doxorubicin), Oncovin (vincristine), Ara-C (cytarabine), prednisone
Multiple myeloma	VBAP	Vincristine, BCNU (carmustine), Adriamycin (doxorubicin), prednisone
	VCAP	Vincristine, Cytoxan (cyclophosphamide), Adriamycin (doxorubicin), prednisone
Non-Hodgkin lymphomas	CHOP	Cytoxan (cyclophosphamide), doxorubicin,* Oncovin, prednisone
	COP	Cytoxan (cyclophosphamide), Oncovin (vincristine), prednisone
Testicular tumors	VB-3	Vinblastine (Velban), bleomycin (Blenoxane)

*The H in this regimen refers to hydroxyldaunorubicin, the chemical synonym for doxorubicin.
Source: Moraca-Sawicki, AM: Antineoplastic chemotherapy. In Kuhn, MA: Pharmacotherapeutics: A Nursing Process Approach, ed 3. FA Davis, Philadelphia, 1994, p 1225, with permission.

cer, and location of the tumor. In many situations, chemotherapy may be the primary or sole form of treatment in neoplastic disease, especially for certain advanced or inoperable tumors or in widely disseminated forms of cancer, such as leukemia or lymphoma.[12] In other situations, chemotherapy is used in combination with other techniques, as an adjuvant to surgery and radiation treatment.[6,31,63] Primary examples of adjuvant cancer chemotherapy include using anticancer drugs following a mastectomy or surgical removal of other carcinomas.[27,36,37,55]

Whether anticancer drugs are used as the primary treatment or as adjuvant therapy, a common general strategy is upheld. To achieve a total cell kill, all reasonable means of dealing with the cancer are employed as early as possible. Cancer is not the type of disease in which a wait-and-see approach can be used. The general strategy is more aligned with the idea that a barrage of anticancer modalities (i.e., surgery, radiation, and a combination of several different antineoplastic drugs) may be necessary to achieve a successful outcome. In addition, a multimodal approach (combining chemotherapy with radiation or using several drugs simultaneously) may produce a synergistic effect between these modalities. For instance, certain drugs may sensitize cancer cells to radiation treatment.[13,25] Likewise, several drugs working together may increase the antineoplastic effects of one another through a synergistic cytotoxic effect.[63]

SUCCESS OF ANTICANCER DRUGS

Various forms of cancer exhibit a broad spectrum of response to antineoplastic medications. Some forms of cancer (choriocarcinoma, Wilms tumor) can be cured in more than 90 percent of the affected patients. In other neoplastic disorders, chemotherapy may not cure the disease but may succeed in mediating remission and prolonging survival in a large percentage of patients. Of course, other factors such as early detection of the cancer and the concomitant use of other interventions (surgery, radiation) will greatly influence the success of chemotherapy drugs.

However, several types of cancer do not respond well to treatment. For example, the majority of metastatic cancers cannot be cured by current chemotherapeutic methods or by any other type of treatment.[23,64] In addition, some of the most common forms of adult neoplastic disease are difficult to treat by using anticancer drugs. As indicated in Table 36–8, the number of deaths associated with colorectal, prostate, and breast cancer is unacceptably high, and the mortality rate for lung cancer and pancreatic cancer is well over 90 percent in both men and women.

Exactly why some forms of cancer are more difficult to treat pharmacologically than others remains unclear. Differences in the biochemistry, genetics, and location of certain cancer cells may make them less sensitive to the toxic effects of anticancer drugs.[23] Resistance to anticancer drugs (see "Resistance to Cancer Chemotherapy Drugs") may also be why certain cancers respond poorly to chemotherapy. Consequently, investigations of how to improve the efficacy of existing agents and the development of new anticancer drugs remain major foci in pharmacologic research. Some of the primary strategies in improving cancer chemotherapy are discussed in "Future Perspectives."

TABLE 36–8 Incidence and Mortality of the Leading Forms of Cancer in Women and Men

Type/Site of Cancer	Number of New Cases	Number of Deaths
Women		
Breast	182,800	40,800
Lung and bronchus	74,600	67,600
Colon and rectum	66,600	28,500
Uterine corpus	36,100	6,500
Non-Hodgkin lymphoma	23,200	12,400
Ovary	23,100	14,000
Pancreas	14,600	14,500
Men		
Prostate	180,400	31,900
Lung and bronchus	89,500	89,300
Colon and rectum	63,600	27,800
Urinary bladder	38,300	8,100
Non-Hodgkin lymphoma	31,700	13,700
Leukemia	16,900	12,100
Pancreas	13,700	13,700

Source: The American Cancer Society Department of Epidemiology and Surveillance Research, estimates for 2000.

RESISTANCE TO CANCER CHEMOTHERAPY DRUGS

As indicated previously, certain cancers do not respond well to cancer chemotherapy. A primary reason is that cancers may develop resistance to a broad range of chemotherapeutic agents (multiple drug resistance), thus rendering these drugs ineffective in treating the cancer.[23,50,56] Cancers can become resistant to drugs through several different mechanisms. One primary mechanism occurs when the cancer cell synthesizes a glycoprotein that acts as a drug efflux pump.[50,56] This glycoprotein pump is inserted into the cancer cell's membrane and effectively expels different types of anticancer drugs from the cancer cell. Thus, cancer chemotherapeutic agents are ineffective because they are removed from the cell before they have a chance to exert cytotoxic effects.

Cancer cells also use other mechanisms to induce drug resistance, including production of specific substances (glutathione, glutathione-S-transferases) that inactivate anticancer drugs within the cancer cell or development of mechanisms that repair DNA that is damaged by anticancer drugs.[28,42,56] Essentially, cancer cells are often capable of developing methods for self-preservation against a broad range of cytotoxic drugs. Hence, various strategies are being explored to prevent or overcome multiple-drug resistance during cancer chemotherapy. These strategies include altering the dosage, timing, and sequence of administration of different medications and using different combinations of medications to combat resistance.[35,47,52] Use of these strategies, along with the development of new anticancer agents that do not cause resistance (e.g., angiogenesis inhibitors; see the next section), should help increase the effectiveness of chemotherapy in certain types of cancer.

FUTURE PERSPECTIVES

Several new strategies are being explored to increase the effectiveness and decrease the toxicity of anticancer drugs.[19] As discussed previously, most of these drugs are toxic not only to tumor cells but also to normal cells. Nonetheless, if the drug can be delivered or targeted specifically for tumor cells, the drug will produce a more selective effect. One way that this targeting can be accomplished is by attaching the drug to another substance that is attracted specifically to tumor cells. For instance, joining the drug with an antibody that recognizes receptors only on cancerous cells may prove to be an effective method of delivering the drug directly to the neoplastic tissues.[62] Drugs may likewise be delivered more effectively to cancerous cells by encapsulating the drug in a microsphere or liposome that becomes lodged in the tumor.[15,26] Drug microspheres or other drug formulations can also be implanted surgically so that the drug remains fairly localized at the tumor site, thereby reducing its systemic effects.[15] Variations on these techniques and other delivery methods continue to be explored and may someday be used on a widespread basis to increase the effectiveness while decreasing the toxicity of anticancer drugs.

Another new and exciting approach to treating cancer is the use of agents that inhibit the development of blood vessels that supply tumors.[24,30,51] Tumors often induce the local vasculature to generate a rich network of blood vessels so that that the tumor can be supplied with oxygen and nutrients to sustain its growth. Because the formation of these new blood vessels (angiogenesis) is essential for tumor growth, agents that inhibit angiogenesis can have a fairly selective effect on the tumor without producing excessive effects on the vascularization of normal tissues.[24,30] These agents, known as angiogenesis inhibitors, can literally starve the tumor of oxygen and nutrients, thereby limiting tumor growth and promoting the death of cancerous cells. Clinical trials of angiogenesis inhibitors are ongoing, and these agents will hopefully become a valuable component in the treatment of various neoplasms.[51]

A number of other experimental strategies that limit the metabolism and proliferation of cancerous cells are likewise being explored. These strategies typically capitalize on some enzymatic process or other unique aspect of cancer cell metabolism so that normal tissues remain largely unaffected by the drug.[19,22,41,54] Additionally, several strategies are being explored to administer drugs that can protect healthy cells from the more traditional anticancer agents.[11,38] Hence, these strategies may ultimately produce chemotherapy regimens that are much more selective for cancerous cells and therefore less toxic to healthy tissues.

Finally, important advances have been made in understanding how the body's immune system can be recruited to help prevent and treat certain cancers. If the body's immune system recognizes the cancer cell as an invader, then various endogenous immune responses can be initiated to combat the cancerous cells. Hence, various strategies are being explored to help stimulate this immunologic response, including genetic modification of the cancer cells to increase their antigenic properties and expose these cells to immune attack.[12,59] These efforts may ultimately lead to anticancer vaccines, whereby the immune system can be sensitized to search out and destroy cancerous cells before they can develop into serious cancers.[19,34] Increased knowledge about the nature of cancer, combined with a better understanding of the endogenous control of cell replication, may ultimately provide drugs that are safe and effective in curing all forms of cancer.

IMPLICATIONS OF CANCER CHEMOTHERAPY IN REHABILITATION PATIENTS

The major way in which antineoplastic drugs will affect physical therapy and occupational therapy is through the adverse side effects of these agents. These drugs are routinely associated with a number of severe toxic effects, including gastrointestinal problems, blood disorders, and profound fatigue. Also, neurotoxic effects including CNS abnormalities (such as convulsions and ataxia) and peripheral neuropathies may be a problem, especially with the plant alkaloids (vinblastine, vincristine). In terms of physical rehabilitation, these side effects typically are a source of frustration to both patient and therapist. On some days, the patient undergoing cancer chemotherapy will simply not be able to tolerate even a relatively mild rehabilitation session. This reality can be especially demoralizing to patients who want to try to overcome their disease and actively participate in therapy as much as possible. Physical therapists and occupational therapists must take into account the debilitating nature of these drugs and be sensitive to the needs of the patient on a day-to-day basis. At certain times, the therapist must simply back off in trying to encourage active participation from the patient. Therapists, however, can often be particularly helpful in providing psychological support to patients undergoing antineoplastic drug treatment. Therapists can reassure the patient that the side effects of these drugs are usually transient and that there will be better days when rehabilitation can be resumed.

Therapists may also be helpful in treating other problems associated with neoplastic disease. In particular, therapists may be involved in reducing the severe pain typically associated with many forms of cancer. Therapists can use transcutaneous electric nerve stimulation (TENS) or other physical agents as a nonpharmacologic means to attenuate pain. Other physical interventions such as massage can also be invaluable in helping decrease the pain and anxiety that often occur in people receiving cancer chemotherapy. These approaches may reduce the need for pain medications, thus reducing the chance that these drugs will cause additional adverse effects and drug interactions with the anticancer drugs.

As previously mentioned, physical therapists and occupational therapists also play a vital role in providing encouragement and support to the patient with cancer. This support can often help immeasurably in improving the quality of life of the cancer patient.

CASE STUDY

CANCER CHEMOTHERAPY

Brief History. R.J. is a 57-year-old woman with metastatic breast cancer, diagnosed 1 year ago, at which time she underwent a modified radical mastectomy followed by antineoplastic drugs. The cancer, however, had evidently metastasized to other tissues, including bone. She recently developed pain in the lumbosacral region that was attributed to metastatic skeletal lesions in the lower lumbar vertebrae. She was admitted to the hospital to pursue a course of radiation treatment to control pain and minimize bony destruction at the site of the skeletal lesion. Her current pharmacologic regimen consists of an antineoplastic antimetabolite (doxorubicin) and an antiestrogen (tamoxifen). She was also given a combination of narcotic and nonnarcotic analgesics (codeine and aspirin) to help control pain. Physical therapy was consulted to help control pain and maintain function in this patient.

Problem/Influence of Medication. The patient began to experience an increase in gastrointestinal side effects, including nausea, vomiting, anorexia, and epigastric pain. These problems may have been caused by the analgesic drugs or by the combination of the analgesics and the antimetabolite. The patient, however, was experiencing adequate pain relief from the aspirin-codeine combination and was reluctant to consider alternative medications. The persistent nausea and anorexia had a general debilitating effect on the patient, and the physical therapist was having difficulty engaging the patient in an active general conditioning program.

Decision/Solution. The therapist instituted a program of local heat (hot packs) and TENS to help control pain in the lumbosacral region. This approach provided a nonpharmacologic means of alleviating pain, thereby decreasing the patient's analgesic drug requirements and related gastrointestinal problems. The patient was able to actively participate in a rehabilitation program throughout the course of her hospitalization, thus maintaining her overall strength and physical condition.

SUMMARY

Antineoplastic drugs typically limit excessive growth and proliferation of cancer cells by impairing DNA synthesis and function or by directly limiting cell division (mitosis). To replicate at a rapid rate, cancer cells must synthesize rather large quantities of DNA and RNA and continually undergo mitosis. Hence, cancer cells tend to be affected by antineoplastic drugs to a somewhat greater extent than normal cells. Normal cells, however, are also frequently affected by these drugs, resulting in a high incidence of adverse side effects. Currently, cancer chemotherapy is effective in reducing and even curing many neoplastic diseases. Other forms of cancer are much more difficult to treat pharmacologically, however. In the future, the development of methods that target the antineoplastic drug directly for cancer cells may improve the efficacy and safety of these agents. Rehabilitation specialists should be aware of the general debilitating nature of these drugs, and therapists must be prepared to adjust their treatment based on the ability of the patient to tolerate the adverse effects of cancer chemotherapy.

REFERENCES

1. Agarwala, SS and Kirkwood, JM: Interferons in the therapy of solid tumors. Oncology 51:129, 1994.
2. Ahnen, DJ: Colon cancer prevention by NSAIDs: What is the mechanism of action? Eur J Surg Suppl 582:111, 1998.
3. Allegra, CJ and Grem, JL: Antimetabolites. In DeVita, VT, Hellman, S, and Rosenberg, SA (eds): Cancer: Principles and Practice of Oncology, ed 5. Lippincott-Raven, Philadelphia, 1997.
4. Auclerc, G, et al: Management of advanced prostate cancer. Oncologist 5:36, 2000.
5. Baines, MJ: Symptom control in advanced gastrointestinal cancer. Eur J Gastroenterol Hepatol 12:375, 2000.
6. Bauer, TW and Spitz, FR: Adjuvant and neoadjuvant chemoradiation therapy for primary colorectal cancer. Surg Oncol 7:175, 1998.
7. Bischoff, PL, et al: Apoptosis at the interface of immunosuppressive and anticancer activities: The examples of two classes of chemical inducers, oxysterols and alkylating agents. Curr Med Chem 7:693, 2000.
8. Boccardo, F: Hormone therapy of prostate cancer: Is there a role for antiandrogen monotherapy? Crit Rev Oncol Hematol 35:121, 2000.
9. Bukowski, RM: Cytokine combinations: therapeutic use in patients with advanced renal cell carcinoma. Semin Oncol 27:204, 2000.
10. Calabresi, P and Chabner, BA: Chemotherapy of neoplastic diseases: Introduction. In Hardman, JG, et al (eds): The Pharmacological Basis of Therapeutics, ed 9. McGraw-Hill, New York, 1996.
11. Capizzi, RL: The preclinical basis for broad-spectrum selective cytoprotection of normal tissues from cytotoxic therapies by amifostine. Semin Oncol 26(Suppl 7):3, 1999.
12. Chabner, BA, et al: Antineoplastic agents. In Hardman, JG, et al (eds): The Pharmacological Basis of Therapeutics, ed 9. McGraw-Hill, New York, 1996.
13. Comis, RL, Friedland, DM, and Good, BC: The role of oral etoposide in non-small cell lung cancer. Drugs 58(Suppl 3):21, 1999.
14. Cotran, RS, Kumar, V, and Robbins, SL: Basic Pathology, ed 6. WB Saunders, Philadelphia, 1999.
15. Dhanikula, AB and Panchagnula, R: Localized paclitaxel delivery. Int J Pharm 183:85, 1999.
16. Eastman, A and Rigas, JR: Modulation of apoptosis signaling pathways and cell cycle regulation. Semin Oncol 26(Suppl 16):7, 1999.
17. Erlichman, C and Loprinzi, CL: Hormonal therapies. In DeVita, VT, Hellman, S, and Rosenberg, SA (eds): Cancer: Principles and Practice of Oncology, ed 5. Lippincott-Raven, Philadelphia, 1997.
18. Fauser, AA, et al: Guidelines for anti-emetic therapy: Acute emesis. Eur J Cancer 35:361, 1999.
19. Ferrante, K, Winograd, B, and Canetta, R: Promising new developments in cancer chemotherapy. Cancer Chemother Pharmacol 43(Suppl):S61, 1999.
20. Foley, KM: Management of cancer pain. In DeVita, VT, Hellman, S, and Rosenberg, SA (eds): Cancer: Principles and Practice of Oncology, ed 5. Lippincott-Raven, Philadelphia, 1997.
21. Gewirtz, DA: A critical evaluation of the mechanisms of action proposed for the antitumor effects of the anthracycline antibiotics adriamycin and daunorubicin. Biochem Pharmacol 57:727, 1999.
22. Giavazzi, R and Taraboletti, G: Preclinical development of metalloproteasis inhibitors in cancer therapy. Crit Rev Oncol Hematol 37:53, 2001.
23. Gottesman, MM: How cancer cells evade chemotherapy. Cancer Res 53:747, 1993.
24. Gourley, M and Williamson, JS: Angiogenesis: New targets for the development of anticancer chemotherapies. Curr Pharm Des 6:417, 2000.
25. Gregoire, V, et al: Chemo-radiotherapy: Radiosensitizing nucleoside analogues. Oncol Rep 6:949, 1999.
26. Harrington, KJ, Lewanski, CR, and Stewart, JS: Liposomes as vehicles for targeted therapy of cancer. Part 2: Clinical development. Clin Oncol (R Coll Radiol) 12:16, 2000.
27. Hortobagyi, G: Adjuvant therapy for breast cancer. Annu Rev Med 51:377, 2000.
28. Johnson, SW, Ozols, RF, and Hamilton, TC: Mechanisms of drug resistance in ovarian cancer. Cancer 71(Suppl 2):644, 1993.
29. Klotz, L: Hormone therapy for patients with prostate carcinoma. Cancer 88(Suppl):3009, 2000.
30. Konno, H, et al: Antiangiogenic therapy for liver metastasis of gastrointestinal malignancies. J Hepatobiliary Pancreat Surg 6:1, 1999.
31. Koutcher, JA, et al: Potentiation of a three drug chemotherapy regimen by radiation. Cancer Res 53:3518, 1993.

32. Kubba, AK: Nonsteroidal anti-inflammatory drugs and colorectal cancer: Is there a way forward? Eur J Cancer 35:892, 1999.

33. Kwon, CH: Metabolism-based anticancer drug design. Arch Pharm Res 22:533, 1999.

34. Laheru, DA and Jaffee, EM: Potential role of tumor vaccines in GI malignancies. Oncology 14:245, 2000.

35. Lauer, SJ, et al: Intensive alternating drug pairs for treatment of high-risk childhood acute lymphoblastic leukemia: A pediatric oncology group pilot study. Cancer 71:2854, 1993.

36. Lee, JH, et al: Outcome of pancreaticoduodenectomy and impact of adjuvant therapy for ampullary carcinomas. Int J Radiat Oncol Biol Phys 47:945, 2000.

37. Lim, CS, et al: Neoadjuvant therapy in the treatment of high risk rectal carcinoma. Surg Oncol 8:1, 1999.

38. Links, M and Lewis, C: Chemoprotectants: A review of their clinical pharmacology and therapeutic efficacy. Drugs 57:293, 1999.

39. Logan, RFA, et al: Effect of aspirin and nonsteroidal anti-inflammatory drugs in colorectal adenomas: Case-control study of subjects participating in the Nottingham faecal occult blood screening programme. BMJ 307:285, 1993.

40. Martin, RF and Rossi, RL: Multidisciplinary considerations for patients with cancer of the pancreas or biliary tract. Surg Clin North Am 80:709, 2000.

41. Nelson, AR, et al: Matrix metalloproteinases: Biologic activity and clinical implications. J Clin Oncol 18:1135, 2000.

42. Nishio, K, et al: Drug resistance in lung cancer. Curr Opin Oncol 11:109, 1999.

43. Osborne, CK, Zhao, H, and Fuqua, SA: Selective estrogen receptor modulators: Structure, function, and clinical use. J Clin Oncol 18:3172, 2000.

44. Osoba, D: Health-related quality-of-life assessment in clinical trials of supportive care in oncology. Support Care Cancer 8:84, 2000.

45. Pereira, MA: Prevention of colon cancer and modulation of aberrant crypt foci, cell proliferation, and apoptosis by retinoids and NSAIDs. Adv Exp Med Biol 470:55, 1999.

46. Perez, EA: 5-HT3 antiemetic therapy for patients with breast cancer. Breast Cancer Res Treat 57:207, 1999.

47. Perez, RP, et al: Mechanisms and modulation of resistance to chemotherapy in ovarian cancer. Cancer 71(Suppl 4):1571, 1993.

48. Pritchard, KI: Current and future directions in medical therapy for breast carcinoma: Endocrine treatment. Cancer 88(Suppl):3065, 2000.

49. Rizk, AN and Hesketh, PJ: Antiemetics for cancer chemotherapy-induced nausea and vomiting. A review of agents in development. Drugs R D 2:229, 1999.

50. Robert, J: Multidrug resistance in oncology: Diagnostic and therapeutic approaches. Eur J Clin Invest 29:536, 1999.

51. Rosen, L: Antiangiogenic strategies and agents in clinical trials. Oncologist 5(Suppl 1):20, 2000.

52. Ross, DD, et al: Enhancement of daunorubicin accumulation, retention, and cytotoxicity by verapamil or cyclosporin-A in blast cells from patients with previously untreated acute myeloid leukemia. Blood 82:1288, 1993.

53. Rubin, E and Farber, JL: Neoplasia. In Rubin, E and Farber, JL (eds): Pathology, ed 3. Lippincott, Philadelphia, 1999.

54. Saijo, N, Tamura, T, and Nishio, K: Problems in the development of target-based drugs. Cancer Chemother Pharmacol 46(Suppl):S43, 2000.

55. Sapunar, F and Smith IE: Neoadjuvant chemotherapy for breast cancer. Ann Med 32:43, 2000.

56. Schneider, E and Cowan, KH: Multiple drug resistance in cancer therapy. Med J Aust 160:371, 1994.

57. Solal-Celigny, P, et al: Recombinant interferon alfa-2b combined with a regimen containing doxorubicin in patients with advanced folliclar lymphoma. N Engl J Med 329:1608, 1993.

58. Suh, O, Mettlin, C, and Petrelli, NJ: Aspirin use, cancer, and polyps of the large bowel. Cancer 72:1171, 1993.

59. Symposium (various authors): Gene therapy for neoplastic diseases. Ann N Y Acad Sci 716:1, 1994.

60. Teicher, BA: Antitumor alkylating agents. In DeVita, VT, Hellman, S, and Rosenberg, SA (eds): Cancer: Principles and Practice of Oncology, ed 5. Lippincott-Raven, Philadelphia, 1997.

61. Thun, MJ, et al: Aspirin use and risk of fatal cancer. Cancer Res 53:1322, 1993.

62. Trail, PA and Bianchi, AB: Monoclonal antibody drug conjugates in the treatment of cancer. Curr Opin Immunol 11:584, 1999.

63. Valley, AW and Balmer, CM: Cancer treatment and chemotherapy. In DiPiro, JT, et al (eds): Pharmacotherapy: A Pathophysiologic Approach, ed 4. Appleton & Lange, Stamford, CT, 1999.

64. Verweij, J and de Jonge, MJ: Achievements and future of chemotherapy. Eur J Cancer 36:1479, 2000.

65. Vokes, EE, Haraf, DJ, and Kies, MS: The use of concurrent chemotherapy and radiotherapy for locoregionally advanced head and neck cancer. Semin Oncol 27(Suppl 8):34, 2000.

66. Walsh, D, et al: Symptom control in advanced cancer: Important drugs and routes of administration. Semin Oncol 27:69, 2000.

CHAPTER 37

Immunomodulating Agents

The immune system is responsible for controlling the body's response to various types of injury and for defending the body from invading pathogens, including bacteria, viruses, and other parasites.[11,19] The importance of this system in maintaining health is illustrated by the devastating effects that can occur in people who lack adequate immune function, such as patients with AIDS. The use of drugs to modify immune responses, or immunomodulating agents, is therefore an important area of pharmacology. For example, it may be helpful to augment immune function if a person's immune system is not functioning adequately. By contrast, it is sometimes necessary to suppress immune function pharmacologically to prevent immune-mediated injury to certain tissues or organs. Following organ transplants and tissue grafts, the immune system may cause rejection of tissues transplanted from other donors (*allografts*) or from other sites in the patient's own body (*autografts*).[5] Likewise, immunosuppression may be helpful when, for some reason, the immune system causes damage to the body's own tissues. Such conditions are often referred to as *autoimmune diseases*. Clinical disorders such as rheumatoid arthritis, myasthenia gravis, and systemic lupus erythematosus are now recognized as having an autoimmune basis.[19]

This chapter addresses immunosuppressive drugs, or **immunosuppressants,** that are currently available to prevent rejection of transplants or to treat specific diseases caused by an autoimmune response. Clearly, these drugs must be used very cautiously because too much suppression of the immune system will increase the susceptibility of the patient to infection from foreign pathogens. Likewise, these drugs are rather toxic and often cause a number of adverse effects to the kidneys, lungs, musculoskeletal system, and other tissues. Nonetheless, immunosuppressive agents are often lifesaving because of their ability to prevent and treat organ rejection and to decrease immune-mediated tissue damage in other diseases.

Drugs that increase immune function, or immunostimulants, are also addressed. This group of agents is rather small, and the clinical use of immunostimulants is limited when compared with the indications for immunosuppressive drugs. Nonetheless, the development and use of immunostimulants is an exciting area of pharmacology, and some insight into the therapeutic use of these drugs is provided.

This chapter begins with a brief overview of the immune response, followed by the drugs that are currently available to suppress or stimulate this response. Physical therapists and occupational therapists may be involved in the rehabilitation of patients who have received organ transplants, skin grafts, or similar procedures that necessitate the use of immunosuppressant drugs. Rehabilitation specialists also often treat patients with autoimmune disorders or immunodeficiency syndromes that affect the musculoskeletal system, and these patients are also likely to be taking immunomodulating drugs. Hence, this chapter will provide therapists with knowledge about the pharmacology of these drugs and how drug effects and side effects can affect physical rehabilitation.

OVERVIEW OF THE IMMUNE RESPONSE

As indicated, one of the primary responsibilities of the immune system is to protect the body from bacteria, viruses, and other foreign pathogens. The immune response consists of two primary components: innate immunity and acquired immunity.[11] Innate immunity involves specific cells (leukocytes) that are present at birth and provide a relatively rapid and nonselective defense against foreign invaders and pathogens throughout the individual's lifetime.[15] Acquired immunity primarily involves certain lymphocytes (T and B lymphocytes) that develop more slowly but retain the ability to recognize specific invading microorganisms and initiate specific steps to attack and destroy the invading cell.[15] The innate and acquired branches of the immune response are both needed for optimal immune function, and there is extensive interaction between innate and acquired immune responses.[10,11,27] The acquired response's ability to recognize and deal with foreign pathogens likewise involves an incredibly complex interaction between various cellular and chemical (humoral) components.[15,19] A detailed description of the intricacies of how these components work together is beyond the scope of this chapter. Additionally, many aspects of the immune response are still being investigated. An overview of key cellular and humoral elements that mediate acquired immunity is illustrated in Figure 37–1, and these elements are described briefly here.

1. *Antigen ingestion, processing, and presentation:*   An invading substance (*antigen*) is engulfed by phagocytes such as macrophages and other antigen-presenting cells (APCs).[15] The APCs then process the antigen by forming a complex between the antigen and specific membrane proteins known as major histocompatibility complex (MHC) proteins. The antigen-MHC complex is placed on the surface of the APC, where this complex can be presented to other lymphocytes such as the T cells. The APCs also synthesize and release chemical mediators such as interleukin-1 (IL-1) and other cytokines, which act on other immune cells (T cells) to amplify the response of these cells to immune mediators.

2. *Antigen recognition and T-cell activation:*   Lymphocytes derived from thymic tissues (hence the term *T cell*) recognize the antigen-MHC complex that is presented to the T cell on the surface of the macrophage. This recognition activates certain T cells (T helper cells), which begin to synthesize and release a number of chemical mediators known as **lymphokines.**[19] These lymphokines are cytokines derived from activated T lymphocytes and include mediators such as interleukin-2 (IL-2), other interleukins, gamma interferon, B-cell growth and differentiation factors, and other chemicals that stimulate the immune system. Certain T cells (T killer cells) are also activated by the APC presentation, and these T killer cells directly destroy targeted antigens.

3. *Proliferation, amplification, and recruitment:*   The T cells continue to replicate and proliferate, thus producing more lymphokines, which further amplify T-cell effects. These lymphokines also recruit lymphocytes derived from bone marrow—that is, B cells.[15] Under the direction of IL-1 and other lymphokines, B cells proliferate and

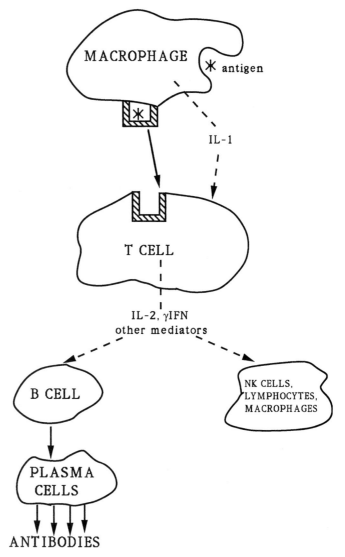

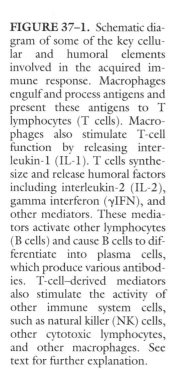

FIGURE 37–1. Schematic diagram of some of the key cellular and humoral elements involved in the acquired immune response. Macrophages engulf and process antigens and present these antigens to T lymphocytes (T cells). Macrophages also stimulate T-cell function by releasing interleukin-1 (IL-1). T cells synthesize and release humoral factors including interleukin-2 (IL-2), gamma interferon (γIFN), and other mediators. These mediators activate other lymphocytes (B cells) and cause B cells to differentiate into plasma cells, which produce various antibodies. T-cell–derived mediators also stimulate the activity of other immune system cells, such as natural killer (NK) cells, other cytotoxic lymphocytes, and other macrophages. See text for further explanation.

differentiate into plasma cells. Plasma cells ultimately release specific antibodies known as *immunoglobulins* (IgG, IgA, IgM, and the like). Likewise, T-cell and macrophage-derived lymphokines recruit additional cellular components, including other macrophages, other cytotoxic lymphocytes (natural killer, or NK, cells), and various other cells that can participate in the destruction of the foreign antigen.

Clearly, the immune response is an intricate sequence of events that involves a complex interaction between a number of cellular and humoral components. The overview provided here is just a brief summary of how some of the primary components participate in mediating acquired immunity. Readers are referred to additional sources for more information on this topic.[15,19]

PHARMACOLOGIC SUPPRESSION
OF THE IMMUNE RESPONSE

Drugs are used to suppress the immune system for two basic reasons (Table 37–1). First, the immune response is often attenuated pharmacologically following transplantation of organs or tissues to prevent rejection of these tissues.[2,32] Sometimes, organs and other tissues can be attacked by the recipient's immune system even if these tissues appear to be cross-matched between donor and recipient. This rejection is often because of membrane proteins on the donor tissue that are recognized as antigens by the host's immune system.[19] Hence, drugs that suppress the cellular and chemical response to these membrane proteins can help prevent these responses from destroying the transplanted tissues and causing additional injury to the host's tissues.

Often, several different types of immunosuppressants are used together in fairly high doses to prevent or treat transplant rejection.[17,29,45] For instance, a glucocorticoid such as betamethasone is often administered with nonsteroidal drugs such as cyclosporine and azathioprine to provide optimal success and viability of the transplant. Of course, giving several powerful drugs at high doses often causes unpleasant or even toxic side effects. These effects must often be tolerated, however, considering the limited number of organs that are available for transplantation and the need to ensure survival of the transplant as much as possible.

A second major indication for these drugs is to limit immune-mediated damage to the body's tissues—that is, suppression of an autoimmune response.[2,24] Autoimmune responses occur when the immune system loses the ability to differentiate the body's own tissues from foreign or pathogenic tissues.[19] Exactly what causes this defect in immune recognition is often unclear, but prior exposure to some pathogen such as a virus may activate the immune response in a way that causes the immune system to mistakenly attack normal tissues while trying to destroy the virus. This autoimmune activation may remain in effect even after the original pathogen has been destroyed, thus leading to chronic immune-mediated injury to the body's tissues.

Autoimmune responses seem to be the underlying basis for a number of diseases, including rheumatoid arthritis, diabetes mellitus, myasthenia gravis, systemic lupus erythematosus, scleroderma, polymyositis/dermatomyositis, and several other disorders.[19] As indicated previously, it is not exactly clear what factors cause autoimmune responses, and why certain individuals are more prone to autoimmune-related diseases remains to be elucidated. Nonetheless, drugs that suppress the immune system can limit damage to various other tissues, and these drugs may produce dramatic improvements in patients with diseases that are caused by an autoimmune response.

SPECIFIC IMMUNOSUPPRESSIVE AGENTS

Drugs commonly used to suppress the immune system are listed in Table 37–1, and the pharmacology of specific agents follows.

Azathioprine

Clinical Use. Azathioprine (Imuran) is a cytotoxic agent that is structurally and functionally similar to certain anticancer drugs, such as mercaptopurine.[7] Azathioprine is used primarily to prevent rejection of transplanted organs, especially in patients with

TABLE 37–1 Common Immunosuppressive Agents

| Generic Name | Trade Name(s) | Primary Indications* | |
		Prevention or Treatment of Transplant Rejection	Diseases That Have an Autoimmune Response
Antibodies	Names vary according to specific lymphocyte targets; see Table 37–2	Bone marrow, other organ transplants (see Table 37–2)	Idiopathic thrombocytic purpura, other hemolytic disorders
Azathioprine	Imuran	Kidney, heart, liver, pancreas	Rheumatoid arthritis, inflammatory bowel disease, myasthenia gravis, systemic lupus erythematosus (SLE), others
Cyclophosphamide	Cytoxan, Neosar	Bone marrow, other organ transplants	Rheumatoid arthritis, multiple sclerosis, SLE, dermatomyositis, glomerulonephritis, hematologic disorders
Cyclosporine	Neoral, Sandimmune	Kidney, liver, heart, lung, pancreas, bone marrow	Psoriasis, rheumatoid arthritis, nephrotic syndrome
Glucocorticoids	See text for listing	Heart, kidney, liver, bone marrow	Multiple sclerosis, rheumatoid arthritis, SLE, inflammatory bowel disease, hemolytic disorders, others
Methotrexate	Folex, Mexate, Rheumatrex	—	Rheumatoid arthritis, psoriasis
Mycophenolate mofetil	CellCept	Heart, kidney	—
Sirolimus	Rapamune	Kidney, heart, liver	Rheumatoid arthritis, psoriasis, SLE
Sulfasalazine	Azulfidine, others	—	Rheumatoid arthritis, inflammatory bowel disease
Tacrolimus	Prograf	Liver, kidney, heart, lung, pancreas	Uveitis

*Indications vary considerably, and many indications listed here are not in the U.S. product labeling for each drug; optimal use of these drugs alone or in combination with each other continues to be investigated.

kidney transplants. Azathioprine may also be used to suppress the immune response in a wide range of other conditions, such as systemic lupus erythematosus, dermatomyositis, inflammatory myopathy, hepatic disease, myasthenia gravis, and ulcerative colitis. As presented in Chapter 16, azathioprine is also used as an antiarthritic disease-modifying agent.

Mechanism of Action. Although the exact mechanism of azathioprine is unknown, this drug probably interferes with DNA synthesis in cells that mediate the immune response. Azathioprine appears to act like the antimetabolite drugs used in cancer chemotherapy (see Chap. 36). The cell normally uses various endogenous substances such as purines as ingredients during DNA synthesis. Azathioprine is structurally similar to these purines, and this drug acts as a false ingredient that competes with the naturally occurring substances to slow down and disrupt DNA synthesis. Impaired nucleic acid synthesis slows down the replication of lymphocytes and other key cellular components that direct the immune response. Thus, azathioprine directly limits cellular proliferation through this inhibitory effect on DNA synthesis and ultimately limits the production of humoral components (antibodies) produced by these cells.

Adverse Effects. The primary side effects of azathioprine are related to suppression of bone marrow function, including leukopenia, megaloblastic anemia, and similar blood dyscrasias. Other side effects include skin rash and gastrointestinal distress (appetite loss, nausea, vomiting), and hepatic dysfunction can also occur when higher doses are used.

Cyclophosphamide

Clinical Use. Cyclophosphamide (Cytoxan) is an anticancer alkylating agent that is commonly used in a variety of neoplastic disorders (see Chap. 36). This drug may also be helpful in suppressing the immune response in certain autoimmune diseases, such as multiple sclerosis, systemic lupus erythematosus, and rheumatoid arthritis.[2] High doses of cyclophosphamide are also used to prevent tissue rejection in patients receiving bone marrow transplants and other organ transplants.

Mechanism of Action. The mechanism of cyclophosphamide as an anticancer alkylating agent was described in Chapter 36. This drug causes strong cross-links to be formed between strands of DNA and RNA, thus inhibiting DNA/RNA replication and function. Cyclophosphamide probably exerts immunosuppressant effects in a similar manner; that is, this drug inhibits DNA and RNA function in lymphocytes and other key cells, thus limiting the rapid proliferation of these cells during the immune response.

Adverse Effects. Cyclophosphamide is used very cautiously as an immunosuppressant because of the possibility of severe side effects, including carcinogenic effects during long-term use. Other serious side effects include hematologic disorders (leukopenia, thrombocytopenia), cardiotoxicity, nephrotoxicity, and pulmonary toxicity.

Cyclosporine

Clinical Use. Cyclosporine (Neoral, Sandimmune) is one of the primary medications used to suppress immune function following organ transplantation.[2,8] This medication can be used alone or combined with glucocorticoids, azathioprine, and other immunosuppressants to prevent rejection of kidney, lung, liver, heart, pancreas, and other organ transplants. Cyclosporine is used to a somewhat lesser extent in treating autoimmune diseases, but it may be helpful in conditions such as psoriasis, rheumatoid arthritis, inflammatory bowel disease, and glomerulonephritis.[2] As discussed in Chapter 32, cyclosporine has also been used in the early stages of type 1 diabetes mellitus to help control immune-mediated destruction of pancreatic beta cells, thus decreasing the severity of this disease in some patients.[4]

Although cyclosporine is one of the most effective immunosuppressants, the traditional form of this drug is associated with unpredictable absorption from the GI tract and potentially severe side effects, such as nephrotoxicity and neurotoxicity.[6,12,31,41] In a newer form of cyclosporine, this drug is modified into microemulsion capsules that disperse more easily within the GI tract, thereby enabling the drug to be absorbed in a more predictable fashion.[22,49] The microemulsion form of cyclosporine appears to be safer because it is not as toxic to the kidneys and other tissues as the regular formulation.[3,23] Hence, this microemulsion formulation (marketed under the trade name Neoral) is often the optimal way to administer cyclosporine following organ transplantation or other situations requiring immunosuppression.[3,12,45]

Mechanism of Action. Cyclosporine inhibits a specific protein (calcineurin) in lymphoid tissues, and this inhibition ultimately inhibits the production of IL-2.[7] IL-2 plays a critical role in the immune response because this substance promotes the growth and proliferation of activated T lymphocytes and other immune cells, such as natural killer (NK) cells (see Fig. 37–1). Thus, cyclosporine is one of the premier immunosuppressants because of its relative selectivity for T cells and inhibition of a key mediator of the immune response (IL-2).[7] This relatively specific inhibition is often advantageous when compared with other nonselective drugs such as azathioprine, cyclophosphamide, and glucocorticoids that inhibit virtually all the cells and chemical mediators involved in the immune response.

Adverse Effects. The primary problem associated with cyclosporine is nephrotoxicity, which can range from mild, asymptomatic cases to severe kidney dysfunction requiring discontinuation of the drug.[6,31] Hypertension is also a common adverse effect, especially when cyclosporine is used for prolonged periods.[38] Other problems include neurotoxicity, gingival hyperplasia, hair growth (hirsutism), and increased infections. These problems, however, tend to be less severe with cyclosporine than with less selective immunosuppressants.

Glucocorticoids

Clinical Use. As described in Chapter 29, glucocorticoids are powerful anti-inflammatory and immunosuppressive drugs. Glucocorticoids exert a rather nonspecific inhibition of virtually all aspects of cell-mediated and chemical-mediated immunity, thus enabling these drugs to be used in a variety of situations when it is necessary to suppress immune function. Hence, these drugs are a mainstay in preventing transplant rejection and in treating various diseases associated with an autoimmune response.[1,39] Glucocorticoids commonly used as immunosuppressants include the following:

- betamethasone (Celestone)
- cortisone (Cortone)
- dexamethasone (Decadron, others)
- hydrocortisone (Cortef)
- methylprednisolone (Medrol)
- prednisolone (Pediapred, Predate, others)
- prednisone (Deltasone, others)
- triamcinolone (Aristocort)

Mechanism of Action. Although their exact mechanism of immunosuppression is unclear, glucocorticoids probably interrupt the immune response by a complex effect at the genomic level of various immune cells.[39,47] These drugs enter immune system cells, where they bind to a cytoplasmic receptor. The drug-receptor complex then migrates to the cell's nucleus, where it acts directly on specific immunoregulatory genes. In particular, glucocorticoids influence the expression of cytokines and other chemicals that orchestrate the immune response; that is, glucocorticoids inhibit the transcription of messenger RNA units that are normally translated into immunostimulatory signals such as interleukin-1, gamma interferon, and other substances that activate the cells responsible for mediating the immune response. Hence, these drugs disrupt the production of chemical signals that activate and control various cellular components of the immune system. See Chapter 29 for more details about how glucocorticoids exert their effects on various cells and tissues.

Adverse Effects. The immunosuppressive effects of these drugs are balanced by several serious side effects. As described in Chapter 29, glucocorticoids typically produce a catabolic effect on collagenous tissues, and breakdown of muscle, bone, skin, and various other tissues is a common adverse effect. Glucocorticoids also produce other side effects including hypertension, adrenocortical suppression, growth retardation in children, increased chance of infection, glaucoma, decreased glucose tolerance, and gastric ulcer. These side effects can be especially problematic when glucocorticoids are used to prevent transplant rejection because these drugs are often given in fairly high doses for extended periods.

Therefore, glucocorticoids typically are combined with other nonsteroidal immunosuppressants such as cyclosporine and azathioprine so that synergistic effects can be obtained and immunosuppression achieved with relatively lower doses of each drug.[45] In addition, efforts are often made to progressively decrease glucocorticoid dosage so that immunosuppression is achieved by using the lowest possible dose. In some cases, the glucocorticoid may even be withdrawn during maintenance immunosuppressive therapy, with nonsteroidal drugs (cyclosporine, tacrolimus, mycophenolate mofetil) used to provide long-term immunosuppression following organ transplantation.[9,14,36]

Methotrexate

Clinical Use. Methotrexate (Folex, Mexate, Rheumatrex) was developed originally as an anticancer agent (see Chap. 36), but this drug is also used occasionally in certain noncancerous conditions that have an autoimmune component.[7] As indicated in Chapter 16, methotrexate is commonly used as a disease-modifying drug in rheumatoid arthritis. Methotrexate is also approved for use in psoriasis. Methotrexate has only mild immunosuppressive effects, however, and this drug is not typically used to treat organ transplants or other conditions that require more extensive immunosuppression.

Mechanism of Action. The pharmacology of methotrexate is described in Chapter 36. This drug acts as an antimetabolite that interferes with the production of DNA and RNA precursors in rapidly proliferating cells. This interference produces a general inhibition of the replication of lymphocytes inherent in the immune response.

Adverse Effects. The major problems associated with methotrexate include hepatic and pulmonary toxicity. These problems are dose-related, however, and serious adverse effects tend to occur less frequently at doses used for immunosuppression than at anticancer doses.

Mycophenolate Mofetil

Clinical Use. Mycophenolate mofetil (CellCept) is used primarily to prevent or treat organ rejection following cardiac and renal transplantation. This drug is typically combined with other immunosuppressants (cyclosporine, glucocorticoids) to provide optimal immunosuppression in people receiving these transplants.[42] Mycophenolate mofetil may also be useful in suppressing the immune response associated with autoimmune conditions such as systemic lupus erythematosus.[13,44]

Mechanism of Action. Mycophenolate mofetil inhibits a specific enzyme (inosine monophosphate dehydrogenase) that is responsible for the synthesis of DNA precursors in T and B lymphocytes.[18,28,42] Because these lymphocytes cannot synthesize adequate amounts of DNA, their ability to replicate and proliferate is impaired, thus blunting the immune response. This drug may also inhibit lymphocyte attraction and adhesion to the vascular endothelium, thereby impairing the ability of these lymphocytes to migrate to the site of the foreign (transplanted) tissues and infiltrate from the bloodstream into these tissues.[28]

Adverse Effects. The primary adverse effects associated with mycophenolate mofetil are blood disorders (anemia, leukopenia, neutropenia) and gastrointestinal problems (abdominal pain, nausea, vomiting, heartburn, diarrhea or constipation).[28] Other side effects of this drug include chest pain, cough, dyspnea, muscle pain, weakness, and cardiovascular problems (hypertension, arrhythmias).

Sulfasalazine

Clinical Use. Sulfasalazine (Azulfidine, other names) has unique properties, with some antibacterial characteristics similar to sulfonamide drugs (see Chap. 33) and some anti-inflammatory characteristics similar to the salicylates (see Chap. 15). This drug is used primarily to suppress the immune response associated with rheumatoid arthritis and inflammatory bowel disease.

Mechanism of Action. The exact mechanism of this drug in immune-related disorders is not fully understood. Sulfasalazine may affect key components in the immune system, including suppression of NK cells. Other effects may be related to the breakdown of this drug into active metabolites, including sulfapyridine and mesalamine, which exert antibiotic and anti-inflammatory effects, respectively.

Adverse Effects. Primary side effects include headache, blood dyscrasias (agranulocytosis, anemia, thrombocytopenia), increased sensitivity to ultraviolet light, and hypersensitivity reactions (fever, skin rashes and itching). Hypersensitivity can be severe or even fatal in susceptible individuals.

Sirolimus

Clinical Use. Sirolimus (Rapamune), one of the newest immunosuppressants, is an antibiotic that also has substantial immunosuppressant effects. This drug is used primarily to prevent organ rejection in people with kidney transplants.[20,25,51] Sirolimus may ultimately be useful in preventing rejection of other organs (heart, liver, and so forth) and in other autoimmune situations such as psoriasis, systemic lupus erythematosus, and rheumatoid arthritis.[2] To provide optimal immunosuppressant effects, sirolimus is typically combined with cyclosporine and glucocorticoids.

Mechanism of Action. Unlike other immunosuppressants (cyclosporine, tacrolimus), sirolimus does not interfere directly with cytokine production. Instead, sirolimus inhibits the ability of T and B lymphocytes to carry out the stimulatory signal from certain cytokines such as interleukin-2 and interleukin-4.[40,46] Sirolimus, for example, binds to specific proteins in T lymphocytes and blocks the ability of cytokines to stimulate T-cell growth and proliferation. This drug also inhibits certain enzymes in B lymphocytes, thereby limiting the ability of cytokines to activate B cells and promote immunoglobulin synthesis.

Adverse Effects. Sirolimus may cause blood lipid disorders, including hypercholesterolemia and hypertriglyceridemia.[14,51] Other side effects include blood disorders (leukopenia, thrombocytopenia), diarrhea, skin rashes, joint and muscle pain, and hypertension.[51]

Tacrolimus

Clinical Use. Tacrolimus (Prograf) is similar to cyclosporine in structure and immunosuppressive effects, but tacrolimus is approximately 10 to 100 times more potent than cyclosporine.[43] Tacrolimus may be somewhat less toxic than cyclosporine and other immunosuppressants, although serious side effects may still occur at higher doses (see "Adverse Effects" in this section). Tacrolimus is used primarily to prevent rejection of kidney and liver transplants. This drug may also be useful in preventing or treating rejection of other organs and tissues including heart, lung, pancreas, and bone marrow transplants.[35,50]

Mechanism of Action. Tacrolimus acts like cyclosporine by binding to specific proteins in lymphoid tissues and inhibiting the production of key immune mediators such as IL-2.[7] This binding provides a somewhat more selective inhibition of immune function than other drugs that exert a general or nonselective inhibition of the immune response.

Adverse Effects. Common side effects of tacrolimus include gastrointestinal disturbances (cramps, nausea, diarrhea or constipation), weakness, fever, and skin rashes and itching. More serious problems include renal toxicity, CNS toxicity (headache, anxiety, nervousness, seizures), and hyperglycemia.[21,50] These effects, however, are generally less severe than those of less selective immunosuppressants such as the glucocorticoids.

Other Methods of Immunosuppression

IMMUNOSUPPRESSANT ANTIBODIES

Immune function can also be suppressed by using antibodies that interact with specific immune system cells and interfere with the function of these cells (Table 37–2).[7,48,52] These antibodies can be obtained from animal sources and cell culture techniques (monoclonal antibodies) to provide a rather selective method of suppressing immune function. For example, antibodies such as Rh(D) immunoglobulin are routinely used to suppress the immune response in mothers who have been exposed to a fetus's incompatible blood type. This immunosuppression prevents the mother from developing antibodies that will be passed on to the fetus or to a fetus in a subsequent pregnancy, thus blocking the production of maternal antibodies that can attack the fetus's blood and cause a potentially fatal condition known as hemolytic anemia of the newborn.[7]

Antibodies have also been developed that are very selective for antigens located on the surface of specific T cells and other lymphocytes, and these antibodies inhibit cell function or cause destruction of the cell.[7,48] These anti–T-cell antibodies are primarily used to help prevent or treat rejection of organ and bone marrow transplants (see Table 37–2).[16,52] Antibodies that block the interleukin-2 receptor, thus preventing interleukin-2 from activating T lymphocytes, have also been developed.[52] These anti–interleukin-2 receptor agents, such as basiliximab (Simulect) and daclizumab (Zenapax), may be helpful in reducing the incidence of acute transplant rejection.[34,53] For more information on the use of specific antibodies in specific disorders, refer to other sources on this topic.[2,7]

TABLE 37–2 Antibody Reagents Used as Immunosuppressants

Generic Name	Trade Name	Primary Indication(s)
Anti-CD2 monoclonal antibody	Medi-507	Prevention of rejection of kidney transplants
Anti-CD45 monoclonal antibody	—	Prevention of acute graft rejection of human organ transplants
Antithymocyte globulin	Nashville Rabbit Anti-thymocyte Serum	Treatment of rejection of kidney, heart, liver, lung, pancreas, and bone marrow transplants
CD5-T lymphocyte immunotoxin	Xomazyme-H65	Treatment of graft-versus-host disease or rejection following bone marrow transplant
Muromonab-CD3 monoclonal antibody	Orthoclone OKT3	Acute rejection of heart, liver, and kidney transplants
$Rh_O(D)$ immune globulin	Gamulin Rh, RhoGAM, others	Prevention of Rh hemolytic disease of the newborn
Interleukin-1 receptor antagonists		
Basiliximab	Simulect	Prevention of acute rejection of kidney transplants
Daclizumab	Zenapax	Prevention of acute rejection of kidney transplants

MISCELLANEOUS IMMUNOSUPPRESSANTS

A variety of other agents with cytotoxic effects can also be used to suppress the immune system. These drugs include chlorambucil (Leukeran), dactinomycin (Cosmegen), mercaptopurine (Purinethol), vinblastine (Velban), and vincristine (Oncovin, Vincasar).[7] These agents are similar to methotrexate; they exert cytotoxic effects that interfere with the proliferation of immune system cellular components. Hence, these drugs are used primarily as anticancer agents, but they may be helpful in certain autoimmune disorders or to prevent rejection of tissue and organ transplants. The pharmacology of antineoplastic drugs that also have immunosuppressive effects is described in more detail in Chapter 36.

Finally, thalidomide can be used as an immunosuppressant in conditions such as systemic lupus erythematosus (SLE)[44] and in preventing graft-versus-host disease following bone marrow transplantation.[7] This drug was developed originally as a sedative but was later discovered to produce severe birth defects when administered to women during pregnancy. Nonetheless, thalidomide may help blunt immunologic responses by regulating the genes that express tumor necrosis factor-alpha.[26] Decreased production of this factor results in diminished activation of neutrophils and other immune components, thereby reducing the severity of immunologic reactions.

IMMUNOSTIMULANTS

A number of agents can suppress the immune system. There has been considerable interest, however, in developing pharmacologic methods to modify or even stimulate immune function in specific situations. In particular, agents that have a positive immunomodulating effect could be beneficial to people with compromised immune function (people with AIDS or certain cancers) or chronic infections.[7] Development of immunostimulants, however, is understandably a complex and potentially dangerous proposition. Excessive or incorrect immune activation could trigger myriad problems that resemble autoimmune diseases. Likewise, it may be difficult to selectively stimulate certain aspects of the immune system to treat a specific problem without also causing a more widespread and systemic immunologic response. Nonetheless, a few strategies are currently available to modify or stimulate immune function in a limited number of situations.

Bacille Calmette-Guérin

Clinical Use. Bacille Calmette-Guérin (BCG, TheraCys) is an active bacterial strain that can be administered systemically as a vaccine against tuberculosis. This agent may also stimulate immune function and has been administered locally within the bladder (intravesicularly) to treat certain forms of superficial bladder cancer.[30,33]

Mechanism of Action. The exact reason that this agent is effective in treating cancer is not known. Some evidence suggests that it may activate macrophages locally at the site of the cancer and that these macrophages engulf and destroy tumor cells.[2,54]

Adverse Effects. When it is administered directly into the bladder, common side effects include bladder irritation and infection. Systemic administration (immunization) may also cause dermatologic reactions (peeling or scaling of the skin), allergic reactions, inflammation of lymph nodes, and local irritation or ulceration at the injection site.

Immune Globulin

Clinical Use. Immune globulin (Gamimune, Gammagard, other trade names) is prepared by extracting immunoglobulins from donated human blood.[7] These preparations contain all subclasses of immunoglobulin (Ig) but consist primarily of IgG. Immune globulin is administered intravenously to boost immune function in several conditions, including primary immunodeficiency syndromes (congenital agammaglobulinemia, common variable immunodeficiency, and severe combined immunodeficiency), idiopathic thrombocytopenic purpura, Kawasaki disease, chronic lymphocytic leukemia, and human immunodeficiency virus infection in children.[37] Other potential indications for immune globulin include dermatomyositis, Guillain-Barré syndrome, demyelinating polyneuropathies, Lambert-Eaton myasthenia syndrome, and relapsing-remitting multiple sclerosis.

Mechanism of Action. Commercial preparations of immune globulin mimic the normal role of endogenous immunoglobulins. These preparations therefore act directly as antibodies against infectious agents. They can also help modulate the activity of T lymphocytes, macrophages, and other immune system cells to maintain competence of the immune system.[37]

Adverse Effects. Immune globulin may cause several bothersome side effects, such as joint and muscle pain, headache, general malaise, and gastrointestinal disturbances (nausea, vomiting). Although rare, allergic reactions including anaphylaxis can occur in some individuals. Because immune globulin is obtained from human blood, care must also be taken to prevent transmission of hepatitis and human immunodeficiency virus from infected donors.

Levamisole

Clinical Use. Levamisole (Ergamisol) is used primarily to treat colorectal carcinoma. Specifically, this drug is administered with fluorouracil (see Chap. 36) to prevent recurrence of colorectal cancer after surgical removal of the primary tumor.

Mechanism of Action. Although the exact effects are not known, levamisole may augment immune function by activating macrophages that selectively engulf and destroy any residual cancerous cells.[2]

Adverse Effects. Levamisole may cause blood disorders such as agranulocytosis, leukopenia, or thrombocytopenia. Other side effects include nausea, diarrhea, and a metallic taste in the mouth.

OTHER IMMUNOMODULATORS

Because of their ability to act as immunoregulatory chemicals, cytokines are a potential way to modify the immune system in several situations. For example, cytokines such as interferon-alpha and interleukin-2 can be administered to treat certain forms of cancer (see Chap. 36). Likewise, certain interferons can help control viral infections, and interferon-beta may also be helpful in autoimmune diseases such as multiple sclerosis (see Chap. 34).

Roquinimex (Linomide) is another potential immunostimulant. Although the details are unclear, this drug may stimulate T and B lymphocytes and can be used to sustain immune function in patients receiving bone marrow transplants.[2] A number of other drugs are also being evaluated for their potential effects on immune function. Most of these drugs are still experimental, and the development of additional immune system modulators may be forthcoming.

SIGNIFICANCE OF IMMUNOMODULATING AGENTS IN REHABILITATION

Physical therapists and occupational therapists are often involved in the physical rehabilitation of patients who have received heart, liver, kidney, and other organ transplants. Therapists also frequently deal with patients who have received autologous grafts, such as skin grafts for treating burns, and bone marrow transplants during treatment of certain cancers. Hence, therapists frequently deal with patients taking drugs to prevent tissue rejection.

Therapists also deal with the rehabilitation of musculoskeletal disorders that are caused by an autoimmune response. Many such diseases attack connective tissues, and autoimmune diseases such as rheumatoid arthritis, dermatomyositis, and systemic lupus erythematosus are often the primary reason that patients are undergoing rehabilitation. Patients with a compromised immune system may develop many musculoskeletal problems related to their immunodeficient state. Hence, immunomodulating drugs are frequently used in many patients receiving physical therapy and occupational therapy.

The most significant impact of these drugs on rehabilitation is related to the side effects of these agents, especially the immunosuppressants. These drugs are typically used in high doses to produce immunosuppressive effects, and these effects are often achieved at the expense of serious and toxic side effects. Many immunosuppressants, especially the glucocorticoids, exert catabolic effects on bone, muscle, and other tissues. Other immunosuppressants, such as cyclosporine and tacrolimus, are neurotoxic and may cause peripheral neuropathies and CNS-related problems in balance and posture.

Hence, rehabilitation specialists can play a critical role in offsetting some of these adverse effects. Therapists can institute strengthening and general conditioning exercises to prevent breakdown of muscle, bone, and other tissues, as well as to maintain cardiovascular function. Problems associated with peripheral neuropathies, such as pain and weakness, may respond to TENS and other electrotherapeutic treatments. Balance and gait training may help patients overcome problems caused by CNS toxicity and vestibular problems. Thus, therapists can implement specific strategies as required to help patients cope with adverse drug effects associated with immunomodulating agents.

CASE STUDY

IMMUNOMODULATING AGENTS

Brief History. A.S. is a 47-year-old concert musician who experienced a progressive decline in renal function that ultimately led to renal failure. Kidney function was maintained artificially through renal dialysis until a suitable kidney transplant became available from a donor who died in an automobile accident. The kidney was transplanted successfully, and A.S. was placed on a prophylactic regimen of three different immunosuppressive drugs to prevent rejection of the transplanted kidney. At the time of the transplant, cyclosporine was initiated at a dose of 10 mg per kilogram of body weight each day. After 15 days, cyclosporine dosage was decreased to 8 mg/kg per day, and dosage was progressively decreased over the next 2 months until a maintenance dosage of 2 mg/kg per day was achieved. On the day of surgery, he also received an intravenous dose of 0.5 g of methylprednisolone. Oral doses of methylprednisolone were then administered in dosages of 16 mg/day for the first 3 months, 12 mg/day for the next 3 months, and 8 mg/day thereafter. Azathioprine was administered at a dosage of 1 mg/kg per day throughout the posttransplant period. Physical therapy was initiated in the intensive care unit (ICU) 1 day after the transplant to increase strength and facilitate recovery from the surgery.

Problem/Influence of Medication. The therapist noted that several drugs were being used to prevent rejection, including rather high doses of methylprednisolone, a glucocorticoid agent. Glucocorticoids are notorious for their catabolic effects, and the therapist was aware that a program of strengthening and weight-bearing exercise would help offset the breakdown of muscle and bone that can often occur with prolonged glucocorticoid administration.

Decision/Solution. Gentle resistance exercises were initiated in the ICU as soon as the patient was alert and could follow basic instructions. Strengthening exercises were progressively increased using manual resistance, and various weights and exercise machines were incorporated into the strengthening regimen as tolerated by the patient. The therapist also initiated weight-bearing activities as soon as the patient was able to tolerate standing in the ICU. Weight-bearing activities were progressively increased, and the patient was able to walk independently for distances up to 1000 feet and climb two flights of stairs at the time of discharge. The therapist also worked closely with the patient and the patient's family to make sure that strengthening exercises and a progressive ambulation program were continued in the patient's home. The patient did not experience any problems related to tissue rejection, and he was able to resume his musical career and maintain an active lifestyle that included daily walks and regular visits to a health club, where he participated in a supervised program of strength training.

SUMMARY

Our knowledge of how the immune system functions in normal and disease states has increased dramatically over the last several decades, and we now have drugs that can moderate the effects of the immune response in certain clinical situations. Immunosuppressants are a mainstay in preventing tissue rejection, and much of the current success of organ transplants is due to the judicious use of immunosuppressive drugs. These drugs are also beneficial in a number of diseases that have an autoimmune basis, and immunosuppressants can help alleviate symptoms or possibly even reverse the sequelae of certain diseases such as rheumatoid arthritis. A few agents are also available that can augment or stimulate immune function in certain situations. The use of these immunostimulants will continue to expand as more is learned about how we can enhance the immune response in conditions such as cancer and certain immunocompromised states. Immunomodulating drugs are not without problems, however, because many agents cause a rather nonspecific effect on immune function, which leads to serious side effects. As more is learned about the details of immune function, it is hoped that new drugs will be developed that are more selective in their ability to modify immune responses without causing a generalized suppression or activation of the immune system.

REFERENCES

1. Almawi, WY, Hess, DA, and Rieder, MJ: Multiplicity of glucocorticoid action in inhibiting allograft rejection. Cell Transplant 7:511, 1998.
2. Barbuto, JA, Akporiaye, ET, and Hersh, EM: Immunopharmacology. In Katzung, BG (ed): Basic and Clinical Pharmacology, ed 7. Appleton & Lange, Stamford, CT, 1998.
3. Belitsky, P: Neoral use in the renal transplant recipient. Transplant Proc 32(Suppl 3A):10S, 2000.
4. Bertera, S, et al: Immunology of type 1 diabetes. Intervention and prevention strategies. Endocrinol Metab Clin North Am 28:841, 1999.
5. Bush, WW: Overview of transplant immunology and the pharmacology of adult solid organ recipients: Focus on immunosuppression. AACN Clin Issues 10:253, 1999.
6. De Mattos, AM, Olyaei, AJ, and Bennett, WM: Nephrotoxicity of immunosuppressive drugs: Long-term consequences and challenges for the future. Am J Kidney Dis 35:333, 2000.
7. Diasio, RB and LoBuglio, AF: Immunomodulators: Immunosuppressive agents and immunostimulants. In Hardman JG, et al (eds): The Pharmacologic Basis of Therapeutics, ed 9. McGraw-Hill, New York, 1996.
8. Dumont, RJ and Ensom, MH: Methods for clinical monitoring of cyclosporine in transplant patients. Clin Pharmacokinet 38:427, 2000.
9. Everson, GT, et al: Early steroid withdrawal in liver transplantation is safe and beneficial. Liver Transpl Surg 5(Suppl 1):S48, 1999.
10. Fearon, DT and Locksley, RM: The instructive role of innate immunity in the acquired immune response. Science 272:50, 1996.
11. Fleisher, TA and Bleesing, JJ: Immune function. Pediatr Clin North Am 47:1197, 2000.
12. Frei, U: Overview of the clinical experience with Neoral in transplantation. Transplant Proc 31:1669, 1999.
13. Godfrey, T, Khamashta, MA, and Hughes, GR: Therapeutic advances in systemic lupus erythematosus. Curr Opin Rheumatol 10:435, 1998.
14. Gonin, JM: Maintenance immunosuppression: New agents and persistent dilemmas. Adv Ren Replace Ther 7:95, 2000.

15. Hall, PD and Karlix, JL: Function and evaluation of the immune system. In DiPiro, JT, et al (eds): Pharmacotherapy: A Pathophysiologic Approach, ed 4. Appleton & Lange, Stamford, CT, 1999.
16. Hiscott, A and McLellan, DS: Graft-versus-host disease in allogeneic bone marrow transplantation: The role of monoclonal antibodies in prevention and treatment. Br J Biomed Sci 57:163, 2000.
17. Hong, JC and Kahan, BD: Immunosuppressive agents in organ transplantation: Past, present, and future. Semin Nephrol 20:108, 2000.
18. Ishikawa, H: Mizoribine and mycophenolate mofetil. Curr Med Chem 6:575, 1999.
19. Johnson, KJ, Chensue, SW, and Ward, PA: Immunopathology. In Rubin, E and Farber, JL (eds): Pathology, ed 3. Lippincott-Raven, Philadelphia, 1999.
20. Kahan, BD: Rapamycin: Personal algorithms for use based on 250 treated renal allograft recipients. Transplant Proc 30:2185, 1998.
21. Laskow, DA, et al: The role of tacrolimus in adult kidney transplantation: A review. Clin Transplant 12:489, 1998.
22. Levy, GA: Neoral use in the liver transplant recipient. Transplant Proc 32(Suppl 3A):2S, 2000.
23. Levy, GA: Neoral/cyclosporine-based immunosuppression. Liver Transpl Surg 5(Suppl 1):S37, 1999.
24. Luqmani, R, Gordon, C, and Bacon, P: Clinical pharmacology and modification of autoimmunity and inflammation in rheumatoid disease. Drugs 47:259, 1994.
25. MacDonald, A, et al: Clinical pharmacokinetics and therapeutic drug monitoring of sirolimus. Clin Ther 22(Suppl B):B101, 2000.
26. McHugh, SM and Rowland, TL: Thalidomide derivatives: Immunological investigation of tumour necrosis factor-alpha (TNF-alpha) inhibition suggest drugs capable of selective gene regulation. Clin Exp Immunol 110:151, 1997.
27. Medzhitov, R and Janeway, CA: Innate immune recognition and control of adaptive immune responses. Semin Immunol 10:351, 1998.
28. Mele, TA and Halloran, PF: The use of mycophenolate mofetil in transplant recipients. Immunopharmacology 47:215, 2000.
29. Montagnino, G, et al: A randomized trial comparing triple-drug and double-drug therapy in renal transplantation. Transplantation 58:149, 1994.
30. Nseyo, UO and Lamm, DL: Immunotherapy of bladder cancer. Semin Surg Oncol 13:342, 1997.
31. Olyaei, AJ, de Mattos, AM, and Bennett, WM: Immunosuppressant-induced nephropathy: Pathophysiology, incidence, and management. Drug Saf 21:471, 1999.
32. Opelz, G: Effect of the maintenance immunosuppressive drug regimen on kidney transplant outcome. Transplantation 58:443, 1994.
33. Patard, JJ, et al: Immune response following intravesical bacillus Calmette-Guerin instillations in superficial bladder cancer: A review. Urol Res 26:155, 1998.
34. Ponticelli, C and Tarantino, A: Promising new agents in the prevention of transplant rejection. Drugs R D 1:55, 1999.
35. Przepiorka, D, et al: Practical considerations in the use of tacrolimus for allogeneic marrow transplantation. Bone Marrow Transplant 24:1053, 1999.
36. Reding, R: Steroid withdrawal in liver transplantation: Benefits, risks, and unanswered questions. Transplantation 70:405, 2000.
37. Rhoades, CJ, et al: Monocyte-macrophage system and targets for immunomodulation by intravenous immunoglobulin. Blood Rev 14:14, 2000.
38. Scherrer, U, et al: Cyclosporine-induced sympathetic activation and hypertension after heart transplantation. N Engl J Med 323:693, 1990.
39. Schimmer, BP and Parker, KL: Adrenocorticotropic hormone; adrenocortical steroids and their synthetic analogs; inhibitors of the synthesis and actions of adrenocortical hormones. In Hardman, JG, et al (eds): The Pharmacological Basis of Therapeutics, ed 9. McGraw-Hill, New York, 1996.
40. Sehgal, SN: Rapamune (RAPA, rapamycin, sirolimus): Mechanism of action immunosuppressive effect results from blockade of signal transduction and inhibition of cell cycle progression. Clin Biochem 31:335, 1998.
41. Shah, AK: Cyclosporine A neurotoxicity among bone marrow transplant recipients. Clin Neuropharmacol 22:67, 1999.
42. Sievers, TM, et al: Mycophenolate mofetil. Pharmacotherapy 17:1178, 1997.
43. Singh, N, et al: Infectious complications in liver transplant recipients on tacrolimus. Transplantation 58:774, 1994.
44. Strand, V: Biologic agents and innovative interventional approaches in the management of systemic lupus erythematosus. Curr Opin Rheumatol 11:330, 1999.
45. Stratta, RJ: Immunosuppression in pancreas transplantation: Progress, problems, and perspective. Transpl Immunol 6:69, 1998.
46. Suthanthiran, M and Strom, TB: Immunoregulatory drugs: Mechanistic basis for use in organ transplantation. Pediatr Nephrol 11:651, 1997.
47. Tsai, M-J, et al: Mechanisms of action of hormones that act as transcription-regulatory factors. In Wilson, JD, et al (eds): Textbook of Endocrinology, ed 9. WB Saunders, Philadelphia, 1998.
48. Tse, JC and Moore, TB: Monoclonal antibodies in the treatment of steroid-resistant acute graft-versus-host disease. Pharmacotherapy 18:988, 1998.

49. Valantine, H: Neoral use in the cardiac transplant recipient. Transplant Proc 32(Suppl 3A):27S, 2000.

50. Van Hooff, JP and Christiaans, MH: Use of tacrolimus in renal transplantation. Transplant Proc 31:3298, 1999.

51. Vasquez, EM: Sirolimus: A new agent for prevention of renal allograft rejection. Am J Health Syst Pharm 57:437, 2000.

52. Wall, WJ: Use of antilymphocyte induction therapy in liver transplantation. Liver Transpl Surg 5(Suppl 1):S64, 1999.

53. Wiseman, LR and Faulds, D: Daclizumab: A review of its use in the prevention of acute rejection in renal transplant recipients. Drugs 58:1029, 1999.

54. Zlotta, AR and Schulman, CC: Biological response modifiers for the treatment of superficial bladder tumors. Eur Urol 37(Suppl 3):10, 2000.

Drugs Administered by Iontophoresis and Phonophoresis

Listed here are some drugs that may be administered by iontophoresis and phonophoresis. Administration of these agents by these techniques is largely empirical. Use of these substances in the conditions listed is based primarily on clinical observation and anecdotal reports in the literature. Likewise, the preparation strengths given here are merely suggestions based on currently available information.

Drug	Principal Indication(s)	Treatment Rationale	Iontophoresis	Phonophoresis
Acetic acid	Calcific tendinitis	Acetate is believed to increase solubility of calcium deposits in tendons and other soft tissues	2–5% aqueous solution from negative pole	—
Calcium chloride	Skeletal muscle spasms	Calcium stabilizes excitable membranes; appears to decrease the excitability of peripheral nerves and skeletal muscle	2% aqueous solution from positive pole	—
Dexamethasone	Inflammation	Synthetic steroidal anti-inflammatory agent (see Chap. 29)	4 mg/mL in aqueous solution from negative pole	0.4% ointment
Hydrocortisone	Inflammation	Anti-inflammatory steroid (see Chap. 29)	0.5% ointment from positive pole	0.5–1.0% ointment
Iodine	Adhesive capsulitis and other soft-tissue adhesions; microbial infections	Iodine is a broad-spectrum antibiotic, hence its use in infections, etc.; the sclerolytic actions of iodine are not fully understood	5–10% solution or ointment from negative pole	10% ointment
Lidocaine	Soft-tissue pain and inflammation (e.g., bursitis, tenosynovitis)	Local anesthetic effects (see Chap. 12)	4–5% solution or ointment from positive pole	5% ointment
Magnesium sulfate	Skeletal muscle spasms; myositis	Muscle relaxant effect may be caused by decreased excitability of the skeletal muscle membrane and decreased transmission at the neuromuscular junction	2% aqueous solution or ointment from positive pole	2% ointment
Hyaluronidase	Local edema (subacute and chronic stage)	Hyaluronidase appears to increase permeability in connective tissue by hydrolyzing hyaluronic acid, thus decreasing encapsulation and allowing dispersion of local edema	Reconstitute with 0.9% sodium chloride to provide a 150 mg/mL solution from positive pole	—
Salicylates	Muscle and joint pain in acute and chronic conditions (e.g., overuse injuries, rheumatoid arthritis)	Aspirin-like drugs with analgesic and anti-inflammatory effects (see Chap. 15)	10% trolamine salicylate ointment or 2–3% sodium salicylate solution from negative pole	10% trolamine salicylate ointment or 3% sodium salicylate ointment
Tolazoline hydrochloride	Indolent cutaneous ulcers	Tolazoline increases local blood flow and tissue healing by inhibiting vascular smooth muscle contraction	2% aqueous solution or ointment from positive pole	—
Zinc oxide	Skin ulcers, other dermatologic disorders	Zinc acts as a general antiseptic; may increase tissue healing	20% ointment from positive pole	20% ointment

APPENDIX B

Potential Interactions between Physical Agents and Therapeutic Drugs

Listed here are some potential interactions between physical agents used in rehabilitation and various pharmacologic agents. It is impossible to list all the possible relationships between the vast array of therapeutic drugs and the procedures used in physical and occupational therapy. However, some of the more common interactions are identified here.

Modality	Desired Therapeutic Effect	Drugs with Complementary/ Synergistic Effects	Drugs with Antagonistic Effects	Other Drug-Modality Interactions
Cryotherapy Cold/ice packs Ice massage Cold bath Vapocoolant sprays	Decreased pain, edema, and inflammation	Anti-inflammatory steroids (glucocorticoids); nonsteroidal anti-inflammatory analgesics (aspirin and similar NSAIDs)	Peripheral vasodilators may exacerbate acute local edema	Some forms of cryotherapy may produce local vasoconstriction that temporarily impedes diffusion of drugs to the site of inflammation
	Muscle relaxation and decreased spasticity	Skeletal muscle relaxants	Nonselective cholinergic agonists may stimulate the neuromuscular junction	—
Superficial and deep heat local application	Decreased muscle/joint pain and stiffness	NSAIDs; opioid analgesics; local anesthetics	—	—
Hot packs Paraffin Infrared	Decreased muscle spasms	Skeletal muscle relaxants	Nonselective cholinergic agonists may stimulate the neuromuscular junction	—
Fluidotherapy Diathermy Ultrasound	Increased blood flow to improve tissue healing	Peripheral vasodilators	Systemic vasoconstrictors (e.g., alpha-1 agonists) may decrease perfusion of peripheral tissues	—
Systemic heat Large whirlpool Hubbard tank	Decreased muscle/joint stiffness in large areas of the body	Opioid and nonopioid analgesics; skeletal muscle relaxants	—	Severe hypotension may occur if systemic hot whirlpool is administered to patients taking peripheral vasodilators and some antihypertensive drugs (e.g., alpha-1 antagonists, nitrates, direct-acting vasodilators, calcium channel blockers)

(continued)

Modality	Desired Therapeutic Effect	Drugs with Complementary/ Synergistic Effects	Drugs with Antagonistic Effects	Other Drug-Modality Interactions
Ultraviolet radiation	Increased wound healing	Various systemic and topical antibiotics	—	Antibacterial drugs generally increase cutaneous sensitivity to ultraviolet light (i.e., photosensitivity)
	Management of skin disorders (acne, rashes)	Systemic and topical antibiotics and anti-inflammatory steroids (glucocorticoids)	Many drugs may cause hyper-sensitivity reactions that result in skin rashes, itching	Photosensitivity with antibacterial drugs
Transcutaneous electrical nerve stimulation (TENS)	Decreased pain	Opioid and nonopioid analgesics	Opioid antagonists (naloxone)	—
Functional neuromuscular electrical stimulation	Increased skeletal muscle strength and endurance	—	Skeletal muscle relaxants	—
	Decreased spasticity and muscle spasms	Skeletal muscle relaxants	Nonselective cholinergic agonists may stimulate the neuromuscular junction	—

Use of the *Physicians' Desk Reference*

Several drug indexes are available that can supplement this text by serving as a detailed source of information about individual drugs. One of the most readily available and frequently used indexes is the *Physicians' Desk Reference*, or *PDR*. The *PDR* is published annually by Medical Economics Company, Inc., Montvale, NJ, 07645-1742.

Basically, drug manufacturers submit information about the indications, dosage, adverse effects, and so on, of individual agents for inclusion into the *PDR*. The *PDR* is then published annually, providing a relatively current source of information. The *PDR* is also updated within a given year through periodic supplements.

The *PDR* begins by listing all the manufacturers who submitted information to the *PDR* in the Manufacturers' Index. Immediately following the Manufacturers' Index, drugs are listed according to the Brand and Generic Name Index and the Product Category Index. These listings are followed by detailed descriptions of the drugs in the Product Information Section, which constitutes the bulk of the *PDR*.

Using the *PDR* for the first time can be somewhat confusing because drugs are listed in several different ways. The brief outline provided here may help individuals use the *PDR* more effectively to obtain information about specific agents.

1. If the Trade Name or Brand Name of the Drug Is Known. Begin by looking in the Brand and Generic Name Index in the front of the *PDR*, easily found by locating the PINK pages. Drugs are listed alphabetically according to the name given by the drug manufacturer (trade or brand name) as well as by the generic name (see section 2). Each trade name is followed by the name of the manufacturer (in parentheses) and by a page number, which indicates where the drug is described in the Product Information section. Some trade names are preceded by a small diamond and will usually have two page numbers following the name. This diamond indicates that a color photograph of the actual medication is provided in the special section of the *PDR* known as the Product Identification Guide. The first page number following the drug name is the page that illustrates a picture of the drug, and the second page number identifies where the written information can be found.

Many drugs listed in the Brand and Generic Name Index have several variations on the trade name, depending on different forms of the drug and routes of administration.

For example, a drug that is available in tablets, capsules, and injectable forms may have slight variations on the trade name that reflect these different preparations.

2. If the Generic or Chemical Name Is Known. If you are using an edition of the *PDR* published in 1994 or later, begin by looking in the Brand and Generic Name Index (PINK pages). This section integrates generic names into the alphabetical listing of trade names. The generic name of each drug is followed by the trade name, manufacturer (in parentheses), and pages where the drug is illustrated and described. Often the generic heading in this section is followed by several different trade names, indicating that several different manufacturers market the drug.

Older editions of the *PDR* (1993 and earlier) list generic and chemical names in a separate section called the Generic and Chemical Name Index, marked by YELLOW pages. If you are using an older edition, consult this section if you know only the generic name.

3. To Find Out What Drugs Are Available to Treat a Given Disorder. The best place to begin is the Product Category Index located in the BLUE pages. Here, drugs are listed according to the principal pharmacologic classifications, such as anesthetics, laxatives, and sedatives. Major categories in this section are often subdivided into more specific subcategories. For example, cardiovascular preparations are subdivided into antiarrhythmics, beta-adrenergic blocking agents, vasodilators, and others. Drugs in each category (or subcategory) are listed according to their trade name, followed by the manufacturer (in parentheses) and pages on which the drug is illustrated and described.

4. If You Want to Contact the Manufacturer for More Information about the Drug. Look in the Manufacturers' Index located in the WHITE pages at the very beginning of the PDR. Manufacturers who have contributed to the *PDR* are listed alphabetically, with an address and phone number that serve as a source for inquiries. Also, a partial listing of the products available from each manufacturer is included following the manufacturer's name and address.

5. If You Want to Identify the Name of a Specific Pill, Capsule, or Tablet. Locate the Product Identification Guide, which contains glossy color photographs of many of the drugs. Drugs are categorized alphabetically according to their manufacturer. Often, individual pills, tablets, and other forms have the name of the manufacturer scored or printed directly on the medication. An unknown medication can be identified by matching the drug to the pictures listed under that manufacturer.

APPENDIX D

Drugs of Abuse

Some of the more frequently abused drugs are listed here. Agents such as cocaine, the cannabinoids, and the psychedelics are illicit drugs with no major pharmacotherapeutic value. Other drugs such as the barbiturates, benzodiazepines, and opioids are routinely used for therapeutic reasons but have a strong potential for abuse when taken indiscriminately. Finally, drugs such as alcohol, caffeine, and nicotine are readily available in various commercial products but may also be considered drugs of abuse when consumed in large quantities for prolonged periods.

Drug(s)	Classification/ Action	Route/Method of Administration	Effect Desired by User	Principal Adverse Effects	Additional Information
Alcohol	Sedative-hypnotic	Oral, from various beverages (wine, beer, other alcoholic drinks)	Euphoria; relaxed inhibitions; decreased anxiety; sense of escape	Physical dependence; impaired motor skills; chronic degenerative changes in brain, liver, and other organs	See Chapter 6
Barbiturates Nembutal Seconal Others	Sedative-hypnotic	Oral or injected (IM, IV)	Relaxation and a sense of calmness; drowsiness	Physical dependence; possible death from overdose; behavior changes (irritability, psychosis) following prolonged use	See Chapter 6
Benzodiazepines Valium Librium Others	Similar to barbiturates	Similar to barbiturates	Similar to barbiturates	Similar to barbiturates	Similar to barbiturates
Caffeine	CNS stimulant	Oral, from coffee, tea, other beverages	Increased alertness; decreased fatigue; improved work capacity	Sleep disturbances; irritability; nervousness; cardiac arrhythmias	See Chapter 26
Cannabinoids Hashish Marijuana	Psychoactive drugs with mixed (stimulant and depressant) activity	Smoked; possible oral ingestion	Initial response: euphoria, excitement, increased perception; later response: relaxation, stupor, dreamlike state	Possible endocrine changes (decreased testosterone in males) and changes in respiratory function with heavy use; similar to chronic cigarette smoking	—

Cocaine	CNS stimulant (when taken systemically)	"Snorted" (absorbed via nasal mucosa); smoked (in crystalline form)	Euphoria; excitement; feelings of intense pleasure and well-being	Physical dependence; acute CNS and cardiac toxicity; profound mood swings	See Chapter 12
Narcotics Demerol Morphine Heroin Others	Natural and synthetic opioids; analgesics	Oral or injected (IM, IV)	Relaxation; euphoria; feelings of tranquility; prevent onset of opiate withdrawal	Physical dependence; respiratory depression; high potential for death by overdose	See Chapter 14
Nicotine	CNS toxin: production of variable effects via somatic and autonomic nervous system interaction	Smoked or absorbed from tobacco products (cigarettes, cigars, chewing tobacco)	Relaxation; calming effect; decreased irritability	Physical dependence; possible carcinogen; associated with pathologic changes in respiratory function during long-term tobacco use	—
Psychedelics LSD Mescaline Phencyclidine (PCP) Psilocybin	Hallucinogens	Oral; possibly also smoked or inhaled	Altered perception and insight; distorted senses; disinhibition	Severe hallucinations; panic reaction; acute psychotic reactions	—

659

Common Drug Suffixes

Medications that are chemically and functionally similar often have generic names that share a common ending or suffix. Listed here are some drug classes that contain groups of drugs that share a common suffix. Please note that some members of a drug class may have a suffix that is different from the one indicated; for instance, not all benzodiazepines end with "-epam" or "-olam."

Drug Class	Suffix	Common Examples	Primary Indication or Desired Effect (Chapter in Parentheses)
Angiotensin-converting enzyme (ACE) inhibitors	-pril	Captopril, enalapril	Antihypertensive (21), congestive heart failure (24)
Azole antifungals	-azole	Fluconazole, miconazole	Fungal infections (35)
Barbiturates	-barbital	Phenobarbital, secobarbital	Sedative-hypnotic (6), antiseizure (9), anesthetic (11)
Benzodiazepines	-epam or -olam	Diazepam, temazepam, alprazolam, triazolam	Sedative-hypnotic (6), antianxiety (6), antiseizure (9), anesthetic (11)
Beta blockers	-olol	Metoprolol, propranolol	Antihypertensive (21), antianginal (22), antiarrhythmic (23), congestive heart failure (24)
Bronchodilators (adrenergic)	-erol	Albuterol, pirbuterol	Bronchodilation (26)
Bronchodilators (xanthine derivatives)	-phylline	Theophylline, aminophylline	Bronchodilation (26)
Calcium channel blockers (dihydropyridine group)	-ipine	Nifedipine, nicardipine	Antihypertensive (21), antianginal (22)
Glucocorticoids	-sone or -olone*	Cortisone, dexamethasone, prednisone, prednisolone, triamcinolone	Anti-inflammatory (16, 29), immunosuppressants (37)
Histamine H_2-receptor blockers	-idine	Cimetidine, ranitidine	Gastric ulcers (27)
HMG-CoA reductase inhibitors (statins)	-statin	Pravastatin, simvastatin	Hyperlipidemia (25)
Local anesthetics	-caine	Lidocaine, bupivacaine	Local anesthetic (12), antiarrhythmics (23)
Low-molecular-weight heparins	-parin	Dalteparin, enoxaparin	Anticoagulants (25)
Oral antidiabetics (sulfonylurea group)	-amide	Chlorpropamide, tolbutamide	Antidiabetic (type 2 diabetes mellitus) (32)
Penicillin antibiotics	-cillin	Penicillin, ampicillin, amoxicillin	Bacterial infections (33)
Tetracycline antibiotics	-cycline	Tetracycline, doxycycline	Bacterial infections (33)
Various other antibacterials	-micin or -mycin†	Streptomycin, gentamicin, erythromycin	Bacterial infections (33)

*Some anabolic steroids also end with -olone, e.g., nandrolone, oxymetholone (Chap. 30).
†Some antibiotics ending with "-mycin" or "-rubicin" are used as antineoplastics (Chap. 36).

Glossary

Listed here are some common terms related to pharmacology and a brief definition of each term. Synonyms (SYN), antonyms (ANT), and common abbreviations (ABBR) are also included, whenever applicable.

Acetylcholine: A neurotransmitter in the somatic and autonomic nervous systems; principal synapses using acetylcholine include the skeletal neuromuscular junction, autonomic ganglia, and certain pathways in the brain.

Adenylate cyclase: An enzyme located on the inner surface of many cell membranes; it is important in mediating biochemical changes in the cell in response to drug and hormone stimulation (SYN: adenyl cyclase).

Adrenergic: Refers to synapses or physiologic responses involving epinephrine and norepinephrine.

Adrenocorticosteroids: The group of steroid hormones produced by the adrenal cortex. These drugs include the glucocorticoids (cortisol, cortisone), mineralocorticoids (aldosterone), and the sex hormones (androgens, estrogens, and progestins).

Affinity: The mutual attraction between a drug and a specific cellular receptor.

Agonist: A drug that binds to a receptor and causes some change in cell function (ANT: antagonist).

Akathisia: A feeling of extreme motor restlessness and an inability to sit still; may occur as a result of antipsychotic drug therapy.

Allergy: A state of hypersensitivity to foreign substances (e.g., environmental antigens and certain drugs), manifested by an exaggerated response of the immune system.

Alpha receptors: A primary class of the receptors that are responsive to epinephrine and norepinephrine. Alpha receptors are subclassified into alpha-1 and alpha-2 receptors based on their sensitivity to various drugs.

Anabolic steroids: Natural and synthetic male hormones that may be misused in an attempt to increase muscle size and improve athletic performance (SYN: androgens).

Analgesia: To lessen or relieve pain. Drugs with this ability are known as *analgesics*.

Androgen: A male steroid such as testosterone.

Angina pectoris: Severe pain and constriction in the chest region, usually associated with myocardial ischemia.

Antagonist: A drug that binds to a receptor but does not cause a change in cell activity (SYN: blocker).

Anthelmintic: A drug that destroys parasitic worms (e.g., tapeworms, roundworms) in the gastrointestinal tract and elsewhere in the body.

Anticholinergic: Drugs that decrease activity at acetylcholine synapses. These agents are often used to diminish activity in the parasympathetic nervous system (SYN: parasympatholytic).

Anticoagulation: A decrease in the capacity of the blood to coagulate (clot). Drugs with this ability are known as *anticoagulants.*

Antimetabolite: The general term for drugs that impair function in harmful cells and microorganisms by antagonizing or replacing normal metabolic substrates in those cells. Certain anti-infectious and antineoplastic agents function as antimetabolites.

Antineoplastic: A drug that prevents or attenuates the growth and proliferation of cancerous cells.

Antipyresis: The reduction of fever. Drugs with this ability are known as *antipyretics.*

Antitussive: A drug that reduces coughing.

Asthma: A chronic disease of the respiratory system characterized by bronchoconstriction, airway inflammation, and formation of mucous plugs in the airway.

Bactericidal: An agent that kills or destroys bacteria.

Bacteriostatic: An agent that inhibits the growth and proliferation of bacteria.

Beta receptor: A primary class of the receptors that are responsive to epinephrine and (to a lesser extent) norepinephrine. Beta receptors are subclassified into beta-1 and beta-2 receptors based on their sensitivity to various drugs.

Bioavailability: The extent to which a drug reaches the systemic circulation following administration by various routes.

Biotransformation: Biochemical changes that occur to the drug within the body, usually resulting in breakdown and inactivation of the drug (SYN: drug metabolism).

Bipolar syndrome: A psychological disorder characterized by mood swings from excitable (manic) periods to periods of depression (SYN: manic-depression).

Blood-brain barrier: The specialized anatomic arrangement of cerebral capillary walls that serves to restrict the passage of some drugs into the brain.

Blood dyscrasia: A pathologic condition of the blood, usually referring to a defect in one or more of the cellular elements of the blood.

Carcinogen: Any substance that produces cancer or increases the risk of developing cancer.

Catecholamine: A group of chemically similar compounds that are important in the modulation of cardiovascular activity and many other physiologic functions. Common catecholamines include epinephrine, norepinephrine, and dopamine.

Cathartic: An agent that causes a relatively rapid evacuation of the bowels.

Ceiling effect: The point at which no further increase in response occurs as drug dose is progressively increased; this effect is represented by a plateau on the drug's dose-response curve (SYN: maximal efficacy).

Chemical name: The drug name that is derived from the specific chemical structure of the compound. Chemical names are not used clinically but are shortened in some way to form the drug's generic name.

Chemotherapy: The use of chemical agents to treat infectious or neoplastic disease.

Cholinergic: Refers to synapses or physiologic responses involving acetylcholine.

Cholinesterase: The enzyme that breaks down acetylcholine (SYN: acetylcholinesterase).

Clearance: The process by which the active form of the drug is removed from the bloodstream by either metabolism or excretion.

Congestive heart failure: A clinical syndrome of cardiac disease that is marked by decreased myocardial contractility, peripheral edema, shortness of breath, and decreased tolerance for physical exertion.

Cretinism: A congenital syndrome of mental retardation, decreased metabolism, and impaired physical development secondary to insufficient production of thyroid hormones.

Cyclic adenosine monophosphate (ABBR: cAMP): The ring-shaped conformation of adenosine monophosphate, which is important in acting as a second messenger in mediating the intracellular response to drug stimulation.

Cyclooxygenase (ABBR: COX): The key enzyme involved in prostaglandin biosynthesis. This enzyme converts arachadonic acid into prostaglandin G_2, thereby providing the precursor for the cell to synthesize additional prostaglandins.

Cytokine: The general term used to describe proteins produced by various immune and inflammatory cells. These proteins act as intercellular chemical signals that help orchestrate immune and inflammatory responses. Common cytokines include the interferons, interleukins, and certain growth factors.

Demand dose: Amount of drug administered when a patient activates certain drug delivery systems, such as those used during patient-controlled analgesia.

Desensitization: A fairly brief and transient decrease in the responsiveness of cellular receptors to drug effects.

Diabetes insipidus: A disease marked by increased urination (polyuria) and excessive thirst (polydipsia) due to inadequate production of antidiuretic hormone (ADH) and/or a decrease in the renal response to ADH.

Diabetes mellitus: A disease marked by abnormal metabolism of glucose and other energy substrates caused by a defect in the production of insulin and/or a decrease in the peripheral response to insulin.

Diuretic: A drug that increases the formation and excretion of urine.

Dopa decarboxylase: The enzyme that converts dihydroxyphenylalanine (dopa) into dopamine.

Dopamine: A neurotransmitter located in the CNS that is important in motor control as well as certain aspects of behavior. The presence of endogenous or exogenous dopamine in the periphery also affects cardiovascular function.

Dosage: The amount of medication that is appropriate for treating a given condition or illness.

Dose: The amount of medication that is administered at one time.

Dose-response curve: The relationship between incremental doses of a drug and the magnitude of the reaction that those doses will cause.

Down-regulation: A prolonged decrease in the number and/or sensitivity of drug receptors, usually occurring as a compensatory response to overstimulation of the receptor.

Drug holiday: A period of several days to several weeks in which medications are withdrawn from the patient to allow recovery from drug tolerance or toxicity; sometimes used in patients with advanced cases of Parkinson disease.

Drug microsomal metabolizing system (ABBR: DMMS): A series of enzymes located on the smooth endoplasmic reticulum that are important in catalyzing drug biotransformation.

Dysentery: The general term for severe gastrointestinal distress (diarrhea, cramps, bloody stools) usually associated with the presence of infectious microorganisms in the intestines.

Eicosanoids: The general term for the group of 20-carbon fatty acids that includes the prostaglandins, thromboxanes, and leukotrienes. These substances are involved in mediating inflammation and other pathologic responses.

Emetic: A drug that initiates or facilitates vomiting.

End-of-dose akinesia: A phenomenon in Parkinson disease in which the effectiveness of the medication wears off toward the end of the dosing interval, resulting in a virtual lack of volitional movement from the patient.

Enteral administration: Administration of drugs by way of the alimentary canal.

Enzyme induction: The process wherein some drugs provoke cells to synthesize more drug-metabolizing enzymes, thus leading to accelerated drug biotransformation.

Epidural nerve block: Administration of local anesthesia into the spinal canal between the bony vertebral column and the dura mater (i.e., the injection does not penetrate the spinal membranes but remains above the dura).

Epilepsy: A chronic neurologic disorder characterized by recurrent seizures that are manifested as brief periods of altered consciousness, involuntary motor activity, or vivid sensory phenomena.

Epinephrine: A hormone synthesized primarily in the adrenal medulla, mimicking the peripheral effects of norepinephrine. Epinephrine is involved in the sympathetic nervous system response to stress and is especially effective in stimulating cardiovascular function (SYN: adrenaline).

Estrogens: The general term for the natural and synthetic female hormones such as estradiol and estrone.

Expectorant: A drug that facilitates the production and discharge of mucous secretions from the respiratory tract.

First-pass effect: The phenomenon in which drugs absorbed from the stomach and small intestine must pass through the liver before reaching the systemic circulation. Certain drugs undergo extensive hepatic metabolism because of this first pass through the liver.

Food and Drug Administration (ABBR: FDA): The official government agency involved in regulating the pharmaceutical industry in the United States.

Gamma-aminobutyric acid (ABBR: GABA): An inhibitory neurotransmitter in the brain and spinal cord.

Generic name: The name applied to a drug, which is not protected by a trademark; usually a shortened version of the drug's chemical name (SYN: nonproprietary name).

Glucocorticoid: The general class of steroid agents that affect glucose metabolism and are used pharmacologically to decrease inflammation and suppress the immune system. Principle examples include cortisol and corticosterone.

Glycosuria: The presence of glucose in the urine.

Gonadotropin: A hormone that produces a stimulatory effect on the gonads (ovaries and testes); primary gonadotropins include luteinizing hormone (LH) and follicle-stimulating hormone (FSH).

G proteins: Proteins that bind with guanine nucleotides and regulate cell activity. G proteins often serve as a link between surface receptors and intracellular enzymes such as adenylate cyclase.

Half-life: The time required to eliminate 50 percent of the drug existing in the body.

Histamine: A chemical produced by various cells in the body, which is involved in the modulation of certain physiologic responses (e.g., secretion of gastric acid), as well as in the mediation of hypersensitivity (allergic) responses.

Hypercalcemia: An excessive concentration of calcium in the bloodstream (ANT: hypocalcemia).

Hyperglycemia: An excessive concentration of glucose in the bloodstream (ANT: hypoglycemia).

Hypersensitivity: An exaggerated response of the immune system to a foreign substance (SYN: allergic response).

Hypertension: A pathologic condition characterized by a sustained, reproducible increase in blood pressure.

Hypnotic: A drug that initiates or maintains a relatively normal state of sleep.

Hypokalemia: An abnormally low concentration of potassium in the bloodstream (ANT: hyperkalemia).

Hyponatremia: An abnormally low concentration of sodium in the bloodstream (ANT: hypernatremia).

Immunosuppressant: A drug used to attenuate the body's immune response. These agents are often used to prevent rejection of organ transplants or to treat diseases caused by overactivity in the immune system (ANT: immunostimulant).

Interferon: A member of the group of proteins that exert a number of physiologic and pharmacologic effects, including antiviral and antineoplastic activity.

Intrathecal: Administration of substances within a sheath; typically refers to injection into the subarachnoid space surrounding the spinal cord.

Laxative: An agent that promotes peristalsis and evacuation of the bowel in a relatively slow manner (as opposed to a cathartic).

Leukotriene: One of the 20-carbon fatty acid compounds (eicosanoids) formed from arachadonic acid by the lipoxygenase enzyme. Leukotrienes are important in mediating certain allergic and inflammatory responses, especially in respiratory tissues.

Lipoxygenase (ABBR: LOX): The enzyme that initiates leukotriene biosynthesis. This enzyme converts arachadonic acid into precursors that the cell uses to synthesize specific leukotrienes.

Loading dose: Amount of drug administered at the onset of treatment to rapidly bring the amount of drug in the body to therapeutic levels.

Lockout interval: The minimum amount of time that must expire between each dose of medication that is administered by patient-controlled analgesia (PCA). The PCA pump is inactivated during the lockout interval so that the patient cannot self-administer excessive amounts of drugs.

Lymphokines: Chemicals released from activated lymphocytes that help mediate various aspects of the immune response. Common lymphokines include the interleukins and gamma interferon.

Malignancy: A term usually applied to cancerous tumors, which tend to become progressively worse.

Maximal efficacy: The maximum response a drug can produce; the point at which the response does not increase even if dosage continues to increase (SYN: ceiling effect).

Median effective dose (ABBR: ED_{50}): The drug dosage that produces a specific therapeutic response in 50 percent of the patients in whom it is tested.

Median lethal dose (ABBR: LD_{50}): The drug dosage that causes death in 50 percent of the experimental animals in which it is tested.

Median toxic dose (ABBR: TD_{50}): The drug dosage that produces a specific adverse (toxic) response in 50 percent of the patients in whom it is tested.

Metabolite: The compound that is formed when the drug undergoes biotransformation and is chemically altered by some metabolic process.

Metastasize: The transfer or spread of diseased (i.e., cancerous) cells from a primary location to other sites in the body.

Mineralocorticoid: A steroid hormone (e.g., aldosterone) that is important in regulating fluid and electrolyte balance by increasing the reabsorption of sodium from the kidneys.

Monoamine oxidase (ABBR: MAO): An enzyme that breaks down monoamine neurotransmitters such as dopamine, norepinephrine, and serotonin.

Mucolytic: A drug that decreases the viscosity and increases the fluidity of mucous secretions in the respiratory tract, thus making it easier for the patient to cough up secretions.

Muscarinic receptor: A primary class of cholinergic receptors that are named according to their affinity for the muscarine toxin. Certain cholinergic agonists and antagonists also have a relatively selective affinity for muscarinic receptors.

Myxedema: The adult or acquired form of hypothyroidism characterized by decreased metabolic rate, lethargy, decreased mental alertness, weight gain, and other somatic changes.

Neuroleptic: A term frequently used to describe antipsychotic drugs, referring to the tendency of these drugs to produce a behavioral syndrome of apathy, sedation, decreased initiative, and decreased responsiveness (SYN: antipsychotic).

Nicotinic receptor: A primary class of cholinergic receptors, named according to their affinity for nicotine, as well as certain other cholinergic agonists and antagonists.

Norepinephrine: A neurotransmitter that is important in certain brain pathways and in the terminal synapses of the sympathetic nervous system (SYN: noradrenaline).

On-off phenomenon: The fluctuation in response seen in certain patients with Parkinson disease, in which the effectiveness of the medications may suddenly diminish at some point between dosages.

Opioid: An analgesic drug with morphinelike effects; commonly refers to the synthetic forms of these analgesics (SYN: narcotic).

Orthostatic hypotension: A sudden fall in blood pressure that occurs when the patient stands erect; this is a frequent side effect of many medications.

Ototoxicity: The harmful side effect of some drugs and toxins influencing the hearing and balance functions of the ear.

Over-the-counter drugs (ABBR: OTC): Drugs that can be purchased directly by the consumer without a prescription (SYN: nonprescription drugs).

Parenteral administration: Administration of drugs by routes other than via the alimentary canal: by injection, transdermally, topically, and so on.

Parkinson disease or **parkinsonism:** The clinical syndrome of bradykinesia, rigidity, resting tremor, and postural instability associated with neurotransmitter abnormalities within the basal ganglia.

Pharmacodynamics: The study of how drugs affect the body; that is, the physiologic and biochemical mechanisms of drug action.

Pharmacokinetics: The study of how the body handles drugs; that is, the manner in which drugs are absorbed, distributed, metabolized, and excreted.

Pharmacologic dose: An amount of drug given that is much greater than the amount of a similar substance produced within the body; this increased dosage is used to exaggerate the beneficial effects normally provided by the endogenous compound.

Pharmacotherapeutics: The study of how drugs are used in the prevention and treatment of disease.

Pharmacy: The professional discipline dealing with the preparation and dispensing of medications.

Physical dependence: A phenomenon that develops during prolonged use of addictive substances, signified by the onset of withdrawal symptoms when the drug is discontinued.

Physiologic dose: The amount of drug given that is roughly equivalent to the amount of a similar substance normally produced within the body; this dosage is typically used to replace the endogenous substance when the body is no longer able to produce the substance.

Placebo: A medication that contains inert or inactive ingredients that is used to pacify a patient or test the patient's psychophysiologic response to treatment.

Potency: The dosage of a drug that produces a given response in a specific amplitude. When two drugs are compared, the more potent drug will produce a given response at a lower dosage.

Progestins: The general term for the natural and synthetic female hormones such as progesterone.

Prostaglandin: A member of the family of 20-carbon fatty acid compounds (eicosanoids) formed from arachadonic acid by the cyclooxygenase enzyme. Prostaglandins help regulate normal cell activity, and may also help mediate certain pathologic responses, including pain, inflammation, fever, and abnormal blood coagulation.

Psychosis: A relatively severe form of mental illness characterized by marked thought disturbances and an impaired perception of reality.

Receptor: The component of the cell (usually a protein) to which the drug binds, thus initiating a change in cell function.

Salicylate: The chemical term commonly used to denote compounds such as aspirin that have anti-inflammatory, analgesic, antipyretic, and anticoagulant properties.

Second messenger: The term applied to compounds formed within the cell, such as cyclic AMP. The second messenger initiates a series of biochemical changes within the cell following stimulation of a receptor on the cell's outer surface by drugs, hormones, and so on.

Sedative: A drug that produces a calming effect and serves to pacify the patient. These agents are sometimes referred to as *minor tranquilizers.*

Seizure: A sudden attack of symptoms usually associated with diseases such as epilepsy. Epileptic seizures are due to the random, uncontrolled firing of a group of cerebral neurons, which results in a variety of sensory and motor manifestations.

Selective toxicity: A desired effect of antineoplastic and anti-infectious agents, wherein the drug kills the pathogenic organism or cells without damaging healthy tissues.

Serotonin: A neurotransmitter located in the CNS that is important in many functions, including mood, arousal, and inhibition of painful stimuli (SYN: 5-hydroxytryptamine).

Side effect: Any effect produced by a drug that occurs in addition to the principal therapeutic response.

Spinal nerve block: Administration of local anesthesia into the spinal canal between the arachnoid membrane and the pia mater (i.e., the subarachnoid space).

Status epilepticus: An emergency situation characterized by a rapid series of epileptic seizures that occur without any appreciable recovery between seizures.

Steroid: The general term used to describe a group of hormones and their analogs that have a common chemical configuration but are divided into several categories depending on their primary physiologic effects. Common types of steroids include the glucocorticoids (cortisone, prednisone, many others), mineralocorticoids (aldosterone), androgens/anabolic steroids (testosterone), and steroids related to female physiologic function (estrogen, progesterone).

Supersensitivity: An increased response to drugs and endogenous compounds caused by an increase in the number and/or sensitivity of receptors for that drug.

Sympatholytics: Drugs that inhibit or antagonize function within the sympathetic nervous system.

Sympathomimetics: Drugs that facilitate or increase activity within the sympathetic nervous system.

Tardive dyskinesia: A movement disorder characterized by involuntary, fragmented movements of the mouth, face, and jaw (i.e., chewing, sucking, tongue protrusion, and the like). This disorder may occur during the prolonged administration of antipsychotic drugs.

Therapeutic index (ABBR: TI): A ratio used to represent the relative safety of a particular drug; the larger the therapeutic index, the safer the drug. It is calculated as the median toxic dose divided by the median effective dose. (In animal trials, the median lethal dose is often substituted for the median toxic dose.)

Therapeutic window: The range of drug concentrations in the body that will promote optimal beneficial effects. Drug concentrations less than the lower end of this range will be ineffective, and concentrations greater than the upper end of this range will create excessive side effects.

Thyrotoxicosis: Abnormally high production of thyroid hormones resulting in symptoms such as nervousness, weight loss, and tachycardia (SYN: hyperthryoidism).

Tolerance: The acquired phenomenon associated with some drugs, in which larger doses of the drug are needed to achieve a given effect when the drug is used for prolonged periods.

Toxicology: The study of the harmful effects of drugs and other chemicals.

Trade name: The name given to a drug by the pharmaceutical company; it is protected by a trademark and used by the company for marketing the drug (SYN: proprietary name).

Vaccine: A substance typically consisting of a modified infectious microorganism that is administered to help prevent disease by stimulating the endogenous immune defense mechanisms against infection.

Viscosupplementation: Injection of a polysaccharide (hyaluronin) into osteoarthritic joints to help restore the viscosity of synovial fluid.

Volume of distribution (ABBR: V_d): A ratio used to estimate the distribution of a drug within the body relative to the total amount of fluid in the body. It is calculated as the amount of drug administered divided by the plasma concentration of the drug.

Withdrawal syndrome: The clinical syndrome of somatic and psychologic manifestations that occur when a drug is removed from a patient who has become physically dependent on the drug (SYN: abstinence syndrome).

Index

An "f" following a page number indicates a figure; a "t" following a page number indicates a table.